D1509070

Kidney Diseases in the Developing World and Ethnic Minorities

Kidney Diseases in the Developing World and Ethnic Minorities

Edited by
Meguid El Nahas
Sheffield Kidney Institute
University of Sheffield
Sheffield, U.K.

Associate Editors
Rashad S. Barsoum
John Dirks
Giuseppe Remuzzi

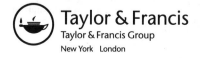
Taylor & Francis
Taylor & Francis Group
New York   London

Published in 2005 by
Taylor & Francis Group
270 Madison Avenue
New York, NY 10016

© 2005 by Taylor & Francis Group, LLC

No claim to original U.S. Government works
Printed in the United States of America on acid-free paper
10 9 8 7 6 5 4 3 2 1

International Standard Book Number-10: 0-8247-2863-7 (Hardcover)
International Standard Book Number-13: 978-0-8247-2863-2 (Hardcover)

Library of Congress Cataloging-in-Publication Data

Catalog record is available from the Library of Congress

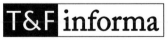

Taylor & Francis Group
is the Academic Division of T&F Informa plc.

Visit the Taylor & Francis Web site at
http://www.taylorandfrancis.com

Foreword

Noncommunicable diseases have taken over from infectious diseases as the number one cause of death on all continents except for Africa. As a consequence, sub-specialty medicine disciplines such as nephrology are increasingly important in establishing in emerging countries a basis for teaching, research, and clinical care. In order to be effective and to meet the local need, nephrologists embark on this task in close collaboration with sister disciplines, general practitioners, and community healthcare workers.

Since its inception in 1960, the International Society of Nephrology (ISN) has pursued its mission to advance nephrology worldwide along three main avenues: the dissemination of basic and clinical scientific progress by means of the society journal *Kidney International*; the establishment of a forum for scientific discussions at the ISN International Congresses; and the development of a global outreach program based on a fellowship and senior scholar exchange program combined with a worldwide continued medical education effort, contributions to local and regional meetings, support of local libraries, description of training guidelines, and the establishment of clinical programs aimed at early detection and prevention in combination with epidemiology and clinical research.

For 45 years, the ISN has been active in bringing top science and clinical progress to all parts of the world, aiming at the best possible results for patients and colleagues in the emerging and the industrialized world alike, although it realizes that priorities may contrast sharply. Of the total population of 1,800,000 patients on renal replacement therapy, over 80% are living in the industrialized world. In middle and low income countries, end-stage renal failure implies death for most patients because of a sheer lack of finances needed for renal replacement therapies. End-stage renal failure is a rapidly rising expression of chronic vascular disease worldwide, but most strikingly in the emerging world, where changes in lifestyle in a genetically susceptible population result in high numbers of patients with type 2 diabetes, hypertension, and obesity. Added to specific local needs related to infectious diseases and a high incidence of renal calculus disease, the type 2 diabetes complications ask for new direction of ISN's global outreach programs.

Spearheaded by the Clinical Research Committee of ISN's Commission on Global Advancement of Nephrology (COMGAN), important initiatives have been developed to combine epidemiology programs in the emerging world with early detection and prevention of renal and cardiovascular disease. These programs take advantage of the eminent example set by the Groningen Prevention of Renal Vascular End Stage Disease (PREVEND) study, which has shown the value of measuring albuminuria as an early, cost-effective marker as well as a risk factor and a target for therapy in high risk groups of patients with diabetes and hypertension, as well as in the general population—not only to avert progressive renal disease but vascular disease including heart failure and stroke as well. By working with first line medical personnel such as general practitioners and healthcare workers in close collaboration with diabetologists and cardiologists, the ISN seeks to fight the global epidemic of chronic vascular disease in an effort to advance equity in health worldwide.

This monograph by Prof. Meguid El Nahas and his colleagues gives a comprehensive overview of all the important issues confronting global nephrology, particularly in the field of chronic kidney and cardiovascular disease. Prof. El Nahas is to be complimented for bringing together a truly global team of expert nephrologists who cover a wide array of clinical and educational subjects, all of great interest to anyone interested not only in nephrology in the emerging world, but in global medicine in general.

Jan J. Weening
President
International Society of Nephrology
Amsterdam, The Netherlands

Preface

An increasing number of patients worldwide are affected by chronic kidney disease (CKD). This is reflected, to some extent, in the number of patients requiring renal replacement therapy (RRT) which is increasing globally by around 5–10% annually. It is anticipated that more than two million patients with endstage renal disease (ESRD) will be on RRT by 2010. Unfortunately, the cost of RRT is prohibitive for most health care systems in the developing world. In fact, individuals in 110 of 222 countries do not have any access to RRT, leaving around 600 million at risk of death if they contract CKD and ESRD. Also, socioeconomic deprivation affecting ethnic minorities in developed countries has been implicated in the higher incidence of CKD. With that in mind, a more critical evaluation of health care provision for CKD in the developing world as well as in ethnic minorities is urgently warranted.

This book aims to address the global health care crisis and challenge of CKD. It reviews the epidemiology, causes, and natural history of CKD in the developing world and in ethnic minorities living in developed countries. It highlights the link among diabetes, hypertension, and CKD, as well as the impact of CKD on cardiovascular complications. It addresses health economic issues relevant to the global provision of renal health care. The book also examines successful examples of training and education links and collaboration between developing and developed countries. Finally, it describes several research initiatives undertaken in the developing world aimed at the early detection and prevention of CKD.

The contributors to the book are all leading international experts in their respective fields. They have considerable experience in training, education, and research in nephrology in developing countries as well as in ethnic minorities residing in the West.

v

It is hoped that this monograph will provide many, in the developing as well as developed world, with the information and insights necessary to stem the global tide of CKD with its ravaging consequences.

Meguid El Nahas

Contents

Contributors

Lawrence Agodoa National Institute of Diabetes and Digestive and Kidney Diseases National Institutes of Health, Bethesda, Maryland, U.S.A.

Ejaz Ahmed Sindh Institute of Urology and Transplantation, Dow Medical College, Karachi, Pakistan

Agustina Anabaya Department of Medicine and Transplantation, Asienda Ospedaliera Ospedali Riuniti di Bergamo—'Mario Negri' Institute for Pharmacological Research, Bergamo, Italy

Ebun L. Bamgboye Dialysis and Transplant Unit, St. Nicholas Hospital, Lagos, Nigeria

Rashad S. Barsoum Kasr El Aini Medical School, Cairo University, Cairo, Egypt

William D. Bates Department of Anatomical Pathology, University of Stellenbosch, and National Health Laboratory Service, Cape Town, South Africa

Aminu K. Bello Sheffield Kidney Institute, University of Sheffield, Sheffield, U.K.

John F. Bertram Department of Anatomy & Cell Biology, Monash University, Clayton, Victoria, Australia

Boris T. Bikbov Department of Nephrology Issues of Transplanted Kidney, Research Institute of Transplantology and Artificial Organs, Moscow, Russia

F. P. Cappuccio Community Health Sciences, St. George's, University of London, London, U.K.

Alan Cass   Renal Program, The George Institute for International Health, Sydney, New South Wales, Australia

Srinivas Kondalsamy Chennakesavan   Discipline of Medicine, Centre for Chronic Disease, University of Queensland, Herston, Queensland, Australia

K. S. Chugh   Department of Nephrology, Postgraduate Institute of Medical Education & Research, Chandigarh, India

Igor Codreanu   Department of Hemodialysis and Kidney Transplantation, Republican Clinical Hospital, Chisinau, Moldova

Manjula Datta   Department of Epidemiology, Tamil Nadu Dr. MGR Medical University, Chennai, India

Marc E. De Broe   Department of Nephrology, University of Antwerp, Belgium

Dick de Zeeuw   Department of Clinical Pharmacology Groningen, University Medical Center, Groningen, The Netherlands

John H. Dirks   University of Toronto and Massey College, Toronto, Ontario, Canada

J. B. Eastwood   Departments of Renal Medicine and Transplantation, and Community Health Sciences, St. George's, University of London, London, U.K. and Department of Medicine, Komfo Anokye Teaching Hospital, Kumasi, Ghana

Meguid El Nahas   Sheffield Kidney Institute, University of Sheffield, Sheffield, U.K.

John Feehally   The John Walls Renal Unit, Leicester General Hospital, Leicester, U.K.

Michael Field   Northern Clinical School, University of Sydney, Sydney, Australia

Giovanni Battista Fogazzi   U.O. di Nefrologia e Dialisi, Ospedale Maggiore, IRCCS, Milano, Italy

Agnes B. Fogo   Department of Pathology, Vanderbilt University Medical Center, Nashville, Tennessee, U.S.A.

Aouanou Guy Division de Pédiatrie, Hôpital Saint Jean de Dieu, Benin Republic

Theo L. Hattingh Department of Internal Medicine, University of Stellenbosch and Renal Unit, Tygerberg Academic Hospital, Parrow Cape Town, South Africa

Fanfan Hou Nanfang Hospital, The First Military Medical University, Guangzhou, China

Wendy E. Hoy Discipline of Medicine, Centre for Chronic Disease, University of Queensland, Herston, Queensland, Australia

Michael D. Hughson Department of Pathology, University of Mississippi Medical Center, Jackson, Mississipi, U.S.A.

Vivekanand Jha Department of Nephrology, Postgraduate Institute of Medical Education & Research, Chandigarh, India

Ivor Katz Dumisani Mzamane African Institute of Kidney Disease, Chris Hani Baragwanath Hospital, University of the Witwatersrand, Johannesburg, South Africa

Martin K. Kuhlmann Albert Einstein College of Medicine and Renal Research Institute, New York, New York, U.S.A.

Eduardo Lacson Jr. Clinical Research and Technology Assessment, Medical Department, Fresenius Medical Care, North America, Lexington, Massachusetts, U.S.A.

Norbert Lameire Renal Division, Department of Medicine, University Hospital Ghent, Ghent, Belgium

Nathan W. Levin Albert Einstein College of Medicine and Renal Research Institute, New York, New York, U.S.A.

Liz Lightstone Renal Section, Division of Medicine, Imperial College London, Hammersmith Hospital, London, U.K.

Shanyan Lin Division of Nephrology, Hua Shan Hospital, Fudan University, Jiangwan, Shanghai, China

Bicheng Liu Zhongda Hospital, Southeast University, Nanjing, China

Nomandla Madala   Department of Medicine, University of KwaZulu Natal, Durban, South Africa

M. K. Mani   Apollo Hospital, Chennai, India

Stephen P. McDonald   Nephrology & Transplantation Unit, The Queen Elizabeth Hospital, Adelaide, South Australia, Australia

Sergio Mezzano   Universidad Austral, Valdivia, Chile

M. Rafique Moosa   Department of Internal Medicine, University of Stellenbosch and Renal Unit, Tygerberg Academic Hospital, Parrow Cape Town, South Africa

Saraladevi Naicker   Division of Nephrology, University of the Witwatersrand, Johannesburg, South Africa

S. A. Anwar Naqvi   Sindh Institute of Urology and Transplantation, Dow Medical College, Karachi, Pakistan

Norberto Perico   Department of Medicine and Transplantation, Asienda Ospedaliera Ospedali Riuniti di Bergamo—'Mario Negri' Institute for Pharmacological Research, Bergamo, Italy

J. Plange-Rhule   Departments of Renal Medicine and Transplantation, and Community Health Sciences, St. George's, University of London, London, U.K. and Department of Medicine, Komfo Anokye Teaching Hospital, Kumasi, Ghana

Jiaqi Qian   Renji Hospital, Shanghai Second Medical University, China

Asghar Rastegar   Department of Medicine, Yale University School of Medicine, New Haven, Connecticut, U.S.A.

Giuseppe Remuzzi   Department of Medicine and Transplantation, Asienda Ospedaliera Ospedali Riuniti di Bergamo—'Mario Negri' Institute for Pharmacological Research, Bergamo, Italy

S. Adibul Hasan Rizvi   Sindh Institute of Urology and Transplantation, Dow Medical College, Karachi, Pakistan

Sheila Robinson   University of Toronto and Massey College, Toronto, Ontario, Canada

Bernardo Rodríguez-Iturbe   Hospital Universitario and Universidad del Zulia, FUNDACITE-Zulia, Maracaibo, Venezuela

Piero Ruggenenti Division of Nephrology and Dialysis, Azienda Ospedaliera Ospedali Riuniti di Bergamo—'Mario Negri' Institute for Pharmacological Research, Bergamo, Italy

Arrigo Schieppati Division of Nephrology and Dialysis, Azienda Ospedaliera Ospedali Riuniti di Bergamo—'Mario Negri' Institute for Pharmacological Research, Bergamo, Italy

Mehmet Sukru Sever Department of Nephrology, Istanbul School of Medicine, Istanbul, Turkey

Kunal Shah Renal Research Institute, New York, New York, U.S.A.

Gurmeet R. Singh Menzies School of Health Research, Causuarina, Northern Territory, Australia

Natalia A. Tomilina Department of Nephrology Issues of Transplanted Kidney, Research Institute of Transplantology and Artificial Organs, Moscow, Russia

Wim Van Biesen Renal Division, Department of Medicine, University Hospital Ghent, Ghent, Belgium

Raymond Vanholder Renal Division, Department of Medicine, University Hospital Ghent, Ghent, Belgium

Attolou Vénérand Centre d'Hemodialyse, Centre National Hospitalier Universitaire, Cotonou, Benin Republic

Yihan Wang Department of Pathology, Vanderbilt University Medical Center, Nashville, Tennessee, U.S.A.

Jan Weuts Artsen zonder Grenzen (Médéçins sans Frontières), Brussels, Belgium

Maki Yoshino Renal Research Institute, New York, New York, U.S.A.

1

Epidemiology of ESRD: A Worldwide Perspective

Rashad S. Barsoum

Kasr El Aini Medical School, Cairo University, Cairo, Egypt

INTRODUCTION

Chronic kidney disease (CKD) has recently jumped into the focus of worldwide attention after many decades of desertion. There are four main reasons for this change in attitude: (a) the progressively increasing epidemiological impact, due to the increasing incidence and prevalence of CKD; (b) the incremental financial demand to meet the cost of expensive renal replacement therapy (RRT); (c) the pressing moral conflicts related to kidney donors and patient selection for RRT; (d) the recent promise of effective prevention measures that have been shown to reduce the incidence of CKD and to reduce its progression.

These fundamental features have been a major driving force for ranking epidemiology as an essential component of nephrology. Thus, a lot of progress has been made in our understanding of global CKD over the past couple of decades, involving methods of sampling for epidemiological research, data storage, analysis, presentation and publicity, etc. This advancement has been largely lead and influenced by the U.S. Renal Data System (USRDS), developed in 1988 essentially to look into the causes of lower patient survival on dialysis in the United States as compared to Europe and Japan (1). But USRDS far exceeded this goal, and has become an extremely valuable source of epidemiological data on CKD, not only in the United States but also in many other parts of the world (2).

Other regional registries look into the epidemiology of CKD from different angles. These include the EDTA/ERA registry (3), which was developed many years before USRDS, but has always focused on the end-stage renal disease (ESRD) population rather that the holistic picture of CKD at large. It is limited to Europe and a few non-European Mediterranean countries. The EDTA/ERA model has inspired many parts of the world to develop their own registries, including the regional renal registries in Africa (AFRAN) (4), Asia (APSN) (5), Australia and New Zealand (ANZDATA) (6), the Gulf (SCOT) (7), South America (SLANH) (8) and others. Many countries have also developed their local registries, with variable levels of credibility.

Besides the specialized renal registries, several agents also look into the epidemiology of CKD as a part of regional "health maps." These include the World Health Organization (WHO) (9), the World Bank (10), World Vision (11), the Rockefeller Foundation (12), and others. Epidemiological data are also available to local health authorities, insurance agencies, and charity organizations that share in covering the expenses of renal failure management.

Despite this plethora of registries, there is a striking disagreement about the relevant facts in many parts of the world, particularly the underdeveloped. This is attributed to differences in project designs, sampling size and methodology, exclusivity, response rates, reliability of information, and other factors. Accordingly, students of CKD epidemiology in the developing world often resort to sporadic country or regional reports, questionnaires addressed to leading nephrologists, or even counting the deaths attributed to CKD in a certain community. So, our information on CKD in the developing world is, at best, approximate, challengeable, and changeable. But still, the available data can provide a fair insight into the magnitude of the problem, and serve to outline the major causes of CKD in different communities. With this information alone, it is possible to design effective prevention programs, without waiting for more accurate and reliable data. One of the best examples of this pragmatic approach is what Professor G. Remuzzi's group (13) has accomplished in Bolivia during the past decade.

GLOBAL PREVALENCE

Prevalence is defined as the number of existing patients in a group divided by the number in the general population base. It is influenced by the number of new patients (incidence) on one hand and the number of deaths on the other. The former typically reflects the interaction of genetic and environmental factors, as well as the efficiency of primary healthcare services in the detection and management of CKD in its early stages. Deaths, on the other hand, are directly related to the technical and organizational competence of renal replacement therapy (RRT) programs.

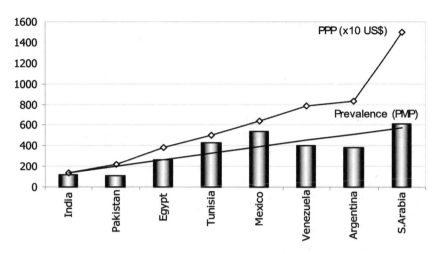

Figure 1 Prevalence of end-stage renal disease in selected developing countries. PPP = purchasing power parity (10). *Source*: From Ref. (16).

With the progressive improvement of RRT worldwide, prevalence curves continue to rise in most countries. In the 2003 USRDS report (14), ESRD prevalence in the United States has reached almost 1400 patients per million population (pmp) in 2001. This figure is close to that reported from Japan (about 1600 pmp), but much higher than in Europe (700–800 cases pmp), which is attributed to lower incidence in the latter continent (15).

In the developing world, prevalence of ESRD is proportionate to national economy (Fig. 1) (16). There are no major differences in incidence between individual developing countries, so the major determinants of prevalence are the capacity and competence of RRT programs, both of which are financially demanding.

GLOBAL INCIDENCE OF ESRD

In 2001, and for 3 years in a row, the incidence of new cases of ESRD in the United States has stabilized at about 330 patients pmp (14). This seems to represent the true incidence among the American population, after correction of many pitfalls in data collection over the previous 18 years.

In the same report (14), Blacks and Native Americans displayed the highest incident rates (988 and 696 pmp), as compared to Asians (395 pmp) and Whites (254 pmp). Those of Hispanic ethnicity had a higher incidence compared to non-Hispanics (470 vs. 325 pmp, respectively). Interestingly, the reported figures for American residents are much higher than those in their countries of origin. The incidence among white Americans is significantly higher than that among European Caucasians (3,15). That among Black

Americans, Asians, and Hispanics is many folds higher than that reported from Africa, Asia, and Latin America, which is generally within the range of 100 to 150 patients pmp (16). While this discrepancy may be attributed to inaccuracy of data collection and reporting from the developing world, it is difficult to accept this explanation when it comes to Western European Caucasians with equally low or even lower rates as in Finland (88.9 pmp), U.K. (97.1 pmp), or Belgium (151.6 pmp) (3). These observations must bring up the case that immigration from native countries to the United States may carry an increased risk of developing CKD.

Indeed, analysis of the regional causes of ESRD shows that diabetes and hypertension are the main determinants of incidence variance in different parts of the world (Fig. 2). Their contribution to the incidence of ESRD in the United States in year 2001 was 238.1 pmp, compared to an average of 45.6 patients pmp in the developing world (16). Such a staggering difference was not seen with any of the other causes of ESRD.

The relatively low incidence of diabetic nephropathy in the developing world is attributed to the low prevalence of diabetes at large, being 2.4% compared to 4.9% in the industrialized world (17), in addition to the relatively short survival of diabetic patients, who often die of other complications before reaching ESRD. This profile is bound to change in the coming couple of decades, as the diabetes pandemic reaches the developing world. Local experience has already shown the trend, while international

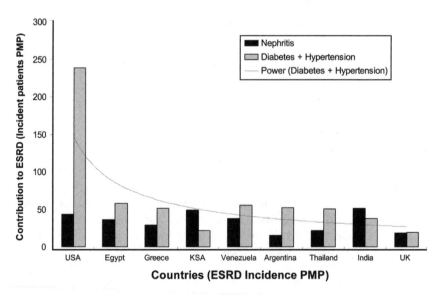

Figure 2 Incidence of new cases of ESRD due to diabetes and hypertension compared to "nephritis" in seven selected developing countries compared to the United States and the U.K.

agencies predict an increase in the global diabetic population from the current 171 millions to 366 millions in 2030 (17). The developing world is expected to be the major contributor to this explosion (Table 1).

Broadly similar implications apply to hypertension, though with some differences in detail. Recent studies have shown a relatively low prevalence of hypertension in the developing world, yet with an extremely low rate of adequate control. An example is the Egyptian National Hypertension study that showed an overall prevalence of 26.3%, of whom only 37.5% were aware of their disease, 23.9% were under treatment, and only 8.0% adequately controlled (18).

It is noteworthy that Blacks constitute a large proportion of the developing world population. Interestingly, the association of skin color to the prevalence and complications of hypertension, including CKD, is controversial. While an Egyptian study has not shown any effect of skin color (19), a South African study showed a higher rate of CKD among hypertensive Blacks (34.6%) compared to Whites (4.3%) and Indians (13.8%) (20), and a Brazilian study attributed the increased risk of complications in Blacks to familial clustering rather than racial factors (21).

Indigenous, non-Black populations constitute significant clusters in the developing world. In addition to their vulnerability to diabetes, they are also prone to significant complications of hypertension, largely involving the kidneys. A typical example is seen in the Australian Aboriginals (22).

Thus, it can be appreciated that the currently low incidence of ESRD in the developing world cannot last for long, as the incidence of diabetes increases, and the survival of diabetic and hypertensive patients improves long enough to develop CKD. As a result of this change alone, it is anticipated that the contribution of patients from the developing world to the global ESRD pool will increase from the current 53% to a figure around 70% in 2030 (Table 2), unless very active preventive measures are adopted to avoid the disaster.

GLOBAL DEMOGRAPHICS OF ESRD

Males predominate in the ESRD populations reported all over the globe. This matches with the known incidence and progression profile of most chronic kidney diseases. However, the male predominance in the developing world is much more striking, suggesting that access to dialysis in those nations may be male-biased, reflecting the generally chauvinistic heritage.

An interesting observation in Western communities is the aging ESRD population, the current average being 58 years. There has been over 13% rise in the median age of patients on RDT in the United States over the past three decades. This observation has been even more remarkable in those of Asian origin. ESRD populations in the emerging nations are generally younger, almost similar to the U.S. profile in the early 1980s. This may be

Table 1 Countries with the Highest Prevalence of Diabetes, 2000; Projections to 2030

	2000			2030			
	Population	Diabetic	Prevalence (%)	Population	Diabetic	Prevalence (%)	Increment (%)
United States	291.044	17.700	6.08	347.590	30.300	8.7	71.2
Japan	127.210	6.800	5.33	115.761	8.900	7.7	30.9
Indonesia	214.471	8.400	3.92	279.446	21.300	7.6	153.6
Pakistan	148.439	5.200	3.50	239.948	13.900	5.8	167.3
India	1,288.400	31.700	2.98	1,403.740	79.400	5.7	150.5
Brazil	176.596	4.600	2.60	226.130	11.300	5.0	145.7
China	1,064.399	20.800	2.39	1,430.831	42.300	3.0	103.4
Bangladesh	138.066	3.200	2.32	196.759	11.100	5.6	246.9

Table 2 Estimated Numbers of ESRD Patients According to Economic Development

| | Current | | | | | 2030 Projections | | | | |
| | Population[a] | | ESRD patients[b] | | | Population[a] | | ESRD patients[c] | | |
	Millions	Global share (%)	Pmp	Total	Global share (%)	Millions	Global share (%)	Pmp	Total	Global share (%)
High-economy countries	902	14.7	1,200	1,082,400	47.0	992.2	12.4	1600	1,587,520	30.1
Medium-economy countries	1,744	28.5	400	697,600	30.3	2,180.00	27.1	800	1,744,000	33.1
Low-economy countries	3,472	56.8	150	520,800	22.6	4,860.8	60.5	400	1,944,320	36.9

[a]World Bank data.
[b]Average estimated according to available reports.
[c]Average projected from past-years evolution and expansion of diabetic populations.

attributed to the general population demographics as well as to the predominant causes of ESRD, which typically occur at a younger age.

As mentioned earlier, although racial and ethnic origins have a major impact on the epidemiology of ESRD in the United States, this cannot be unequivocally documented in the developing world. This is a very interesting aspect in Nephro-epidemiology that will undoubtedly receive adequate attention in the coming years.

REGIONAL ETIOLOGY OF ESRD

The causes of ESRD of epidemiological importance in the developing world are represented in Figure 3. This is based on a questionnaire conducted among many leading nephrologists in Africa, India, South East Asia, and Latin America (16). Despite regional variability, it is clear that chronic glomerulonephritis and interstitial nephritis constitute the principal causes. This reflects the high prevalence of bacterial, viral, and parasitic infections known to affect the kidneys (23). Of the principal bacterial infections, tuberculosis ranks quite high in India and the Arabian Gulf, being associated with ureteric strictures, back pressure, and chronic interstitial nephritis. Streptococcal infections of the throat and skin (complicating scabies) are responsible for chronic glomerular disease in a large number of African children. Of the viral infections, HCV is currently the most important cause of progressive mesangiocapillary (membranoproliferative) glomerulonephritis in many countries, particularly Egypt. Several parasitic infections

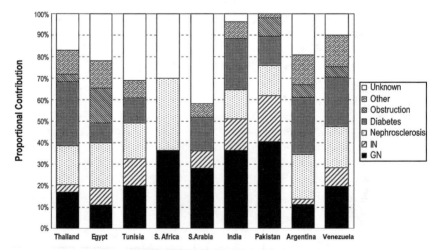

Figure 3 Principal causes of ESRD in selected developing countries. *Source*: From Ref. (16). *Abbreviation*: IN, Chronic interstitial nephritis; GN, Chronic glomerulonephritis.

cause ESRD through ureteric obstruction (e.g., schistosomiasis in most of Africa), interstitial nephritis (e.g., Kala-azar in many African and Asian countries), and glomerulonephritis (e.g., malaria in West Africa, schistosomiasis in Africa and Latin America, filariasis in Nigeria, etc.).

There is a considerable variation in the histological types of glomerulonephritis encountered in the developing world, mirroring the predominant infectious agents as well as genetic predisposition (24). Generally speaking, IgA nephropathy is the predominant type in South East Asia and the Pacific region (35–45%), while being quite rare in Africa (3–4%). In contrast, focal and segmental glomerulosclerosis supervenes among the Black populations in Africa (15–25%), Arabia (40%), India (up to 46%), and South America (up to 43%), probably as a consequence of the low nephron mass. Proliferative forms of glomerulonephritis are more homogeneously spread all over the developing world, being responsible for 25–35% of reported cases.

The contribution of diabetes varies from 9.1% to 29.9% in different reports from the developing world. Over 80% of cases are Type 2. End-stage diabetic nephropathy exhibits a constantly rising trend, attributed to increasing incident cases as well as improved survival on RRT. In a single-center experience in Egypt, diabetics constituted 8.0% of patients on RDT in 1980, 13.3% in 1990, 18.7% in 2000, and 24.3% in 2003 (Barsoum, unpublished data).

The lack of general agreement on the role of primary hypertension in causing ESRD reflects on the statistical reports from most developing countries. Upon standardization of the definition of this disease entity, the prevalence of hypertensive nephrosclerosis among ESRD patients in the developing world was reported between 13% and 21% (Fig. 3) (16).

Other important causes of ESRD in developing countries include urolithiasis with subsequent obstruction and infection, chronic drug abuse, and possibly environmental pollution. The public magnitude of the latter remains questionable, being documented only in occupational exposure to lead, cadmium, and mercury (25).

THE QUESTION OF CKD AS OPPOSED TO ESRD

Epidemiological data from the United States suggest that ESRD constitutes a barely visible tip of an enormous iceberg of chronic kidney disease. According to the NHANES III estimates, 64% of CKD patients are in Stage I, 31% in Stage II, 4.3% in Stage III, 0.2% in stage IV and only 0.02% in stage V (26). There is no room for the term ESRD in the recent CKD classification, being an administrative term referring to those on RRT rather than a medical term implying those in advanced renal insufficiency. Since there is no sharp line under which Stage V patients are enrolled for RRT, the proportion of ESRD to Stage V CKD is variable in different communities.

While the available information on ESRD in the developing world is incomplete, that on CKD at large is simply non-existent. It is only

Table 3 Frequency of Different Histopathological Types of Glomerulonephritis in Asymptomatic Patients, Those with the Nephrotic Syndrome and Those with ESRD [Egyptian Series of 1234 Cases (27)]

	Subnephrotic (%)	Nephrotic (%)	ESRD (%)
Minimal change disease	4.1	19.0	0.0
Focal and segmental sclerosis	17.2	26.1	25.0
Mesangiocapillary (membranoproliferative) GN	19.5	15.5	22.6
Membranous nephropathy	8.3	14.7	17.9
Mesangial proliferative glomerulonephritis	24.0	18.2	14.3
Focal proliferative GN	24.7	3.2	13.1
Nodular glomerulopathy	2.2	1.5	7.1
Diffuse proliferative GN	0.0	1.8	0.0

presumable that the ESRD etiological profile reflects that of CKD at large. But that is an oversimplification, since different kidney diseases progress at different rates, which necessarily implies that the breakdown of causes of Stage I CKD must be different from that in Stage V. A recent large multicenter study published from Egypt (27) emphasizes this point by comparing the histopathological profile of glomerulonephritis in asymptomatic patients, those with the nephrotic syndrome and patients with ESRD (Table 3).

IMPACT OF EPIDEMIOLOGICAL KNOWLEDGE ON THE PREVENTION AND MANAGEMENT OF CKD

Regardless of the supervening etiological profile in early CKD, those predominant in Stage V are more important from the prevention point of view. Thus, a progressive disease like diabetic nephropathy, which is bound to cause ESRD if the patient lives long enough, must receive higher priority in prevention as compared to nephrolithiasis, even if the latter is more common in a particular community.

Other factors of logistic importance in this respect include the availability of evidence-based preventive measures and their affordability. For example, we know very well that the control of diabetes and hypertension by angiotensin converting enzyme inhibitors or angiotensin II receptor I inhibitors slows progression of diabetic nephropathy, but we do not know for sure that the use of unleaded gasoline can reduce the incidence of interstitial nephritis in polluted communities. In such a situation, countries with limited resources must insightfully allocate their funds to the proper control of diabetes and hypertension rather than switching to unleaded gasoline.

Table 4 Healthcare Budgets in Different Parts of the World, Classified According to Economic Development (10)

	% of GDP	Public Percent	US $	Private Percent	US $	Share per capita (US $)
World	9.3	59.4		40.6		482
Low income	4.3	27.1	1.2	72.9	3.1	21
Middle income	5.9	51.8	3.1	48.2	2.9	116
Lower middle income	5.3	49.4	2.6	50.6	2.7	72
Upper middle income	6.6	54.2	3.6	45.8	3.0	309
Low and middle income	5.6	47.6	2.7	52.4	3.0	71
East Asia and Pacific	4.7	38.6	1.8	61.4	2.9	44
Europe and Central Asia	5.5	72.4	3.9	27.6	1.5	108
Latin America and Carib.	7.0	47.6	3.3	52.4	3.7	262
Middle East and N. Africa	4.6	61.9	2.9	38.1	1.8	171
South Asia	4.7	20.8	1.0	79.2	3.7	21
Sub-Saharan Africa	6.0	42.4	2.5	57.6	3.4	29
High income	10.2	62.2	6.3	37.8	3.8	2,736

Adequate prevention needs funding. Unfortunately, the healthcare budgets in most developing countries are extremely limited (Table 4) (10). What is even worse in the low-economy countries is that the public sector expenditure on health is minimal, compared to the private. It is the former that reflects on prevention and primary care, which is all what matters in any attempt to reduce the CKD burden. It is the duty of renal physicians, however, to highlight the importance of CKD, its preventability, cost effectiveness in order to get a bigger piece of the small cake to reduce the incidence and prevalence of ESRD.

In many instances, prevention of CKD can be achieved by collaborating with other medical disciplines with better appeal to the public and the health authorities. Kidney-oriented prevention can be coupled with the early detection and management of diabetes and hypertension, mass control of parasitic diseases as malaria and schistosomiasis, prevention of rheumatic heart disease, combating environmental pollution, etc.

Finally, there are educational aspects in prevention that do not need a lot of funding, such as antismoking campaigns, dodging obesity, encouragement of regular exercise, and avoidance of inadvertent use of medications.

SUMMARY AND CONCLUSION

The prevalence of ESRD is lower in the low- and medium-economy countries than in the United States, Japan, and Europe. This is partly attributed to relatively limited access to RRT, poor outcome of such treatment, as well as to lower incidence of CKD. Under-reporting may be contributing to these observations.

Low incidence of CKD in the developing world is attributed to the relatively low incidence of diabetes and hypertension as compared to the economically better developed communities. Yet there is epidemiological evidence that the diabetes pandemic will undoubtedly hit the developing world even more than the developed, leading to an anticipated increase in the former's global share in the ESRD pool from the current 53% to about 70% in 2030.

The increasing contribution of diabetes will change the relative significance of "nephritis," particularly as the control of infections and environmental pollution achieves better outcomes in the future.

With these future projections in mind, it is obvious that the global mission of nephrologists in the coming three decades should be directed to primary and secondary prevention of CKD. This requires better funding, collaboration with other bodies involved in health care, as well as emphasis on public and medical school education.

REFERENCES

1. Eknoyan G. Meeting the challenges of the new K/DOQI guidelines. Am J Kidney Dis 2003; 41(5 suppl):3–10.
2. United States Renal Data System Website: www.usrds.org.
3. EDTA/ERA Registry Website: www.era-edta-reg.org.
4. African Nephronet: www.sined.com/Annet.
5. Chugh KS, ed. Asian Nephrology. USA: Oxford University Press, 1995.
6. Australian and New Zealand Society of Nephrology Website: www.nephrology. edu.au.
7. Saudi Center for Organ Transplantation Website: www.scot.org.sa.
8. Latin American Society of Nephrology and Hypertension Website: www.slanh.org.
9. World Health Organization Website: www.who.int.
10. World Bank Group Data and Statistics: www.worldbank.org/data.
11. World Vision International Website: www.wvi.org.
12. Rockefeller Foundation Website: www.rockfound.org.
13. Plata R, Silva C, Yahuita J, Perez L, Schieppati A, Remuzzi G. The first clinical and epidemiological programme on renal disease in Bolivia: a model for prevention and early diagnosis of renal diseases in the developing countries. Nephrol Dial Transplant 1998; 13(12):3034–3036.
14. United States Renal Data System Website: http://www.usrds.org/2003.
15. Bommer J. Prevalence and socio-economic aspects of chronic kidney disease. Nephrol Dial Transplant 2002; 17(suppl 11):8–12.
16. Barsoum RS. Overview: end-stage renal disease in the developing world. Artif Organs 2002; 26(9):737–746.

17. Wild S, Roglic G, Green A, Sicree R, King H. Global prevalence of diabetes: estimates for the year 2000 and projections for 2030. Diabetes Care 2004; 27(5):1047–1053.
18. Ibrahim MM, Rizk H, Appel LJ, el Aroussy W, Helmy S, Sharaf Y, Ashour Z, Kandil H, Roccella E, Whelton PK. Hypertension prevalence, awareness, treatment, and control in Egypt. Results from the Egyptian National Hypertension Project (NHP). NHP Investigative Team. Hypertension 1995; 26(6 Pt 1): 886–890.
19. Mosley JD, Appel LJ, Ashour Z, Coresh J, Whelton PK, Ibrahim MM. Relationship between skin color and blood pressure in Egyptian adults: results from the national hypertension project. Hypertension 2000; 36(2): 296–302.
20. Naicker S. End-stage renal disease in sub-Saharan and South Africa. Kidney Int Suppl 2003; 83:S119–S22.
21. Queiroz Madeira EP, da Rosa Santos O, Ferreira Santos SF, Alonso da Silva L, MacIntyre Innocenzi A, Santoro-Lopes G. Familial aggregation of end-stage kidney disease in Brazil. Nephron 2002; 91(4):666–670.
22. Cass A, Cunningham J, Snelling P, Wang Z, Hoy W. Exploring the pathways leading from disadvantage to end-stage renal disease for indigenous Australians. Soc Sci Med 2004; 58(4):767–785.
23. Barsoum R. The kidney in tropical infections. El Nahas AM, Harris KV, Anderson S, eds. Mechanisms and Clinical Management of Chronic Renal Failure. Vol. 2. Oxford: Oxford University Press, 2000:373–400.
24. Barsoum R. Glomerulonephritis in the tropics. Nur Elhuda M, ed. Glomerular Diseases. 1st ed. Dubai: Al Nadwah, 2004:87–162.
25. Barsoum R, Sitprija V. Tropical nephrology. Schrier RW, Gottschalk CW, eds. Diseases of the Kidney. Vol. VI. Boston: Little Brown, 1996:2221–2268.
26. National Health and Nutrition Examination Survey (NHANES III) Website: www.pop.psu.edu/data-archive/daman/nhanes4.htm.
27. Barsoum R, Francis M. Spectrum of glomerulonephritis in Egypt. Saudi J Kidney Dis Transplant 2000; 11(3):1–9.

2

Outcomes and Economics of ESRF

Eduardo Lacson Jr.

*Clinical Research and Technology Assessment, Medical Department,
Fresenius Medical Care, North America, Lexington, Massachusetts, U.S.A.*

Martin K. Kuhlmann and Nathan W. Levin

*Albert Einstein College of Medicine and Renal Research Institute, New York,
New York, U.S.A.*

Kunal Shah and Maki Yoshino

Renal Research Institute, New York, New York, U.S.A.

The exact number of patients with end-stage renal failure (ESRF) globally is unknown because there is neither a global registry nor an official countrywide registry in the majority of nations and sovereign states. However, in a survey of 120 countries with established dialysis programs in 2001, 1.479 million people were estimated to have ESRF (1). Since then, an expanded follow-up survey revealed that ESRF affected 1.681 million people globally by year-end 2003 (2). Of these, only 382,000 (22.7%) received a renal transplant (RTX) and even fewer at 141,000 (8.4%) were on peritoneal dialysis (PD). The majority of patients numbering over 1.158 million (68.9%) received various forms of hemodialysis (HD) treatments to stay alive. These numbers are expected to rise in the near future due to the increasing prevalence of diabetes worldwide and increasing life expectancy. Currently, patients are distributed among 122 countries that reported having programs caring for ESRF patients. These 122 countries have a combined population of 5.8 billion, representing 92.4% of the world's estimated 6.3 billion people at year-end 2003. Although it is tempting to define geographic regions or delineate economic systems and structures as well as to compare outcomes between them, the absence of uniform definitions of processes, systems and outcomes as well as standardized data collection instruments for complete tracking of diagnoses and treatments among these 122 countries preclude direct comparisons. Furthermore, the inability to quantify the impact of local culture and hereditary/genetic/environmental effects on the illness, access to care, population lifespan, patient preferences, available therapeutic strategies, and the outcomes themselves confound the interpretation of any comparison. This chapter will attempt to elucidate key factors confounding clinical outcomes, describe the economics within ESRF management, and review some available "controlled" comparison of clinical outcomes, realizing that the available data are limited mostly to the United States of America (USA), Japan, and the European Union (EU). In addition, since the majority of ESRF patients are provided renal replacement therapy (RRT) via HD, most of the concepts in this chapter are developed with information based on this modality.

DIFFERENTIAL ACCESS TO ESRF CARE

Perhaps the greatest obstacle towards apples-to-apples comparison between countries or regions of the world is unequal access to ESRF diagnosis and RRT. First, consider that there are at least 500 million people from 110 countries or sovereign states without organized ESRF care. Any attempt to compare outcomes will have to exclude them. Second, despite limiting the comparisons to the treatment programs in the remaining 122 countries, it turns out that the majority of them are actually small and limited. In fact, 99% of the global ESRF dialysis population comes from only 75 countries. To narrow it down further, five countries account for 56% of all the global dialysis patients: USA, Japan, Germany, Brazil, and Italy. These five countries represent a mere 12% of the world's population yet they cater to more than half of the patients on dialysis care. Thus, there exists a huge discrepancy among different countries regarding the access to RRT based on the variation of the reported prevalence of dialysis-treated ESRF. This is very evident from Table 1, showing the regional distribution of dialysis patients (HD and PD combined) in comparison to their reported population (2). A key assumption here is that the countries with the largest dialysis populations do not necessarily have populations that are overwhelmingly predisposed to have ESRF, either because of genetic or environmental influences. Given such an assumption, if the entire global population had equal access to ESRF care, such a disproportional distribution of dialysis patients would be highly improbable. This realization poses two important questions: First, how can a balanced comparison be made between the clinical outcomes from a country that treats a miniscule fraction of its ESRF cases against one that treats almost all diagnosed patients? Second, are the reported care processes and clinical outcomes in the countries with the most ESRF patients even applicable to derive projections and conclusions about all the other countries

Table 1 Distribution of ESRF Patients on Dialysis Therapies

Countries ranked by dialysis population	Population (million)	% of world population	Dialysis patients (thousand)	% of total dialysis patients	Prevalence of dialysis (p.m.p.)
USA	292	4.6%	310	24%	1,060
Japan	128	2.0%	242	19%	1,890
Germany	82	1.3%	65	5%	790
Brazil	183	2.9%	64	5%	350
Italy	58	0.9%	45	3%	770
Countries 6 to 15	1,811	28.6%	290	22%	160
Countries 16 to 122	3,306	52.2%	284	22%	85
Countries 123 to 232	476	7.5%	0	0%	0
Total	6,336		1,299		205

Source: From Ref. 2.

of the world? The simplistic answer to the first question is that a balanced comparison is not possible and any attempt towards such a comparison will be subject to major caveats. The simplistic answer to the second question is that we have to rely on data from mature clinical programs in order to define projections for the rest of the world because there is currently no better alternative.

A case in point will be a country like India, with a population count of over 1 billion, roughly 16% of the world's population (more about India in Chapter 19) and a higher population density than that of the USA, Japan, Germany, Brazil, and Italy combined. The estimated number of prevalent patients in India is 14,000 or 13 patients per million population (pmp) (Stefan F. Mueller, personal communication). This stands in contrast to an estimated incidence of ESRF of 100 pmp or about 100,000 to 120,000 new patients per year that would theoretically develop ESRF (3). However, the final "acceptance rate" of patients for RRT (actual incidence) is estimated as 3 to 5 pmp or only 3000 to 5000 patients per year (4,5). The disparity is enormous when comparing to the dialysis patients treated in other nations as reported in the last column of Table 1. If there were 100,000 new patients in a given year, up to 90% or 90,000 incident ESRF patients don't even see the nephrologist (3). Of the remaining 10,000 patients, 1000 (10%) will not be able to afford any dialysis therapy (6). Among the remaining 9000 patients, 0.5% (500 patients) will perform continuous ambulatory PD (CAPD), thus leaving about 8500 new patients on HD annually. Of these 8500 patients, within the first year, 9–13% die, 17–23% gets a kidney transplant, and about 60% are lost to follow-up, presumably because HD is not a cure and it will impoverish the entire patient's family (3). Thus, the small number of HD patients noted in India. Similarly, an estimated 3 to 5 pmp dialysis patients are attributed to China, the highest populated country in the world (7). A caveat for China, if the data were limited only to the economically developed areas (i.e., major cities), the prevalent dialysis estimates are increased up to 102 pmp (8), but this computation does an injustice to the majority of the Chinese population without such access to RRT that is ignored. The situation is not better in many developing nations, some with numbers of patients so low, that you have to present patient counts that are not normalized (per million population) so that the numbers appear plausible.

It is doubtful that a comparison of clinical outcomes or even therapeutic options between India and the USA or countries of the EU will be sensible, let alone fair. However, it may be possible to predict the potential for growth in the ESRF population for a country like India based on experiences from well-developed programs, if the prevailing situation were to change and each and every person were given equal access to care. The world may be heading in that direction as the combined pattern of growth of ESRF patients treated in Asia, Latin America, Middle East, Africa now averages 10% per year over the past few years. This rate is more than twice that for the USA, Japan, and the European Union, each growing annually at approximately 4% annually (2). Although the absolute numbers are less for the developing countries, the relative growth speaks volumes regarding the potential impact that improved access to ESRF care can have in these areas. Furthermore, if the growth pattern continues, there could be a major shift in the number of patients with ESRF receiving RRT towards the developing world within the next decade.

ECONOMICS OF ESRF CARE

It is not unreasonable to postulate that globalization with its associated economic growth may improve access to ESRF care as the individual national healthcare budgets increase and dialysis programs in the developing nations continue to mature. True enough, there appears to be a threshold relationship with a country's per capita income, where the dialysis program's record of ESRF prevalence drops dramatically as the country's per capita income falls below US$10,000 per year, as can be seen from data in Figure 1, obtained from the top 75 countries that service 99% of the world's ESRF population (2). Even within the European continent alone, up to a two-fold or greater difference in the prevalence of treated ESRF patients and a corresponding similar difference in average gross national product (GNP) was noted in the 1990s, exaggerated further when the EU and the former Soviet-bloc Eastern European countries were compared, illustrated in Figure 2 (9,10). More importantly, the break-up of the former Soviet Union brought about socioeconomic changes in the non-EU countries with a profound effect on access to ESRF care illustrated by a dramatic increase of patients treated with HD of 78% and PD of 306% within the first 7 years (10).

It is not difficult to understand why national economics plays a major role in ESRF care. First, general per capita income is a major determinant of the

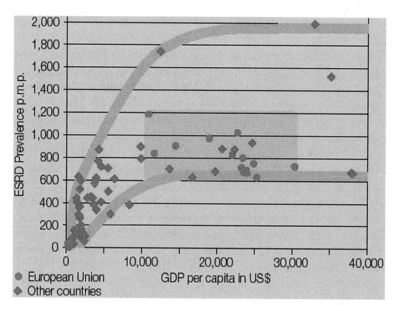

Figure 1 Relationship between GDP per capita and prevalence of ESRF in the top 75 countries with 99% of the world's ESRF population.
Source: From Ref. 2.

purchasing power of both the country and its people. Second, renal replacement therapy for ESRF requires sustained, lifelong therapy by definition. Third, all forms of RRT entail some cost, both initially and for maintenance of the

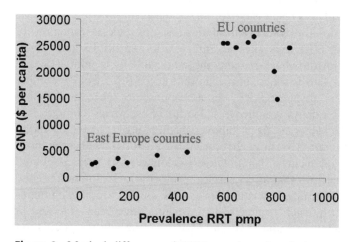

Figure 2 Marked difference of RRT prevalence in relation to per capita income even within the European continent.
Source: From Ref. Dr. Miguel Riella, Curitiba, Brazil.

treatment. Taken together, the cumulative cost of providing RRT to patients with ESRF over time will take its toll as a burgeoning economic burden to society. Although multiple national economic RRT payment models have been described (11) and will be discussed in the subsequent section of this chapter, it is prudent to examine the determinants of cost between modalities of RRT.

The most physiologic form of RRT is RTX, where the lost function from the native kidneys is replaced by another kidney. It is generally accepted as the most cost-effective ESRF treatment in developed countries (12,13). This is the case, even among developing countries (3,14,15). The cost of RTX is much higher than dialysis in the first year because of up-front surgery and hospitalization expenses. Over time, the maintenance costs decline as the expenses are reduced to mostly antirejection medications, rejection episodes, and complications of immune suppression. When the appropriate resources allow for the recommended immunosuppression protocols to be followed, RTX has also been shown to improve survival and quality of life when compared to dialysis therapies for ESRF (16). In developing countries, creative protocols to discontinue the more expensive medications, like cyclosporine, in lieu of less expensive medications, like steroids and azathioprine, further reduce the cost burden (5). Analogous to this in the USA, medication non-compliance has recently emerged as a major factor that can adversely affect clinical outcomes (17). Thus, because of deviation from recommended immunosuppression protocols, it is not surprising that in developing countries such as India, RTX has been reported to have relatively worse clinical outcomes (18).

A potential model for funding RTX in developing countries was adopted in Pakistan that allows for a community–government partnership, where the government is responsible for 40% of costs and the rest is derived from community donations (19). This model develops societal responsibility as the approach to RTX and takes advantage of local attitudes and values. However, the major drawback remains the same globally: a limited supply of donor kidneys. This is the main reason that keeps RTX from becoming the most prevalent form of RRT. As a response to the overwhelming demand for donor kidneys, a controversial industry known as "commercial" transplantation has emerged from impoverished countries, including India. However, the outcomes from such procedures are often worse for both donors (20) and recipients (21,22). These outcomes have been attributed to cost-cutting measures that affect surgical protocols including non-aseptic operating rooms, poor infection control protocols, and sub-optimal immuno-suppression regimen. Such commercial transplants have been outlawed in many nations, including India (23). Until more of the world's population agree to become voluntary kidney donors, kidneys can be grown from renal progenitor cells (24,25) and/or the problems associated with xenotransplantation is solved (25–28), the shortage of donor kidneys will hamper the growth of RTX. Until then and as is the current state of affairs, the bulk of expenditure for ESRF therapy is spent on dialysis.

The costing of dialysis therapies is not as simple as it seems. Different countries with varying payment schemes consider multiple inputs into costing out dialysis therapy. Perhaps what is most commonly considered as part of "basic" or "core" direct dialysis-related costs globally include disposables (e.g., needles, dialyzers, bloodlines, dialysate, water, electricity, or PD solution), hardware (dialysis machine, technical services, water filtration system), and patient care services (nursing care, auxiliary services, or PD catheter insertion). However, apart from these costs, a myriad of components can either be considered as additional direct costs or considered as part of indirect costs as can be seen in Table 2 (29). Therefore, cost comparisons between countries or world regions can be quite complicated. Sample models for cost comparisons between dialysis modalities can thus be contrasted as seen in Figures 3 and 4. One modality may be more expensive than another depending on the approach, although most reports point to PD as the less expensive therapy, especially if the comparison to HD is made with chronic ambulatory PD (CAPD) as opposed to automated PD (APD) (30).

Another key variable in costing out dialysis therapies is the components of the specific therapy. For example, type of dialyzer or "reuse" of dialyzers impacts the potential cost of HD therapy. Using India as a representative of the developing world, it is no surprise that cost-cutting measures are taken to provide the lowest possible cost of HD therapies. Most patients are dialyzed only twice a week, using cheaper cellulosic dialyzer ($1-1.3\,m^2$), with manual reuse of both dialyzer and tubing (4–6 times), formaldehyde cleansing, many

Table 2 Input into Computation of "Dialysis Costs"

Total dialysis cost			
Dialysis treatment: "basic" reimbursement (direct costs)	Disposables Machine/ RO Technical services Nursing care Auxillary care	Catering Laboratory tests Pharmaceuticals Diagnostics Access care	Physician fee Patient training Centre overheads
Dialysis care: "additional" reimbursement (Indirect induced costs)	Transport Home aid Hospital care	Catering Laboratory tests Pharmaceuticals Diagnostics Access care	Physician fee Patient training Centre overheads
Additional cost components (induced costs)	Patient co-payments: Sick leave, Pensions, Unemployment benefit, Home aid		

Source: From Ref. 29.

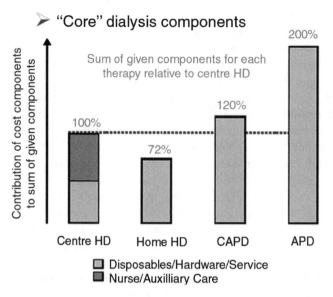

Figure 3 Model comparing modality costs using a "core" direct costing approach commonly considered in many developing countries.
Source: From Ref. 29.

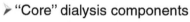
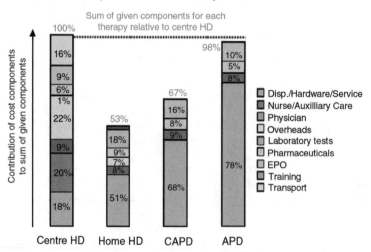

Figure 4 Model comparing modality costs using a direct costing approach often seen in countries with mature dialysis programs.
Source: From Ref. 29.

HD machines have no volumetric ultrafiltration control, almost all facilities have no standardized water quality testing, and acetate dialysate is used in 70–80% of treatments (3,5,31). Therefore, an individual HD treatment in India may cost between US $20–40 (3), which is very low when compared to US $100 to > US $500 per treatment for the USA and the EU (29). At a mean HD treatment cost of around US $30 (between US $20 and US $40) per session, the annual expenditure for the basic or core HD amounts to US $3120 at a frequency of twice weekly or at thrice weekly HD, US $4680 (3,32). This does not include any laboratory testing, drugs (e.g., erythropoietin), or hospital admissions and procedures (e.g., HD vascular access placement). In some countries, however, reuse is forbidden by government edict, even when economics would dictate the opposite.

In general, care should be taken when comparing cost or outcome of HD treatments between countries, because there are substantial differences in regard of technology, mode, and frequency of HD therapies. These differences in the components of HD therapies alone may confound any outcome differences observed between countries.

PAYMENT AND PROVIDER MODELS FOR ESRF CARE

Three main models of healthcare in the USA, EU, and Japan have been described based on their funding (11). The public ("Beveridge") model is based on taxation (e.g., National Health Service) with a network of predominantly public providers. Some examples of countries where this model can be used to describe healthcare systems include the United Kingdom (UK), Italy, Spain, Sweden, Denmark, Norway, Finland, and Canada. The mixed ("Bismarck") model uses a premium-financed social insurance system and is served by a mixture of public and private providers. Representative examples include France, Germany, Austria, Switzerland, Belgium, Holland, and Japan. The private insurance model is reserved for the USA where ESRD care in patients younger than 65 years at start of dialysis is initially the burden of private insurance with the premium-funded social insurance (Medicare) eventually bearing the burden of the program. In contrast, patients older than 65 years at initiation of RRT have Medicare as primary payer. However, based on providers of dialysis care, the preponderance of private providers in Japan tends to group the country with the USA. The providers in the USA are predominantly private and the majority of outpatient dialysis facilities now belong to large corporate chains, with the top 10 dialysis chains providing care to >70% of all dialysis patients (33). Some developing nations may loosely fall under two of the three models described above. Mexico has national coverage (34) and may be classified under the Beveridge model. Other countries such as Pakistan (19,35), Turkey (14), or Brazil (36) fall under the Bismarck model. Other Latin American countries that have been classified under the Bismarck model include Argentina, Chile, Colombia, Uruguay, and Venezuela (37).

The classification models were found to have a correlation with the prevalent modality of treatment, but correlating more with provider type than funding source. Access to dialysis care increases from public provider to mixed provider to private provider models in that order, based on the prevalent ESRF patients at 419 to 572, 600 to 748, 790 to 1150 pmp, respectively, and incident ESRF patients at 60 to 104, 94 to 125, 194 to 214 pmp, respectively (38). This trend is consistent with the number of available dialysis chairs at 45 to 88, 55 to 152, 144 to 468 pmp, from public provider to mixed provider to private provider models, respectively. In the EU, the availability of nephrologists differs between public and mixed as well (e.g., UK = 4 pmp versus Germany = 26 pmp or Italy = 66 pmp). However, there appears to be a reverse trend for improved transplantation rates from 45% to 81%, 20% to 48%, and 0.3% to 26%, with functioning kidney grafts with public > mixed > private providers, respectively. Similarly, strictly stratifying by public or private providers without respect to funding type, the utilization of PD regardless of country was 0–13% for private providers in comparison to 11–47% in public providers (37). An analysis of cost for therapies within the provider models reveal: public in-center HD > private in-center HD > limited-care in-center HD > automated PD > Home HD or CAPD (30). The authors theorized that private providers invest heavily into HD centers such that PD or home HD is likely considered as an adjunct once capacity is reached. In contrast, public providers require low personnel and investment costs although there may be higher variable supply costs. It is interesting that in the USA where there is a fixed reimbursement for dialysis and the profit margin may be slightly in favor of PD, there is still no substantial growth of the PD population (39).

The main problem with these models is that they cannot fully describe the healthcare systems in the developing world. In many countries, there is some form of government-sponsored healthcare that is mostly acute and combined with a largely private fee-for-service provision of medical/surgical care and an open market for medical supplies. Mixed into the system is a variable amount of private insurance and at least two models of community/societal supported care. A trial program in Pakistan allows for a 40% government funded program with charity supporting 60% of costs within one hospital system in the capital, Karachi (19,35). A more established program is found in Singapore, although one can argue that this country should not be classified with its less developed Southeast Asian neighbors and should be compared more with Japan, especially since they treat 750 pmp with RRT. On large, the Singapore model (40) is funded by a partnership between a public foundation and for-profit corporations, while the providers consist of collaboration between the same public foundation and local health institutions.

Perhaps it is best to examine the funding situation in India, the surrogate nation used to describe developing nations in this chapter. The income per capita for this nation of 1 billion people is around US $440 and the government-allocated healthcare expenditure is US $1.80 for the year 2003 (32). Moreover, there is only 0.4 nephrologist and 0.2 dialysis chair, pmp (3). Therefore, it is no surprise that a large portion of patients with ESRF remain unable to get medical attention, not even RRT. Those who are fortunate enough to get RRT end up having to find creative ways to finance it, most with the assistance of family members and many more through the help of employers (63%), loans and asset liquidation (33%), although 4% are left to their own resources (3). Consequently, up to 71% of the patients who initiate therapy withdraw from therapy within 6 months, 88% of whom (~69% of total patients) do so for economic reasons. Therefore, it is not a mystery why the remaining patients on HD therapy in India account for only 13 pmp. Majority of developing countries from all the regions of the world have similar healthcare scenarios for ESRF such as China (8), Nigeria (41), Korea (42), most of Southeast Asia (43) [except Singapore (40)], and sub-Saharan/South Africa (44), among them. It is common to have some government funding for government employees, limited private employer assistance, miniscule role for private insurance, and self-pay/family support is required to support RRT. In South Africa, like in India, government support for RRT is premised on being a candidate for transplantation (44). Therefore, the data for outcomes from many developing countries are fraught with a strong patient selection bias that weighs heavily on wealth or employment, thus further decreasing the ability to ascribe any potential outcome differences between countries or regions to any single treatment-related or practice-related factor. One caveat is that patient selection bias is not confined to developing countries only. For example, provision of RRT for Australian patients is overtly restricted by an expected survival >6 months as well as a clinical indication that the patient's overall condition will be improved by dialysis (45).

From a theoretical perspective, it is plausible to include future costs for related and unrelated medical care and non-medical expenditures within economic evaluations. This is especially the case for ESRD, where prolonging patient life will have a significant effect on future costs for related medical care (i.e., dialysis and transplantation) and for unrelated medical care and non-medical expenditure health economics. Even relatively inexpensive interventions that extend survival of dialysis patients may not be cost effective since, by extending survival, extra outpatient dialysis costs will be large and need to be covered. These theoretical considerations are necessary when discussing the future economics of ESRD care in developing countries but should not be used as arguments against spreading and improving RRT.

As pointed out, a rise in the number of dialysis patients is an economic threat for developing countries. In that regard, slowing the progression of chronic kidney disease can have an important economical impact. Reduction in the progression of CRF could lead to a meaningful decrease in the prevalence and cost of ESRD. Even slowing the rate of decline in GFR by only 10% per year would have a significant cumulative economic impact. Data from Reference 46 for the U.S. Medicare system provide strong support for the development and implementation of intensive reno-protective efforts beginning at the early stages of chronic renal disease and continued throughout its course. This approach will be even more important in economically weaker nations.

CLINICAL OUTCOMES OF ESRF CARE

All the concern generated by the prior discussion regarding differences of access to care (and by default, patient selection for RRT) as well as the impact of economic factors is germane, as we attempt a reasonable comparison of outcomes among different countries. Death being the final outcome of consequence is often the main focus when comparing life-saving therapies. Thus, it was concerning when the available data from almost two decades ago revealed that the death rate in the USA was 15% higher than in Europe and 33% higher than in Japan, despite adjusting for age and the presence of diabetes mellitus (47). The available data were limited and the registry data collection methodologies and classification were variable, thus precluding a more thorough analysis. With the advent of the Dialysis Outcomes and Practice Patterns Study or DOPPS, the limitations of the past have been methodologically eliminated with a more thorough data collection from a representative sample population as well as adjustment for more case-mix variables towards a more robust comparison between countries (48). During the first phase of the DOPPS study, participating countries were limited to the largest dialysis programs in the world (USA, Japan, and EU to include UK, France, Italy, Germany, and Spain), but meanwhile numerous other countries have joined, such as Australia, Canada, New Zealand, Belgium, and Sweden. This data set provides an interesting parallel for the available data from some developing countries. Some demographic variables from DOPPS and selected reports from other countries are shown in Table 3.

Table 3 provides an interesting case study as to why DOPPS is very important. A cursory look at the table may leave the reader with the following impressions:

1. Patients dialyzed in developing countries are younger.
2. Patients dialyzed in developing countries have less diabetes.
3. With the exception of Kenya, the crude death rate for HD patients in developing countries is better than or similar to the top three DOPPS regions.

What is not overtly expressed in similar tables or reviews in the literature are the following potential sources of bias and confounding:

Table 3 Comparative Crude Mortality Rate Between Countries (with Age and Diabetes Information) Obtained from a Sampling of Published Literature. Please Read Text for Critique.

Country or Region	Age (years)	DM+ (%)	Death Rate (crude % / yr)
Jap-DOPPS [48]	58.6	25.6	6.6
EU-DOPPS [48]	60.2	20.1	15.6
USA-DOPPS [48]	60.5	45.7	21.7
Turkey [13]	44.2	–	10.9
India [31]	38.6	13.8	9.7
Korea [42]	53	15	–
Latin America [49]	50.5	16.9	21.1
Yugoslavia [50]	–	7	17.9
Kenya [51]	29.6	–	65
Uruguay [52]	57	15	13.8

a. Sampling method—e.g., "Did the data come from a national registry or a single-center experience?"
b. Definition of terms—e.g., "How was the presence or absence of diabetes determined?"
c. Period of data collection—e.g., "Are the data being compared contemporaneous?"
d. Completeness of the data collection—e.g., "Are all patients treated included in the denominator for computing the crude mortality rate?"

First, single-center experiences may be biased towards any factor and may not be representative of the country. Therefore, it can skew age, diabetes prevalence, and even death rates. That being said, younger dialysis patients appear to be a near universal finding among developing countries. Studies from different period of observation, country of observation, geographic location, and manner of data collection (e.g., survey vs. center data) confirm it. It may be a result of patient survival (e.g., older patients die before seeing the nephrologist), patient selection (e.g., physician gatekeeper projecting outcome), patient/societal attitudes (e.g., younger patients have a full life ahead of them and should be treated aggressively), poor preventive care (e.g., uncontrolled hypertension causing ESRF to present at a younger age), environmental exposure (e.g., schistosomiasis in the active young farmer), or some other unmeasured factor. Second, comparing different time periods can be misleading. The dialysis population has been aging over time such that age data from 1984 will not likely reflect the age of ESRF patients in 2004 (49). The same effect is noted with increasing incidence of diabetic renal disease (50). Consider the experience from Eastern Europe after the break up of the Soviet Union when diabetic renal disease increased from 4.4% to 10.7% within a few years (10). Third, the crude mortality rates may also vary over time. It may also be affected by center as illustrated by the single-center experience with the 65% death rate reported for Kenya in Table 3. The denominator may exclude deaths due to withdrawal from dialysis as illustrated by the example of India (3,31). The crude mortality rate shown for India (9.7%) in Table 3 ignores the fact that 60% of the denominator was excluded because the patients withdrew from dialysis therapy. Finally, assuming that the data obtained are indeed accurate, uniformly collected, contemporaneous, and complete, the influence of age, diabetes, and other factors will need to be defined so that a more balanced or adjusted mortality rate can be obtained. This is the value of having the DOPPS study from which most of the remaining outcomes will be discussed.

One key report from DOPPS allowed for the comparison of mortality outcomes between the three continents now adjusted for age, male gender, black race, diabetes, and 24 other comorbidities (51). The inequalities of the crude mortality rates did not totally balance out and still left mortality rates greatest in the USA > EU > Japan. Health-related quality of life was measured among the three continents in DOPPS and results reveal that the Japanese perceived the heaviest burden, yet had the highest physical function scores (52). Subsequent analyses reveal that a higher PCS score is associated with improved survival (53). However, it is unclear whether or not interventions can significantly increase the physical function score and more importantly, whether or not such an improvement if present, will lead to subsequent improvement in mortality. Other potential predictors of mortality include non-adherence to prescribed therapy (54). Non-adherence was associated with increased mortality, specifically with skipping >1 treatment per month or shortening dialysis sessions by 10 min or more. It is not surprising that these parameters are more prevalent in the USA where mortality rate is the highest. This is very relevant to developing countries, where dialysis treatments are performed twice weekly or even once weekly with higher risk for inadequate dialysis and death. High phosphorus levels >7.5 g/dL and high interdialytic weight gain above 5.7% of dry weight were also associated with mortality and hospitalization risk.

Among surrogate outcomes such as dialysis adequacy, the DOPPS had spKt/V of 1.3 among all continents, thus negating any comparisons (54). When the data were pooled, it raised some concern about the potential need for higher dialysis dose for women (55), consistent with the findings from the recently concluded HEMO study (56). For developing countries like India, for example, Kt/V is often not measured or if done, results show that many patients have spKt/V <1.0 (3). Again, the main concern in developing countries is the provision of HD, sometimes to alleviate emergent fluid or electrolyte problems and with less emphasis on laboratory-based adequacy measurements. There was a large variation between the DOPPS countries when considering anemia management (57). However, there is little to add to currently existing clinical practice guidelines except perhaps to encourage judicious iron replacement (35–40% had transferring saturation <10%) and maintenance of a high index of clinical suspicion for other sources of blood loss or covert infection/inflammation. The findings confirmed that the wide standard deviations of the hemoglobin values made it very difficult to keep hemoglobin within the narrow 11–12 mg/dL range recommended by the Kidney Disease Outcomes Quality Initiative (K/DOQI) guidelines for anemia management (58), consistent with data from Ref. 59. The relevance of this finding to the developing world rests mostly in the lack of funds for the procurement of erythropoietin. The potential need for erythropoietin can be exponentially grown if the access to RRT continues to grow. However, as in the case of India, the cost of erythropoietin may be twice that of the HD treatment itself (3). Medications are often not reimbursed in developing countries and these become out-of-pocket expenses. Therefore, given the choice, most patients would rather save any spare funds to pay for future HD therapy rather than pay for a single dose of erythropoietin, with uncertainty as to when they can get funds for the next dose.

More recently, attention has been given to the correlation between serum bicarbonate and mortality and even hospitalization (60). Pooled results from DOPPS indicate that the target bicarbonate may need to be 20 to 23 meq/L, a range associated with the lowest mortality risk and least hospitalization risk. These numbers are slightly lower than the >22 meq/L value recommended by the K/DOQI guidelines for nutrition (61). Serum bicarbonate is rarely measured in developing countries, but severe acidosis, especially below 17 to 18 meq/L, certainly requires corrective action. Again, similar to erythropoietin, patients in developing countries would rather divert any spare funds to future HD therapy and if needed, life-saving medications, before spending it on additional laboratory tests such as bicarbonate. Finally, one intervention that has recently been identified that is associated with around 16% improved mortality despite adjusting for age, race, gender, vintage, diabetes, and 14 other comorbid conditions in HD patients in DOPPS is the intake of water-soluble multivitamin supplement (62). There is substantial variation in multivitamin intake among DOPPS countries and this may be related to the cost. HD patients in developing countries may be encouraged to buy water-soluble multivitamins containing folate, vitamin B6, vitamin B12, and ascorbic acid, if they are able to get them. However, as with all things, this expense will likely have lower priority than more basic survival needs in the developing world.

Taken together, the DOPPS study shows that dialysis practices are not very different in United States, Japan, and the EU. DOPPS so far has not revealed a satisfactory explanation for the mortality differences between these three continents. Shorter dialysis time, lower rate of native fistulas, higher rate of catheter use, higher UF rates and lower MDxt/P (time a doc-

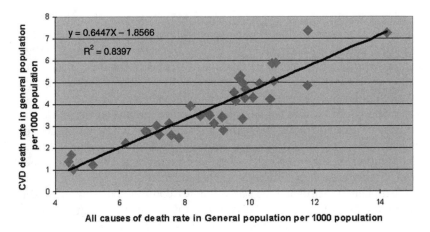

Figure 5 High variability in cardiovascular mortality that correlates with general mortality rates in the population from the World Health Organization [63].

tor spends per patients) are found in the United States, but these potential factors are counteracted by higher dialysis dose and better anemia management. During the recent years, practice patterns in the various countries became more and more similar, but, nevertheless, differences in mortality rates prevailed. This demonstrates that international differences in mortality rates may be influenced by other factors than practice patterns, such as environmental factors and genetic background.

Interestingly, preliminary data show a relationship between cardiovascular and all-cause death rates in the general population of various countries worldwide. Data on cardiovascular and all-cause mortality for 35 countries, as provided by the WHO database (63), are depicted in Figure 5. Cardiovascular death rates are almost seven-fold higher in countries in the upper end compared to the lower end of the spectrum. The highest cardiovascular death rates are observed in Eastern European countries, such as Romania and Hungary, while lower death rates are reported for Southeast Asian countries, which, despite a high incidence of hypertension and diabetes, cluster at the left end of the spectrum. Mediterranean, other Western European countries and the United States assemble in between. These preliminary data demonstrate that there is a variability in cardiovascular death rates worldwide, ranging from 1 to 7 per 1000 population and that this is reflected in all-cause mortality rates. These differences in background general population mortality rates may account for some of the differences observed in international dialysis patient mortality rates. Further studies will compare dialysis mortality with background mortality of specific countries. In the dialysis population, Asians tend to have improved survival even among the different racial categories within the USA (64; A. Collins, personal communication) and this has also been noted in Canada (65).

NUTRITION AND OUTCOME

Another important point that affects survival of dialysis patients in developing countries is the nutritional status. It is well documented that both the prevalence of protein-energy malnutrition (PEM) at initiation of renal replacement therapy, as well as the development of PEM during dialysis are associated with morbidity and mortality in dialysis patients. The prevalence of malnutrition in the ESRD population of developing countries is an estimated 42–77% with an average serum albumin concentration of 2.39 mg/dL at the time of dialysis initiation (66). In Western countries, PEM is mainly due to underlying diseases, depression, or uremia per se, while in developing countries there is a multitude of other reasons for PEM, such as poverty, chronic infections, lack of food supply, or religious practices, which promote abstinence from meat, fish, and eggs (67). It has to be recognized that low serum albumin levels are often due to a chronic inflammatory status. The co-association of malnutrition, inflammation, and atherosclerosis has been described as MIA syndrome, which is prevalent in a large fraction of dialysis patients. Increased levels of C-reactive protein (CRP), a positive acute-phase protein, and low levels of serum albumin, a negative acute-phase protein, are found in patients with chronic inflammation. The acute-phase response is induced by pro-inflammatory cytokines released from activated monocytes and macrophages. Insufficient water quality is a major cause of inflammation and use of ultrapure water for dialysis may be an important step towards less inflammation and better survival in hemodialysis patients (68). The prevalence of MIA syndrome is likely to be high and under-diagnosed in the developing world.

ECONOMICS OF PERITONEAL DIALYSIS IN DEVELOPING COUNTRIES

Countries in Asia vary significantly in culture and socioeconomic status. Dialysis costs and reimbursement structures are significant factors in decisions about the rates and modalities of renal replacement therapy. From a survey of Asian nephrologists conducted in 2001, a number of observations can be made (69). In many developing countries, the annual cost of continuous ambulatory peritoneal dialysis (CAPD) is greater than the per capita gross national income (GNI). The median cost of a 2-L bag of peritoneal dialysis (PD) fluid is around US$5. The absolute cost of PD fluid among countries with significant differences in per capita GNI actually varies very little. Thus, most renal failure patients can be expected to have problems accessing PD therapy in developing countries in Asia. In countries with unequal reimbursement policies for PD versus hemodialysis, a lack of incentive to prescribe PD also exists. Automated PD is nearly non-existent in many developing countries in Asia. Some possible ways to reduce the cost barriers to PD in those countries include individual governments providing more public funding for treating dialysis patients, dialysate-producing companies reducing the cost of their products. This can be achieved by setting up plants for dialysate production in the respective countries. This approach has recently been used in India and already led to a rising number of PD patients:

- physicians using appropriately smaller exchange volumes (3 × 2 L) in some Asian patients with smaller body sizes and with residual renal function;
- reducing the complication rate for PD (for example, peritonitis), thereby reducing the costs required for treatment and hospitalization.

SUMMARY

The outcomes of ESRF in the world remain an estimate at best, especially among the developing world. Direct comparisons of outcomes between countries are fraught with confounders that require astute review and interpretation. The economics of ESRF therapy limit the therapeutic options and influence basic access to RRT. Although RTX is the treatment of choice, the shortage of donor kidneys remains the major hindrance and is a global problem. Therefore, dialytic therapy remains the major RRT worldwide. With increasing economic globalization, there may be improving access to ESRF care in the developing world. The pattern of growth of the ESRF population in Asia, Latin America, Middle East, and Africa is 2.5 times higher than in the USA, EU, or Japan. This may signal a significant shift in the ESRF burden towards the developing world within this decade. The provision of dialysis entails significant cost that is cumulative over time. Therefore, society as a whole, whether within regions, countries, states, cities, or communities, needs to prepare for a potential global epidemic of ESRF. Recent initiatives have been made to increase awareness about kidney disease and to employ preventive measures through global clinical practice guidelines to stem the progress of chronic kidney disease into ESRF (70). Again, the limiting factor for implementing preventive guidelines remains financial (46,70). However, for the sake of patients in the developing world who are near ESRF now, the best way to improve outcomes is for nephrologists and public health practitioners to spur the development of partnerships between citizens of the world, communities, private corporations, and government agencies so that a cooperative approach based on available models (19,40) may be utilized for adequate access to healthcare, support for maintenance therapy, high-quality ESRF care, and adoption of best practices with judicious use of novel technological advancements.

REFERENCES

1. Moeller S, Gioberge S, Brown G. ESRD patients in 2001: global overview of patients, treatment modalities and development trends. Nephrol Dial Transplant 2002; 17:2071–2076.
2. Fresenius Medical Care. ESRD Patients in 2003—a Global Perspective. Fresenius Medical Care Internal Survey, Bad Homburg, Germany, 2004:1–10.
3. Kher V. End-stage renal disease in developing countries. Kidney Int 2002; 62:350–362.
4. Cha V, Chugh KS. Dialysis in developing countries: priorities and obstacles. Nephrology 1996; 2:65–72.
5. Jha V. End-stage renal care in developing countries: the India experience. Ren Fail 2004; 26:201–208.
6. Keshaviah P. Resource limitations and strategies for the treatment of uremia: a dialysis unit in the Himalayan foothills. Blood Purif 2001; 19:44–52.
7. Li L. End stage renal disease in China. Kidney Int 1996; 49:287–301.
8. Lin S. Nephrology in China: a great mission and momentous challenge. Kidney Int 2003; 63(suppl 83):S108–S110.
9. Berthoux F, Jones E, Gellert R, Mendel S, Saker L, Briggs D. Epidemiological data of treated end-stage renal failure in the European Union (EU) during the year 1995: report of the European Renal Association Registry and the National Registries. Nephrol Dial Transplant 1999; 14:2332–2342.
10. Rutkowski B, Ciocalteu A, Djukanovic L, Kiss I, Kovac A, Krivoshiev S, Kveder R, Polenakovic M, Puretic Z, Stanaityte M, Tareyeva I, Teplan V, Zavitz J. Evolution of renal replacement therapy in Central and Eastern Europe 7 years after political and economical liberation. Central and Eastern Europe Advisory Board in Chronic Renal Failure. Nephrol Dial Transplant 1998; 13:860–864.
11. Lameire N, Joffe P, Wiedemann M. Healthcare systems—an international review: an overview. Nephrol Dial Transplant 1999; 14(suppl 6):3–9.
12. Winkelmayer WC, Weinstein MC, Mittleman MA, Glynn RJ, Pliskin JS. Health economic evaluations: the special case of end-stage renal disease treatment. Med Decis Making 2002; 22:417–430.
13. Kaminota M. Cost-effectiveness analysis of dialysis and kidney transplants in Japan. Keio J Med 2001; 50:100–108.
14. Erek E, Sever MS, Akoglu E, Sariyar M, Bozfakioglu S, Apaydin S, Ataman R, Sarsmaz N, Altiparmak MR, Seyahi N, Serdengecti K. Cost of renal replacement therapy in Turkey. Nephrology (Carlton) 2004; 9:33–38.
15. Kalo Z, Jaray J, Nagy J. Economic evaluation of kidney transplantation versus hemodialysis in patients with end-stage renal disease in Hungary. Prog Transplant 2001; 11:188–193.
16. Wolfe RA, Ashby VB, Milford EL, Ojo AO, Ettenger RE, Agodoa LY, Held PJ, Port FK. Comparison of mortality in all patients on dialysis, patients on dialysis awaiting transplantation, and recipients of a first cadaveric transplant. N Engl J Med 1999; 341:1725–1730.
17. Nevins TE, Matas AJ. Medication noncompliance: another iceberg's tip. Transplantation 2004; 77:776–778.

18. Gulati S, Kumar A, Sharma RK, Gupta A, Bhandari M, Kumar A, Srivastava A. Outcome of pediatric renal transplants in a developing country. Pediatr Nephrol 2004; 19:96–100.

19. Rizvi SA. Present state of dialysis and transplantation in Pakistan. Am J Kidney Dis 1998; 31:xlv–xlviii.

20. Goyal M, Mehta RL, Schneiderman LJ, Sehgal AR. Economic and health consequences of selling a kidney in India. JAMA 2002; 288:1589–1593.

21. Anonymous. Commercially motivated renal transplantation: results in 540 patients transplanted in India. The Living Non-Related Renal Transplant Study Group. Clin Transplant 1997; 11:536–544.

22. Sever MS, Kazancioglu R, Yildiz A, Turkmen A, Ecder T, Kayacan SM, Celik V, Sahin S, Aydin AE, Eldegez U, Ark E. Outcome of living unrelated (commercial) renal transplantation. Kidney Int 2001; 60:1477–1483.

23. India Legislature. An Act (No 42 of 1994) to provide for the regulation of removal, storage and transplantation of human organs for therapeutic purposes and for the prevention of commercial dealings in human organs and for matters connected therewith or incidental thereto. Date of Assent by the President: 8 July 1994 (The Transplantation of Human Organs Act, 1994). Int Dig Health Legis 1995; 46:34–38.

24. Steer DL, Nigam SK. Developmental approaches to kidney tissue engineering. Am J Physiol Renal Physiol 2004; 86:F1–F7.

25. Hammerman MR. Organogenesis of kidneys following transplantation of renal progenitor cells. Transplant Immunol 2004; 12:229–239.

26. Lavillette D, Kabat D. Porcine endogenous retroviruses infect cells lacking cognate receptors by an alternative pathway: implications for retrovirus evolution and xenotransplantation. J Virol 2004; 78:8868–8877.

27. Fishman JA, Patience C. Xenotransplantation: infectious risk revisited. Am J Transplant 2004; 4:1383–1390.

28. Yang G. Application of xenogeneic stem cells for induction of transplantation tolerance. : present state and future directions. Springer Semin Immunopathol Sep 11 [Epub ahead of print], 2004.

29. Brown G. Dialysis funding and cost in Europe. Presentation at the World Congress of Nephrology, Berlin, 2003.

30. De Vecchi AF, Dratwa M, Wiedemann ME. Healthcare systems and end-stage renal disease (ESRD) therapies—an international review: costs and reimbursement/funding of ESRD therapies. Nephrol Dial Transplant 1999; 14(suppl 6): 31–41.

31. Rao M, Juneja R, Shirly RB, Jacob CK. Haemodialysis for end-stage renal disease in Southern India—a perspective from a tertiary referral care centre. Nephrol Dial Transplant 1998; 13:2494–2500.

32. Jacob C. Dialysis cost and funding in emerging nations. Presentation at the World Congress of Nephrology, Berlin, 2003.

33. Chartier K. Analysis: ten largest renal providers in 2004. Nephrol News Issues 2004; 18:41.

34. Cueto-Manzano AM. Peritoneal dialysis in Mexico. Kidney Int 2003; 63(suppl 83):S90–S92.

35. Sakhuja V, Sud K. End-stage renal disease in India and Pakistan: burden of disease and management issues. Kidney Int 2003; 63(suppl 83):S115–S118.
36. Zatz R, Romao JE Jr, Noronha IL. Nephrology in Latin America, with special emphasis on Brazil. Kidney Int 2003; 63(suppl 83):S131–S134.
37. Riella M. Dialysis funding and cost in Latin America. Presentation at the World Congress of Nephrology, Berlin, 2003.
38. Horl WH, de Alvaro F, Williams PF. Healthcare systems and end-stage renal disease (ESRD) therapies—an international review: access to ESRD treatments. Nephrol Dial Transplant 1999; 14(suppl 6):10–15.
39. U.S. Renal Data System. USRDS 2003 Annual Data Report: Atlas of End-Stage Renal Disease in the United States. Bethesda, MD: National Institutes of Health:National Institute of Diabetes and Digestive and Kidney Diseases 2003.
40. Ramirez SP, Durai TT, Hsu SI. Paradigms of public–private partnerships in end-stage renal disease care: the National Kidney Foundation Singapore. Kidney Int 2003; 63(suppl 83):S101–S107.
41. Bamgboye EL. Hemodialysis: management problems in developing countries, with Nigeria as a surrogate. Kidney Int 2003; 63(suppl 83):S93–S95.
42. Han H, Bleyer AJ, Houser RF, Jacques PF, Dwyer JT. Dialysis and nutrition practices in Korean hemodialysis centers. J Ren Nutr 2002; 12:42–48.
43. Sitprija V. Nephrology in South East Asia: fact and concept. Kidney Int 2003; 63(suppl 83):S128–S130.
44. Naiker S. End-stage renal disease in sub-Saharan and South Africa. Kidney Int 2003; 63(suppl 83):S119–S122.
45. Health Department of Western Australia. Review of End Stage renal Failure Services. Report of the Working Party. Perth, Australia: Health Department of Western Australia, 1994.
46. Trivedi HS, Pang MM, Campbell A, Saab P. Slowing the progression of chronic renal failure: economic benefits and patients' perspectives. Am J Kidney Dis 2002; 39:721–729.
47. Held PJ, Brunner F, Odaka M, Garcia JR, Port FK, Gaylin DS. Five-year survival for end-stage renal disease patients in the United States, Europe, and Japan, 1982 to 1987. Am J Kidney Dis 1990; 15:451–457.
48. Young EW, Goodkin DA, Mapes DL, Port FK, Keen ML, Chen K, Maroni BL, Wolfe RA, Held PJ. The Dialysis Outcomes and Practice Patterns Study (DOPPS): an international hemodialysis study. Kidney Int 2000; 57(suppl 74): S74–S81.
49. Stack AG, Messana JM. Renal replacement therapy in the elderly: medical, ethical, and psychosocial considerations. Adv Ren Replace Ther 2000; 7:52–62.
50. Harvey JN. Trends in the prevalence of diabetic nephropathy in type 1 and type 2 diabetes. Curr Opin Nephrol Hypertens 2003; 12:317–322.
51. Goodkin DA, Bragg-Gresham JL, Koenig KG, Wolfe RA, Akiba T, Andreucci VE, Saito A, Rayner HC, Kurokawa K, Port FK, Held PJ, Young EW. Association of comorbid conditions and mortality in hemodialysis patients in Europe, Japan, and the United States: the Dialysis Outcomes and Practice Patterns Study (DOPPS). J Am Soc Nephrol 2003; 14:3270–3277.

52. Fukuhara S, Lopes AA, Bragg-Gresham JL, Kurokawa K, Mapes DL, Akizawa T, Bommer J, Canaud BJ, Port FK, Held PJ, Worldwide Dialysis Outcomes, Practice Patterns Study. Health-related quality of life among dialysis patients on three continents: the Dialysis Outcomes and Practice Patterns Study. Kidney Int 2003; 64:1903–1910.

53. Mapes DL, Lopes AA, Satayathum S, McCullough KP, Goodkin DA, Locatelli F, Fukuhara S, Young EW, Kurokawa K, Saito A, Bommer J, Wolfe RA, Held PJ, Port FK. Health-related quality of life as a predictor of mortality and hospitalization: the Dialysis Outcomes and Practice Patterns Study (DOPPS). Kidney Int 2003; 64:339–349.

54. Saran R, Bragg-Gresham JL, Rayner HC, Goodkin DA, Keen ML, Van Dijk PC, Kurokawa K, Piera L, Saito A, Fukuhara S, Young EW, Held PJ, Port FK. Nonadherence in hemodialysis: associations with mortality, hospitalization, and practice patterns in the DOPPS. Kidney Int 2003; 64:254–262.

55. Port FK, Wolfe RA, Hulbert-Shearon TE, McCullough KP, Ashby VB, Held PJ. High dialysis dose is associated with lower mortality among women but not among men. Am J Kidney Dis 2004; 43:1014–1023.

56. Depner T, Daugirdas J, Greene T, Allon M, Beck G, Chumlea C, Delmez J, Gotch F, Kusek J, Levin N, Macon E, Milford E, Owen W, Star R, Toto R, Eknoyan G, Hemodialysis Study Group. Dialysis dose and the effect of gender and body size on outcome in the HEMO Study. Kidney Int 2004; 65:1386–1394.

57. Pisoni RL, Bragg-Gresham JL, Young EW, Akizawa T, Asano Y, Locatelli F, Bommer J, Cruz JM, Kerr PG, Mendelssohn DC, Held PJ, Port FK. Anemia management and outcomes from 12 countries in the Dialysis Outcomes and Practice Patterns Study (DOPPS). Am J Kidney Dis 2004; 44:94–111.

58. National Kidney Foundation. IV. NKF-K/DOQI clinical practice guidelines for anemia of chronic kidney disease: update 2000. Am J Kidney Dis 2001; 37(1 suppl 1):S182–S238.

59. Lacson E Jr, Ofsthun N, Lazarus JM. Effect of variability in anemia management on hemoglobin outcomes in ESRD. Am J Kidney Dis 2003; 41:111–124.

60. Bommer J, Locatelli F, Satayathum S, Keen ML, Goodkin DA, Saito A, Akiba T, Port FK, Young EW. Association of predialysis serum bicarbonate levels with risk of mortality and hospitalization in the Dialysis Outcomes and Practice Patterns Study (DOPPS). Am J Kidney Dis 2004; 44:661–671.

61. National Kidney Foundation. Clinical practice guidelines for nutrition in chronic renal failure. K/DOQI, National Kidney Foundation. Am J Kidney Dis 2000; 35(6 suppl 2):S1–S140.

62. Fissell RB, Bragg-Gresham JL, Gillespie BW, Goodkin DA, Bommer J, Saito A, Akiba T, Port FK, Young EW. International variation in vitamin prescription and association with mortality in the Dialysis Outcomes and Practice Patterns Study (DOPPS). Am J Kidney Dis 2004; 44:293–299.

63. http//www.who.int/research/en/

64. Wong JS, Port FK, Hulbert-Shearon TE, Carroll CE, Wolfe RA, Agodoa LY, Daugirdas JT. Survival advantage in Asian American end-stage renal disease patients. Kidney Int 1999; 55:2515–2523.

65. Pei YP, Greenwood CM, Chery AL, Wu GG. Racial differences in survival of patients on dialysis. Kidney Int 2000; 58:1293–1299.

66. Saxena S, Jayaraj PM, Mittal R. Clinical and laboratory features of patients with chronic renal failure at the start of dialysis in North India. Indian J Nephrol 1995; 5:4–8.
67. Abraham G, Varsha P, Mathew M, Sairam VK, Gupta A. Malnutrition and nutritional therapy of chronic kidney disease in developing countries: the Asian perspective. Adv Ren Replace Ther 2003; 10:213–221.
68. Pecoits-Filho R, Lindholm B, Stenvinkel P. The malnutrition, inflammation, and atherosclerosis (MIA) syndrome—the heart of the matter. Nephrol Dial Transplant 2002; 17(suppl 11):28–31.
69. Li PK, Chow KM. The cost barrier to peritoneal dialysis in the developing world—an Asian perspective. Perit Dial Int 2001; 21(suppl 3):S307–S313.
70. Eknoyan G, Lameire N, Barsoum R, Eckardt K, Levin A, Levin N, Locatelli F, Macleod A, Vanholder R, Walker R, Wang H. The burden of kidney disease: improving global outcomes. Kidney Int 2004; 66:1310–1314.

3

Economics of ESRD in Developing Countries: India

Vivekanand Jha and K. S. Chugh
*Department of Nephrology, Postgraduate Institute of
Medical Education & Research, Chandigarh, India*

The benefits of renal replacement therapy (RRT) for end-stage renal disease (ESRD) are firmly established. In the advanced countries, it is offered uniformly to all patients who need it; the availability is still limited in the developing world (1). Nissenson et al. (2) drew attention to the strong influence of non-medical, especially economic, factors on the quality and quantity of ESRD care. Their findings were limited to the industrialized North American and European nations, but are also applicable to the large part of the world dubbed "developing."

The World Bank (3) divides all the nations into three major economic groups on the basis of their annual per capita gross national income (GNI) and purchasing power parity (Table 1). The low (per capita GNI < US $735) and middle-income (per capita GNI US $736–9075) economies are clubbed together and referred to as "developing countries." In general, the standard of living in these countries is lower compared to the developed world (per capita GNI > US $9076) and access to goods and services is limited. Currently, there are over 160 developing countries (125 with populations of over 1 million), comprising approximately 85% of the world population. Most of these are in Asia, Africa, and South America. It is estimated that about 1.3 billion people live on less than US $1/day and another 2 billion are only slightly better off. In general, these countries score lower on the scale in all

Table 1 Economic Classification of All Countries

Group	Number of countries	Countries with population >1 million	Total population (billions)	Annual per capita GNI[a] (US $)	Purchasing power parity (US $)
High	53	26	0.96	26,490	26,480
Middle	125	67	2.4	1,400	5,800
Upper middle	95		0.3	5,110	9,550
Low middle	30		2.4	1,200	5,290
Low income	61	58	2.5	430	2,110
Highly indebted poor countries	49	39	0.66	320	
India			1.05	470	2,650

[a]GNI: Gross national income (World Bank Atlas Method).
Source: From Ref. 3.

the indices used by the World Bank (3) and the World Health Organization (4) to measure social or health status (Table 2). The use of the term "developing countries" is convenient; it is not intended to imply that all economies in the group have identical development status. In fact, vast differences are apparent in the scale of economic development amongst the various developing countries. Countries like Argentina, Brazil, China, India, Indonesia, Mexico, Pakistan, Russia, Thailand, and Turkey account for about 60% of the developing world's GNI, whereas sub-Saharan Africa constitutes 10.4% of the world population but contributes only 1.1% of the world GNI.

As an example, India has one of the largest trained scientific and technical workforce in the world and is considered one of the leading nations in

Table 2 Selected Social and Health Indicators of Developed and Developing Countries in 2002

Parameter	Developed countries	Developing countries	India
Population (billions)	0.96	5.2	1.05
Urban (%)	77	41	28
Female literacy rate (%)	100	68	44
Death rate (per 1000)	8.8	9.9	9.5
Fertility rate (births per woman/year)	1.7	2.9	3.1
Infant mortality rate (per 1000 live births/year)	5	60	65
Life expectancy at birth (years)	78	65	63
Population growth (%)	1	1.2	1.8

Source: From Ref. 3,4.

information technology, but about 40% of the population is still illiterate. An economic disparity is also apparent amongst its people. About 2% of the Indian population earns US $1000 or more in a year; and 0.5% are rich enough to afford a lifestyle similar to that in the advanced nations. There is a large and rapidly expanding middle class that is increasingly getting used to the consumer culture. However, a vast majority of the impoverished population lives either in rural areas or in slums in large cities. Over 35% survive on an annual income of less than US $105, the official definition of poverty line (5).

HEALTH CARE DELIVERY SYSTEMS

The economic, human, and technical resources required for ESRD treatment pose a major economical and political challenge. A three-tier healthcare delivery system is prevalent throughout the developing world. India, for example, is divided into 35 administrative units, called states and union territories. The Union Government decides broad policies, but each state finalizes its own healthcare priorities and budgeting. The public sector health care is organized in the shape of a pyramid, with primary health centers at the bottom, followed by block and district level hospitals, and referral hospitals at the top. ESRD care is available only at the major referral hospitals. There is no established system of referral to these facilities and patients go directly to the referral hospitals, bypassing the lower levels. At the time of gaining independence (1947), the government had envisaged spending 12% of GNI on health. According to the latest estimates, the actual figure is 0.9% (6). Most of this amount is spent on the national health programs like control of infectious diseases, family planning, nutrition, salaries, and maintenance of basic hospital infrastructure. Patients are not charged for physician advice, hospitalization, investigations, or surgical procedures. The budget, however, does not usually provide drugs or disposables and the patients have to pay for these out of their own funds. The hospitals are usually overcrowded, and the waiting times for specialized procedures like dialysis or kidney transplantation can stretch to several months.

The inability of the states to provide adequate health care has led to proliferation of the "for-profit" private hospitals. There are enormous variations in the quality of service provided by these hospitals, but in general the larger corporate hospitals provide better comfort levels to the patients, and many advertise international standards. The available equipment is modern and better maintained than most government hospitals. The treatment costs are often quite high and only the rich or those whose healthcare expenses are covered by their employers can afford treatment here. Recent estimates put the private sector healthcare spending at 4.7% of GNI. Hospitals run by charitable organizations offer treatment at subsidized costs (7).

Indigenous healthcare delivery systems are still popular in rural Africa and Asia, and patients are frequently treated by witch doctors with herb and potions (8).

EPIDEMIOLOGY

Incidence and Prevalence

The prevalence of chronic kidney disease (CKD) and the number of patients requiring RRT in developing countries are not known. Patients often travel to far off places to seek specialized care, even to different states and countries. Data from these hospitals, therefore, do not necessarily reflect the incidence and prevalence of ESRD in the geographic areas where the hospitals are located. Attempts have been made to collect this information indirectly, such as from the reported causes of death collected by the government in Egypt and through the Institute for Social Security in Mexico (9). Such sources, however, are considered flawed since the data are obtained only from a minority of the population and the information provided is mostly inaccurate. Periodic efforts have also been made to get this information through questionnaires from nephrologists, but the response is usually inadequate and incomplete. The currently available data, therefore, are at best approximations based on the individual experiences.

According to a recent survey carried out by Barsoum (9), the incidence of new ESRD cases varies from 40 patients per million population (pmp) in Pakistan to 340 pmp in Mexico. In a study conducted amongst expatriate Indians living in two different areas in U.K., the annual incidence of ESRD ranged between 120 and 200 pmp (10). This means that approximately 120,000 to 200,000 people develop ESRD every year in India. A large proportion of patients living in rural areas in India do not seek specialist advice because of ignorance and poverty, and hence are excluded from the estimates. The "acceptance rate" of patients for RRT is less than 20 pmp/year.

In the developing countries, particularly in those where RRT is supported by the government, the prevalence rates (number of ESRD patients alive at a point of time on different RRT modalities) seem to be more reliable as the data are collected from well-defined sources like renal units or central financing bodies. The figures vary widely, from an estimated 50 pmp in India to about 500 pmp in Mexico. The Latin American Society of Nephrology has set a minimum target of 400 pmp patients on RRT, but the current prevalence figures are less than 50% of this standard (11). The reported ESRD prevalence rates from some developing countries are given in Figure 1.

The precise incidence and prevalence of CKD can be determined only through community-based detection programs. Such organized programs do not exist in the developing world. The primary care physicians are hardly

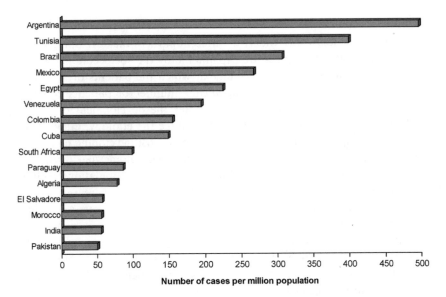

Figure 1 ESRD Prevalence in different developing countries.

aware of the magnitude of the CKD burden and its possible long-term impact on the public health (12). Even the need for screening high-risk groups, e.g., diabetics, hypertensives, and those with family history of kidney disease, is not well appreciated.

Some community-based data have recently become available in India with the help of non-governmental organizations. In a survey carried out during a medical camp held in the predominantly tribal area of Jharkhand (India) by one of us (V. J.), 6.7% of 3540 patients were found to be hypertensive, and 2.9% were diabetic. Interestingly, out of those who were already aware of these diagnoses, only 23% had undergone a urinalysis, and serum creatinine had been estimated in a mere 8%. Despite treatment, the blood pressure was above 140/90 mm Hg in over 60%. Another study is being conducted by Kidney Help Trust covering six villages near Chennai in the state of Tamil Nadu. The entire population of the villages was initially screened through a questionnaire, BP measurement, and urinalysis, and subjects with abnormalities were then seen and investigated by a doctor. About 5% of the population was found to be hypertensive, with an annual incidence of 0.55% and 3.6% were diabetic, with an annual incidence of 0.33%. About 1.2% was found to have CKD or urological disorders (12). The prevalence of hypertension in the developing countries ranges from 9% to 26%. Data from Egypt showed that only about one-third of these subjects was aware of the diagnosis, and the blood pressure was controlled in a mere 11% (13).

Etiology

The etiology of CKD varies widely in different parts of the developing world (Fig. 2). Partly, the differences are explainable by the socioeconomic status of the population represented, the stage at which the patients present, and the available diagnostic tools. A significant number of patients come to medical attention for the first time only after the development of ESRD at which time it is impossible to accurately judge the etiology. Glomerulo-nephritis still tops the list of causes of ESRD in most developing countries. On a closer analysis, the proportion of patients with glomerular diseases is found to be bigger in low-income countries with large populations such as China, India, Pakistan, South Africa, Nigeria, and Sudan, whereas its impact is less prominent in the medium-economy countries like Egypt, Argentina, and Saudi Arabia (9,14–16). Proliferative glomerulonephritis constitutes the bulk of these cases in contrast to its remarkably low frequency in the developed world. The high prevalence is linked to the prevalence of strepto-coccal throat and skin infections (Indian sub-continent and Sub-Saharan Africa), hepatosplenic schistosomiasis (North, East, and West Africa, Arabia, South and Central America), quartan malaria (British Guyana, Uganda, Kenya, Madagascar, Nigeria, Ivory Coast, Sumatra, and Yemen), hepatitis B and C (East Asia, South Africa, Zimbabwe, and Namibia), and human immunodeficiency virus (black Africa) (17–23). Focal segmental glomerulosclerosis is common in South Africa and IgA nephropathy in the Pacific rim countries (24). Amyloidosis secondary to tuberculosis, schisto-somiasis, and familial Mediterranean fever are fairly common in certain

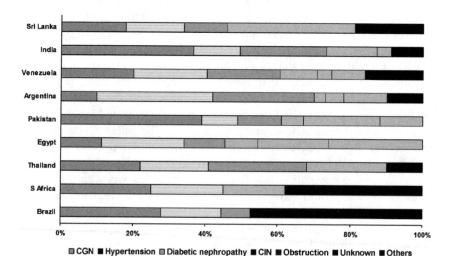

Figure 2   Causes of ESRD in different developing countries.

geographical areas (9,25). Interstitial nephritis, related to congenital and acquired structural abnormalities of the urinary tract, environmental or industrial nephrotoxins, or ingestion of herbal medicines, is prevalent in some geographic regions. Urolithiasis is the commonest cause of ESRD in North Africa (26). In most cases, the stones are related to the high prevalence of metabolic abnormalities such as renal tubular function defects and hyperoxaluria.

Diabetic nephropathy, the commonest cause of ESRD in the developed world, is also common in the middle-income countries. In the low-income nations, this disease is encountered with increasing frequency amongst the relatively well off, who present to private hospitals and in persons above the age of 40 (27). Registry figures from Egypt suggest that diabetic nephropathy is responsible for ESRD in 9% of patients (28), but hospital-based data indicate a much higher incidence (29). Li (30) reported a higher incidence of glomerulonephritis in the less developed regions of China, and an increase in diabetes-related renal diseases amongst the more affluent sections of the society. Diabetic nephropathy is also common in certain indigenous populations living in the Danagla region of Sudan and Durango of Mexico (31,32).

Hypertensive nephrosclerosis accounted for 13–21% in the survey reported by Bursoum (9), whereas other reports put the frequency at 4% and 43% (33,34). Such large differences are likely due to variation in the diagnostic criteria for the classification of this condition.

Referral Patterns

The impact of the time of referral on the outcome of ESRD is receiving a lot of attention in the developed world. Due to lack of resources in the developing world, pre-dialysis care is almost non-existent outside a few selected institutions. To study the quality of CKD care, one of us (V. J.) analyzed the medical history and records of all patients referred to our institute with a diagnosis of ESRD. Out of a total of 469 patients who came to the outpatients or emergency departments over a 7-month period, the interval between the first medical visit and diagnosis of ESRD was less than 1 month in about 60% cases, and 1 to 3 months in another 14%. Out of the 26% in whom the CKD had been diagnosed since more than 3 months, only 9% had received regular pre-dialysis care. About 75% of patients had presented with fluid overload, hyperkalemia, metabolic acidosis or uremic encephalopathy, necessitating dialysis within 24 hours of arrival. About 50% came with uncontrolled hypertension. The presentation of patients with advanced renal failure makes the primary diagnosis a guesswork at best. In a hospital-based survey from West Africa, the serum creatinine was above 2 mg/dL in about 3.3% of all hospital admissions, whereas urinalysis had shown >3+ albumin in about 1%. It was considered that most patients, even after diagnosis, are unlikely to receive adequate medical care because of lack of finances (35).

ESRD patients in developing countries are younger compared to their western counterparts, with an average age of 25 to 45 years. Most of them are in the prime of their lives and are the bread-earners of their families. In some countries, 70–80% of dialysis population is in the age range of 20 to 50 years (15). Delay in the detection and failure to institute timely preventive measures in patients with progressive renal disease contributes to the faster rate of deterioration and progression to ESRD at a relatively young age. Children are usually under-represented in the dialysis population because of lack of pediatric dialysis units (1,7,9).

AVAILABILITY OF NEPHROLOGISTS AND RRT FACILITIES

Compared to the developed nations, developing countries have far fewer nephrologists and facilities providing RRT (Fig. 3). The number of units providing RRT varies from 0.9 to 30 pmp, with an average of 5.2 pmp (9). Similarly, the number of nephrologists ranges between 0.1 and 10 pmp. India has approximately 650 practicing nephrologists (0.6 pmp), 950 dialysis units, and 75 transplant centers. About one-third of the hospitals are in public sector, whereas the remainder is managed privately. Neither the government nor the professional societies have laid down any norms or minimum standards for setting up dialysis units. Majority of dialysis units are small minimal care facilities with less than five dialysis stations. A few dialysis units have been set up by entrepreneurs, and are being managed by general practitioners and in

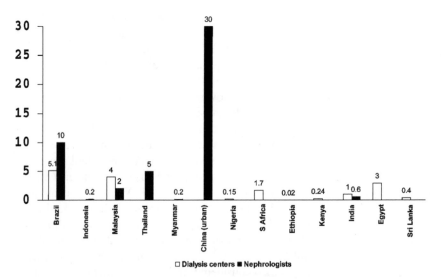

Figure 3 Number of dialysis centers and nephrologists per million population in different developing countries.

some cases, by technologists alone. This is in contrast to countries like Brazil, where the RRT program is universal and government sponsored, and there are formal sets of rules for setting up dialysis centers (36).

Some countries have a small pool of units that provides only peritoneal dialysis. There is a strong correlation between the number of dialysis facilities and the per capita GNI (9). Even in the same country, different states exhibit different levels of economic development. The more industrialized Western and Southern Indian states have more nephrologists and dialysis and transplant centers, whereas the least developed eastern part of India has the fewest nephrologists and RRT facilities. Another remarkable feature is the concentration of nephrologists and RRT facilities in a few large cities. By contrast, about 60–80% of the population lives in rural areas. The lack of specialists is a major contributor to the poor quality of CKD care in the rural areas. The need to travel long distances to seek specialized treatment discourages patients until complications arise and RRT becomes unavoidable. At our center, patients come from as far as 1000–2000 km for ESRD treatment. Because of strong emotional ties, family members usually accompany the patient. The treatment is usually prolonged, and such temporarily relocation leads to loss of livelihood of several family members. Because of social inequalities, ESRD treatment facilities are not available uniformly to all sections of the society; women and the elderly often bear the brunt of this discrimination. Lack of expertise and equipment prevents small children from getting dialysis or transplantation.

Some West and Central African countries are still struggling to establish the basic facilities required for diagnosis and management of CKD. According to a recent report from the West African nations of Benin and Togo, even urinalysis, urine culture, and electrolyte estimations were not available to the general population, and needed support of voluntary organizations (35) (see Chapter 21).

Retention of trained manpower by developing countries is a major challenge. Opportunities of more comfortable lifestyle and better financial as well as academic fulfillment prompt large number of trained doctors, nurses, and technical staff to move to the more affluent Western countries. We estimate that about 20% of nephrologists trained in India have permanently relocated to the West. Similar trends have been reported from other developing countries.

DIALYSIS EQUIPMENT

Most HD units in the developing world are equipped with individual proportionating dialysis machines. Central proportioning systems installed earlier in some centers have been mostly phased out. Private sector units have modern machines with volumetric ultrafiltration and microprocessor-based controls and provision for bicarbonate dialysis. Economic constraints force units with limited funding to use old machines that have been considered out-dated and obsolete and discarded in favor of more efficient models in the Western world. As these are still in working order, they are sent as donation to the developing countries. Some units also use refurbished machines (1,7,15). About two-thirds of the machines have volumetric control, but the proportion varies from about 30% to 100% in different countries. A major problem with the use of these machines is the lack of locally available spares and trained engineers. As a result, once a machine breaks down, it remains out of action for long periods of time. Erratic power supply, inefficient organization and insufficient funds for maintenance contribute to the frequent breakdowns of these machines. In contrast to the West, acetate dialysis is still widely used in several parts of developing world. About 80% units in South Africa and 60% in India use this buffer (7,16). Facilities for individualizing the dialysis to suit the needs of a patient by sodium or ultrafiltration profiling are available only in a minority of units.

Similarly, despite the universal use of newer biocompatible membranes in the rest of the world, membranes made of cuprophane are used in a vast majority of units in the developing world, especially in the government-funded hospitals. Dialyzer reuse is widespread and helps bring down the costs. The number of reuses is higher in private units with intent to increase the prof-its. Dialyzers are usually reprocessed manually, and the level of contaminants or the fiber bundle volume is rarely measured. This results in delivery of inade-quate dialysis, frequent occurrence of pyrogenic reactions, and even sepsis following dialysis. In some countries like China and Egypt reuse is prohibited by law, whereas countries like Togo and Benin do not reuse dialyzers because of poor facilities (35).

In several developing countries of Latin America, changes in the govern-ment policies have allowed use of modern machines, and most centers have switched exclusively to newer synthetic membranes (11,36).

WATER TREATMENT FOR DIALYSIS

Facilities for purifying the water to a level suitable for use in HD are grossly inadequate throughout the developing world. The quality of municipal water is highly unpredictable. Water transported in tankers is used for dialysis in areas where the supply is irregular (37). Water treatment plants are not regu-larly serviced, and replacement of spent filters and cartridges is infrequent. This leads to substantial risk of exposure of patients to a number of contami-nants. An example of this was seen in Brazil, when 50 patients dialyzed during a 4-day period in 1996 using water from tank trucks developed visual distur-bances, nausea, and vomiting. Over the next 4 months, several patients died of liver failure. Investigations established contamination by a toxin named "microcystin-LR," produced by an alga of the family *Cyanobacteriaceae*. The toxin was detected in the samples obtained from the source of water (a lake), the truck used for transporting water, dialysis filters, and the liver tissue of the affected patients. Investigations also revealed that the filters and cartridges in the water treatment plant had not been replaced on stipulated dates. In a survey carried out in 1999, only about 20% of all centers were found to be using some form of water purification system in India (38).

MAINTENANCE HEMODIALYSIS

Long-term HD is available to everyone who needs it in most Latin American countries with the help of government funding. In contrast, mass-based HD programs are almost non-existent in most developing countries of Asia and Africa, and only a few rich patients are known to be on long-term maintenance dialysis. Government hospitals are constantly burdened with a large load of patients with acute renal failure, which limits the number of ESRD patients who can be taken for long-term dialysis. Setting up new units or expansion of existing units is difficult because of high cost of dialysis machines and water treatment systems. There is no consensus on the dialysis frequency or prescription. Many units routinely dialyze their patients only once or twice a week. The frequency is mostly decided by symptomatology of the patient and financial considerations. It is not uncommon for patients to reduce the frequency of dialysis even more as financial resources dwindle, culminating in discontinuation of dialysis or death (7). About 5–25% of patients are on once-a-week dialysis schedule in countries like Thailand, Tunisia, India, South Africa, and Mexico. Data on the adequacy of such dialysis schedules are not available. Some nephrologists believe that satisfactory clearances can be achieved in Indian ESRD patients by two 4-hours dialysis sessions/week (39). This has been attributed to the lower protein content of the diet with consequent less generation of uremic toxins and to the smaller body weight. This assumption, however, needs to be tested in rigorous clinical trials. It is our experience that most patients continue to suffer from uremic symptoms on such dialysis schedules and there are few long-term survivors. The mean duration of HD was only 1 month amongst a cohort of 436 patients dialyzed at a large referral hospital over a 1-year period (40). About 10% patients died in hospital and another 60% left the program and were lost to follow-up. Only 3.6% continued HD for over 6 months, comprising mostly of the patients who were waiting for a transplant. The proportion of dialysis patients who are able to return to work varies from 0% to 20% in India and South Africa and about 50% in Malaysia (41–43).

The well being of patients on maintenance HD also depends upon adequate management of comorbid conditions. The exact prevalence of these conditions is not known. Infection remains the second most important cause of morbidity and mortality after the complications of under-dialysis. Most patients are not routinely screened for cardiovascular complications.

Erythropoietin is not used routinely in developing countries. According to the survey (9), less than 25% of dialysis patients are on erythropoietin. Most patients receive inadequate dose of the drug, leading to a sub-optimal response. Other reasons for poor response include infrequent use of parenteral iron, deficiencies of other nutrients, frequent infections, and inadequate control of secondary hyperparathyroidism.

CHRONIC PERITONEAL DIALYSIS (CPD)

In advanced countries, CPD is cheaper than HD and is the preferred form of RRT where the ESRD treatment programs are nationalized and the governments do not want to spend vast amounts of money in setting up new HD units (2). An increasing proportion of patients are being initiated on CPD rather than HD in the United Kingdom, Australia, and New Zealand, where dialysis services are funded by the government. In the developing countries, since the labor costs and staff salaries are low, CPD is expected to be even cheaper. It has the added advantage of bringing dialysis to the homes of those living in remote areas where HD is not available. The ambulatory nature of the treatment and less frequent visits to the nephrologists after the initial training period make CPD ideally suited for the developing world.

Great disparities are observed, however, in the CPD utilization amongst various developing nations. Whereas 50–90% of dialysis patients are on CPD in Mexico (44,45), its use in other developing countries is much less common. CPD is 1.5 to 3 times more expensive than HD in the Asian countries including Thailand and India (7). The chief reason for this paradox is the lack of facilities to manufacture PD bags locally, with consequent need to import PD fluid bags from the industrialized nations. One bag of PD fluid costs around US$3.2 in India. The high cost has prevented the growth of this promising modality in the developing world and precludes the use of more sophisticated systems of PD. Presently, there are about 4250 patients on PD in India (*source*: Baxter India Ltd). The major manufacturers of CPD bags in India have recently started an initiative in which a patient is assured of lifetime supply of PD bags and disposables upon making a one-time payment of approximately US $7800 (3 exchanges/day) or US $10,800 (4 exchanges/day). Such schemes are helpful in increasing patient recruitment (Fig. 4), but the critical mass would be achieved only when the PD cost becomes comparable to HD.

As with HD, the PD prescription is dictated by the patient's economic situation. Most patients are on 3 exchanges/day and cycler-assisted peritoneal dialysis is practiced rarely. Although the number of patients being initiated on CPD has increased rapidly in recent years, the dropout rates also remain high. Factors contributing to the dismal success rates include poor patient training and compliance; increased risk of infections due to hot and humid climate and poor hygienic conditions; and lack of trained

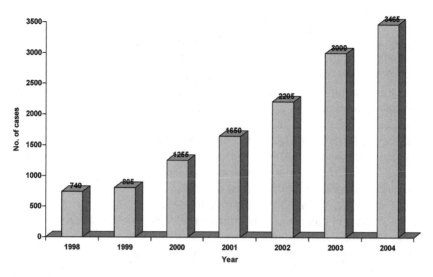

Figure 4 Prevalence of cases on CPD in India.

social workers, dedicated nurses, and dieticians. Peritonitis rates, high in the initial years, have come down significantly in the last couple of years since most patients have been switched to double-bag system. Adequacy data are limited. Most studies are small and were done at the time of initiation, when the residual renal function contributes significantly to the total clearance. In a study of 55 patients, Abraham et al. (46) found the combined weekly creatinine clearances to be 70 L. As the residual renal function dwindles with time, the efficacy of dialysis is likely to decrease. The patients, however, refuse to increase the dialysis dose because of resource constrains, leading to reappearance of uremic symptoms and eventually increased mortality. Long-term survival is still far below that reported from the West. The long-term results of CPD continue to be poor in the developing countries. Nephrologists in Mexico, that has the highest CAPD penetration rate amongst developing nations, are having a second look at the procedure. Driven by the promise of the technique, the marketing was aggressive in the initial years, and PD procedures were soon being performed by non-nephrologists. In less than 5 years, over 90% of all ESRD patients were on CAPD (47). Such rampant use of CAPD by general practitioners without attention to quality was associated with disastrous results. Survival was less than 2 years in 85% out of over 7500 cases, and the overall peritonitis mortality rate exceeded 60%. The rates were less than 20% at centers where CAPD was supervised by nephrologists. A modification program that aims at strengthening HD facilities and emphasizes correct patients selection for CAPD was proposed by the Mexican Institute for Social Security in 1996.

KIDNEY TRANSPLANTATION

Kidney transplantation is currently the best and in most cases the only viable alternative for long-term survival of ESRD patients in the developing nations. Many countries do not have adequate legislations for regulation of organ transplantation. Cadaver transplant programs are by and large rudimentary, and transplants are almost exclusively done using living donors (48). The shortage of donors and success of genetically unmatched transplants following the introduction of cyclosporine led to the widespread practice of trafficking in kidneys in the 1980s (49). Despite being condemned by professional societies around the world and enactment of legislation banning this activity by several countries, sale and purchase of kidneys continues in some form in different parts of the developing world even today. Discussion of the ethical and medical aspects of commercial transplants (48–50) is beyond the scope of this review. Even after getting a transplant, financial considerations preclude continuation of optimum lifelong immunosuppression in a large number of patients. Until recently, it was a common practice to stop cyclosporine and switch over to azathioprine and prednisolone after the first 12 months. This conversion was often indiscriminate and led to acute rejection in about a third of the patients (51). The introduction of powerful but safe immunosuppressive drugs such as IL-2 receptor antagonists, tacrolimus, mycophenolate mofetil, and sirolimus has presented the transplant community of developing countries with the agonizing dilemma of findings ways to balance the use of these drugs with the economic realities. Other difficult situations arise when complications such as cytomegalovirus infection or post-transplant lymphoproliferative disorder develop, which require expensive drugs like ganciclovir or rituximab. As a functioning graft is considered the only hope of long-term survival, heavy immunosuppression is often continued even in the face of life-threatening infections, jeopardizing the life of the patient.

RRT COSTS

The exact cost of RRT in developing countries is hard to estimate. A rough estimate of hemodialysis costs in different developing countries is presented in Figure 5. The cost of treatment varies with the prescription and the way a unit is set up. The exact proportion of cost that is formed by the subsidy provided by government hospitals is very difficult to calculate. The expense incurred in setting up and maintenance of the units and the salaries paid to the physicians, nursing, and other staff are included in the global hospital budget, and separate information is generally not available. This amount can vary widely depending upon the size and location of the hospital, number of dialysis machines in the unit, and hospital affiliation. The charges in private profit-making centers vary widely depending upon the hospital

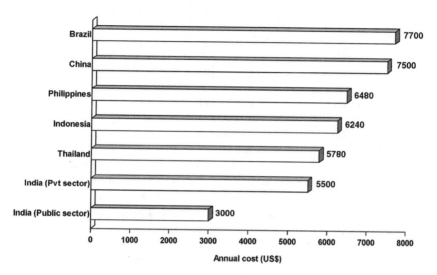

Figure 5 Annual hemodialysis costs in selected developing countries.

size, type (uni- or multi-specialty), location, reputation, and additional facilities for patients and their relatives.

Setting up a modern dialysis unit requires significant capital investment, which normally requires the support of either the government or the industry. The Sind Institute of Urology and Transplantation, Karachi (Pakistan), represents a successful model of active recruitment of the community to set up an institution for providing quality RRT services without charging the patients (52). The initial effort for raising finances were limited to individuals and philanthropic organizations, but seeing the success, even the government and major pharmaceutical companies have started contributing to the endeavor.

When a head-to-head comparison is made with the developed countries, the RRT costs appear to be far less in developing countries due to the lower staff salaries and the lower cost of drugs, but are still 10 to 20 times higher than the per capita GNI, and therefore out of reach of a majority of the population (10). The cost estimates do not include the cost of drugs like erythropoietin and Vitamin D analogues, now considered an essential part of CKD management. These drugs raise the RRT costs by over 100% and are the exclusive preserve of the rich. Another prominent missing factor is the cost of patient hospitalizations. The poor clinical status of the patients necessitates frequent and often long-term hospitalizations. Treatment is prolonged and represents an additional financial burden. Also not included are the cost of transport to and from HD center and loss of patient and family income due to missing workdays.

Unlike the Western nations, the concept of health insurance is in a primitive stage in the developing countries. In China, most people employed by the government in major cities are covered by government-sponsored health insurance (53). However, those living in the rural areas do not have this cover. Similarly, government-funded social security programs now cover RRT costs in several Latin American countries like Venezuela and Uruguay (11,54); but this scheme is available only to people holding regular employments. The costs of RRT, therefore, have to be borne by the majority of patients out of their own funds. A few government and private organizations in India reimburse the cost of treatment of employees or their dependants. The reimbursement policies vary tremendously in terms of the amount and duration of coverage. Most organizations reimburse the hospitalization costs, but only a few cover outpatient treatment. This effectively eliminates outpatient hemodialysis, chronic peritoneal dialysis, and post-transplant immunosuppressive therapy from the ambit of reimbursement. Also, the process of reimbursement is slow, and patients have to wait for months or even years to recover the large sums of money that they may have borrowed. Most large public hospitals have active transplant programs, and preferentially accept for dialysis patients who are thought suitable for transplant. The others are put on a wait list and need to get dialysis in the more expensive private hospitals. In recent times, some organizations have negotiated reimbursement rates for their employees with private hospitals. Charitable organizations and government administered "relief funds" provide limited assistance to some poor patients. Such assistance can usually take care of a couple of month's treatment. One study on the psychosocial aspects of chronic renal failure in India found that 63% of patients took help from employers or accepted charity, 30% sold property or family valuables such as jewelry, and 26% took loans to cover the cost of RRT (55). Most patients raised funds in more than one way. Only 4% were able to cover the cost from within the family resources.

In Philippines, patients undergo a thorough financial evaluation and those found suitable can get discounts on treatment in government hospitals from the Medical Social Service. Another source is "Philippine Charity Sweepstakes," which provides grants for certain number of dialysis sessions (A. Estrella, personal communication). Other novel ways of raising finances are encountered in some societies. For example, social gatherings called "harambee" (pull-together) are organized in Kenya to raise money for treatment. Presided over by a local dignitary, these are attended by friends and well wishers of the patients, who contribute towards the treatment fund. However, the collections depend upon the popularity and social influence of the person for whom the event is held, and a poor farmer has much less chance of success than a person holding an important position in the society. Despite the limitations, this is thought to be responsible for partial success of renal transplant program in Kenya (56).

In conclusion, the healthcare issues of CKD patients and the problems related to ESRD treatment have not yet attracted the attention of healthcare policy planners in most parts of the developing world. Although rough estimates are now available about the populations with ESRD, the exact magnitude of CKD problem is not known. Even amongst the medical community, there is little awareness of the long-term dangers posed by CKD. Programs for prevention, screening and detection of CKD are virtually non-existent even in high-risk groups. There is a severe shortage of trained manpower equipped to treat CKD patients. Instruments for provision of uremia therapy are inadequate, unregulated, and inaccessible to a large part of the populations. RRT is expensive and there is no organized reimbursement system. Government apathy has prevented the growth of long-term dialysis programs. Successful kidney transplantation represents the only hope of survival of these patients. The financial burden of RRT impacts on the lifestyle and future of entire families, and extracts a cost far higher than the actual amount of money spent on treatment.

REFERENCES

1. Jha V, Chugh KS. Dialysis in developing countries: priorities and obstacles. Nephrology 1996; 2:65–72.
2. Nissenson AR, Prichard SB, Cheng IKP, Gokal R, Kubota M, Maiorca R, Reilla MC, Rottembourg J, Stewart JH. Non-medical factors that impact on ESRD modality selection. Kidney Int 1993; 43(suppl 40):S120–S127.
3. World Development Report 2004. http://www.worldbank.org/data/ (accessed on July 12, 2004).
4. World Health Report 1999. The World Health Organization, Geneva, 1999.
5. http://indiabudget.nic.in/es97-98/chap101.pdf (accessed on July 12, 2004).
6. Times of India, New Delhi, July 8, 2004.
7. Jha V, Chugh KS. The practice of dialysis in the developing countries. Hemodial Int 2003; 7:239–249.
8. Jha V, Chugh KS. Nephropathy associated with animal, plant, and chemical toxins in the tropics. Semin Nephrol 2003; 23:49–65.
9. Barsoum RS. Overview: end-stage renal disease in the developing world. Artif Organs 2002; 26:737–746.
10. Jha V. End-stage renal disease in the developing world: the Indian perspective. Ren Fail 2004; 26:201–208.
11. Bellorin-Font E, Milanes CL, Rodriguez-Iturbe B. End-stage renal disease and its treatment in Venezuela. Artif Organs 2002; 26:747–749.
12. Mani MK. Prevention of chronic renal failure at the community level. Kidney Int 2003; 63(suppl 83):S86–S89.
13. El-Khashab O. Hypertension and end-stage renal disease in the developing world. Artif Organs 2002; 26:765–766.
14. Sakhuja V, Sud K. End-stage renal disease in India and Pakistan: burden of disease and management issues. Kidney Int 2003; 63(suppl 83):S115–S118.

15. Bamgboye EL. Hemodialysis: management problems in developing countries, with Nigeria as a surrogate. Kidney Int 2003; 63(suppl 83):S93–S95.
16. Naicker S. End-stage renal disease in sub-Saharan and South Africa. Kidney Int 2003; 63(suppl 83):S119–S122.
17. Tewodros W, Muhe L, Daniel E, Schalen C, Kronvall G. A one-year study of streptococcal infections and their complications among Ethiopian children. Epidemiol Infect 1992; 109:211–225.
18. Barsoum R. Schistosomal glomerulopathies. Kidney Int 1993; 44:1–12.
19. Chugh KS, Sakhuja V. Tropical glomerulopathies. Med Int 1991; 86: 3548–3552.
20. Bhimma R, Coovadia HM, Adhikari M. Hepatitis B virus-associated nephropathy in black South African children. Pediatr Nephrol 1998; 12:479–484.
21. Seggie J, Nathhoo K, Davies PG. Association of hepatitis-B (HBs) antigenemia and membranous glomerulonephritis in Zimbabwean children. Nephron 1984; 38:115–119.
22. van Buuren AJ, Bates WD, Muller N. Nephrotic syndrome in Namibian children. S Afr Med J 1999; 89:1088–1091.
23. Diallo AD, Nochy D, Niamkey E, Yao Beda B. Etiologic aspects of nephrotic syndrome in black African adults in a hospital setting in Abidjan. Bull Soc Pathol Exot 1997; 90:342–345.
24. Sitprija V. Nephrology in South East Asia: fact and concept. Kidney Int 2003; 63(suppl 83):S128–S130.
25. Chugh KS, Datta BN, Singhal PC, Jain SK, Sakhuja V, Dash SC. Pattern of renal amyloidosis in Indian patients. Postgrad Med J 1981; 57:31–35.
26. Barsoum RS. End-stage renal disease in north Africa. Kidney Int 2003; 63(suppl 83):S111–S114.
27. Sakhuja V, Jha V, Ghosh AK, Ahmed S, Saha TK. Chronic renal failure in India. Nephrol Dial Transplant 1994; 9:871–872.
28. The Third Annual Report of the Egyptian Society of Nephrology. Available at http://163.121.19.91/esnnew/ data.htm (accessed on 12 July 2004).
29. Essamie MA, Soliman A, Fayad TM, Barsoum S, Kjellstrand CM. Serious renal disease in Egypt. Int J Artif Organs 1995; 18:254–260.
30. Li L. End stage renal disease in China. Kidney Int 1996; 49:287–301.
31. Elbagir MN, Eltom MA, Elmahadi EM, Kadam IM, Berne C. A high prevalence of diabetes mellitus and impaired glucose tolerance in the Danagla community in northern Sudan. Diabet Med 1998; 15:164–169.
32. Guerrero-Romero F, Rodriguez-Moran M, Sandoval-Herrera F. Prevalence of NIDDM in indigenous communities of Durango, Mexico. Diabetes Care 1996; 19:547–548.
33. Abboud O. Special problems and challenges with dialysis: Sudan [abstr]. Saudi Kidney Dis Transplant Bull 1993; 4(suppl 1):35.
34. Ojogwu LI. The pathological basis of endstage renal disease in Nigerians: experience from Benin City. West Afr J Med 1990; 9:193–196.
35. Fogazzi GB, Attolou V, Kadiri S, Fenili D, Priuli F. A nephrological program in Benin and Togo (West Africa). Kidney Int 2003; 63(suppl 83):S55–S60.
36. Zatz R, Romao JE Jr, Noronha IL. Nephrology in Latin America, with special emphasis on Brazil. Kidney Int 2003; 63(suppl 83):S131–S134.

37. Jochimsen EM, Carmichael WW, An J, Cardo DM, Cookson ST, Holmes CEM, de C, Antunes MB, de Melo Filho DA, Lyra TM, Barreto VST, Azevedo SMFO, Jarvis WR. Liver failure and death after exposure to microcystins at a hemodialysis center in Brazil. N Engl J Med 1998; 338:873–878.
38. Kripalani AL, Madhav K. Current practices in water treatment for hemodialysis in India. Indian J Nephrol 2001; 11(suppl):S10–S12.
39. Desai JD, Shah BV, Sirsat KA. Urea kinetics: a guide to dialysis prescription [abstr]. Indian J Nephrol 1991; 1:41.
40. Rao M, Juneja R, Shirly RB, Jacob CK. Haemodialysis for end-stage renal disease in Southern India—a perspective from a tertiary referral care centre. Nephrol Dial Transplant 1998; 13:2494–2500.
41. Chugh KS, Jha V. Differences in the care of ESRD patients worldwide: required resources and future outlook. Kidney Int 1995; 48(suppl 50):S7–S13.
42. Naicker S. Nephrology in South Africa. Nephrol Dial Transplant 1996; 11:30–31.
43. Lim TO, Lim YN. 4th Report of the Malaysian Dialysis and Transplant Registry, Malaysian Society of Nephrology, 1996.
44. Cueto-Manzano AM. Peritoneal dialysis in Mexico. Kidney Int 2003; 63(suppl 83):S90–S92.
45. Santiago-Delpin EA, Cangiano JL. Renal disease and dialysis in Latin America. Transplant Proc 1991; 23:1851–1854.
46. Abraham G, Bhaskaran S, Soundarajan P, Ravi R, Nitya S, Padma G, Jayanthi V. Continuous ambulatory peritoneal dialysis. J Assoc Physicians India 1996; 44: 599–601.
47. Trevino-Becerra A, Maimone MA. Peritoneal dialysis in the developing world: the Mexican scenario. Artif Organs 2002; 26:750–752.
48. Jha V. Paid transplants in India: the grim reality. Nephrol Dial Transplant 2004; 19:541–543.
49. Chugh KS, Jha V. Commerce in transplantation in Third World countries. Kidney Int 1996; 49:1181–1186.
50. Chugh KS, Jha V. Problems and outcomes of living unrelated donor transplants in the developing countries. Kidney Int 2000; 57(suppl 74):S131–S135.
51. Jha V, Muthukumar T, Kohli HS, Sud K, Gupta KL, Sakhuja V. Impact of cyclosporine withdrawal on living related renal transplants: a single-center experience. Am J Kidney Dis 2001; 37:119–124.
52. Rizvi A, Aziz R, Ahmed E, Naqvi R, Akhtar F, Naqvi A. Recruiting the community for supporting end-stage renal disease management in the developing world. Artif Organs 2002; 26:782–784.
53. Lin S. Nephrology in China: a great mission and momentous challenge. Kidney Int 2003; 63(suppl 83):S90–S92.
54. Fernandez JM, Schwedt E, Ambrosoni P, Gonzalez F, Mazzuchi N. Eleven years of chronic hemodialysis in Uruguay: mortality time course. Kidney Int 1995; 47(6):1721–1725.
55. Bapat U. A Study on the Psychosocial Aspects of Chronic Renal Failure. A project report for the MA degree in social work, Tata Institute of Social Sciences, Bombay, 1984.
56. Were AJ, McLigeyo SO. Cost consideration in renal replacement therapy in Kenya. East Afr Med J 1995; 72:69–71.

4

Infections and Kidney Diseases: A Continuing Global Challenge

Bernardo Rodríguez-Iturbe

Hospital Universitario and Universidad del Zulia, FUNDACITE-Zulia, Maracaibo, Venezuela

Sergio Mezzano

Universidad Austral, Valdivia, Chile

INTRODUCTION

This chapter will discuss two specific renal conditions associated with bacterial infections: acute post-streptococcal glomerulonephritis (PSGN) and the hemolytic uremic syndrome. The etiology, pathogenesis, clinical and pathological characteristics, and the treatment of these conditions are well covered in textbooks of nephrology and outside the boundaries of this revision. This chapter will examine the epidemiology of these two conditions from a global perspective.

The incidence of glomerulonephritis associated with streptococcal infections has experienced a worldwide reduction in the last 2 to 3 decades, but, nevertheless, this form of acute glomerulonephritis remains an important cause of hospital admissions in pediatric services of developing countries. Furthermore, epidemic outbreaks of this disease continue to occur in rural and aboriginal communities, particularly in America and Australia. The hemolytic uremic syndrome resulting from infections with verotoxin-producing *Escherichia coli* and *Shigella* species is a disease with a worldwide distribution and a particularly high incidence in Argentina. In many countries in Latin America and Asia, it is a frequent cause of acute renal failure in the pediatric population.

POST-STREPTOCOCCAL GLOMERULONEPHRITIS

The association of streptococcal infections and glomerulonephritis is one of the oldest clinical observations that guided investigations on the etiology of parenchymal kidney disease. The histological picture is that of a typical diffuse endocapillary glomerulonephritis (Fig. 1). As far back as the 18th century, "dark and scanty urine" was noted to be a complication of the convalescent period of scarlet fever (1) and the pathological description of post-scarlatinal glomerulonephritis (2) actually preceded by two decades the identification of group A beta hemolytic streptococcus as the etiologic agent of scarlatina (3). Shortly thereafter, the association between acute glomerulonephritis and upper respiratory (4,5) and skin infections (6) with this bacteria were firmly established in the medical literature. More recently, ingestion of unpasteurized milk contaminated with group C streptococcus (*Streptococcus zooepidemicus*) has caused clusters of cases (7,8) and at least one large epidemic (9). The pathogenesis of PSGN was outlined nearly a century ago in seminal papers that defined this disease as a non-infectious

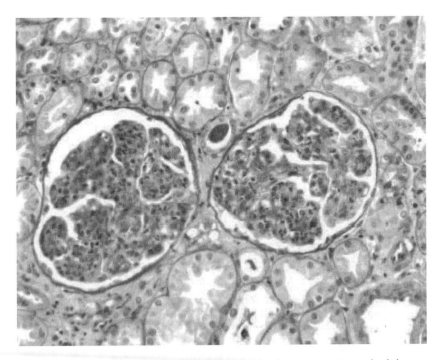

Figure 1   Acute endocapillary glomerulonephritis of post-streptococcal etiology.

complication resulting from "altered reactivity or allergy" to serum antibodies developed during the convalescence (10,11). Since second attacks
of PSGN are extremely rare, it is likely that the responsible antigen in this
disease is shared by nephritogenic streptococci and confers a long-lasting
immunity. Several streptococcal components, including M protein, have
been evaluated as potential nephritogens, but results are still a matter of
debate (12). The lack of an accepted animal model of the disease and the
difficulty in localizing putative antigens in the glomeruli are some of the
reasons for the continuing controversy (12). At the present time, two streptococcal antigens are being actively investigated. Both these antigens are
claimed to be consistently demonstrable in the glomeruli of early biopsies
of PSGN, both antigens are reported to induce an antibody response that
is characteristically found in convalescent sera of patients with nephritis
and is absent in non-nephritogenic streptococcal infections.

These antigens are the glyceraldehyde-phosphate dehydrogenase
plasmin receptor (GAPDH or NAPlr) (13) and the cysteine cationic pro-
teinase exotoxin B and its zymogen precursor (SPE B/zymogen) (14,15).
Hopefully, some insight will be gained in the future by back to back testing
of both these antigens in the same serum samples and biopsies to compare
the relative consistency of the positive findings.

There has been a reduction in the number of cases as well as changes
in the epidemiologic characteristics of PSGN in industrialized countries, but
streptococcal infections remains a significant cause of glomerulonephritis in
some communities where it may represent a risk factor that contributes to
their high incidence of chronic renal failure.

Changing Epidemiology of Post-streptococcal Nephritis

Epidemics of PSGN have appeared regularly in the literature since the
classic report of the Banbridge epidemic in military recruits (16). The distribution of the epidemics is worldwide (Table 1).

Recurrent epidemics have been studied in the Red Lake Indian
Reservation in Minnesota (18), in San Fernando, Trinidad (20), and in
Maracaibo, Venezuela (22,24), and recent outbreaks are reported from
Armenia (34) and Nova Serrana, Brazil (9; R. Sesso, personal communica-
tion, 2004). Clusters of cases have recently been documented in Aboriginal
communities in Australia (8,32) and in Peru (35) (Table 1).

Nephritis classically follows specific group A streptococci. Traditionally recognized strains associated with nephritis are 1, 4, 12 (throat), and
45, 49, and 52 (skin). Yet nephritogenicity is not restricted to these strains
and many of the bacteria isolated from nephritic patients are not M typable.
Furthermore, nephritis may result from infections of streptococci of different groups. Specifically, the nephritogenicity in group C streptococci has
been demonstrated by the occurrence of several outbreaks (7,8) and one

Table 1 Epidemics of Post-streptococcal Glomerulonephritis

Year	Location	Population affected	Site of infection	Number of cases	Streptococcal type	References
1951–1952	Bainbridge, MA, USA	Military recruits	Throat	180	M12	16
1952	Nova Scotia, Canada	Rural	Throat	22	ND	17
1953	Red Lake, MN, USA	Aboriginal	Skin	63	M49	18
1960	Memphis, TN, USA	City dwellers	Skin	57	M1, M12, M49	19
1964–1965	San Fernando, Trinidad, WI	Rural and city	Skin	760	M55, M49	20
1966	Red Lake, MN, USA	Aboriginal	Skin	27	M49	21
1968	Maracaibo, Venezuela	City dwellers	Throat	384	ND	22
1967–1968	San Fernando, Trinidad, WI	Rural and city	Skin	540	M49, M60	23
1974	Maracaibo, Venezuela	City dwellers	Skin	200	ND	24
1974	Baracoa, Guantánamo, Cuba	Rural	Skin and throat	295	ND	25
1975–1977	Alaska, USA	Eskimo children	Skin	75	ND	26
1984–1989	Santiago, Chile	City dwellers	Skin and throat	83	ND	27
1980	Guayacan 4, Las Tunas, Cuba	Rural	Skin	12	M49, M12	28

1990–1998	Northern Territory, Australia	Rural	Skin and throat	Clusters of cases	ND	29
1982–1983	Belgrade, Yugoslavia	Military academy	Throat	Clusters of 6–24 cases	ND	30
1883	North Yorkshire, UK	Rural	Unpasteurized milk	Clusters of cases	*S. zooepidemicus*	7
1986	San Fernando, Trinidad, WI	Rural and city	Skin	181	M73, 48, 55, 57, 59	31
1992	Saga, Japan	Rural	Throat	42	M1	32
1993	North Queensland	Aborigines	Skin	58	ND	33
1993	Brisbane, Australia	Rural	Unpasteurized milk	Clusters of cases	*S. zooepidemicus*	8
1995	Yerevan, Armenia	City and rural	Throat	196	ND	34
1995	San José, Costa Rica	City and rural	Skin and throat	103	ND	R. Lou[a]
1998	Nova Serrana, Brazil	Rural	Unpasteurized milk	135	*S. zooepidemicus*	9
1998–2001	Lima, Perú	City	Throat	186 (in clusters)	ND	35
2003–2004	Guaranesia, Minas Gerais, Brazil	City and rural	Upper respiratory	80	In progress	R. Sesso[a]

[a]Personal communication, 2004.

large epidemic (9) caused by the consumption of unpasteurized milk and cheese obtained from cows with mastitis (Table 1). These outbreaks emphasize the fact that nephritogenic antigen(s) are more widely distributed among streptococcal strains than traditionally accepted.

Sporadic cases of PSGN are becoming increasingly rare. The reduction in the incidence and prevalence of the disease was recognized for more than two decades in the industrialized countries (36) and it has practically disappeared in certain regions of central Europe (37). The decrease in frequency of PSGN has been documented in Memphis, where the incidence decreased from 31 patients per year between 1961 and 1970, to 9.5 patients per year between 1979 and 1988 (38). In the period 1987–1993, PSGN represented only 2.6–3.7% of all primary glomerulonephritis in the Italian Registry, with an incidence of 0.7 cases per million population (39) and in the period 1992–1994, out of 432 kidney biopsies in children younger than 15 years of age, there were only nine cases of post-infectious glomerulonephritis, corresponding to 0.35 per million children under the age of 15, consulting pediatric nephrology services (40). In China, a reduction in the attack rate of PSGN has been observed since 1956 (41) and even though is still the most common form of glomerulonephritis in Singapore, its frequency is diminishing (42). In Chile, where an epidemic outbreak in 1986–1988 affected 13.2 patients per 100,000 inhabitants, the incidence of PSGN decreased progressively since that time. The most prevalent streptococcal serotypes were T14-MO and T1-M1 in the cases that followed upper respiratory infection (about 30%), while T1-mp19-MO was the most common in post-pyoderma cases (60% of the cases) (27,43). Since 1999, PSGN has practically disappeared in Chile (27).

A decrease in the incidence of PSGN has also been documented in Guadalajara, Mexico, where the combined data from two hospitals show a progressive decrease in PSGN from 27 cases in 1992 to six cases in 2003 (G. Garcia, A. Arevalo, M. L. Salazar, S. Ramirez, G. Pérez, personal communication, 2004). In Maracaibo, Venezuela, the incidence of PSGN has dropped from 90 to 110 patients per year in the early 1980s (24) to 20 to 25 patients per year in the last 5 years.

The reduction in the incidence of PSGN is less evident in restricted aboriginal, rural, and low-income communities; for instance, it remains a common disease in aboriginal communities in Australia (44) and is the cause of 70% of the hospital admission in pediatric nephrology services in Valencia, Venezuela (45). In Bolivia, 47.3% of the pediatric nephrology admissions in 2003 were PSGN (D. Bocángel, personal communication, 2004).

An additional epidemiologic change is that PSGN, traditionally a disease of children with a 2:1 predominance in the male sex, is now affecting elderly individuals, particularly alcoholics, diabetics, and intravenous drug users (46). In the Italian biopsy registry (40), acute post-streptococcal glomerulonephritis is now more common after the age of 60 years than before this age (0.9 patients per million vs. 0.4 PMP). This tendency of shifting

Table 2 Acute Post-infectious Glomerulonephritis as a Cause of Acute Renal Failure in the Pediatric Population (1990–2003)

City, country	Patients with acute renal failure (n)	Incidence of post-infectious glomerulonephritis (%)	References
New Delhi, India	255	13.0	48
Istambul, Turkey	530	30.0	49
Casablanca, Maroc	89	51.6	50
Lagos, Nigeria	175	4.6	51
Bombay, India	48	27.0	52
Lucknow, India	52	19.2	53
Asunción, Paraguay	520	33.0	54
Lima, Perú	403	5.2	55
Varanasi, India	891	9.3[a]	56

[a]Endocapillary proliferative glomerulonephritis, post-streptococcal etiology not established.

frequency towards older population groups has been also observed in less affluent societies; for instance, in India post-infectious glomerulonephritis represent 73% of the acute glomerulonephritis affecting elderly populations (47).

Despite the reduction in the incidence of PSGN, the disease still presents an unsolved health problem in many third-world countries, where a significant proportion of the patients with acute renal failure in pediatric nephrology hospital wards are still PSGN. Table 2 shows that in series reported since 1990, an average of 21% of the cases of acute renal failure (range 4.6–51.6%) are due to post-infectious glomerulonephritis.

Guidelines in the Prevention and Management PSGN

Early treatment of streptococcal infection may prevent the development of PSGN. Prophylactic treatment with antibiotics may be used in household members of index cases because of the very high incidence of cross-infection among family members (57). The reports implicating milk contaminated with *S. zooepidemicus* as a cause of PSGN in rural communities make it worthwhile to emphasize the need for consuming only pasteurized milk.

Early antibiotic treatment in patients with sore throat is possible if a positive result is obtained with the use of rapid colorimetric high-sensitivity immunoabsorbent assay (Testpack Strep A plus, Abbot Laboratories); however, culture confirmation of negative results are advisable.

Patients with the acute nephritic syndrome should have restricted sodium and water intake. A safe practice is to withhold oral intake for 12 to 24 hours after admission to establish the severity of oliguria and to achieve an early negative balance. Patients with edema may benefit of therapy with intravenous furosemide, which may induce several-fold increments in urine output. Antihypertensive drugs (oral nifedipine, IV hidralazine, or diazoxide) may be required during the first 48 hours if significant hypertension is present. Medications that are better avoided because of potential adverse effects include digitalis preparations (ineffective in this condition), spironolactone (hyperkalemia), angiotensin converting enzyme inhibitors (hyperkalemia), propanolol (hyperkalemia and possible congestive heart failure), and alpha methyldopa (usually ineffective and risk of oversedation). The value of bed rest is unproven, but it appears wise to prescribe a moderate restriction of activities in the acute phase. Emergency treatment for hypertensive encephalopathy may require sodium nitroprusside, and dialysis for uremia or hyperkalemia may be required in adult patients with acute glomerulonephritis but rarely in children.

PSGN and End-Stage Renal Disease: Prognostic Factors

It is well known that the immediate mortality of children with acute PSGN is very low but the long-term prognosis of PSGN has been a subject of controversy (57). Initial studies in the 1930s based their optimistic outlook on relatively short follow-up and subsequent studies have given widely different figures; for instance, proteinuria was found in only 3.5% of the patients followed in Trinidad (58), while it was found in 60% of the patients followed in New York (59). Abnormal renal biopsy findings are relatively frequent (22,59,60), but they do not necessarily mean progressive renal disease. Several characteristics worsen the likelihood of subsequent development of abnormal renal function, proteinuria, and hypertension, among them are the age at the time of the acute attack and the presentation with proteinuria in the nephrotic range. In contrast with children, adult patients with acute PSGN may present azotemia (60–70%), congestive heart failure (40%), nephritic proteinuria (20%), and significant early mortality (25%). A particularly severe prognosis is found in older patients with massive proteinuria; as many as 77% of these sub-group of patients develop chronic renal failure (61).

Specific communities may have a worse long-term prognosis. For example, Australian Aborigines from the Northern Territory who had PSGN had an increased risk for albuminuria (adjusted odds ratio 6.1%, 95% CI 2.2–16.9) and hematuria (OR 3.7, 95% CI 1.8–8.0) when compared to controls who had not suffered PSGN (62). In Nova Serrana, Brazil, the most recent follow-up study of 56 adults found that hypertension, reduced creatinine clearance, and microalbumniuria were present in 30%, 49%, in 22%, respectively (63; R. Sesso, personal communication, 2004).

White et al. (62) have raised an additional aspect worth considering when analyzing the long-term follow-up of patients with PSGN. Residual damage from PSGN may be sub-clinical and therefore the reduction of functioning nephrons may not be detected by an increase in serum creatinine nor even by a significant reduction in the glomerular filtration rate. This condition may only be manifested by impairment in the capacity to increase the creatinine clearance after a protein meal (64,65).

Nevertheless, such a reduction in nephron units, if associated with other conditions independently capable of decreasing nephron numbers, could result in progressive renal damage that eventually will reach end-stage renal disease. This possibility merits consideration in specific Aboriginal communities that have additional risks factors for progression of renal damage; among them are low birth weight, diabetes, and features of syndrome X (66–68). The cooperation of all these risk factors may facilitate the access to the one-way road of single nephron hyperfiltration towards chronic renal failure (69).

In specific high-risk communities as well as in patients with known risk factors, it is advisable to maintain yearly follow-up evaluations after recovery from the acute attack. The early detection of hypertension or proteinuria requires active drug treatment to control these conditions that are known to be associated with progression to end-stage renal damage.

HEMOLYTIC UREMIC SYNDROME

In 1955, Gasser et al. (70) described four infants with a syndrome characterized by hemolysis and uremia and subsequent studies demonstrated the association between *E. coli* infections and the hemolytic uremic syndrome (HUS) and the role of the verotoxins in the pathogenesis of the disease (71,72).

The HUS is a thrombotic microangiopathy (Fig. 2) that may present two different clinical entities: the classical form, associated with gastroenteritis (D+ HUS) and the atypical or idiopathic form, not associated with diarrhea (D– HUS), which includes genetic forms of thrombotic microangiopathy (73). The various conditions associated with thrombotic microangiopathy trigger a sequence of events that is largely a common pathogenetic pathway that includes endothelial injury, leukocyte and platelet activation, complement consumption, hemolysis, microthrombosis, and thrombocytopenia. Several bacteria and viral infections have been associated with HUS. The bacterial infections reported in association with the HUS are shown in Table 3.

In this section, we will only be concerned with the epidemiological characteristics of the classical D+ HUS, resulting from gastrointestinal infections with *E. coli* and *Shigella*. The clinical picture of this syndrome is well recognized (reviewed in Ref. 74) and in the reported outbreaks of *E. Coli* 0157:H7 (the most common serotype causing HUS) in the United States, 25% of the patients have needed hospitalization, 6% developed HUS or thrombotic thrombocytopenic purpura, and 1% died (75).

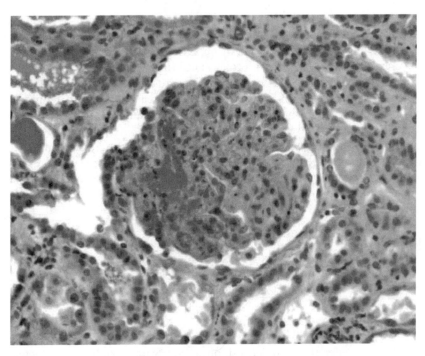

Figure 2 Renal biopsy of a patient with the hemolytic uremic syndrome showing a thrombus in the glomerular capillaries. (Courtesy of Dr. Daniel Carpio, Pathology Department, Valdivia, Chile.)

Worldwide Distribution of the Hemolytic Uremic Syndrome

E. coli infections have increased and are likely to continue to increase in humans (72) and, therefore, the risk of HUS could be assumed to increase also. HUS usually results from the ingestion of undercooked meat contaminated with the *E. coli*, but other foods such as milk, fruits, vegetables, apple

Table 3 Bacteria Associated with Hemolytic Uremic Syndrome

Escherichia coli
Shigella dysenteriae
Streptococcus pneumoniae
Salmonella typhi
Group A streptococcus
Campilobacter jejuni
Clostridium dificile
Clostridium septicum
Fusobacterium necroforum
Bacteroides fragilis

cider, and even water may be contaminated and cause the disease. Infants and adults can be affected, but the majority of cases are children between 6 months and 4 years of age. The disease has a worldwide distribution (Table 4) and highest incidence of sporadic cases is reported in Argentina where 350 new cases are reported every year (76,96). The usual enteropathogenic *E. coli* type causing HUS is the 0157:H7 (Table 4) and in sporadic cases in Central Europe (Belgium, The Netherlands, Germany) verocytotoxin-2 is the most frequently produced toxin (74).

Small clusters of cases have been reported after the consumption of unpasteurized milk contaminated with *E. coli* 026 (97), swallowing water while swimming in a Connecticut lake contaminated with *E. coli* 0121: H19 (98), and gastroenteritis caused by *E. coli* 0111 (99). There is an increased risk in family members of children with D+ HUS, which has led to the suggestion that siblings of affected children should be kept under surveillance (100).

The Afro-American race has been reported to be 10 times less frequently affected by the HUS in Alabama (91), while Black children in Johannesburg have an increased prevalence of *Shigella* type I-induced HUS (101).

Clusters of cases and epidemics have been reported from all over the world. Table 5 shows the outbreaks reported since 1991.

Immediate and Long-Term Outcome of the SUH

The immediate mortality of the HUS was reduced from nearly 50% to 2–4% with the use of peritoneal dialysis (118). Older patients and patients who had infection with *Shigella dysenteriae* type 1 appear to have a worse immediate prognosis. The reasons for this are unclear and the fact that malnourished patients in poor communities have more frequently shigella-associated HUS may be a partial explanation.

The long-term outcome in Inuit survivors of an epidemic of HUS evaluated after 4 years was reported as excellent (102). However, Western European series report complete recovery in only 64% of the patients. Renal insufficiency and hypertension was found in 4% of the patients and end-stage renal disease in 9% (73). Spizzirri et al. (119) followed 118 patients at yearly intervals for 10 to 19 years and found complete recovery in 62.7%, proteinuria with or without hypertension in 17.7%, reduced creatinine clearance in 16.1%, and end-stage renal failure in 3.4% of the patients. Exeni et al. (76) in a follow-up of 152 patients in Argentina (107 patients for more than 10 years) report essentially the same findings. Evaluation of 288 patients followed for at least 1 year in Chile found chronic renal failure in 12%, proteinuria with normal renal function in 6%, and normal renal function in 82% (85). These studies indicate the need for continued surveillance of the patients that had HUS, as emphasized in a recent study in the United Kingdom (120).

Table 4 Worldwide Distribution of Hemolytic Uremic Syndrome

Country	Incidence/prevalence	References
Argentina (Mendoza)	10.2 cases/100,000 children <15 years	76
	350 new cases/year	77
	12 cases/year (1994–1996)	
Austria	0.4/100,000 children/year	78
Belgium	4.3 cases/100,000 children <5 years	79
	1.8 cases/100,000 children <15 years	
	0.42 cases/100,000 population	
Canada	3.2 cases/1,000,000 population/year	80–82
	1.44 cases/100,000 children <15 years old	
	31.4% risk after infection with E. coli 0157:H7	
	(Reginal variations: In Alberta 8.1% risk after infection with E. coli 0157:H7)	
Chile (Santiago)	17 cases/year (1991–1993), E. coli 0157:H7	83, 84
Chile	472 cases (1990–2002), 90% D(+), E. Coli the most frequent isolated agent, mortality 4.3%, CRF 12%	85
Czech Republic (Prague)	Five cases/year (1988–1995), 52% are E. coli 0157:H7 and 026:H11	86
Germany	0.7/100,000 children/year	78
India		
Lucknow	30% of the patients with acute renal failure in a pediatric population	48, 52, 53, 56, 87
Varanasi	39% of the patients with acute renal failure in a pediatric population	

Location	Description	Ref.
Bombay	10% of the patients with acute renal failure in a pediatric population	
New Delhi	36% of the patients with acute renal failure in a pediatric population. 8.1 cases/year (1980–1988)	80, 88
Italy	0.28 cases/100,000 pop/year, 15% of the children with infection with *E. coli* 0157:H7	
Kuwait (Safat)	Five cases/year in pediatric nephrology services	89
Maroc (Casablanca)	13.5% of the patients with acute renal failure in a pediatric population	50
Paraguay (Asunción)	0.96% of the patients with acute renal failure in the pediatric population	54
Perú (Lima)	10.6% of the patients with acute renal failure in a pediatric population	90
United Kingdom	2.2 cases/1,000,000 pop/year	80
USA	6.5 cases/1,000,000 pop/year	91
Alabama	0.45 cases/100,000 White children; 0.043 cases/100,000 Afro-American children	91
California	0.67/100,000 children; >80% due to *E. coli* 0157:H7	92
Minneapolis	Increase from 0.5 cases/100,000 child-years in 1979 to 2.0 in 1988	93, 94
Utah	1.42 cases /100,000 children 7 years (20-year population-based study)	95

Table 5 Outbreaks (>10 Cases) of Hemolytic Uremic Syndrome (1990–2003)

Year	Country (city)	Cases (origin)	Bacteria	References
1991	Alaska	18 cases	*E. coli* 0157:H7	102
1991	USA (Massachussets)	18 cases (consumption of apple cider)	*E. coli* 0157:H7	103
1992	Canada (Arviat, Inuit community)	19 cases out of 84 cases with diarrhea	*E. coli* 0157:H7	104
1992	Italy (Lombardia)	Nine cases	*E. coli* 011	105
1992–1993	USA (several states)	45 cases out of 501 patients with diarrhea (hamburger consumption in a fast-food chain)	*E. coli* 0157:H7	106
1993	USA (Washington State)	278 children	*E. coli* 0157:H7	107
1993	USA (San Diego, California)	Nine cases out of 34 cases with diarrhea (hamburger patties from food chain)	*E. coli* 0157:H7	108
1994	USA (Trenton, New Jersey)	23 cases	*E. coli* 0157:H7	109
1994–1995	South Africa (KwaZulu/Natal)	130 cases	*S. dysenteriae*	110
1995	Saudi Arabia	12 cases of hospitalized patients with dysentery		111
1995	Australia	23 cases in South Australia		112
1996	United Kingdom (Lanarkshire, Scotland)	34 cases out of 120 with diarrhea	*E. coli* 0157:H7	113
1995–1996	Germany (Bavaria)	28 cases (sausage consumption)	*E. coli* 0157:H-	114
1998	USA (Alpine, Wyoming)	157 cases (waterborne infection)	*E. coli* 0157:H7	115
2000	Zimbabwe (Bulawayo)	14 cases out of 91 with diarrhea		116
2003	France (Paris)	11 children (index case returning from Senegal)	*S. dysenteriae* Type 1	117

Patients with HUS that progress to end-stage renal disease are frequently transplanted. The idiopathic and genetic forms of HUS/thrombotic microangiopathy frequently recur in the transplanted kidney; in contrast, the D+ HUS rarely, if ever, has a post-transplant recurrence.

General Treatment Guidelines and Prevention Measures

Several treatments have been used in the management of the HUS. Plasmapheresis, anticoagulants, antiplatelet agents, fibrinolytics, prostacyclin, steroids, and intravenous gammaglobulin have all tried in this condition, but their usefulness has not been proved. In general, the following guidelines of treatment may be recommended:

1. Once the diagnosis is made, the patient should be admitted to the hospital, a report should be made to local health authorities, and the family should be kept under surveillance.
2. If enterocolitis is present, oral intake should be avoided and electrolyte imbalance and dehydration should be corrected with appropriate IV therapy. Enteric isolation precautions should be enforced. Antibiotic therapy should be avoided and be aware about possible complications that require surgical intervention, such as toxic megacolon or perforation.
3. After the onset of the HUS, acute renal failure usually develops with oliguria and overhydration. In most circumstances, diuretic therapy and volume expansion are ineffective and contraindicated. Complications of acute renal failure, such as azotemia, acidosis, and hyperkalemia are an indication of dialysis. Peritoneal dialysis is the usual modality employed in children, but hemodialysis may also be used.
4. Transfusions of packed red cells are indicated when the hematocrit falls to 20% or less and usually multiple transfusions are necessary. Platelet transfusions may be used only in patients who require surgical intervention or present active gastrointestinal bleeding.
5. Hypertension frequently follows transfusions and usually requires drug therapy: nifedipine, diazoxide and, in extreme cases, sodium nitroprusside may be used. Convulsions, if present, may be controlled with IV diazepam.

In Argentina, where the HUS is the first cause of acute renal failure in children younger than 5 years and the third cause of renal transplantation in children, the following recommendations for the general public have been issued in the official publication of the Latin American Pediatric Nephrology Association (121):

- All foods may be contaminated but in particular, meat and visceral organs. Keep vegetables and fruits separate from meat to avoid potential cross-contamination. Avoid using the same kitchen utensils in raw meat and the rest of the food.
- Keep in mind the need to maintain the temperature at less than 4°C in the meats and dairy products prior to their consumption. Meat and dairy products that remain for more than 2 hr (cumulative) at temperatures ranging between 4°C and 60°C are to be considered contaminated and should be discarded.
- Bacteria are destroyed at a temperature of 70°C or higher. Make sure that this temperature is reached in the cooking and the center of the meat does not remain red (raw). Ground meat needs to be closely examined to assure that complete cooking has been achieved. It may be necessary to complement the cooking with 2–3 min of microwave oven.
- Do not consume red meat in places where you are in doubt about its correct handling and care.

The widespread awareness of the problem and the use of these recommendations should result in a substantial decrease in the incidence of the disease in the underdeveloped world.

ACKNOWLEDGMENTS

The authors want to recognize the help and data provided by the following colleagues: Guillermo García, Angélica Arevalo, Maria Luisa Salazar, Santa Ramirez, and Gustavo Pérez from Hospital Civil (AA, GG), Hospital Civil Juan Menchaca (MLS, GP), and Centro Médico Nacional (SR), Guadalajara, Mexico; Gustavo Gordillo (Hospital Angeles del Pedregal, México, DF); Francisco Santacruz (Universidad de Paraguay, La Asunción, Paraguay); Randall Lou (FUNDANIER, Ciudad de Guatemala, Guatemala); José Grunberg (Sanatorios Evangélico y Español, Montevideo, Uruguay); Ramón Exeni (Hospital de Niños San Justo, Buenos Aires, Argentina); Abdías Hurtado and Elizabeth Escudero (Universidad Cayetano Heredia, Lima, Peru); Ricardo Sesso (Ecola Paulista de Medicina, Sao Paulo, Brazil); Deisy Bocángel (Universidad Mayor de San Andres) and Raúl Plata (Instituto de Nefrología, La Paz, Bolivia); Jorge Alfonzo and Miguel Almaguer (Instituto Nacional de Nefrología, La Habana Cuba).

REFERENCES

1. von Plenciz MA. Tractatus II de Scarlatina. Viena, JA Trattner, 1792. Cited by Becker CG, Murphy GE. The experimental production of glomerulonephritis like that in man by infection with group A streptococcus. J Exp Med 1968; 127:1–23.
2. Reichel H. Uber nephritis bei Scharlach. Z Heilk 1905; 6:72–80.

3. Dochez AR, Sherman L. The significance of *Streptococcus hemolyticus* in scarlet fever and the preparation of specific antiscarlatinal serum by immunization of the horse to *Streptococcus hemolyticus* scarlatinae. J Am Med Assoc 1924; 82:542–544.

4. Longcope WT. The pathogenesis of glomerulonephritis. Bull Johns Hopkins Hosp 1929; 45:335.

5. Lyttle JD, Seegal D, Loeb EN, Jost EL. The serum anti-streptolysin titer in acute glomerulonephritis. J Clin Invest 1938; 17:631–639.

6. Futcher PH. Glomerular nephritis following skin infections. Arch Intern Med 1940; 65:1192–1210.

7. Barnham M, Thornton TJ, Lange K. Nephritis caused by *Streptococcus zooepidemicus* (Lancefield group C). Lancet 1983; 1:945–948.

8. Francis AJ, Nimmo GR, Efstratiou A, Galanis V, Nuttall N. Investigation of milk-borne *Streptococcus zooepidemicus* infection associated with glomerulonephritis in Australia. J Infect 1993; 27:317–323.

9. Balter S, Benin A, Pinto SW, Teixeira LM, Alvim GG, Luna E, Jackson D, LaClaire L, Elliott J, Facklam R, Schuchat A. Epidemic nephritis in Nova Serrana, Brazil. Lancet 2000; 355:1776–1780.

10. Schick B. Die Nachkrankheiten des Scharlach. Jahrb Kinderheilk 1907; 65(suppl):132–173.

11. Von Pirquet CE. Allergy. Arch Intern Med 1911; 7:259–288, 382–436.

12. Rodríguez-Iturbe B. Nephritis-associated streptococcal antigens: where are we now? J Am Soc Nephrol 2004; 15:1961–1962.

13. Yoshisawa N, Yamakami K, Fujino M, Oda T, Tamura K, Matsumoto K, Sugisaki T, Boyle MDP. Nephritis associated plasmin receptor and acute glomerulonephritis: characterization of the antigen and associated antibody immune response. J Am Soc Nephrol 2004; 15:1785–1793.

14. Poon-King T, Bannan J, Viteri A, Cu G, Zabriskie JB. Identification of an exracellular plasmin binding protein from nephritogenic streptococci. J Exp Med 1993; 178:759–763.

15. Parra G, Rodriguez-Iturbe B, Batsford S, Vogt A, Mezzano S, Olavarria F, Exeni R, Lasso M, Orta N. Antibody response to *Streptococcal zymogen* in the serum of patients with acute glomerulonephritis: a multicentric study. Kidney Int 1998; 54:509–517.

16. Stetson CA, Rammelkamp CH, Krause RA, Kohen RJ, Perry WD. Epidemic acute nephritis: studies on etiology, natural history and prevention. Medicine 1955; 34:431–450.

17. Reed RW. An epidemic of acute nephritis. Can Med Assoc J 1953; 68: 48–455.

18. Reinstein CR. Epidemic nephritis in Red Lake Minnesota. J Pediatr 1955; 47:25–34.

19. Bisno AL, Pierce IA, Wall HP, Moody MD, Stollerman GH. Contrasting epidemiology of acute rheumatic fever and acute glomerulonephritis. N Engl J Med 1970; 283:561–565.

20. Poon-King T, Mohammed I, Cox R, Potter EV, Simon NM, Siegel AC, Earle DP. Recurrent epidemic nephritis in South Trinidad. N Engl J Med 1967; 277:728–732.

21. Kaplan EL, Anthony BF, Chapman SS, Wannamaker LW. Epidemic acute glomerulonephritis associated with type 49 *Streptococcal pyoderma* I. Clinical and laboratory findings. Am J Med 1970; 48:9–27.

22. Rodriguez-Iturbe B, García R, Rubio L, Cuenca L, Treser G, Lange K. Epidemic glomerulonephritis in Maracaibo. Clin Nephrol 1976; 5:197–206.

23. Potter EV, Ortiz JS, Sharrett R, Burt EG, Bray JP, Finklea JF, Poon-King T, Earle DP. Changing types of nephritogenic streptococci in Trinidad. J Clin Invest 1971; 50:1197–1205.

24. Rodriguez-Iturbe B, Garcia R, Rubio L, Cuenca L. Características clínicas y epidemiológicas de la glomerulonefritis postestreptocóccica en la región zuliana. Invest Clin 1985; 26(3):191–211.

25. Dávalos C, Valle C. Tesis de grado. Havana, Cuba: Instituto Nacional de Nefrología, 1975.

26. Margolis HS, Lum MKW, Bender TH, Elliot SI, Fitzgerald MA, Harpster AP. Acute glomerulonephritis and streptococcal skin lesions in Eskimo children. Am J Dis Child 1980; 134:681–685.

27. Berrios X, Lagomarsino E, Solar E, Sandoval G, Guzmán B, Riedel. Post-streptococcal acute glomerulonephritis in Chile: 20 years of experience. Pediatr Nephrol 2004; 19:306–312.

28. Zuazo J, Almaguer M, Cabrera MS, Texidor MEM. Estudio epidemiológico de un brote de nefritis aguda postestreptocóccica. Rev Cub Hygiene Epidemiol 1986; 24:363–269.

29. Johnston F, Carapetis J, Patel MS, Wallace T, Spillane P. Evaluating the use of penicillin to control outbreaks of acute poststreptococcal glomerulonephritis. Pediatr Infect Dis J 1999; 18:327–332.

30. Jovanovic D, Maric M, Kovacevic Z, Skataric V, Jokovic B. Epidemiology of poststreptococcal glomerulonephritis in the military population. Srp Arh Celok Lek 1996; 124(suppl 1):187–189.

31. Reid HF, Bassett DC, Gaworzewska E, Colman G, Poon-King T. Streptococcal serotypes newly associated with epidemic post-streptococcal acute glomerulonephritis. J Med Microbiol 1990; 32:111–114.

32. Masuyama T, Ishii E, Muraoka K, Honjo S, Yamaguchi H, Hara T, Shimazaki K, Koga T, Moriya K, Ide M, Miyazaki S. Outbreak of acute glomerulonephritis in children: observed association with the T1 subtype of group A streptococcal infection in northern Kyushu, Japan. Acta Paediatr Jpn 1996; 38:128–131.

33. Streeton CL, Hanna JN, Messer RD, Merianos A. An epidemic of acute post-streptococcal glomerulonephritis among aboriginal children. J Paediatr Child Health 1995; 31:245–248.

34. Sarkissian A, Papazian M, Azatian G, Arikiants N, Babloyan A, Leumann E. An epidemic of acute postinfectious glomerulonephritis in Armenia. Arch Dis Child 1997; 77:342–344.

35. López V, Sekihara G, Pimentel G, Mendoza A, Asmat K. Abstracts of the National Peruvian Congress of Nephrology, 2002.

36. McCarty M. The streptococcus and human disease. Am J Med 1978; 65: 717–718.

37. Simon P, Ramee MP, Autuly V, Laruelle E, Charasse C, Cam G, Ang KS. Epidemiology of primary glomerular diseases in a French region. Variations according to period and age. Kidney Int 1994; 46:1192–1198.
38. Roy S, Stapleton FB. Changing perspectives in children hospitalized with poststreptococcal acute glomerulonephritis. Pediatr Nephrol 1990; 4:585–588.
39. Schena FP. Survey of the Italian Registry of renal biopsies. Frequency of the renal diseases for 7 consecutive years. Nephrol Dial Transplant 1997; 12: 418–426.
40. Coppo R, Gianoglio B, Porcellini MG, Maringhini S. Frequency of renal diseases and clinical indications for renal biopsies in children (Report of the Italian National registry of Renal Biopsies in Children). Nephrol Dial Transplant 1998; 13:293–297.
41. Zhang Y, Shen Y, Feld LG, Stapleton FB. Changing pattern of glomerular disease in Biejing Children's Hospital. Clin Pediatr 1994; 33:542–547.
42. Yap HK, Chia KS, Murugasu B, Saw AH, Tay JS, Ikshuvanam M, Tan KW, Cheng HK, Tan CL, Lim CH. Acute glomerulonephritis-changing patterns in Singapore children. Pediatr Nephrol 1990; 4:482–484.
43. Berrios X, Quesney F, Morales A, Blazquez J, Lagomarsino E, Bisno AL. Acute rheumatic fever and poststreptococcal glomerulonephritis in an open population: comparative studies of epidemiology and bacteriology. J Lab Clin Med 1986; 108:535–542.
44. Currie B, Brewster DR. Childhood infections in the tropical north of Australia. J Paediatr Child Health 2001; 37:326–330.
45. Orta N, Moriyón JC. Epidemiología de las enfermedades renales en niños en Venezuela. Arch Venez Puericult Pediatr 2001; 64:76–83.
46. Montseny JJ, Meyrier A, Kleinknecht D, Callard P. The current spectrum of infectious glomerulonephritis. Experience with 76 patients and review of the literature. Medicine (Baltimore) 1995; 74:63–73.
47. Prakash J, Saxena RK, Sharma OP. Spectrum of renal diseases in the elderly: single center experience from a developing country. Int Urol Nephrol 2001; 33:227–233.
48. Srivastava RN, Bagga A, Moudgil A. Acute renal failure in north Indian children. Indian J Med Res 1990; 92:404–408.
49. Gokcay G, Emre S, Tanman F, Sirin A, Elcioglu N, Dolunay G. An epidemiological approach to acute renal failure in children. J Trop Pediatr 1991; 3:191–193.
50. Bourquia A, Zaid D. Acute renal insufficiency in children: a retrospective study of 89 cases. Ann Pediatr (Paris) 1993; 40:603–608.
51. Bamgboye EL, Mabayoje MO, Odutola TA, Mabadeje AF. Ren Fail 1993; 15: 77–80.
52. Kandoth PW, Agarwal GJ, Dharnidharka VR. Acute renal failure in children requiring dialysis therapy. Indian Pediatr 1994; 31:305–309.
53. Arora P, Kher V, Gupta A, Kohli HS, Gulati S, Rai PK, Kumar P, Sharma RK. Pattern of acute renal failure at a referral hospital. Indian Pediatr 1994; 31:1047–1053.
54. Florentin de Merech L. Prevalencia de la insuficiencia renal aguda y de sus etiologías más frecuentes en pacientes nefrológicos pediátricos. Arch Argent Pediatr 2001; 99:219–227.

55. López V, Sakihara G, Pimentel G, Mendoza A, Asmat K. Glomerulonefritis aguda difusa postinfecciosa (GNDAPI). Abstracts of the Peruvian Nacional Congreso of Nephrology, 2002.

56. Prakash J, send, Kumar NS, Kumar H, Tripathi LK, Saxena RK. Acute renal failure due to intrinsic renal diseases: review of 112 cases. Ren Fail 2003; 25:225–233.

57. Rodriguez-Iturbe B. Epidemic poststreptococcal glomerulonephritis (Nephrology Forum). Kidney Int 1984; 25:129–136.

58. Potter EV, Lipschultz SA, Abidh S, Poon-King T, Earle DP. Twelve to seventeen-year follow-up of patients with poststreptococcal acute glomerulonephritis in Trinidad. N Engl J Med 1982; 307:725–729.

59. Baldwin DS, Gluck MC, Schacht RG, Gallo G. The long-term course of poststreptococcal glomerulonephritis. Ann Intern Med 1974; 80:342–358.

60. Gallo GR, Feiner HD, Steele JM Jr, Schacht RG, Gluck MC, Baldwin DS. Role of intrarenal vascular sclerosis in progression of poststreptococcal glomerulonephritis. Clin Nephrol 1980; 13:49–57.

61. Vogl W, Renke M, Mayer-Eichberger D, Schmitt H, Bohle A. Long-term prognosis for endocapillary glomerulonephritis of poststreptococcal type in children and adults. Nephron 1986; 44:58–65.

62. White AV, Hoy WE, McCredie DA. Childhood post-streptococcal glomerulonephritis as a risk for chronic renal disease in later life. Med J Aust 2001; 174:492–496.

63. Sesso R, Wynton S. Follow up of patients with epidemic glomerulonephritis. Am J Kidney Dis 2001; 38:249–255.

64. Rodriguez-Iturbe B, Herrera J, Garcia R. Response to acute protein load in kidney donors an in apparently normal postacute glomerulonephritis patients: evidence for glomerular hyperfiltration. Lancet 1985; 2:461–464.

65. Cleper R, Davidovitz M, Halevi R, Eisenstein B. Renal functional reserve after acute poststreptococcal glomerulonephritis. Pediatr Nephrol 1997; 11:473–476.

66. Spencer JL, Silva DT, Snelling P, Hoy WE. An epidemic of renal failure among Australian Aboriginals. Med J Aust 1998; 168:537–541.

67. Hoy WE, Mathews JD, McCredie DA, Pugsley DJ, Hayhurst BG, Rees M, Kile E, Walker KA, Wang Z. The multidimensional nature of renal disease: rates and association of albuminuria in the Australian Aboriginal community. Kidney Int 1998; 54:1296–1304.

68. Hoy WE, Rees M, Kile E, Mathews JD, Wang Z. A new dimension to the Barker hypothesis: low birthweight an susceptibility to renal disease. Kidney Int 1999; 56:1072–1077.

69. Nenov V, Maarten WT, Sakharova OV, Brenner BM. Multi-hit nature of chronic renal disease. Curr Opin Nephrol Hypertens 2000; 9:85–97.

70. Gasser C, Gauthier C, Steck A. Hemolytisch Uremische Syndrome. Med Wochenschr 1955; 85:905–909.

71. Karmali M, Steele B, Petric M, Lim C. Sporadic cases of hemolytic uremic syndrome associated with fecal cytotoxin producing *E. coli* in stools. Lancet 1983; 1:619–620.

72. Karmali M, Petric M, Lim C, Fleming P, Arbus GS, Lior H. Association between idiopathic hemolytic uremic syndrome and the infection by verotoxin-producing *Escherichia coli*. J Infect Dis 1985; 151:775–782.
73. Kaplan BS, Meyers KW, Shulman SL. The pathogenesis and treatment of the hemolytic uremic syndrome. J Am Soc Nephrol 1998; 9:1126–1133.
74. van de Kar NC, Roelofs HG, Muytjens HL, Tolboom JJ, Roth B, Proesmans W, Reitsma-Bierens WC, Wolff ED, Karmali MA, Chart H, Monnens LA. Verocytotoxin-producing *Escherichia coli* infection in hemolytic uremic syndrome in part of Western Europe. Eur J Pediatr 1996; 155:592–595.
75. Besser RE, Griffin PM, Slutsker L. *Escherichia coli* 0157:H7 gastroenteritis and the hemolytic uremic syndrome: an emerging infectious disease. Ann Rev Med 1999; 50:355–367.
76. Exeni R. Exeni A, Exeni C. Sindrome urémico hemolítico. In: García Nieto V, Santos F, Rodríguez-Iturbe B, eds. Nefrología Pediátrica. 2nd ed. Madrid: Aula Médica. In press.
77. Rivas M, Balbi L, Miliwebsky ES, Garcia B, Tous MI, Leardini NA, Prieto MA, Chillemi GM, de Principi ME. Hemolytic uremic syndrome in children of Mendoza, Argentina: association with Shiga toxin-producing *Escherichia coli* infection. Medicina (Buenos Aires) 1998; 58:1–7.
78. Gerber A, Karch H, Allerberger F, Verweyen HM, Zimmerhackl LB. Clinical course and the role of shiga toxin-producing *Escherichia coli* infection in the hemolytic-uremic syndrome in pediatric patients, 1997–2000, I Germany and Austria: a prospective study. J Infect Dis 2002; 186:493–500.
79. Cornu G, Proesmans W, Dediste A, Jacobs F, Van de Walle J, Mertens A, Ramet J, Lauwers S. Hemolytic uremic syndrome in Belgium: incidence and association with verocytotoxin-producing *Escherichia coli*. Clin Microbiol Infect 1999; 5:16–22.
80. Miller DP, Kaye JA, Shea K, Zyyadeh N, Cali C, Black C, Walker AM. Incidence of thrombotic thrombocytopenic purpura/hemolytic uremic syndrome. Epidemiology 2004; 15:208–215.
81. Rowe PC, Orrbine E, Lior H, Wells GA, Yetisir E, Clulow M, McLaine PN. Risk of hemolytic uremic syndrome after sporadic *Escherichia coli* 0157:H7 infection: results of a Canadian collaborative study. J Pediatr 1998; 132: 777–782.
82. Rowe PC, Orrbine E, Wells GA, McLaine PN. Epidemiology of hemolytic-uremic syndrome in Canadian children from 1986 to 1988. The Canadian Pediatric Kidney Disease Reference Center. J Pediatr 1991; 119:218–224.
83. Prado V, Cordero J, Garreaud C, Olguin H, Arellano C, Nachar CL, Misraji A, Martinez J, Tous M, Rivas M. Enterohemorrhagic *Escherichia coli* in hemolytic uremic syndrome in Chilean children. Evaluation of different techniques in the diagnosis of infection. Rev Med Chil 1995; 123:13–22.
84. Cordero J, Baeza J, Fielbaum O, Saieh C, Varela M, Rodriguez E, Olivos P, Hernandez C, Gonzalez J. Hemolytic uremic syndrome. Experience with 154 cases. Rev Chil Pediatr 1990; 61:235–242.
85. Zambrano P, Delucchi A, Pilar H, et al. Hemolytic uremic syndrome in Chile: follow-up of renal function and prognostic features. ERA-EDTA, XLI Congress, Lisbon, Portugal, 2004.

86. Bielaszewska M, Janda J, Blahova K, Feber J, Potuznik V, Souckova A. Verocytotoxin-producing *Escherichia coli* in children with hemolytic uremic syndrome in the Czech Republic. Clin Nephrol 1996; 46:42–44.

87. Srivastava RN, Moudgil A, Bagga A, Vasudev AS. Hemolytic uremic syndrome in children in northern India. Pediatr Nephrol 1991; 5:284–288.

88. Chiurchiu C, Firrincieli A, Santostefano M, Fusaroli M, Remuzzi G, Ruggenentti P. Adult nondiarrhea hemolytic uremic syndrome associated with Shiga toxin *Escherichia coli* 0157:H7 bacteremia and urinary infection. Am J Kidney Dis 2003; 41:EA.

89. Al-Eisa A, Al.Hajeri M. Hemolytic uremic syndrome in Kuwaiti Arab children. Pediatr Nephrol 2001; 16:1093–1098.

90. Encinas M, Guevara C, Lopez M, Sakihara G, Mendoza A, Lopez V, Pimentel G, Valdivia V. Abstracts of the National Congress of Nephrology, Lima, Peru, 2002.

91. Jernigan SM, Waldo FB. Racial incidence of hemolytic uremic syndrome. Pediatr Nephrol 1994; 8:545–547.

92. Cummings KC, Mohle-Boetani JC, Werner SB, Vugia DJ. Population-based trends in pediatric hemolytic uremic syndrome in California 1994–1999: substantial underreporting and public health implications. Am J Epidemiol 2002; 155:941–948.

93. Banatvala N, Griffin PM, Greene KD, Barrett TJ, Bibb WF, Greem JH, Wells JG. Hemolytic Uremic Syndrome Study Collaborators. The United States National Prospective Hemolytic Uremic Syndrome Study: microbiologic, serologic, clinical and epidemiologic findings. J Infect Dis 2001; 183:1063–1070.

94. Martin DL, MacDonald KL, White KE, Soler JT, Osterholm MT. The epidemiology and clinical aspects of the hemolytic uremic syndrome in Minnesota. N Engl J Med 1990; 323:1161–1167.

95. Siegler RL, Pavia AT, Christofferson RD, Milligan MK. A 20-year population-based study of postdiarrheal hemolytic uremic syndrome in Utah. Pediatrics 1994; 94:35–40.

96. Voyer LE, Wainsztein RE, Quadri BE, Corti SE. Hemolytic uremic syndrome in families—an Argentinian experience. Pediatr Nephrol 1996; 10:70–72.

97. Allergerger F, Friederich AW, Grif K, Dierich MP, Dornbusch HJ, Mache CJ, Machbaur E, Freilinger M, Rieck P, Wagner M, Caprioli A, Karch H, Zimmerhackl LB. Hemolytic-uremic syndrome associated with enterohemorrhagic *Escherichia coli* 026:H infection and consumption of unpasteurized cow's milk. Int J Infect Dis 2003; 7:42–45.

98. McCarthy TA, Barrett NL, Hadler JL, Salsbury B, Howard RT, Dingman DW, brinkman CD, Bibb WF, Cartter ML. Hemolytic-uremic syndrome and *Escherichia coli* 0121 at a lake in Connecticut, 1999. Pediatrics 2001; 108:E59.

99. Banatvala N, Debeukelaer MM, Griffin PM, Barrett TJ, Greene KD, green JH, Wells JG. Shiga-like toxin-producing *Escherichia coli* 0111 and associated hemolytic uremic syndrome: a family outbreak. Pediatr Infect Dis J 1996; 15:1008–1011.

100. Siegler RL, Sherbotie JR, Denkers ND, Pavia AT. Clustering of post-diarrheal (Shiga toxin mediated) hemolytic uremic syndrome in families. Clin Nephrol 2003; 60:74–79.

101. Thompson PD. Renal problems in black South Africans children. Pediatr Nephrol 1997; 11:508–512.

102. Ogborn MR, Hamiwka L, Orrbine E, Newburg DS, Sharma A, McLaine PN, Orr P, Rowe P. Renal function in Inuit survivors of epidemic hemolytic-uremic syndrome. Pediatr Nephrol 1998; 12:458–488.

103. Besser RE, Lett SM, Weber JT, Doyke MP. An outbreak of diarrhea and hemolytic uremic syndrome from *Escherichia coli* 0157:H7 in fresh-pressed apple cider. JAMA 1993; 269:2217–2220.

104. Rowe PC, Orrbine E, Ogborn M, Wells GA, Winther W, Lior H, Manuel D, McLaine PN. Epidemic *Escherichia coli* 0157:H/gastroenteritis and hemolytic-uremic syndrome in Canadian Inuit community: intestinal illness in family members as a risk factor. J Pediatr 1994; 124:21–26.

105. Caprioli A, Luzzi I, Rosmini F, Resti C, Edefonti A, Perfumo F, Farina C, Golglio A, Gianviti A, Rizzoni G. Community-wide outbreak of hemolytic-uremic syndrome associated with non-0157 verocytotoxin-producing *Escherichia coli*. J Infect Dis 1994; 169:208–211.

106. Bell BP, Goldoft M, Griffin PM, Davis MA, Gordon DC, Tarr PI, Bartleson CA, Lewis JH, Barrett TJ, Wells JG. A multistate outbreak of *Escherichia coli* 057:H7-associated bloody diarrhea and hemolytic uremic syndrome from hamburgers. The Washington experience. JAMA 1994; 272: 1349–1353.

107. Bell BP, Griffin PM, Lozano P, Christie DL, Kobayashi JM, Tarr PI. Predictors of hemolytic uremic syndrome in children during a large outbreak of *Escherichia coli* 0157:H7 infections. Pediatrics 1997; 100:E12.

108. Shefer AM, Koo D, Werner SB, Mintz ED, Baron R, Wells JG, Barrett TJ, Ginsberg M, Bryant R, Abbott S, griffin PM. A cluster of *Escherichia coli* 0157:H7 infections with hemolytic uremic syndrome and death in California. A mandate for improved surveillance. East J Med 1996; 165:15–19.

109. Genese CA, Brook J, Spitalny K. Hemolytic uremic syndrome in New Jersey. N J Med 1995; 92:29–32.

110. Bhimma R, Coovadia HM, Adhikari M, Connolly CA. Re-evaluating criteria for peritoneal dialysis in "classical" (D+) hemolytic uremic syndrome. Clin Nephrol 2001; 55:133–142.

111. Al-Qarawi S, Fontaine RE, Al-Qahtani MS. An outbreak of hemolytic uremic syndrome associated with antibiotic treatment of hospital inpatients for dysentery. Emerg Infect Dis 1995; 1:138–140.

112. South Australian Communicable Disease Control Unit. Community outbreak of hemolytic uremic syndrome attributable to *Escherichia coli* 0111:NM-South Australia 1995. MMWR Morb Mortal Wkly Rep 1995; 44:550–551, 557–558.

113. Dundas S, Todd WT, Stewart AI, Murdoch PS, Chaudhuri AK, Hutchinson SJ. The central Scotland *Escherichia coli* 0157:H7 outbreak: risk factors for hemolytic uremic syndrome. Clin Infect Dis 2001; 33:923–931.

114. Ammon A, Petersen LR, Karch H. A large outbreak of hemolytic uremic syndrome caused by an unusual sorbitol-fermenting strain of *Escherichia coli* 0157:H-. J Infect Dis 1999; 179:1274–1277.

115. Olsen SJ, Miller G, Breuer T, Kennedy M, Higgings C, Walford J, McKee G, Fox K, Bibb W, Mead P. A waterborne ourbreak of *Escherichia coli* 0157:H7

infections and the hemolytic uremic syndrome: implications for rural water systems. Emerg Infect Dis 2002; 8:370–375.

116. Oneko M, Nyathi MN, Doehring E. Post-dysenteric hemolytic uremic syndrome in Bulawayo, Zimbabwe. Pediatr Nephrol 2001; 16:1142–1145.

117. Houdin V, Doit C, Mariani P, Brahimi N, Lorita C, Bourrillon A, Bingen E. A pediatric cluster of *Shigella dysenteriae* serotype 1 diarrhea with hemolytic uremic syndrome. Clin Infect Dis 2004; 38:e96–e99.

118. Gianantonio C, Vitaco M, mendilaharzu F, Gallo G, Sojo E. Hemolytic uremic syndrome. J Pediatr 1964; 64:478–491.

119. Spizzirri FD, Rahman RC, Bibiloni N, Ruscasso JD, Amoreo OR. Childhood hemolytic uremic syndrome in Argentina: long-term follow-up and prognostic features. Pediatr Nephrol 1997; 11:156–160.

120. Small G, Watson AR, Evans JH, Gallager J. Hemolytic uremic syndrome: defining the need for long-term follow-up. Clin Nephrol 1999; 52:352–356.

121. Exeni A. Recomendaciones para la prevención del syndrome urémico hemolítico. Arch Latinoamer Nefrol Pediatr 2003; 3:98–100.

5

Viral Infections and the Kidney: A Major Problem in Developing Countries

M. Rafique Moosa and Theo L. Hattingh
Department of Internal Medicine, University of Stellenbosch and Renal Unit, Tygerberg Academic Hospital, Parrow Cape Town, South Africa

William D. Bates
Department of Anatomical Pathology, University of Stellenbosch, and National Health Laboratory Service, Cape Town, South Africa

Viruses are the most common cause of human infections—as well as the most deadly and most feared. Despite this, it is reassuring that the number of viral infections that result in kidney disease is relatively small. The spectrum of kidney diseases associated with viral infections includes acute tubulointerstitial nephritis, glomerulonephritis, hemolytic-uremic syndrome, nephrotic syndrome, and acute tubular necrosis. However, establishing a causal relationship between viral infections and kidney disease is often difficult and based on recognition of the clinical syndrome, serological evidence, identification of specific viral antigenemia, and the detection of viral antigens and host antibodies in glomerular and other renal structures (1). The resolution of the disease with clearance of the suspect antigen is an additional criterion. The mechanisms whereby viral infections may induce glomerular disease are summarized in Table 1. The most common viral infections causing chronic glomerular disease [human immunodeficiency virus (HIV), hepatitis B virus (HBV), and hepatitis C virus (HCV)] all have in common the inability of the body to eradicate the virus resulting in viral

Table 1 Mechanisms of Viral-Induced Glomerular Injury (1)

- Circulating immune complexes involving:
  - Viral antigens and host antiviral antibodies (2)
  - Endogenous antigens modified by viral injury and host auto-antibodies (3)
- In situ immune-mediated mechanisms involving viral antigens bound to glomerular structures (4,5)
- Expression of viral proteins or abnormal host proteins in tissue inducing:
  - Cell death through necrosis or apoptosis or cell dysfunction (6)
  - Increased matrix synthesis and/or decreased matrix degradation
  - Release of cytokines, chemokines and adhesion molecules, growth factors (7)
- Direct cytopathogenic effect of glomerular cells with undefined mechanisms (9)

persistence not thwarted by what is often a vigorous immune response (8). The kidney diseases associated with these viruses and other less common viral infections are summarized in Table 2.

INTRODUCTION: THE SCOURGE OF HUMAN IMMUNODEFICIENCY VIRUS (HIV) INFECTION

Worldwide infection with the human immunodeficiency virus (HIV) has reached pandemic proportions never before experienced in the history of humankind. The pandemic has been particularly rampant in inhabitants of developing countries and shows no signs of abating. Of the 40 million people living with HIV/acquired immunodeficiency syndrome (AIDS) at

Table 2 Kidney Diseases Associated with Viral Infections

Virus	Associated renal disease(s)
Hepatitis A	Acute tubular necrosis, interstitial nephritis, immune complex glomerulonephritis (9–11)
Hepatitis B virus (HBV)	Membranous GN, mesangiocapillary GN, IgA nephropathy (see text for details)
Hepatitis C (HCV)	Mesangiocapillary GN, others (see text for details)
HIV	HIVAN, ICN, thrombotic thrombocytopenic purpura/hemolytic-uremic syndrome (TTP/HUS) (see text for details)
Parvovirus B19	Non-HIV collapsing glomerulopathy, FSGS, immune complex glomerulonephritis (12–15)
Cytomegalovirus	IgA (?), transplant glomerulopathy (16–19)
Coxsackie B virus	IgA nephropathy (20,21), hemolytic-uremic syndrome
Polyoma virus BK	Tubulo-interstitial nephritis (renal allograft) (22,23)
Hantavirus	Tubulo-interstitial nephritis, (hemorrhagic fever with renal failure syndrome) (24,25)

Abbreviation: HIV, human immunodeficiency virus.

Table 3 The Global HIV–AIDS Pandemic, End of 2003

Region	People living with HIV–AIDS	New Infections in 2003	Adult prevalence (%)	Deaths from AIDS
Sub-Saharan Africa	28,000,000	3,400,000	8.5	2,400,000
Caribbean	590,000	80,000	3.1	50,000
Eastern Europe and Central Asia	1,600,000	280,000	0.9	37,000
South and South East Asia	8,200,000	1,100,000	0.8	590,000
Latin America	1,900,000	180,000	0.7	70,000
North America	1,200,000	54,000	0.7	18,000
North Africa and Middle East	730,000	67,000	0.4	50,000
Western Europe	680,000	40,000	0.3	3,400
East Asia and Pacific	1,300,000	270,000	0.1	58,000
Australia and New Zealand	18,000	1000	0.1	<100
Total	40,000,000	5,000,000	1.1	3,000,000

Source: From Ref. (26). Data are from the UNAIDS AIDS Epidemic Update, 2003.

the end of 2003, over 95% were in developing countries (Table 3). The most severely affected region is sub-Saharan Africa which is home to 70% of all HIV-infected adults and children; more specifically, 30% of all cases of HIV/AIDS worldwide occur in Southern Africa, which has less than 2% of the world population (26). It has been estimated that by 2010 life expectancy in some sub-Saharan countries will fall to near 30 years, levels not seen since the end of the 19th century (27). The disease is spreading in all developing countries to a greater or lesser degree but of concern is that the disease is making major inroads into regions previously relatively spared, including China, Vietnam, and Indonesia. In the Caribbean, East Europe (especially the Russian Federation, Baltic States, and Ukraine), and Central Asia, the disease continues to spread rapidly. In contrast to the dismal situation prevailing in developing countries, the death rate from HIV–AIDS in developed countries has become negligible following widespread access to antiretroviral agents in these regions and is proof that with the correct intervention the disease can be controlled (26).

Renal disease is a well-recognized complication of HIV infection. With rampant HIV infection in developing countries, HIV-associated renal disease can be expected to add a significant health burden to regions that are already struggling under the yoke of other health problems. HIV-related renal diseases is the third most common cause of end-stage renal failure among Black adults in the United States, despite the introduction of highly active antiretroviral therapy (HAART) (28). Projections are that the exponential increase in the number of people living with HIV infection will result in a commensurate increase in the number of patients with HIV-associated renal disease and ultimately end-stage renal failure (ESRF) (29). The prevalence of renal disease in patients varies widely depending on the ethnic makeup of the region but in certain centers HIV associated nephropathy (HIVAN) has been reported to be present in up to 10% of AIDS patients (30).

HIV-RENAL SYNDROMES

A spectrum of renal syndromes has been associated with HIV (Table 4). These include acute renal failure (ARF) and chronic renal failure. The etiology of acute renal syndromes can be classified as in uninfected patients, into pre-renal, intrinsic renal, and obstructive (intrarenal and extrarenal) causes (31,32). Pre-renal azotemia is due to circulatory volume depletion caused by loss of fluids from the gastrointestinal tract, hypotensive septic shock, inadequate fluid intake as a result of mental obtundation and finally, fluid may be sequestered in the third space as a result of hypoalbuminemia associated with malnutrition (33).

Inadequately managed, pre-renal causes of renal failure may progress to acute tubular necrosis (ATN), which is the most common cause of renal failure in HIV disease. The incidence of ARF in hospitalized patients ranges between 6% and 20%. The main causes are hypovolemia, sepsis, antimicrobials, radiocontrast material (34), but more recent reports note the increased incidence of HIV-associated thrombotic microangiopathies and rhabdomyolysis (34). The severity of ATN can vary from mild to severe and the prognosis varies accordingly. The management of ATN is the same as that for HIV-negative patients. The overall prognosis is not influenced by the patient's HIV status (35). In patients who survive ATN, renal function recovers even in gravely ill patients.

Table 4 Renal Syndromes in HIV-Infected Patients

Acute renal failure	Chronic renal failure
Prerenal azotaemia	HIVAN
Acute tubular necrosis	HIV-associated immune-complex nephritis
Interstitial nephritis	Mesangial proliferative GN
Glomerulonephritis	Diffuse proliferative GN
Vasculitis	IgA nephropathy
Cryoglobulinemia	Membranous nephropathy
Urinary tract obstruction	Other glomerular lesions
	HIV-associated thrombotic microangiopathies

HIV-infected patients are also susceptible to allergic interstitial nephritis, which can be caused by a host of medications, many of which are used widely. These include trimethoprim-sulfamethoxazole, cephalosporins, rifampicin, and epanutin. Protease inhibitors have also been associated with the development of ARF by various pathogenic mechanisms (31,36,37).

Extrarenal obstruction is a rare cause of renal failure and may be due to tumors or lymph nodes; intrarenal obstruction can result from the deposition of crystals, complicating the administration of certain drugs. Drugs commonly used in HIV/AIDS patients that may lead to crystalluria include sulphonamides, acyclovir, and protease inhibitors (35,38).

The choice of acute dialysis treatment depends on availability and patient tolerability rather than the HIV status of the patient. With the high mortality of ARF and the high cost of treatment (where available), every attempt should be made to prevent the disease by ensuring adequate hydration, avoiding nephrotoxins, and adjusting the dosages of medication appropriate for the degree of renal failure. Cognizance should also be taken of the fact that certain drugs such as aminoglycoside antibiotics accumulate in the kidney and recurrent exposure should be avoided.

Each of the three principal chronic renal syndromes in HIV-infected patients has a unique clinical pattern.

HIVAN

Frequency

The true incidence of HIVAN is unknown and will remain so until estimates, derived from large population-based cohorts that have been followed with sufficient attention to renal involvement, become available. Until then, the best estimates are derived from postmortem studies that suggest that up to 12% of American patients dying from HIV-1 infection have histologically proven HIVAN (39). The frequency of HIVAN in natives of other countries seems to vary: it is uncommon in Thailand (40), Italy (41), Brazil (42), but common in Indians (43). There are no data from Africa but indications are that FSGS is now becoming the most common cause of nephrotic syndrome in a study of renal biopsies performed between 1986 and 1989 in place of minimal change glomerulonephritis and amyloid, which had been the most common causes prior to the AIDS pandemic (44). It has been estimated that in South Africa with some 6.5 million people living with HIV infection and assuming a similar HIVAN rate as North America, 650,000 people may have renal disease (45). In sub-Saharan Africa, there should be an estimated 1 to 3.4 million prevalent cases. It is likely that the lack of published literature in Africa is related to multiple factors including lack of surveillance and reporting of renal disease. HIVAN is possibly a late manifestation of HIV infection (46); therefore, it is likely that many Africans with AIDS die of opportunistic infections before HIVAN becomes clinically evident.

Epidemiology

There are marked ethnic differences in the propensity to develop HIVAN. In most regions, HIVAN occurs predominantly in Black patients. In the United States, almost 90% of patients are African Americans (47); it has been calculated that the relative risk of HIVAN is 18-fold greater in African Americans (48). Among Black adults, HIVAN is now the third most common cause of ESRF in the United States (28). Susceptibility to the disease is supported by reports from Brazil and France, where the disease also occurs predominantly in Black patients (42,49). A recent report that included only HIVAN cases proven on biopsy confirms that over 95% of patients with HIVAN are blacks (50), suggesting that genetic and environmental cofactors may contribute to the pathogenesis of renal disease, although these cofactors remain to be elucidated (47). Also of concern is that the disease in Black patients appears to follow a more aggressive course (30). The initial descriptions of HIVAN were mainly in intravenous drug users (IVDU) (51), but the disease has subsequently been described with all forms of HIV acquisition (52). In sub-Saharan Africa, where IVDU and homosexuality are less common than in United States and Europe, most cases of HIVAN are in patients who have acquired the disease through heterosexual transmission (Bates, unpublished data).

Men account for some 80% of HIVAN (52,53), but the incidence of HIV infection is increasing so rapidly in women (54) that there are predictions that HIVAN may become more common in women (47,55). The mean age of patients with HIVAN is 33 years (35).

Clinical Presentation

The clinical course of HIVAN has changed little from its early description. Most of the patients present with progressive proteinuria and renal failure with normal to enlarged echogenic kidneys despite significant renal failure (51). The proteinuria may be modest but nephrotic range proteinuria develops in 90%. The renal failure advances rapidly and end-stage renal disease invariably develops, often within 4 to 6 months from the initial discovery of proteinuria (35). The median time to end-stage renal disease had increased to 16.6 months with the introduction of highly active antiretroviral treatment (HAART) (56). It is uncertain whether markers of early nephropathy may be present prior to the onset of clinically significant proteinuria or renal failure. Microalbuminuria has been identified in 20% of HIV-infected patients and is inversely correlated with the CD4 count; however, no prospective information is available regarding progression to clinically significant renal disease in these patients (57). The clinical picture is diagnostic of HIVAN in only 55–60% of cases, which is why a renal biopsy is important to confirm the diagnosis.

Certain clinical findings may be more suggestive of HIVAN than other common forms of nephropathy: hypertension and hematuria as well as peripheral edema and hypercholesterolemia are uncommon despite nephrotic range proteinuria (35,53,58–62). Whether such findings represent distinctive characteristics of the nephropathy or are simply indicative of the poor overall health and nutritional status of patients with advanced HIV disease is uncertain. Evidence suggests HIVAN is a late manifestation of HIV-1 infection: most patients either have signs defining AIDS or have CD4 counts less than 200 cells/μL (46,47). Alternatively, it may be that patients with lower CD4 counts manifest a more aggressive course of disease. Approximately, 50% of patients with HIVAN are asymptomatic with regard to their HIV-1 infection and suffer no opportunistic infections (46).

Pathology (Fig. 1) and Pathogenesis of HIVAN (Fig. 2)

Characteristically, the pathology of HIVAN involves all components of the nephron and the main features are illustrated in the series of images in Figure 1.

HIVAN is a direct result of infection of the kidney with HIV-1 and the resultant expression of viral gene products (63). The virus has been demonstrated in all cells of the nephron including the mesangial cells, tubules, glomerular endothelial, and epithelial cells as well as infiltrating leucocytes (61,64–67). The mechanism whereby the virus enters the renal cells is still unknown since CD4, the receptor for HIV and major co-receptors, CCR5 and CXR4, which are required for infection, do not appear to be expressed on intrinsic renal cells (68).

The virus is present in the kidney irrespective of whether there is clinical or histological evidence of renal disease (61). However, support for the role of HIV protein comes from observations in several animal models: FSGS has been observed in rhesus monkeys with simian AIDS; cats with feline immunodeficiency viral infection may develop a nephropathy closely resembling HIVAN. In a pivotal experiment, Bruggeman et al. (69) showed that HIVAN developed in kidneys transplanted from transgenic mice into normal mice but not in normal kidneys transplanted into transgenic littermates. This observation suggests that the development of renal disease is dependent upon HIV-1 expression within the kidney itself. Such findings fail to explain the predilection of HIVAN in Black patients. It is known that Blacks are at increased risk of developing a variety of other renal diseases such as lupus nephritis, heroin nephropathy and diabetic nephropathy implying that there is an underlying genetic pre-disposition to severe renal dysfunction in this group that is independent of disease (60,70). The observation that HIV is present in patients without FSGS suggests that some additional "trigger" is required such as genetic pre-disposition. That HIV is present in patients without FSGS can, alternatively, reflect the difference between

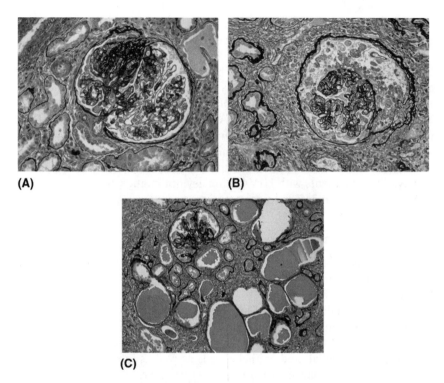

Figure 1 Pathology. The key histopathological features of HIVAN are the presence, firstly, of focal segmental sclerosis, glomerular collapse (collapsing glomerulopathy, although typical, is not diagnostic) and finally microcystic tubulointerstitial disease. There is often an infiltrate of chronic inflammatory cells in the interstitium. The combination of these features establishes the diagnosis of HIVAN. (**A**) This shows an established focal segmental sclerosing glomerular lesion with prominent mesangial sclerosis and tuft collapse. A capsular adhesion is evident at a 12 o'clock position (silver-methenamine stain; X400). (**B**) It depicts a prominent visceral epithelial cell reaction, with pseudo-crescent formation, overlying an evolving collapsing glomerulopathy. There is peri-glomerular fibrosis and inflammation (silver-methenamine stain; X400). (**C**) It shows cystically dilated tubular profiles surrounding collapsing glomerulopathy and an interstitial inflammatory cell component (silver-methenamine stain; X200). (*Courtesy Professor Stewart Goetsch, Department of Pathology, University of Witwatersrand, Johannesburg, South Africa.*)

latent infection and the actual expression of viral peptides. Observations of viral genome in kidney tissue of AIDS without evidence of renal disease raises the possibility that this material could be an "innocent" bystander with no casual relationship to the development of tissue damage (61).

The mechanisms by which HIV-1 infection leads to renal disease are not established. An attractive hypothesis is that HIV-1 infection of renal

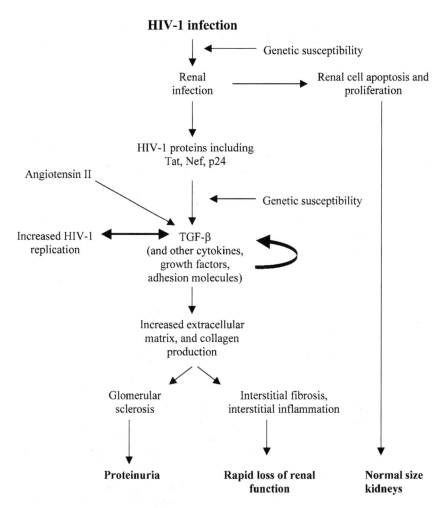

Figure 2 Pathogenesis of HIVAN. HIVAN results from a complex interplay of direct viral infection, modulation of HIV proteins as well as genetic factors. See text for details. Solid arrows indicate positive feedback.

cells leads to the synthesis of HIV-1 proteins in genetically susceptible individuals, which may induce FSGS by stimulating the release of cytokines, growth factors, chemokines, and adhesion molecules. The cellular response mediated by these substances, modulated by host genetic factors, leads to varying degrees of inflammation combined with sclerotic, fibrotic, and apoptotic responses that ultimately result in HIVAN (33). Transforming growth factor (TGF)-β in particular is a very important mediator of HIVAN by virtue of its capacity to cause matrix accumulation, fibrosis, and tubular injury (71,72). TGF-β production by macrophages may be stimulated by the viral protein Tat (73). TGF-β increases deposition of extracellular matrix in the kidney and is fibrogenic by stimulating collagen production. TGF-β has two other remarkable properties: firstly, it stimulates its own synthesis and secondly, it promotes HIV-1 viral replication by increasing expression of the HIV-1 LTR promoter (72,74). Renal infection with HIV-1 may initiate accelerated production of TGF-β and other cytokines. A vicious cycle is established whereby viral replication is rapidly increased within the kidney and extracellular matrix formation is driven by ever higher levels of TGF-β. Such a scheme would account for the widespread glomerular and interstitial sclerosis seen in kidneys with HIVAN and the rapid progression of renal failure (Fig. 1) (30,72). Angiotensin II increases synthesis of TGF-β and blockade of the renin-angiotensin system may be an important therapeutic option (75).

Treatment

In developing countries, a sense of therapeutic helplessness exists in regard to the management of HIVAN. In part, this is due to the rapid progression to end-stage renal disease limiting the time available for treatment regimens, and in part to the reluctance on the part of clinicians to expose already immunocompromised HIV-infected patients to therapeutic regimens involving further immunosuppression. The unavailability (due mainly to costs) of antiretroviral therapy and the late presentation of third-world patients are additional problems with which physicians have to contend. The medical management of HIV patients is of crucial importance in developing countries, where, unlike in developed countries, the option of renal replacement treatment does not exist for the majority of patients. As survival improves in the genetically susceptible populations of Africa and the Caribbean, the development of HIVAN will take its human toll and the medical management of this disease will assume increasing global importance (76).

Appropriate treatment of HIVAN can only be realized with an understanding of the pathophysiology of HIVAN; therefore, many of the treatment approaches are empiric. In principle, treatment of HIVAN should consist of reducing viral replication, retarding the progression of renal failure and preparing the patient for renal replacement treatment if appropriate (77). Inflammation plays an important role and therefore early reports [before the availability of HAART] of a benefit from corticosteroid therapy were not unexpected. However, the benefits were not sustained and associated with serious adverse effects (78). More recent studies in which steroids and HAART were used concomitantly suggested an improved outcome and fewer complications (76,77,79). The mechanism whereby steroids exert their effect on HIVAN is uncertain, but it has been postulated that they may act on interstitial immune cells (80,81). Angiotensin converting enzyme inhibitors (ACEI) were shown to be of benefit before the introduction of HAART treatment (82,83). ACEI improve long-term outcome in patients with HIVAN if initiated before the onset of severe renal failure (84). The beneficial effects of ACEI were confirmed in HIV-1 transgenic mice (85). The direct mechanism whereby ACEI are protective remains uncertain but possibilities include changes in renal hemodynamics, a reduction in the transglomerular passage of protein, and an antiproliferative effect mediated by inhibiting TGF-β or interference with ACE-mediated pathways involved in antigen processing and presentation between macrophages and T-lymphocytes. ACEI may reduce generation of tissue cytokines such as TGF-β and may influence interstitial cellular function (3,77,81,82). Experience with HAART in HIVAN is still empiric, based on anecdotal reports or uncontrolled studies (60,77). There are to date no randomized controlled studies proving that HAART therapy is beneficial. Nevertheless, some of the reports show dramatic responses to treatment with improvement not only in renal function but also in renal pathological abnormalities (65,86), although the kidney remains a reservoir of infection (65). Other evidence of the possible benefit of HAART comes from epidemiological data showing a decline in the incidence of HIVAN since 1996 coinciding with the introduction of HAART therapy in the United States and parallels similar improvements in the rate of opportunistic infections and HIV mortality (28).

In South Africa and possibly in many developing countries, renal replacement is currently not an option for patients with terminal uremia due to HIVAN. The reason for this is that transplantation cannot be offered to these patients because of the scarcity of organs, which it is felt should be reserved for uninfected patients.

However, with the increasing access to HAART and improvement in the life expectancy of HIV-infected patients, this issue may need to be revisited. The outcome of patients treated with dialysis was initially quite dismal (32,87) but has improved with the introduction of HAART in the mid-1990s; improvements in dialysis techniques, anemia management, and other factors could have contributed as well (Fig. 3) (33,88–91). There are data suggesting that hemodialysis may have detrimental effects on patient survival by inducing the release of various cytokines which promote viral replication (92–95). However, the majority of patients on hemodialysis had undetectable viral loads (96). The jury is therefore still out on the impact of dialysis on patient survival. Survival rates are similar between patients on hemodialysis and peritoneal dialysis (91). The mode of dialysis should be determined by patient preference and availability of resources. It is unclear whether HIV-infected patients have higher overall rates of peritonitis, although peritonitis due to fungi and *Pseudomonas* are more common (97). An additional consideration is that the spent dialysis fluid may contain viable HIV and the dialysate must be disposed of with caution. The costs of

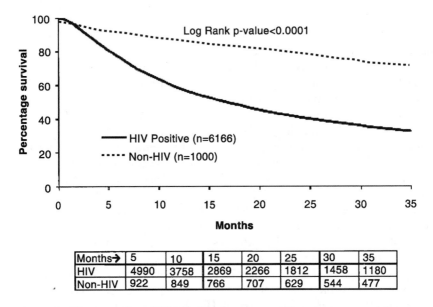

Figure 3 The mortality of HIV-infected patients with end-stage renal failure on dialysis is considerably higher than those who are HIV-negative (88).

treating HIV patients have not been assessed, but with the increased risk of complications in these patients it is likely costs are substantially higher than that required to treat the average patient on hemodialysis, an important consideration in treating patients in developing countries.

In most centers outside the United States, renal transplantation is usually not recommended for HIV-infected patients with end-stage renal disease. In part, this is because of the perception that immunosuppressive therapy may enhance progression of the viral illness (although there are some tantalizing reports in abstract form to the contrary), and that the life-span of the recipients is limited (33). However, studies to evaluate renal transplantation in these patients are underway. Patients with end-stage renal disease who would be considered eligible for transplantation would have to have undetectable viral load, be on stable HAART treatment, with no evidence of neoplasms or opportunistic infections, CD4 counts >200/mL, and a suitable living donor (98).

HIV-ASSOCIATED IMMUNE-COMPLEX NEPHRITIS

The HIV-associated immune-complex nephritides (ICN) are much less common than HIVAN and occur predominantly in non-Black patients. In regions where the predominant population is Caucasian, ICN may account for up to one-third of cases in renal biopsy series in HIV patients

(33,49,99,100). Biopsy series confirm that Caucasian and Asian patients typically develop ICN while patients of African origin from the same center have HIVAN (41,49,101–103). A recent biopsy report from Thailand confirmed that Asian patients had ICN and failed to develop HIVAN (40). These racial differences in the manifestation of HIV renal disease strongly support a genetic basis (63). The HIV-associated renal diseases in this category include IgA nephropathy, lupus-like syndrome, and mixed sclerotic/proliferative forms (49). Secondly, co-infection with hepatitis B and/or C is common in the setting of mesangiocapillary glomerulonephritis, membranous glomerulonephritis, and postinfectious glomerulonephritis, calling into question the pathogenic role of HIV (33); these patterns may be the consequence of response to infection in patients with dysfunctional humoral immunity (63,104). Finally, the renal disease may be a coincidental finding, especially in a developing country setting where primary nephritides are still rife (105). The clinical presentation of ICN is not as dramatic as that of HIVAN. Patients with IgA nephropathy, for example, have an indolent course characterized by hematuria, proteinuria, and mild renal failure that seldom progresses to ESRF (33,63). No controlled studies have been performed to assess the benefit of different treatment strategies but anecdotal reports have documented the benefit of HAART, ACEI, and steroids on ICN (29,106,107).

HIV-ASSOCIATED THROMBOTIC MICROANGIOGRAPHIES (TM)

Recent reports have highlighted an increase in the incidence of HIV-TM (108,109). Reports of this disease are confined to developed countries. The extent of the problem in developing countries remains to be elucidated. The disease is likely the result of endothelial dysfunction mediated by HIV proteins (3,110–113). Clinically, HIV-TM is characterized by the pentad of fever, neurological deficits, thrombocytopenia, microangiopathic hemolytic anemia and renal failure. Hematuria is present but nephrotic range proteinuria usually suggests coexistent HIVAN or ICN (3,80,114,115). Treatment is primarily with plasmapharesis/plasma exchange and plasma infusions, with specific therapy of the underlying HIV infection. In addition, treatment with corticosteroids, antiplatelet agents, immunoglobulin infusions, vincristine, and splenectomy (for refractory cases) has enjoyed varying degrees of success. The prognosis is poor with one-third dying in the acute phase of the disease despite aggressive therapy (113,114,116,117).

RECOMMENDED MANAGEMENT

Nephrologists should be working very closely with infectious diseases specialists to screen HIV-positive patients for renal disease. It would seem appropriate to screen patients for proteinuria by urinalysis performed at the initial visit. Thereafter, high-risk patients such as Black patients should have annual follow-up visits. If proteinuria is present, further evaluation should consist of quantification of the proteinuria by 24 hour urine collection or the urinary protein to creatinine ratio. In addition, patients should be screened for the presence of secondary renal diseases associated with HBV, hepatitis C virus, and syphilis. As a significant number of patients who have proteinuria have disease other than HIVAN, it is advisable to perform a renal biopsy to guide therapy. Indications include those used in other renal diseases, including nephrotic-range proteinuria and progressive loss of renal function (118,119). On the basis of observational evidence, the use of HAART and ACEI appears to benefit the patient with HIV-related disease by slowing the progression of decline in renal function and decreasing the level of proteinuria. Because the use of prednisone is associated with an increased risk of infectious complications consideration regarding its use should be given only after these other measures fail to stabilize renal function (118). The lowest level of proteinuria that warrants biopsy, we would suggest, should be 1 g/day. Current evidence supports the use of ACEI, but randomized studies are needed to confirm the benefit of this treatment. Collaborative studies will be necessary to include sufficient numbers of patients (77).

HEPATITIS C VIRUS

The hepatitis C virus (HCV) is a single-stranded RNA virus of the *Flaviridae* family. HCV infection is both a cause of glomerular disease and a complication of renal replacement therapy. The World Health Organization estimates that 170 million people (approximately 3% of the world's population) are infected with HCV (120). The prevalence of HCV in the economically developed world is less than 1–2% (121). The sharp decline in incidence of acute HCV infection in the 1990s is attributed to screening of blood products and safer needle practices among intravenous drug users (122,123). The highest prevalence of HCV is found in developing countries with estimated prevalence rates in sub-Saharan Africa of 3%, west Africa 2.4%, and central Africa 6% (121). An exceptionally high 20–30% prevalence of HCV in Egypt has been attributed to the parenteral treatment of schistosomiasis in the 1960s and 1970s (121,124).

EPIDEMIOLOGY

Transmission of HCV is mainly through contact with blood or blood products. Intravenous drug use has become the most common risk factor in developing countries. Iatrogenic exposure, sexual spread, and mother-to-child transmission are rare (121,123,125,126). The high prevalence in many African countries may be explained by the lack of routine screening of donated blood and high-risk activities (121). The prevalence of HCV in dialysis units varies considerably between countries and even between units within the same country, ranging between 1% and 63% (127). Seroprevalence in hemodialysis patients is 21% in South Africa, 25% in Western India, and 5% in Kenya (128–130). Patients are at risk of acquiring infection from reuse of unsterilized dialysis equipment and failure of standard infection control principles (122,125).

Although acute infection with HCV is asymptomatic in the majority of patients, the main problem associated with HCV is that chronic infection develops in 80% of those infected; once established, spontaneous clearance of HCV is rare (131). Infected patients develop chronic hepatitis with varying degrees of inflammation and fibrosis. HCV elicits an immune response that is sufficient to cause hepatic injury, but insufficient to eradicate the virus. Cirrhosis develops 30 years after the primary infection in 15–20% of patients and the annual incidence of hepatocellular carcinoma is 1–4% in patients with established cirrhosis (120,131). The numerous extrahepatic manifestations of HCV infection, of which glomerular disease is an important one, are mostly associated with autoimmune or lymphoproliferative states (131,132).

PATHOGENESIS

The pathogenesis of HCV-induced renal disease remains ill-defined. Glomerular injury is likely caused by deposition of circulating immune complexes containing HCV antigens, anti-HCV antibodies (IgG or IgM), complement (mainly C3), and rheumatoid factors (133,134). It is not clear whether autoantibodies to glomerular antigens contribute to glomerular disease (133,134). There are six HCV genotypes and the natural history of HCV infection is similar for all genotypes. An individual is infected with only one genotype; ongoing mutations are responsible for a heterogeneous population (quasispecies) of virus with different nucleotide sequences that change with time (123,135). Quasispecies permit HCV to escape immune surveillance and thereby establish chronic infection (135).

Circulating cryoglobulins, which appear to play an important role in the pathogenesis of HCV renal disease, are detected in over 50% of HCV-infected individuals, and are thought to be a consequence of chronic B cell exposure to HCV (127). Mixed cryoglobulinemia (MC), previously called "essential" mixed cryoglobulinemia, is associated with HCV in more than 90% of cases, but is only symptomatic in 2–3% of cases (126,136–138). It is likely that other unknown genetic and environmental co-factors are also required for the development of autoimmunity (136). Mixed cryoglobulins are composed of polyclonal IgG bound to immunoglobulins with anti-IgG rheumatoid factor activity. In type II MC, the antiglobulin component is a monoclonal (usually IgM) rheumatoid factor, and in type III MC it is polyclonal (139). Cryoglobulinemic glomerulonephritis occurs mostly in type II MC with monoclonal IgMκ rheumatoid factor. The monoclonal IgMκ is produced by an HCV-infected B-cell clone. It is unknown if circulating IgMκ–IgG complexes are deposited in the kidney, or if IgMκ is deposited alone with subsequent in situ binding of IgG (139).

GLOMERULAR DISEASE

The most common glomerular diseases associated with HCV are type I mesangiocapillary glomerulonephritis (MCGN), with or without cryoglobulinemia, and less frequently membranous nephropathy (MN) (134,139–146). Although diffuse proliferative glomerulonephritis, focal segmental glomerulosclerosis, fibrillary glomerulonephritis, and immunotactoid glomerulopathy have been described, the association with HCV remains uncertain (133,147–151). The prevalence of HCV in patients with type I MCGN varies widely. HCV infection was reported in up to 60% of MCGN cases in Japan, in 10% of patients in the United States and Brazil, but none in a recent South African series (140,152–154).

HCV-related MCGN typically occurs in adults with chronic HCV infection and mild sub-clinical liver disease (127). Patients have microscopic hematuria and proteinuria, mild-to-moderate renal impairment (50%), nephrotic syndrome (25%), or acute nephritis (20%) (133). Hypertension is present in 80% (147). The systemic signs of mixed cryoglobulinemia suggests an immune complex-type vasculitis with purpura, arthralgia, weakness, and peripheral neuropathy, which may precede cryoglobulinemic MCGN by several years. The associated HCV infection is diagnosed by highly sensitive and specific enzyme immunoassays that detect antibodies to multiple HCV antigens. Other laboratory findings include the presence of very low serum C4 levels, moderately reduced or normal serum C3, and elevated serum rheumatoid factor (136). Cryoglobulins are detected in 50–70% of patients (127). Serum transaminases are elevated more frequently (two-thirds of cases) in MCGN than other HCV-related glomerulopathies (147). Membranous nephropathy associated with HCV presents with nephrotic syndrome in 80% of cases, and in the remainder with isolated non-nephrotic range proteinuria. Renal function and serum complement levels are normal or only mildly impaired. Circulating cryoglobulins and rheumatoid factor are absent (145).

Pathology

Light microscopy of MCGN shows lobular accentuation of glomerular tufts, increased mesangial matrix and cellularity, and reduplication of capillary basement membranes. In cryoglobulinemic MCGN, there is greater glomerular hypercellularity due to heavy leukocyte infiltration. Prominent intracapillary eosinophilic deposits representing precipitated immune complexes or cryoglobulins may also be present. Sub-endothelial deposits are seen by electron microscopy; mesangial and glomerular capillary wall deposits containing IgM, IgG, and C3 by immunofluorescence. Sub-endothelial deposits may have an organized fibrillar or cylindrical structure in cryoglobulinemic MCGN. One-third of patients with cryoglobulinemic MCGN may also have necrotizing vasculitis of small- and medium-sized renal arteries (127,133,139,147). The MN is similar to the idiopathic form: there is thickening of the capillary wall, sub-epithelial electron-dense deposits, and IgG and C3 diffuse granular deposits along the basement membrane (144).

Treatment

The optimal treatment of HCV-related renal disease has not been established. Not only is the course of the disease unknown but also current therapeutic strategies are based on experience in small numbers of patients. Treatment may be directed at eradication of the virus or at suppression of the immune response. In three controlled trials, interferon alpha was associated with clinical improvement and reduced levels of HCV RNA, serum cryoglobulins, rheumatoid factor, and creatinine (155–157). The usefulness of interferon alpha is limited by the low response rate, the high rate of relapse on withdrawal of treatment, and frequency of side effects (136). Higher doses of interferon alpha or the addition of ribavirin may improve virological response rates, but most patients still relapse when therapy is discontinued (127,134,158–161). Combination therapy of pegylated interferon and ribavirin produce the best sustained virological response rates (55%) in the treatment of HCV liver disease (162,163). Identifying the genotype or serotype (genotype-specific antibodies) helps predict sustained response—genotypes 2 and 3 respond much better to pegylated interferon and ribavirin than genotypes 1, 4, 5, and 6 (126). The efficacy of this regimen has not yet been established for HCV-related cryoglobulinemia or HCV-related renal disease. Interferon alpha alone or in combination with ribavirin leads to variable improvement in proteinuria and renal function, particularly in patients with sustained virological response (164–174). Interferon alpha may reduce proteinuria in patients with MN, but this effect is not consistently present (146,169,175). Prospective studies are required to confirm the indications as well as the efficacy and safety of antiviral therapy in patients with HCV-induced renal disease (134).

In acute flares of glomerulonephritis, interferon alpha does not prevent progression of renal damage (176). Immunosuppressive therapy using corticosteroids and cyclophosphamide with or without plasmapheresis may control symptoms and limit renal damage in patients with severe cryoglobulinemic systemic vasculitis, or rapidly progressive glomerulonephritis (134). Relapses are common and therefore viral eradication should also be attempted (176).

RENAL TRANSPLANTATION

HCV infection in transplant recipients may be present before transplantation, or may be transmitted by organs from infected donors. The presence of HCV infection does not adversely affect patient or graft survival during the first 5 years post-transplantation (177). Beyond 10 years, however, patient and graft survival is significantly reduced in HCV-positive patients. Chronic liver disease develops in 50% of recipients from HCV-positive donors (178). Cirrhosis, hepatocellular carcinoma, and sepsis are the major causes of increased patient morbidity and mortality in the second decade after transplantation (179). Graft survival is influenced by the risk of recurrence HCV-related glomerular disease and possibly by a greater likelihood of chronic allograft nephropathy (127,177). MCGN as well as MN may recur after transplantation (180). There is no safe and effective treatment of HCV-induced liver or renal disease in transplant patients. Of note is that interferon alpha enhances the risk of acute rejection (181).

Routine screening of organ donors for antibodies to HCV is performed by most organ procurement organizations to prevent viral transmission. Current opinion holds that organs from HCV-positive donors be restricted to life-saving heart, liver or lung transplants (182). The use of kidneys from HCV-positive donors in HCV RNA-positive recipients does not increase the post-transplantation prevalence of liver disease and does not adversely affect patient or graft survival when compared to organs from HCV-negative donors (183–185). Superinfection with a new genotype is possible, but did not influence short-term outcome (186).

HEPATITIS C IN DIALYSIS PATIENTS

The effect of dialysis on the natural history of chronic liver disease in HCV-positive patients has not been established (187). An increased mortality is observed in HCV-positive hemodialysis patients and has been linked to the development of liver cirrhosis and hepatocellular carcinoma (188,189). Despite its long-term complications, renal transplantation remains the best form of replacement therapy in HCV-positive patients with end-stage renal disease. Patient survival is superior in transplanted patients compared to those who remain on maintenance dialysis (179,190). The ideal pre-transplant management of HCV-positive candidates has not been established, but logic dictates that achieving viral clearance may benefit post-transplant outcome. Interferon alpha monotherapy achieves a sustained virological response in 40% of treated end-stage renal disease patients and this response usually persists after transplantation (127). Adverse events are more frequent in renal failure, necessitating early discontinuation in a quarter of patients. The efficacy of peginterferon is unsubstantiated (127). Ribavirin accumulates in renal failure and causes life-threatening dose-related hemolysis. The addition of low-dose ribavirin to interferon regimens is currently under investigation (127).

Liver biopsy is the most reliable method of determining the degree of liver damage and is indicated in renal transplant candidates, who do not have any evidence of cirrhosis or portal hypertension (187,191). Decompensated cirrhosis precludes isolated kidney transplantation, but combined liver and kidney transplantation may be considered. Patients with chronic hepatitis without cirrhosis should be offered 12 months interferon monotherapy. Those with compensated cirrhosis should also receive antiviral treatment, but proceed to transplantation only if a sustained virological response is achieved (191). Lack of access to costly antiviral drugs in developing countries represents a barrier to transplantation of HCV-positive patients. In this situation, it might be reasonable to proceed with transplantation in patients with HCV-induced chronic hepatitis, but to exclude all patients with cirrhosis.

Finally, the prevention of HCV spread in hemodialysis units is essential. The Centers for Disease Control and Prevention (CDC) recommend six monthly HCV serological testing and dialysis unit-specific precautions to control the spread of HCV. The isolation of HCV patients, the use of dedicated machines, and the exclusion of dialyzer reuse are not currently recommended by the CDC (122,192).

HEPATITIS B VIRUS INFECTION

Infection with the hepatitis B virus (HBV) continues to be a major problem and cause of renal disease in developing countries. HBV infection is endemic in sub-Saharan Africa, Eastern Europe, and Asia but uncommon in North America and Western Europe. The carrier state constitutes the reservoir of infection and varies from 0.1% to over 15% in different regions of the world. The probability of becoming a chronic carrier is greater following infection during infancy and early childhood. About 25–40% of carriers will die from complications of the infection such as cirrhosis and hepatocellular carcinoma (193).

The three principal HBV antigens have all been implicated in the development of glomerulonephritis. Hepatitis B surface antigen (HBsAg) from the outer surface of the intact virus is present in all active infections, but the core antigen (HBcAg) and particularly the e-antigen (HBeAg), associated with the viral nucleocapsid, may be more important in the pathogenesis of membranous glomerulonephritis (MGN), the most frequent associated glomerulonephritis (194). In contrast to the rising incidence of human immunodeficiency virus associated renal diseases, HBV-MGN is occurring less frequently. Urbanization, associated with lower HBV carrier rates, and HBV vaccination have contributed to this decrease (195,196).

HBV-ASSOCIATED MEMBRANOUS GN (HBV-MGN)

Although HBV-MGN was first documented in 1971 in a 53-year-old man (197), over the last three decades the association of the HBV carrier state with membranous glomerulonephritis has been established more prominently in children than adults. In areas with low HBV prevalence (0.1–1.0%), such as the United States and Western Europe, HBV-associated MGN forms a lower proportion of childhood MGN cases (20–60%), whereas in countries with high HBV carrier rates the proportion rises to 57–100% (194). In a study from our center of 281 childhood nephrotics seen from 1973 to 1993, the HBV-MGN group formed 93% of MGN patients (66/71) and 23% (66/281) of all nephrotics (198,199).

The frequency of HBsAg carrier state in adults with MGN is significant but less than in children and ranges from 0% to 4% in low HBV prevalence areas like the U.K. to 43% in Hong Kong with a carrier rate of 5–10% (194,200,201). The lower proportion in adults is due both to fewer HBV-MGN cases in adults and the diluting effect of larger numbers of idiopathic MGN. In our experience, HBV-positive patients accounted for 9.5% of 126 cases of membranous nephropathy seen over 16 years at our center in Cape Town, South Africa. The carrier rate in our population is between 5% and 10%.

Clinical Presentation

In children, the virus appears to be acquired by vertical transmission from infected mothers but, possibly more frequently, by horizontal transmission from infected siblings and other young children (194,202). HBV-MGN has a more marked male predominance than does idiopathic MGN with 80–100% affected children being boys. Children with HBV-MGN usually present between the ages of 2 and 12 years (mean of 6 years) with nephrotic syndrome, or proteinuria and microscopic hematuria. Renal failure is uncommon but hypertension is present in up to 25% of cases (194). Children with HBV-MGN generally have no history or clinical evidence of chronic liver disease although most have mildly raised liver enzymes (203,204). Adults with HBV-MGN are more likely to have a history of acute hepatitis, 6 months to several years prior to the onset of the renal disease (194,197). The liver pathology in children with HBV-MGN is usually mild, showing chronic persistent hepatitis or minimal abnormalities (194,205). By contrast, the typical liver pathology in adults is chronic active hepatitis, although a range has been described (194,206,207).

Immunopathology and Pathogenesis

HBeAg occurs in the serum of 65–80% patients with HBV-MGN with the remainder having antibodies (202–204,208–211). Unusually, patients may be positive for both HBeAg and anti-HBe or both HBs and anti-HBs (212). Serum C3 and C4 levels may be reduced in between 15% and 60% of cases (203,208). Immunofluorescent staining in the glomeruli is usually positive for IgG and C3 with lower levels for IgM and IgA (194,203). In addition to the characteristic sub-epithelial deposits of idiopathic MGN, there are often deposits in mesangial and sub-endothelial areas, and mesangial interposition (a characteristic feature of the mesangiocapillary pattern) in HBV-MGN (208,213). Virus-like particles and tubuloreticular inclusions are typically present (205,214). Although HBsAg was identified in the first case of HBV-MGN, it subsequently became apparent that HBe was more important in the development of HBV-MGN. Circulating HBeAg frequently correlates with the activity of the disease, its elimination being linked to remission of disease; it is also the main antigen in the immune deposits and biopsies negative for HBeAg occur late in the disease (194,204,208,215). Local formation of antigen–antibody complexes, as opposed to circulating immune complexes, appears to be the more likely mechanism of sub-epithelial deposits, characteristic of HBV-MGN (194).

Course in Children

HBV-MGN often resolves spontaneously between 6 months and 2 years in children (216). This resolution usually coincides with disappearance of HBV antigens and appearance of the corresponding antibodies, particularly to HBeAg, but occasionally HBsAg. Clinical resolution may be associated with partial or total resolution of deposits (217,218). Other factors such as age, duration of renal disease, and quantity of immune complex deposition may influence remission (219). A summation of a number of large published series produced remission rates of 65% at 1 year, 85% at 2 years, and 95% at 5 to 7 years (203,215–217,219–221). These included series from Taiwan, Japan, France, Zimbabwe, United States, and Poland.

Remission rates from South Africa with extended follow-up confirm a very high cumulative remission rate of 85%, with 90% being asymptomatic, at 9 years, similar to the 92% remission rate at 9 years observed by Hsu (210,219). Chronic renal failure is uncommon. In more than 300 children from Southern Africa with HBV-associated MGN, only 11 (3.6%) have developed chronic renal failure (199,211,220,222–225).

Course in Adults

The natural course of adult HBV-MGN is less well documented. A landmark series from Hong Kong in 1991 evaluated the clinical features and outcome over a mean of 60 months in a group of 21 patients. The adults had acquired chronic HBV infection in childhood. HBeAg was present in the serum of 17 patients (81%). In contrast to the experience in children, spontaneous remission in adults in this study was uncommon with 29%

developing progressive renal failure and 10% requiring dialysis (226). The experience at our center has been similar, with none of 12 HBV-MGN adult patients (13 years of age and over) seen between 1985 and 2002 remitting. Of the eight followed for 2 years, one had died, two were in renal failure, and the remaining five remained proteinuric.

Treatment

The high spontaneous remission rate in children suggests that conservative support is sufficient and that steroids or cytotoxic therapy will add minimal benefit (194,217,220,221). Indeed, a prospective trial found that predniso-lone had deleterious effects, inducing viral replication in the liver (227). Various studies of small numbers of HBV-MGN patients treated with alpha interferon showed encouraging results, usually with clearance of HBeAg and partial or complete clinical remission (228–230). A study of 24 Black South African children with biopsy-proven HBV-MGN found that, compared to 20 controls, those treated with interferon alpha 2b for 16 weeks had accelerated clearance of HBeAg with remission of proteinuria. The interferon was also well tolerated (231). In adults, spontaneous resolution of HBV-MGN is rare, while complications related to the nephrotic syndrome are common. This situation makes it worthwhile considering active treatment although reported results indicate variable benefit (226,230).

HBV ASSOCIATED WITH OTHER FORMS OF GN

Mesangiocapillary GN has also been reported in carriers of HBsAg, although not as frequently as MGN (194,216,232). Several studies have noted that both adults and children with mesangiocapillary GN have a markedly higher carrier rate of HBsAg than the general population (202,232,233). The usual pattern of HBV-MGN often has mesangiocapillary elements (sub-endothelial deposits and mesangial interposition) and these could cause diagnostic difficulty and overlap. Patients present with nephritic syndrome and microhematuria (194). In one series, hypertension was reported in 45% and renal insufficiency in 20% (232). In our series of 36 HBV adult patients, five showed mesangiocapillary GN (14%), compared to 33% with MGN. Mesangial proliferative GN, with increased mesangial cell hypercellularity and deposition of IgG and/or IgM, has also been documented (194,204). Other forms of glomeruloneophritis, including IgA and systemic lupus erythematosis have been reported to be more frequent in HBV carriers, but these associations remain controversial (234–236).

HBV-ASSOCIATED POLYARTERITIS NODOSA (HBV-PAN)

The association of PAN and hepatitis was recognized by 1947 and following the description of HBV in 1964 PAN was more firmly linked to HBV. The frequency of HBsAg is between 0% and 54% of cases of PAN (194). HBV-PAN has been documented more commonly in Europe and the United States where adult carrier rates are higher than in children and HBV is often acquired parenterally. By contrast, in Asia and Africa where overall carrier rates are higher especially in children, HBV-PAN is less common (194). This assessment fits with our experience in South Africa where HBV-associated glomerular disease is relatively frequent especially in children, but PAN associated with HBV is rare.

REFERENCES

1. di Belgiojoso GB, Ferrario F, Landriani N. Virus-related glomerular diseases: histological and clinical aspects. J Nephrol 2002; 15(5):469–479.
2. Glassock RJ. Immune complex-induced glomerular injury in viral diseases: an overview. Kidney Int Suppl 1991; 35:S5–S7.
3. Kimmel PL. The nephropathies of HIV infection: pathogenesis and treatment. Curr Opin Nephrol Hypertens 2000; 9(2):117–122.
4. Couser WG. Mechanisms of glomerular injury in immune-complex disease. Kidney Int 1985; 28(3):569–583.
5. Golbus SM, Wilson CB. Experimental glomerulonephritis induced by in situ formation of immune complexes in glomerular capillary wall. Kidney Int 1979; 16(2):148–157.
6. Conaldi PG, Biancone L, Bottelli A, Wade-Evans A, Racusen LC, Boccellino M, et al. HIV-1 kills renal tubular epithelial cells in vitro by triggering an apoptotic pathway involving caspase activation and Fas upregulation. J Clin Invest 1998; 102(12):2041–2049.
7. Segerer S, Nelson PJ, Schlondorff D. Chemokines, chemokine receptors, and renal disease: from basic science to pathophysiologic and therapeutic studies. J Am Soc Nephrol 2000; 11(1):152–176.
8. Johnson WE, Desrosiers RC. Viral persistance: HIV's strategies of immune system evasion. Annu Rev Med 2002; 53:499–518.
9. Malbrain ML, De MX, Wilmer AP, Frans E, Peeters J, Nevens F. Another case of acute renal failure (ARF) due to acute tubular necrosis (ATN), proven by renal biopsy in non-fulminant hepatitis A virus (HAV) infection. Nephrol Dial Transplant 1997; 12(7):1543–1544.
10. Vaboe AL, Leh S, Forslund T. Interstitial nephritis, acute renal failure in a patient with non-fulminant hepatitis A infection. Clin Nephrol 2002; 57(2): 149–153.
11. Garel D, Vasmant D, Mougenot B, Bensman A. Glomerular nephropathy with mesangial proliferation and acute hepatitis A virus infection. 2 cases. Ann Pediatr (Paris) 1986; 33(3):185–188.

12. Moudgil A, Nast CC, Bagga A, Wei L, Nurmamet A, Cohen AH, et al. Association of parvovirus B19 infection with idiopathic collapsing glomerulopathy. Kidney Int 2001; 59(6):2126–2133.

13. Tanawattanacharoen S, Falk RJ, Jennette JC, Kopp JB. Parvovirus B19 DNA in kidney tissue of patients with focal segmental glomerulosclerosis. Am J Kidney Dis 2000; 35(6):1166–1174.

14. Komatsuda A, Ohtani H, Nimura T, Yamaguchi A, Wakui H, Imai H, et al. Endocapillary proliferative glomerulonephritis in a patient with parvovirus B19 infection. Am J Kidney Dis 2000; 36(4):851–854.

15. Nakazawa T, Tomosugi N, Sakamoto K, Asaka M, Yuri T, Ishikawa I, et al. Acute glomerulonephritis after human parvovirus B19 infection. Am J Kidney Dis 2000; 35(6):E31.

16. Park JS, Song JH, Yang WS, Kim SB, Kim YK, Hong CD. Cytomegalovirus is not specifically associated with immunoglobulin A nephropathy. J Am Soc Nephrol 1994; 4(8):1623–1626.

17. Kanahara K, Taniguchi Y, Yorioka N, Yamakido M. In situ hybridization analysis of cytomegalovirus and adenovirus DNA in immunoglobulin A nephropathy. Nephron 1992; 62(2):166–168.

18. Kashyap R, Shapiro R, Jordan M, Randhawa PS. The clinical significance of cytomegaloviral inclusions in the allograft kidney. Transplantation 1999; 67(1):98–103.

19. Boyce NW, Hayes K, Gee D, Holdsworth SR, Thomson NM, Scott D, et al. Cytomegalovirus infection complicating renal transplantation and its relationship to acute transplant glomerulopathy. Transplantation 1988; 45(4):706–709.

20. Yoshida K, Suzuki J, Suzuki S, Kume K, Mutoh S, Kato K, et al. Experimental IgA nephropathy induced by coxsackie B4 virus in mice. Am J Nephrol 1997; 17(1):81–88.

21. Conaldi PG, Biancone L, Bottelli A, De Martino A, Camussi G, Toniolo A. Distinct pathogenic effects of group B coxsackieviruses on human glomerular and tubular kidney cells. J Virol 1997; 71(12):9180–9187.

22. Nickeleit V, Hirsch HH, Zeiler M, Gudat F, Prince O, Thiel G, et al. BK-virus nephropathy in renal transplants-tubular necrosis, MHC-class II expression and rejection in a puzzling game. Nephrol Dial Transplant 2000; 15(3):324–332.

23. Nebuloni M, Tosoni A, Boldorini R, Monga G, Carsana L, Bonetto S, et al. BK virus renal infection in a patient with the acquired immunodeficiency syndrome. Arch Pathol Lab Med 1999; 123(9):807–811.

24. Cosgriff TM, Lewis RM. Mechanisms of disease in hemorrhagic fever with renal syndrome. Kidney Int Suppl 1991; 35:S72–S79.

25. Grcevska L, Polenakovic M, Oncevski A, Zografski D, Gligic A. Different pathohistological presentations of acute renal involvement in Hantaan virus infection: report of two cases. Clin Nephrol 1990; 34(5):197–201.

26. Anonymous. AIDS epidemic update: December 2003. 1–39. 2004. UNAIDS/WHO.

27. Steinbrook R. Beyond Barcelona—the global response to HIV. N Engl J Med 2002; 347(8):553–554.

28. United States Renal Data System. 2003 Annual Data Report/Atlas. http://www.usrds.org/adr.htm. 2004. Bethesda, MD, National Institutes of Health, National Institutes of Diabetes and Digestive Diseases. 2–17–0040.

29. Schwartz EJ, Szczech LA, Winston JA, Klotman PE. Effect of HAART on HIV-associated nephropathy [abstr]. J Am Soc Nephrol 2000; 11:165A.

30. Humphreys MH. Human immunodeficiency virus-associated glomerulosclerosis. Kidney Int 1995; 48(2):311–320.

31. Rao TK. Acute renal failure syndromes in human immunodeficiency virus infection. Semin Nephrol 1998; 18(4):378–395.

32. Rao TK, Friedman EA, Nicastri AD. The types of renal disease in the acquired immunodeficiency syndrome. N Engl J Med 1987; 316(17):1062–1068.

33. Weiner NJ, Goodman JW, Kimmel PL. The HIV-associated renal diseases: current insight into pathogenesis and treatment. Kidney Int 2003; 63(5): 1618–1631.

34. Joshi MK, Liu HH. Acute rhabdomyolysis and renal failure in HIV-infected patients: risk factors, presentation, and pathophysiology. AIDS Patient Care STDS 2000; 14(10):541–548.

35. Rao TK. Human immunodeficiency virus (HIV) associated nephropathy. Annu Rev Med 1991; 42:391–401.

36. Benveniste O, Longuet P, Duval X, Le MV, Leport C, Vilde JL. Two episodes of acute renal failure, rhabdomyolysis, and severe hepatitis in an AIDS patient successively treated with ritonavir and indinavir. Clin Infect Dis 1999; 28(5):1180–1181.

37. Kopp JB, Falloon J, Filie A, Abati A, King C, Hortin GL, et al. Indinavir-associated interstitial nephritis and urothelial inflammation: clinical and cytologic findings. Clin Infect Dis 2002; 34(8):1122–1128.

38. Rao TK. Renal complications in HIV disease. Med Clin North Am 1996; 80(6):1437–1451.

39. Shahinian V, Rajaraman S, Borucki M, Grady J, Hollander WM, Ahuja TS. Prevalence of HIV-associated nephropathy in autopsies of HIV-infected patients. Am J Kidney Dis 2000; 35(5):884–888.

40. Praditpornsilpa K, Napathorn S, Yenrudi S, Wankrairot P, Tungsaga K, Sitprija V. Renal pathology and HIV infection in Thailand. Am J Kidney Dis 1999; 33(2):282–286.

41. Casanova S, Mazzucco G, Barbiano DB, Motta M, Boldorini R, Genderini A, et al. Pattern of glomerular involvement in human immunodeficiency virus-infected patients: an Italian study. Am J Kidney Dis 1995; 26(3):446–453.

42. Lopes GS, Marques LP, Rioja LS, Basilio-de-Oliveira CA, Oliveira AV, Nery AC, et al. Glomerular disease and human immunodeficiency virus infection in Brazil. Am J Nephrol 1992; 12(5):281–287.

43. Madiwale C, Venkataseshan VS. Renal lesions in AIDS: a biopsy and autopsy study. Indian J Pathol Microbiol 1999; 42(1):45–54.

44. Pakasa M, Mangani N, Dikassa L. Focal and segmental glomerulosclerosis in nephrotic syndrome: a new profile of adult nephrotic syndrome in Zaire. Mod Pathol 1993; 6(2):125–128.

45. Bihl G. HIV-related renal diseases: a clinical and practical approach in the South African context. The Specialist Forum, Cape Town, South Africa 2002, September 38–41.
46. Winston JA, Klotman ME, Klotman PE. HIV-associated nephropathy is a late, not early, manifestation of HIV-1 infection. Kidney Int 1999; 55(3):1036–1040.
47. Winston JA, Burns GC, Klotman PE. The human immunodeficiency virus (HIV) epidemic and HIV-associated nephropathy. Semin Nephrol 1998; 18(4): 373–377.
48. Kopp JB, Winkler C. HIV-associated nephropathy in African Americans. Kidney Int Suppl 2003;(83):S43–S49.
49. Nochy D, Glotz D, Dosquet P, Pruna A, Guettier C, Weiss L, et al. Renal disease associated with HIV infection: a multicentric study of 60 patients from Paris hospitals. Nephrol Dial Transplant 1993; 8(1):11–19.
50. Bourgoignie JJ, Ortiz-Interian C, Green DF, Roth D. Race, a cofactor in HIV-1-associated nephropathy. Transplant Proc 1989; 21(6):3899–3901.
51. Rao TK, Filippone EJ, Nicastri AD, Landesman SH, Frank E, Chen CK, et al. Associated focal and segmental glomerulosclerosis in the acquired immunodeficiency syndrome. N Engl J Med 1984; 310(11):669–673.
52. Cohen AH. HIV-associated nephropathy: current concepts. Nephrol Dial Transplant 1998; 13(3):540–542.
53. Mokrzycki MH, Oo TN, Patel K, Chang CJ. Human immunodeficiency virus-associated nephropathy in the Bronx: low prevalence in a predominantly Hispanic population. Am J Nephrol 1998; 18(6):508–512.
54. Hader SL, Smith DK, Moore JS, Holmberg SD. HIV infection in women in the United States: status at the Millennium. JAMA 2001; 285(9): 1186–1192.
55. Stringer EM, Sinkala M, Kumwenda R, Chapman V, Mwale A, Vermund SH, et al. Personal risk perception, HIV knowledge and risk avoidance behavior, and their relationships to actual HIV serostatus in an urban African obstetric population. J Acquir Immune Defic Syndr 2004; 35(1):60–66.
56. Laradi A, Mallet A, Beaufils H, Allouache M, Martinez F. HIV-associated nephropathy: outcome and prognosis factors. Groupe d' Etudes Nephrologiques d'Ile de France. J Am Soc Nephrol 1998; 9(12):2327–2335.
57. Luke DR, Sarnoski TP, Dennis S. Incidence of microalbuminuria in ambulatory patients with acquired immunodeficiency syndrome. Clin Nephrol 1992; 38(2):69–74.
58. Glassock RJ, Cohen AH, Danovitch G, Parsa KP. Human immunodeficiency virus (HIV) infection and the kidney. Ann Intern Med 1990; 112(1):35–49.
59. Seney FD Jr, Burns DK, Silva FG. Acquired immunodeficiency syndrome and the kidney. Am J Kidney Dis 1990; 16(1):1–13.
60. Klotman PE. HIV-associated nephropathy. Kidney Int 1999; 56(3):1161–1176.
61. Kimmel PL, Ferreira-Centeno A, Farkas-Szallasi T, Abraham AA, Garrett CT. Viral DNA in microdissected renal biopsy tissue from HIV infected patients with nephrotic syndrome. Kidney Int 1993; 43(6):1347–1352.
62. Bourgoignie JJ, Pardo V. The nephropathology in human immunodeficiency virus (HIV-1) infection. Kidney Int Suppl 1991; 35:S19–S23.

63. Kimmel PL, Barisoni L, Kopp JB. Pathogenesis and treatment of HIV-associated renal diseases: lessons from clinical and animal studies, molecular pathologic correlations, and genetic investigations. Ann Intern Med 2003; 139(3):214–226.
64. Cohen AH, Sun NC, Shapshak P, Imagawa DT. Demonstration of human immunodeficiency virus in renal epithelium in HIV-associated nephropathy. Mod Pathol 1989; 2(2):125–128.
65. Winston JA, Bruggeman LA, Ross MD, Jacobson J, Ross L, D'Agati VD, et al. Nephropathy and establishment of a renal reservoir of HIV type 1 during primary infection. N Engl J Med 2001; 344(26):1979–1984.
66. Green DF, Resnick L, Bourgoignie JJ. HIV infects glomerular endothelial and mesangial but not epithelial cells in vitro. Kidney Int 1992; 41(4): 956–960.
67. Bruggeman LA, Ross MD, Tanji N, Cara A, Dikman S, Gordon RE, et al. Renal epithelium is a previously unrecognized site of HIV-1 infection. J Am Soc Nephrol 2000; 11(11):2079–2087.
68. Eitner F, Cui Y, Hudkins KL, Stokes MB, Segerer S, Mack M, et al. Chemokine receptor CCR5 and CXCR4 expression in HIV-associated kidney disease. J Am Soc Nephrol 2000; 11(5):856–867.
69. Bruggeman LA, Dikman S, Meng C, Quaggin SE, Coffman TM, Klotman PE. Nephropathy in human immunodeficiency virus-1 transgenic mice is due to renal transgene expression. J Clin Invest 1997; 100(1):84–92.
70. Smith SR, Svetkey LP, Dennis VW. Racial differences in the incidence and progression of renal diseases. Kidney Int 1991; 40(5):815–822.
71. Ray PE, Bruggeman LA, Weeks BS, Kopp JB, Bryant JL, Owens JW, et al. bFGF and its low affinity receptors in the pathogenesis of HIV-associated nephropathy in transgenic mice. Kidney Int 1994; 46(3):759–772.
72. Yamamoto T, Noble NA, Miller DE, Gold LI, Hishida A, Nagase M, et al. Increased levels of transforming growth factor-beta in HIV-associated nephropathy. Kidney Int 1999; 55(2):579–592.
73. Schwartz EJ, Klotman PE. Pathogenesis of human immunodeficiency virus (HIV)-associated nephropathy. Semin Nephrol 1998; 18(4):436–445.
74. Shukla RR, Kumar A, Kimmel PL. Transforming growth factor beta increases the expression of HIV-1 gene in transfected human mesangial cells. Kidney Int 1993; 44(5):1022–1029.
75. Li J, Zhou C, Yu L, Wang H. Renal protective effects of blocking the intrarenal renin-angiotensin system. Hypertens Res 1999; 22(3):223–228.
76. Eustace JA, Nuermberger E, Choi M, Scheel PJ Jr, Moore R, Briggs WA. Cohort study of the treatment of severe HIV-associated nephropathy with corticosteroids. Kidney Int 2000; 58(3):1253–1260.
77. Winston JA, Burns GC, Klotman PE. Treatment of HIV-associated nephropathy. Semin Nephrol 2000; 20(3):293–298.
78. Smith MC, Austen JL, Carey JT, Emancipator SN, Herbener T, Gripshover B, et al. Prednisone improves renal function and proteinuria in human immunodeficiency virus-associated nephropathy. Am J Med 1996; 101(1):41–48.
79. Sothinathan R, Briggs WA, Eustace JA. Treatment of HIV-associated nephropathy. AIDS Patient Care STDS 2001; 15(7):363–371.

80. Briggs WA, Tanawattanacharoen S, Choi MJ, Scheel PJ Jr, Nadasdy T, Racusen L. Clinicopathologic correlates of prednisone treatment of human immunodeficiency virus-associated nephropathy. Am J Kidney Dis 1996; 28(4):618–621.

81. Kimmel PL, Bosch JP, Vassalotti JA. Treatment of human immunodeficiency virus (HIV)-associated nephropathy. Semin Nephrol 1998; 18(4):446–458.

82. Kimmel PL, Mishkin GJ, Umana WO. Captopril and renal survival in patients with human immunodeficiency virus nephropathy. Am J Kidney Dis 1996; 28(2):202–208.

83. Burns GC, Paul SK, Toth IR, Sivak SL. Effect of angiotensin-converting enzyme inhibition in HIV-associated nephropathy. J Am Soc Nephrol 1997; 8(7):1140–1146.

84. Wei A, Burns GC, Williams BA, Mohammed NB, Visintainer P, Sivak SL. Long-term renal survival in HIV-associated nephropathy with angiotensin-converting enzyme inhibition. Kidney Int 2003; 64(4):1462–1471.

85. Bird JE, Durham SK, Giancarli MR, Gitlitz PH, Pandya DG, Dambach DM, et al. Captopril prevents nephropathy in HIV-transgenic mice. J Am Soc Nephrol 1998; 9(8):1441–1447.

86. Wali RK, Drachenberg CI, Papadimitriou JC, Keay S, Ramos E. HIV-1-associated nephropathy and response to highly-active antiretroviral therapy. Lancet 1998; 352(9130):783–784.

87. Ortiz C, Meneses R, Jaffe D, Fernandez JA, Perez G, Bourgoignie JJ. Outcome of patients with human immunodeficiency virus on maintenance hemodialysis. Kidney Int 1988; 34(2):248–253.

88. Ahuja TS, Grady J, Khan S. Changing trends in the survival of dialysis patients with human immunodeficiency virus in the United States. J Am Soc Nephrol 2002; 13(7):1889–1893.

89. Ifudu O, Mayers JD, Matthew JJ, Macey LJ, Brezsnyak W, Reydel C, et al. Uremia therapy in patients with end-stage renal disease and human immunodeficiency virus infection: has the outcome changed in the 1990s? Am J Kidney Dis 1997; 29(4):549–552.

90. Mazbar SA, Schoenfeld PY, Humphreys MH. Renal involvement in patients infected with HIV: experience at San Francisco General Hospital. Kidney Int 1990; 37(5):1325–1332.

91. Kimmel PL, Umana WO, Simmens SJ, Watson J, Bosch JP. Continuous ambulatory peritoneal dialysis and survival of HIV infected patients with end-stage renal disease. Kidney Int 1993; 44(2):373–378.

92. Bingel M, Lonnemann G, Koch KM, Dinarello CA, Shaldon S. Plasma interleukin-1 activity during hemodialysis: the influence of dialysis membranes. Nephron 1988; 50(4):273–276.

93. Herbelin A, Nguyen AT, Zingraff J, Urena P, Descamps-Latscha B. Influence of uremia and hemodialysis on circulating interleukin-1 and tumor necrosis factor alpha. Kidney Int 1990; 37(1):116–125.

94. Varela MP, Kimmel PL, Phillips TM, Mishkin GJ, Lew SQ, Bosch JP. Biocompatibility of hemodialysis membranes: interrelations between plasma complement and cytokine levels. Blood Purif 2001; 19(4):370–379.

95. Osborn L, Kunkel S, Nabel GJ. Tumor necrosis factor alpha and interleukin 1 stimulate the human immunodeficiency virus enhancer by activation of the nuclear factor kappa B. Proc Natl Acad Sci USA 1989; 86(7):2336–2340.

96. Ahuja TS, Borucki M, Grady J. Highly active antiretroviral therapy improves survival of HIV-infected hemodialysis patients. Am J Kidney Dis 2000; 36(3): 574–580.

97. Dressler R, Peters AT, Lynn RI. Pseudomonal and candidal peritonitis as a complication of continuous ambulatory peritoneal dialysis in human immunodeficiency virus-infected patients. Am J Med 1989; 86(6):787–790.

98. Monahan M, Klotman PE. Renal Diseases Associated with HIV Infection. Primer on Kidney Diseases. Academic Press, San Diego, California 2001: 230–202.

99. Kimmel PL, Phillips TM, Ferreira-Centeno A, Farkas-Szallasi T, Abraham AA, Garrett CT. HIV-associated immune-mediated renal disease. Kidney Int 1993; 44(6):1327–1340.

100. D'Agati V, Appel GB. HIV infection and the kidney. J Am Soc Nephrol 1997; 8(1):138–152.

101. Hailemariam S, Walder M, Burger HR, Cathomas G, Mihatsch M, Binswanger U, et al. Renal pathology and premortem clinical presentation of Caucasian patients with AIDS: an autopsy study from the era prior to antiretroviral therapy. Swiss Med Wkly 2001; 131(27–28):412–417.

102. Connolly JO, Weston CE, Hendry BM. HIV-associated renal disease in London hospitals. Q J Med 1995; 88(9):627–634.

103. Williams DI, Williams DJ, Williams IG, Unwin RJ, Griffiths MH, Miller RF. Presentation, pathology, and outcome of HIV associated renal disease in a specialist centre for HIV/AIDS. Sex Transm Infect 1998; 74(3):179–184.

104. Korbet SM, Schwartz MM. Human immunodeficiency virus infection and nephrotic syndrome. Am J Kidney Dis 1992; 20(1):97–103.

105. Kimmel PL, Phillips TM. Immune complex glomerulonephritis associated with renal disease in a specialist for HIV/AIDS. Kimmel PL, Berns JS, Stein JH, eds. Renal and Urologic Aspects of HIV Infection. New York: Churchill Livingstone, 1995:77–110.

106. Gorriz JL, Rovira E, Sancho A, Ferrer R, Paricio A, Pallardo LM. IgA nephropathy associated with human immuno deficiency virus infection: anti-proteinuric effect of captopril. Nephrol Dial Transplant 1997; 12(12): 2796–2797.

107. Mattana J, Siegal FP, Schwarzwald E, Molho L, Sankaran RT, Gooneratne R, et al. AIDS-associated membranous nephropathy with advanced renal failure: response to prednisone. Am J Kidney Dis 1997; 30(1):116–119.

108. Peraldi MN, Maslo C, Akposso K, Mougenot B, Rondeau E, Sraer JD. Acute renal failure in the course of HIV infection: a single-institution retrospective study of ninety-two patients and sixty renal biopsies. Nephrol Dial Transplant 1999; 14(6):1578–1585.

109. Perazella MA. Acute renal failure in HIV-infected patients: a brief review of common causes. Am J Med Sci 2000; 319(6):385–391.

110. Alpers CE. Light at the end of the TUNEL: HIV-associated thrombotic microangiopathy. Kidney Int 2003; 63(1):385–396.

111. Mitra D, Kim J, MacLow C, Karsan A, Laurence J. Role of caspases 1 and 3 and Bcl-2-related molecules in endothelial cell apoptosis associated with thrombotic microangiopathies. Am J Hematol 1998; 59(4):279–287.

112. Eitner F, Cui Y, Hudkins KL, Schmidt A, Birkebak T, Agy MB, et al. Thrombotic microangiopathy in the HIV-2-infected macaque. Am J Pathol 1999; 155(2):649–661.

113. Hymes KB, Karpatkin S. Human immunodeficiency virus infection and thrombotic microangiopathy. Semin Hematol 1997; 34(2):117–125.

114. Bottieau E, Colebunders R, Bosmans JL. Favourable outcome of haemolytic uraemic syndrome in an HIV-infected patient treated only with prednisone. J Infect 2000; 41(1):108–109.

115. Sacristán Lista F, Saavedra Alonso AJ, Oliver Morales J, Vázquez Martul E. Nephrotic syndrome due to thrombotic microangiopathy (TMA) as the first manifestation of human immunodeficiency virus infection: recovery before antiretroviral therapy without specific treatment against TMA. Clin Nephrol 2001; 55(5):404–407.

116. Abraham B, Baud O, Bonnet E, Roger PM, Chossat I, Merle C, et al. Thrombotic microangiopathy during HIV infection. A retrospective study performed in infectious diseases units in southern France. Presse Med 2001; 30(12):581–585.

117. Gruszecki AC, Wehrli G, Ragland BD, Reddy VV, Nabell L, Garcia-Hernandez A, et al. Management of a patient with HIV infection-induced anemia and thrombocytopenia who presented with thrombotic thrombocytopenic purpura. Am J Hematol 2002; 69(3):228–231.

118. Szczech LA. Renal diseases associated with human immunodeficiency virus infection: epidemiology, clinical course, and management. Clin Infect Dis 2001; 33(1):115–119.

119. Olatinwo T, Hewitt RG, Venuto RC. Human immunodeficiency virus-associated nephropathy: a primary care perspective. Arch Intern Med 2004; 164(3):333–336.

120. Global surveillance and control of hepatitis C. Report of a WHO Consultation organized in collaboration with the Viral Hepatitis Prevention Board, Antwerp, Belgium. J Viral Hepat 1999; 6(1):35–47.

121. Madhava V, Burgess C, Drucker E. Epidemiology of chronic hepatitis C virus infection in sub-Saharan Africa. Lancet Infect Dis 2002; 2(5):293–302.

122. Yen T, Keeffe EB, Ahmed A. The epidemiology of hepatitis C virus infection. J Clin Gastroenterol 2003; 36(1):47–53.

123. Flamm SL. Chronic hepatitis C virus infection. JAMA 2003; 289(18): 2413–2417.

124. Sabry AA, Sobh MA, Irving WL, Grabowska A, Wagner BE, Fox S, et al. A comprehensive study of the association between hepatitis C virus and glomerulopathy. Nephrol Dial Transplant 2002; 17(2):239–245.

125. Bruguera M, Sanchez Tapias JM. Epidemiology of hepatitis C virus infection. Nephrol Dial Transplant 2000; 15(suppl 8):12–14.

126. Poynard T, Yuen MF, Ratziu V, Lai CL. Viral hepatitis C. Lancet 2003; 362(9401):2095–2100.

127. Meyers CM, Seeff LB, Stehman-Breen CO, Hoofnagle JH. Hepatitis C and renal disease: an update. Am J Kidney Dis 2003; 42(4):631–657.

128. Otedo AE, Mc'Ligeyo SO, Okoth FA, Kayima JK. Seroprevalence of hepatitis B and C in maintenance dialysis in a public hospital in a developing country. S Afr Med J 2003; 93(5):380–384.

129. Cassidy MJ, Jankelson D, Becker M, Dunne T, Walzl G, Moosa MR. The prevalence of antibodies to hepatitis C virus at two haemodialysis units in South Africa. S Afr Med J 1995; 85(10):996–998.

130. Arankalle VA, Chadha MS, Jha J, Amrapurkar DN, Banerjee K. Prevalence of anti-HCV antibodies in western India. Indian J Med Res 1995; 101:91–93.

131. Lauer GM, Walker BD. Hepatitis C virus infection. N Engl J Med 2001; 345(1):41–52.

132. Gumber SC, Chopra S. Hepatitis C: a multifaceted disease. Review of extra-hepatic manifestations. Ann Intern Med 1995; 123(8):615–620.

133. Daghestani L, Pomeroy C. Renal manifestations of hepatitis C infection. Am J Med 1999; 106(3):347–354.

134. Philipneri M, Bastani B. Kidney disease in patients with chronic hepatitis C. Curr Gastroenterol Rep 2001; 3(1):79–83.

135. Rodes J, Sanchez Tapias JM. Hepatitis C. Nephrol Dial Transplant 2000; 15(suppl 8):2–11.

136. Ferri C, Zignego AL, Pileri SA. Cryoglobulins. J Clin Pathol 2002; 55(1): 4–13.

137. Ferri C, Greco F, Longombardo G, Palla P, Marzo E, Moretti A. Hepatitis C virus antibodies in mixed cryoglobulinemia. Clin Exp Rheumatol 1991; 9(1): 95–96.

138. Agnello V, Chung RT, Kaplan LM. A role for hepatitis C virus infection in type II cryoglobulinemia. N Engl J Med 1992; 327(21):1490–1495.

139. D'Amico G. Renal involvement in hepatitis C infection: cryoglobulinemic glomerulonephritis. Kidney Int 1998; 54(2):650–671.

140. Johnson RJ, Gretch DR, Yamabe H, Hart J, Bacchi CE, Hartwell P, et al. Membranoproliferative glomerulonephritis associated with hepatitis C virus infection. N Engl J Med 1993; 328(7):465–470.

141. Doutrelepont JM, Adler M, Willems M, Durez P, Yap SH. Hepatitis C infection and membranoproliferative glomerulonephritis. Lancet 1993; 341(8840):317.

142. Rollino C, Roccatello D, Giachino O, Basolo B, Piccoli G. Hepatitis C virus infection and membranous glomerulonephritis. Nephron 1991; 59(2):319–320.

143. Davda R, Peterson J, Weiner R, Croker B, Lau JY. Membranous glomerulo-nephritis in association with hepatitis C virus infection. Am J Kidney Dis 1993; 22(3):452–455.

144. Morales JM, Campistol JM, Andres A, Rodicio JL. Glomerular diseases in patients with hepatitis C virus infection after renal transplantation. Curr Opin Nephrol Hypertens 1997; 6(6):511–515.

145. Romas E, Power DA, Machet D, Powell H, d'Apice AJ. Membranous glomer-ulonephritis associated with hepatitis C virus infection in an adolescent. Pathology 1994; 26(4):399–402.

146. Stehman-Breen C, Alpers CE, Couser WG, Willson R, Johnson RJ. Hepatitis C virus associated membranous glomerulonephritis. Clin Nephrol 1995; 44(3):141–147.

147. Pouteil-Noble C, Maiza H, Dijoud F, MacGregor B. Glomerular disease associated with hepatitis C virus infection in native kidneys. Nephrol Dial Transplant 2000; 15(suppl 8):28–33.
148. Coroneos E, Truong L, Olivero J. Fibrillary glomerulonephritis associated with hepatitis C viral infection. Am J Kidney Dis 1997; 29(1):132–135.
149. Markowitz GS, Cheng JT, Colvin RB, Trebbin WM, D'Agati VD. Hepatitis C viral infection is associated with fibrillary glomerulonephritis and immunotactoid glomerulopathy. J Am Soc Nephrol 1998; 9(12):2244–2252.
150. Horikoshi S, Okada T, Shirato I, Inokuchi S, Ohmuro H, Tomino Y, et al. Diffuse proliferative glomerulonephritis with hepatitis C virus-like particles in paramesangial dense deposits in a patient with chronic hepatitis C virus hepatitis. Nephron 1993; 64(3):462–464.
151. Stehman-Breen C, Alpers CE, Fleet WP, Johnson RJ. Focal segmental glomerular sclerosis among patients infected with hepatitis C virus. Nephron 1999; 81(1):37–40.
152. Yamabe H, Johnson RJ, Gretch DR, Fukushi K, Osawa H, Miyata M, et al. Hepatitis C virus infection and membranoproliferative glomerulonephritis in Japan. J Am Soc Nephrol 1995; 6(2):220–223.
153. Madala ND, Naicker S, Singh B, Naidoo M, Smith AN, Rughubar K. The pathogenesis of membranoproliferative glomerulonephritis in KwaZulu-Natal, South Africa is unrelated to hepatitis C virus infection. Clin Nephrol 2003; 60(2):69–73.
154. Lopes LM, Lopes EP, Silva E, Kirsztajn GM, Pereira AB, Sesso RC, et al. Prevalence of hepatitis C virus antibodies in primary glomerulonephritis in Brazil. Am J Nephrol 1998; 18(6):495–497.
155. Ferri C, Marzo E, Longombardo G, Lombardini F, La Civita L, Vanacore R, et al. Interferon-alpha in mixed cryoglobulinemia patients: a randomized, crossover-controlled trial. Blood 1993; 81(5):1132–1136.
156. Misiani R, Bellavita P, Fenili D, Vicari O, Marchesi D, Sironi PL, et al. Interferon alfa-2a therapy in cryoglobulinemia associated with hepatitis C virus. N Engl J Med 1994; 330(11):751–756.
157. Dammacco F, Sansonno D, Han JH, Shyamala V, Cornacchiulo V, Iacobelli AR, et al. Natural interferon-alpha versus its combination with 6-methyl-prednisolone in the therapy of type II mixed cryoglobulinemia: a long-term, randomized, controlled study. Blood 1994; 84(10):3336–3343.
158. Misiani R, Bellavita P, Baio P, Caldara R, Ferruzzi S, Rossi P, et al. Successful treatment of HCV-associated cryoglobulinaemic glomerulonephritis with a combination of interferon-alpha and ribavirin. Nephrol Dial Transplant 1999; 14(6):1558–1560.
159. Casato M, Agnello V, Pucillo LP, Knight GB, Leoni M, Del Vecchio S, et al. Predictors of long-term response to high-dose interferon therapy in type II cryoglobulinemia associated with hepatitis C virus infection. Blood 1997; 90(10):3865–3873.
160. Zuckerman E, Keren D, Slobodin G, Rosner I, Rozenbaum M, Toubi E, et al. Treatment of refractory, symptomatic, hepatitis C virus related mixed cryoglobulinemia with ribavirin and interferon-alpha. J Rheumatol 2000; 27(9):2172–2178.

161. Calleja JL, Albillos A, Moreno-Otero R, Rossi I, Cacho G, Domper F, et al. Sustained response to interferon-alpha or to interferon-alpha plus ribavirin in hepatitis C virus-associated symptomatic mixed cryoglobulinaemia. Aliment Pharmacol Ther 1999; 13(9):1179–1186.
162. Manns MP, McHutchison JG, Gordon SC, Rustgi VK, Shiffman M, Reindollar R, et al. Peginterferon alfa-2b plus ribavirin compared with interferon alfa-2b plus ribavirin for initial treatment of chronic hepatitis C: a randomised trial. Lancet 2001; 358(9286):958–965.
163. Fried MW, Shiffman ML, Reddy KR, Smith C, Marinos G, Goncales FL Jr, et al. Peginterferon alfa-2a plus ribavirin for chronic hepatitis C virus infection. N Engl J Med 2002; 347(13):975–982.
164. Alric L, Plaisier E, Thebault S, Peron JM, Rostaing L, Pourrat J, et al. Influence of antiviral therapy in hepatitis C virus-associated cryoglobulinemic MPGN. Am J Kidney Dis 2004; 43(4):617–623.
165. Lopes EP, Valente LM, Silva AE, Kirsztajn GM, Cruz CN, Ferraz ML. Therapy with interferon-alpha plus ribavirin for membranoproliferative glomerulonephritis induced by hepatitis C virus. Braz J Infect Dis 2003; 7(5):353–357.
166. Bruchfeld A, Lindahl K, Stahle L, Soderberg M, Schvarcz R. Interferon and ribavirin treatment in patients with hepatitis C-associated renal disease and renal insufficiency. Nephrol Dial Transplant 2003; 18(8):1573–1580.
167. Rossi P, Bertani T, Baio P, Caldara R, Luliri P, Tengattini F, et al. Hepatitis C virus-related cryoglobulinemic glomerulonephritis: long-term remission after antiviral therapy. Kidney Int 2003; 63(6):2236–2241.
168. Loustaud-Ratti V, Liozon E, Karaaslan H, Alain S, Paraf F, Le Meur Y, et al. Interferon alpha and ribavirin for membranoproliferative glomerulonephritis and hepatitis C infection. Am J Med 2002; 113(6):516–519.
169. Sabry AA, Sobh MA, Sheaashaa HA, Kudesia G, Wild G, Fox S, et al. Effect of combination therapy (ribavirin and interferon) in HCV-related glomerulopathy. Nephrol Dial Transplant 2002; 17(11):1924–1930.
170. Nishi S, Ueno M, Shimada H, Oosawa Y, Iino N, Iguchi S, et al. Treatment of membranoproliferative glomerulonephritis associated with hepatitis C virus infection. Niigata Research Group of Glomerulonephritis and Nephrotic Syndrome. Intern Med 2000; 39(10):788–793.
171. Johnson RJ, Gretch DR, Couser WG, Alpers CE, Wilson J, Chung M, et al. Hepatitis C virus-associated glomerulonephritis. Effect of alpha-interferon therapy. Kidney Int 1994; 46(6):1700–1704.
172. Sarac E, Bastacky S, Johnson JP. Response to high-dose interferon-alpha after failure of standard therapy in MPGN associated with hepatitis C virus infection. Am J Kidney Dis 1997; 30(1):113–115.
173. Yamabe H, Johnson RJ, Gretch DR, Osawa H, Inuma H, Sasaki T, et al. Membranoproliferative glomerulonephritis associated with hepatitis C virus infection responsive to interferon-alpha. Am J Kidney Dis 1995; 25(1):67–69.
174. Laganovic M, Jelakovic B, Kuzmanic D, Scukanec-Spoljar M, Roncevic T, Cuzic S, et al. Complete remission of cryoglobulinemic glomerulonephritis (HCV-positive) after high dose interferon therapy. Wien Klin Wochenschr 2000; 112(13):596–600.

175. Fabrizi F, Pozzi C, Farina M, Dattolo P, Lunghi G, Badalamenti S, et al. Hepatitis C virus infection and acute or chronic glomerulonephritis: an epidemiological and clinical appraisal. Nephrol Dial Transplant 1998; 13(8): 1991–1997.

176. Giannico G, Manno C, Schena FP. Treatment of glomerulonephritides associated with hepatitis C virus infection. Nephrol Dial Transplant 2000; 15(suppl 8):34–38.

177. First MR. Hepatitis C virus infection in the renal transplant recipient. Nephrol Dial Transplant 2000; 15(suppl 8):60–64.

178. Pereira BJ, Wright TL, Schmid CH, Bryan CF, Cheung RC, Cooper ES, et al. Screening and confirmatory testing of cadaver organ donors for hepatitis C virus infection: a U.S. National Collaborative Study. Kidney Int 1994; 46(3): 886–892.

179. Knoll GA, Tankersley MR, Lee JY, Julian BA, Curtis JJ. The impact of renal transplantation on survival in hepatitis C-positive end-stage renal disease patients. Am J Kidney Dis 1997; 29(4):608–614.

180. Morales JM. Hepatitis C virus infection and renal disease after renal transplantation. Transplant Proc 2004; 36(3):760–762.

181. Rostaing L. Treatment of hepatitis C virus infection after renal transplantation: new insights. Nephrol Dial Transplant 2000; 15(suppl 8):74–76.

182. Natov SN. Transmission of viral hepatitis by kidney transplantation: donor evaluation and transplant policies (Part 1: hepatitis B virus). Transplant Infect Dis 2002; 4(3):124–131.

183. Morales JM, Campistol JM, Andres A, Dominguez-Gil B, Esforzado N, Munoz MA, et al. Policies concerning the use of kidneys from donors infected with hepatitis C virus. Nephrol Dial Transplant 2000; 15(suppl 8):71–73.

184. Morales JM, Campistol JM, Castellano G, Andres A, Colina F, Fuertes A, et al. Transplantation of kidneys from donors with hepatitis C antibody into recipients with pre-transplantation anti-HCV. Kidney Int 1995; 47(1): 236–240.

185. Ali MK, Light JA, Barhyte DY, Sasaki TM, Currier CB Jr, Grandas O, et al. Donor hepatitis C virus status does not adversely affect short-term outcomes in HCV+ recipients in renal transplantation. Transplantation 1998; 66(12): 1694–1697.

186. Widell A, Mansson S, Persson NH, Thysell H, Hermodsson S, Blohme I. Hepatitis C superinfection in hepatitis C virus (HCV)-infected patients transplanted with an HCV-infected kidney. Transplantation 1995; 60(7):642–647.

187. Barril G. Hepatitis C virus-induced liver disease in dialysis patients. Nephrol Dial Transplant 2000; 15(suppl 8):42–45.

188. Nakayama E, Akiba T, Marumo F, Sato C. Prognosis of anti-hepatitis C virus antibody-positive patients on regular hemodialysis therapy. J Am Soc Nephrol 2000; 11(10):1896–1902.

189. Stehman-Breen CO, Emerson S, Gretch D, Johnson RJ. Risk of death among chronic dialysis patients infected with hepatitis C virus. Am J Kidney Dis 1998; 32(4):629–634.

190. Pereira BJ, Natov SN, Bouthot BA, Murthy BV, Ruthazer R, Schmid CH, et al. Effects of hepatitis C infection and renal transplantation on survival in

end-stage renal disease. The New England Organ Bank Hepatitis C Study Group. Kidney Int 1998; 53(5):1374–1381.

191. Gane E, Pilmore H. Management of chronic viral hepatitis before and after renal transplantation. Transplantation 2002; 74(4):427–437.

192. Alter MJ, Margolis HS, Bell BP, Bice SD, Burrington J, Mary Chamberland M, et al. Recommendations for prevention and control of hepatitis C virus (HCV) infection and HCV-related chronic disease. Centers for Disease Control and Prevention. MMWR Recomm Rep 1998; 47(RR-19):1–39.

193. Levy M, Chen N. Worldwide perspective of hepatitis B-associated glomerulonephritis in the 80s. Kidney Int Suppl 1991; 35:S24–S33.

194. Johnson RJ, Couser WG. Hepatitis B infection and renal disease: clinical, immunopathogenetic and therapeutic considerations. Kidney Int 1990; 37(2): 663–676.

195. DiBisceglie AM, Kew MC, Dusheiko GM, Berger EL, Song E, Paterson AC, et al. Prevalence of hepatitis B virus infection among black children in Soweto. Br Med J (Clin Res Ed) 1986; 292(6533):1440–1442.

196. Bhimma R, Coovadia HM, Adhikari M, Connolly CA. The impact of the hepatitis B virus vaccine on the incidence of hepatitis B virus-associated membranous nephropathy. Arch Pediatr Adolesc Med 2003; 157(10):1025–1030.

197. Combes B, Shorey J, Barrera A, Stastny P, Eigenbrodt EH, Hull AR, et al. Glomerulonephritis with deposition of Australia antigen-antibody complexes in glomerular basement membrane. Lancet 1971; 2(7718):234–237.

198. Bates WD, Muller N, van Buuren AJ, Steyn DW. Pregnancy in partially remitted hepatitis B-associated membranous glomerulonephritis. Int J Gynaecol Obstet 1996; 52(2):163–165.

199. van Buuren AJ, Bates WD, Muller N. Nephrotic syndrome in Namibian children. S Afr Med J 1999; 89(10):1088–1091.

200. Rashid H, Morley AR, Ward MK, Kerr DN, Codd AA. Hepatitis B infection in glomerulonephritis. Br Med J (Clin Res Ed) 1981; 283(6297):948–949.

201. Lai KN, Lai FM, Chan KW, Chow CB, Tong KL, Vallance-Owen J. The clinico-pathologic features of hepatitis B virus-associated glomerulonephritis. Q J Med 1987; 63(240):323–333.

202. Takekoshi Y, Tanaka M, Shida N, Satake Y, Saheki Y, Matsumoto S. Strong association between membranous nephropathy and hepatitis-B surface antigenaemia in Japanese children. Lancet 1978; 2(8099):1065–1068.

203. Hogg JR, Silva FG, Cavallo T, Krous HF, Walker P, Roy S, et al. Hepatitis B surface antigenemia in North American children with membranous glomerulonephropathy. Southwest Pediatric Nephrology Study Group. J Pediatr 1985; 106(4):571–578.

204. Wiggelinkhuizen J, Sinclair-Smith C, Stannard LM, Smuts H. Hepatitis B virus associated membranous glomerulonephritis. Arch Dis Child 1983; 58(7):488–496.

205. Hsu HC, Lin GH, Chang MH, Chen CH. Association of hepatitis B surface (HBs) antigenemia and membranous nephropathy in children in Taiwan. Clin Nephrol 1983; 20(3):121–129.

206. Kohler PF, Cronin RE, Hammond WS, Olin D, Carr RI. Chronic membranous glomerulonephritis caused by hepatitis B antigen–antibody immune complexes. Ann Intern Med 1974; 81(4):448–451.

207. Collins AB, Bhan AK, Dienstag JL, Colvin RB, Haupert GT Jr, Mushahwar IK, et al. Hepatitis B immune complex glomerulonephritis: simultaneous glomerular deposition of hepatitis B surface and e antigens. Clin Immunol Immunopathol 1983; 26(1):137–153.

208. Yoshikawa N, Ito H, Yamada Y, Hashimoto H, Katayama Y, Matsuyama S, et al. Membranous glomerulonephritis associated with hepatitis B antigen in children: a comparison with idiopathic membranous glomerulonephritis. Clin Nephrol 1985; 23(1):28–34.

209. Gregorek H, Jung H, Ulanowicz G, Madalinski K. Immune complexes in sera of children with HBV-mediated glomerulonephritis. Arch Immunol Ther Exp (Warsz) 1986; 34(1):73–83.

210. Gilbert RD, Wiggelinkhuizen J. The clinical course of hepatitis B virus-associated nephropathy. Pediatr Nephrol 1994; 8(1):11–14.

211. Bhimma R, Coovadia HM, Adhikari M. Hepatitis B virus-associated nephropathy in black South African children. Pediatr Nephrol 1998; 12(6): 479–484.

212. Wiggelinkhuizen J, Sinclair-Smith C. Membranous glomerulonephropathy in childhood. S Afr Med J 1987; 72(3):184–187.

213. Wrzolkowa T, Zurowska A, Uszycka-Karcz M, Picken MM. Hepatitis B virus-associated glomerulonephritis: electron microscopic studies in 98 children. Am J Kidney Dis 1991; 18(3):306–312.

214. Mills AE, Emms M. Frequent occurrence of microtubuloreticular complexes encountered during routine ultrastructural examination at a children's hospital. Ultrastruct Pathol 1988; 12(6):599–604.

215. Ito H, Hattori S, Matusda I, Amamiya S, Hajikano H, Yoshizawa H, et al. Hepatitis B e antigen-mediated membranous glomerulonephritis. Correlation of ultrastructural changes with HBeAg in the serum and glomeruli. Lab Invest 1981; 44(3):214–220.

216. Venkataseshan VS, Lieberman K, Kim DU, Thung SN, Dikman S, D'Agati V, et al. Hepatitis-B-associated glomerulonephritis: pathology, pathogenesis, and clinical course. Medicine (Baltimore) 1990; 69(4):200–216.

217. Kleinknecht C, Levy M, Peix A, Broyer M, Courtecuisse V. Membranous glomerulonephritis and hepatitis B surface antigen in children. J Pediatr 1979; 95(6):946–952.

218. Nagata K, Fujita M, Aoyama R, Miyakawa Y, Yoshizawa K, Mayumi M. A case of membranous glomerulonephritis in which positive to negative change of hepatitis B e antigen in glomeruli was observed. Int J Pediatr Nephrol 1981; 2(2):103–108.

219. Hsu HC, Wu CY, Lin CY, Lin GJ, Chen CH, Huang FY. Membranous nephropathy in 52 hepatitis B surface antigen (HBsAg) carrier children in Taiwan. Kidney Int 1989; 36(6):1103–1107.

220. Seggie J, Nathoo K, Davies PG. Association of hepatitis B (HBs) antigenaemia and membranous glomerulonephritis in Zimbabwean children. Nephron 1984; 38(2):115–119.

221. Wyszynska T, Jung H, Madalinski K, Morzycka M. Hepatitis B mediated glomerulonephritis in children. Int J Pediatr Nephrol 1984; 5(3):147–158.

222. Dreyer L. The frequency of hepatitis B surface antigen in membranous nephropathy in black and white South Africans. S Afr Med J 1984; 65(5): 166–168.
223. Milner LS, Dusheiko GM, Jacobs D, Kala U, Thomson PD, Ninin DT, et al. Biochemical and serological characteristics of children with membranous nephropathy due to hepatitis B virus infection: correlation with hepatitis B e antigen, hepatitis B DNA and hepatitis D. Nephron 1988; 49(3):184–189.
224. Thomson PD. Renal problems in black South African children. Pediatr Nephrol 1997; 11(4):508–512.
225. Seggie J, Davies PG, Ninin D, Henry J. Patterns of glomerulonephritis in Zimbabwe: survey of disease characterised by nephrotic proteinuria. Q J Med 1984; 53(209):109–118.
226. Lai KN, Li PK, Lui SF, Au TC, Tam JS, Tong KL, et al. Membranous nephropathy related to hepatitis B virus in adults. N Engl J Med 1991; 324(21):1457–1463.
227. Lai KN, Tam JS, Lin HJ, Lai FM. The therapeutic dilemma of the usage of corticosteroid in patients with membranous nephropathy and persistent hepatitis B virus surface antigenaemia. Nephron 1990; 54(1):12–17.
228. Mizushima N, Kanai K, Matsuda H, Matsumoto M, Tamakoshi K, Ishii H, et al. Improvement of proteinuria in a case of hepatitis B-associated glomerulonephritis after treatment with interferon. Gastroenterology 1987; 92(2): 524–526.
229. de Man RA, Schalm SW, van der Heijden AJ, ten Kate FW, Wolff ED, Heijtink RA. Improvement of hepatitis B-associated glomerulonephritis after antiviral combination therapy. J Hepatol 1989; 8(3):367–372.
230. Lisker-Melman M, Webb D, Di Bisceglie AM, Kassianides C, Martin P, Rustgi V, et al. Glomerulonephritis caused by chronic hepatitis B virus infection: treatment with recombinant human alpha-interferon. Ann Intern Med 1989; 111(6):479–483.
231. Bhimma R, Coovadia HM, Kramvis A, Adhikari M, Kew MC. Treatment of hepatitis B virus-associated nephropathy in Black children. Pediatr Nephrol 2002; 17:393–399.
232. Lee HS, Choi Y, Yu SH, Koh HI, Kim MJ, Ko KW. A renal biopsy study of hepatitis B virus-associated nephropathy in Korea. Kidney Int 1988; 34(4): 537–543.
233. Brzosko WJ, Krawczynski K, Nazarewicz T, Morzycka M, Nowoslawski A. Glomerulonephritis associated with hepatitis-B surface antigen immune complexes in children. Lancet 1974; 2(7879):477–482.
234. Lai KN, Lai FM, Lo S, Leung A. Is there a pathogenetic role of hepatitis B virus in lupus nephritis?. Arch Pathol Lab Med 1987; 111:185–188.
235. Lai KN, Lai FM, Lo S, Ho CP, Chan KW. IgA nephropathy associated with hepatitis B virus antigenemia. Nephron 1987; 47(2):141–143.
236. Lai KN, Lai FM, Tam JS. IgA nephropathy associated with chronic hepatitis B virus infection in adults: the pathogenetic role of HBsAG. J Pathol 1989; 157(4):321–327.

6

Acute Renal Failure and Toxic Nephropathies in the Developing World

Marc E. De Broe

Department of Nephrology, University of Antwerp, Belgium

INTRODUCTION

There is a striking difference between the etiology of acute renal failure (ARF) in the developed world compared to that of developing countries. ARF in Western societies is now largely the consequence of cardiovascular surgery, drugs, multiorgan failure, consequences of traffic and industrial accidences, and more specifically renal transplantation rejection. In the developing world, medical causes remain the dominant sub-group of ARF. In this context, herbal medicines and infections remain the most common etiological factors in the medical sub-group in black Africa and remained so when studied over a decade (Table 1) (1). In India, infectious diarrheal disease, malaria, leptospirosis, intravascular hemolysis due to G6PD-deficiency, snakebites, and insect stings constitute over 60% of ARF (2). In Nigeria, herbs are involved in 50% of ARF cases of which 60% necessitates hemodialysis.

Excellent reviews dealing with herbal remedies and their effect on the kidney have recently been published (3,4) (Table 2).

In this short review, some particular forms of acute and toxic nephropathies observed in the developing world will be discussed.

Dropsy

J. Prakash reported ARF complicating epidemic dropsy. Dropsy, resembling bery bery, is caused by ingestion of mustard oil adulterated with seeds

Table 1   Etiology of ARF in South Africa (1978, 1986–1988)

	1978		1986–1988	
Etiology	N	%	N	%
Medical	98	65	174	77
Nephrotoxins	53	35	46	20.4
Herbal	50		44	
Non-herbal	3	17	4	30.1
Infections	28		89	
Typhoid fever	5		18	
E. coli septicemia	6		15	
Pneumonia (various)	—		14	
Klebsiella pneumoniae	6		4	
Malaria	2		9	
Obstructive uropathy from				
Schistosomiasis	3		—	
Septicemia (culture negative)	—		3	
Acute pyelonephritis	2		1	
Tetanus	2		1	
Hepatitis virus	1		—	
Acute bacterial endocarditis	1		—	
Pseudomonas septicemia	—		1	
Streptococcus pyogenes septicemia	—		2	
Gastroenteritis	5		21	
Other causes	12		29	
Acute pancreatitis	2		3	
Other causes	10		—	
Rhabdomyolysis	—		12	
No etiological factor	—		24	
Gynecological	26	17	12	5.3
Self-induced abortion	24		8	
Others	2		4	
Obstetrical	11	7	21	9.3
Antepartum hemorrhage	5		4	
Eclampsia	4		9	
Post-partum hemorrhage	2		2	
After caesarean section	—		4	
Intra-uterine death	—		1	
Puerperal sepsis	—		1	
Surgical	15	10	19	8.4
Motor vehicle accidents with				
Crush injuries	11		6	
Post-laparotomy	—		7	
Stab abdomen	—		4	
Gunshot injury	—		1	
Post-cardiac arrest	1		—	
Post-prostatectomy	3		1	
Total	150		226	

Source: From Ref. 1.

Table 2 Examples of Kidney Syndromes Induced by Herbal Medicines

Hypertension	• *Glycyrrhiza* species (Chinese herbal teas, gancao, Boui-ougi-tou) • *Ephedra* species (*Ma huang*)
Acute tubular necrosis	• Traditional African medicine: toxic plants (*Securida longe pedunculata, Euphoria metabelensis, C. laureola, Cape aloes*) or adulteration by dichromate • Chinese medicine: *Taxus celebica* • Marocco: *Takaout roumia* (paraphenylenediamine)
Acute interstitial nephritis	• Peruvian medicine (*Uno degatta*) • Tung Shueh pills (adulterated by mefenamic acid)
Fanconi's syndrome	• Chinese herbs containing Aas (*Akebia* species, *Boui, Mokutsu*) • Chinese herbs adulterated by cadmium
Papillary necrosis	• Chinese herbs adulterated by phenylbutazone
Chronic interstitial renal fibrosis	• Chinese herbs or Kampo containing Aas (*Aristolochia* species, *Akebia* species, *Mu-tong, Boui, Mokutsu*)
Urinary retention	• Datura species, *Rhododendron molle* (atropine, scopolamine)
Kidney stones	• *Ma huang* (ephedrine) • Cranberry juice (oxalate)
Urinary tract carcinoma	• Chinese herbs containing AAs

Source: From Ref. 3.

of *Argemone mexicana*, occurring in an epidemic or endemic form, mostly in India although also observed in Mauritius and South Africa (5). The disease is characterized by gastrointestinal disturbances, edema, heart failure, pyrexia, glaucoma, cutaneous pigmentation and nodular eruption. Sanguinarine is a toxic alkaloid from oil obtained from the seeds of *A. mexicana*. This substance interferes with the oxidation of pyruvic acid, which accumulates and causes dilatation of capillaries and small arterioles. Pasricha and colleagues (6) showed that toxicity of contaminated mustard oil could be eliminated by heating to 240°C for 15 minutes. The product is absorbed by the skin and contaminated oil used for massage has been reported to cause dropsy (7). Extensive vascular dilatation in the deeper layer of the skin is characteristic in dropsy. The basic lesion is a proliferation of capillaries below the skin due to producing the mottling and blanching (8). Similar changes are observed in the lungs, cervix, ovaries, intestines, and liver. Disturbances of the heart and circulation are prominent in nearly all cases. ARF in epidemic dropsy is most likely the result of renal hypoperfusion caused by marked peripheral vascular dilatation, heart failure, and volume depletion as a consequence of diarrhea and vomiting. The widespread capillary damage of internal organ is a common feature in dropsy. The possibility of intrarenal capillaries and glomeruli damage cannot be ruled out (5).

Djenkolism

Djenkol (jering) trees, *Pithecolobium lobatum*, family Mimosaceae, grow in Indonesia, Malaysia, Southern Thailand, and Miramar. Most cases have been reported from Java and Sumatra in the Dutch literature. Recently, several cases were reported in other areas where this tree grows (9). Djenkol beans, considered a local delicacy, are consumed raw, fried, or roasted. When consumed in large amounts, they may cause poisoning, particularly if associated with dehydration or low fluid intake. The bean contains djenkolic acid, a sulfur-rich amino acid with precipitate as needle-like crystals in concentrated and acidic urine causing intratubular obstruction. It is not surprising that in view of this pathophysiological mechanism there is a large variation observed in individual susceptibility to the toxic effect. A single animal study reported that acute tubular necrosis was observed in rats and mice. Crystals were detected only in a limited number of the renal tissue of the animals (10). On the other hand, typical crystals are observed in the urine of all animals ingesting djenkol (11). Symptoms may occur immediately after consuming the fruits or at late as 36 hours after consumption. They include dysuria, lumbar and lower abdominal pain, hypertension, hematuria, and oligo-anuria (9). Urine analysis shows presence of needles-shaped crystals of djenkolic acid. High fluid intake and alkalinization of the urine helps in dissolving the crystals and prevents the formation of tubular obstruction. Finally, djenkolism can be prevented by pre-treatment of the beans by boiling or consumption of small amounts of the raw beans, associated with liberal fluid intake.

While not addressed as frequently in the literature, the safety of herbal medicine used in developing countries is a major concern (3). In South Africa, it is estimated that between 60% and 80% of the native population use traditional medicines, usually in combinations. Cases of acute poisoning due to traditional medicine are not uncommon. Many of which have resulted in significant morbidity and mortality, which mortality has been estimated has to be as high as 10,000/year (12,13).

Venter and Joubert (14) found that poisoning with traditional medicines resulted in the highest mortality, accounting for 51.7% of all deaths that were due to acute poisoning. Traditional healers were the main source of the medicines and in some cases substances were bought at a shop for African remedies. The study by Stewart et al. (15) found that African traditional remedies were involved in 43% of the poisoning cases.

Callilepis laureola—Impila

The ox-eye daisy, *Callilepis laureola*, is a herb and used as traditional remedy by the Zulus of the North-East of South Africa (Fig. 1). It is known to be very poisonous and has been responsible for several deaths among the Zulu. The plant is commonly known as impila, which ironically is the Zulu word for health. Although there are no approved medical uses of impila from a health regulatory standpoint, the plant is widely used and appears to serve as multipurpose remedy for the treatment of stomach problems, tape worm infestations, impotence, and to induce fertility. The greatest and most

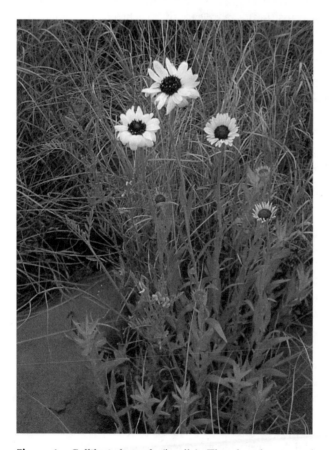

Figure 1 *Callilepis laureola* (impila). The plant bears a tuberous root, similar to a potato with characteristic bulbous shape and pungent odor. During the months of August to November, *C. laureola* yields solitary creamy white flowers with a purple disc. (Photograph taken in the Northern KwaZulu-Natal region, courtesy of Geoff Nichols, Silverglen Medicinal Plant Nursery, Durban, South Africa.) *Source*: From Ref. 16.

valued attribute of this plant, however, appears to lie in his protective powers in warding off "evil spirits." It is suspected that these magical beliefs are the primary reason for the use of impila in young children and the high-impila rate mortality in these children. An extract of the rootstock is used either orally or given as an enema. Renal failure is an early finding preceding the hepatoxic effects of these extracts (2). The clinical manifestations are abdominal pain, vomiting, and hypoglycemia. Although the precise mechanism of renal failure is not clear, a direct nephrotoxicity has been attributed to atractyloside. Atractyloside is a hypoglycemic agent and the product itself or a not yet identified metabolite targets mitochondria, inhibiting oxidative phosphorylation. The mechanism appears to involve opening of the mitochondrial permeability transition pore, release of cytochrome C and caspase activation (16–18). Glutathion depletion is also an early and critical event in the mechanism of the impila-induced cytotoxicity (16). The majority of cases are fatal, particularly in children (up to 90%). Sixty-three percent die within 24 hours due to hypoglycemia, at 5 days due to acute renal failure combined with hepatotoxicity. There is no antidote available.

Raw Carp Bile

The raw carp bile of fresh water or grass carps (*Ctenopharyngodon idella*) is used to improve failing vision and rheumatism in the rural areas of Taiwan, China, Japan, and South Korea (2). Recently, it has been reported as an unconventional remedy for diabetes mellitus in Saudi Arabia (19). Raw gall bladder of the Indian carp (*Labeo rohita*) has also been used as a traditional remedy for various ailments in certain parts of India. Symptoms such as abdominal pain, nausea, vomiting, watery diarrhea occur very quickly within 12 hours following ingestion. ARF occurs later but within 48 hours and is oliguric (20). Hypotension and hemolysis may be responsible for the development of ARF although a direct nephrotoxic effect could be additional factors. Recently, Kyon Choi and colleagues (21) found that grass carp bile inhibit the release of renal dipeptidase from the proximal tubules by nitric oxide generation. Kidney biopsies revealed interstitial edema. The duration of renal failure ranges from 2 to 3 weeks and up to now does not show a high mortality rate (2).

Copper Sulfate

The extensive use of copper sulfate in the leather industry because of its low cost and easy availability were the main reasons for its widespread use as a mode of suicide amongst the poor groups in India. Chugh et al. (22) observed a decreasing trend in their study lasting cross-sectional observations over a 10-year period.

Spiritual water or green water is a solution that is used in many Nigerian rituals as a cathartic agent (23). It is given by church leaders to their members to induce emesis, signifying the purging of ones problem and impurities. Their severe hemolysis and ARF was also described in several cases by Akintonwa et al. (24). Within minutes of ingestion, the patients develop severe abdominal pain, vomiting, fever, nausea, a metallic taste in the mouth. They may also develop diarrhea, hematemesis, and melena. In the case of severe poisoning, hypotension, convulsions, and coma may develop. Hypovolemia due to fluid loss, direct nephrotoxicity, and severe hemolysis are the main pathogenic factors in the development of ARF. Depending on the severity of the poisoning, renal failure develops in a substantial percentage of the cases (23). The copper is thought to induce hemolysis by disrupting intracellular enzymatic activity, reducing erythrocyte glutathione concentration and further sensitizing the cells to the effect of oxidants (25). Although hemoglobin unlike myoglobin is not thought to be nephrotoxic in itself, severe hemolysis has been associated with decreased renal function, in particularly in the presence of concomitant factors such as shock and dehydration, which is the case in copper sulfate poisoning. In addition, the role of hemoglobin as an inhibitor of both baseline and stimulated endothelium-derived relaxing factor activity has been elucidated in various vascular systems. Inhibition of nitric oxide by free hemoglobin is a possible pathogenic mechanism for the vasospasm observed in copper sulfate poisoning (26). The frequently observed among Black Africans gluco-6-phosphate dehydrogenese deficiency may predispose these patients to the toxic effects of copper.

Gastric lavage should be done using 1% potassium ferrocyanide solutions leading to formation of insoluble cupric ferrocyanide. Emesis should not be induced, volume deficit should be corrected, and patients with hemolysis should receive blood transfusion. Obviously, hyperkalemia is often severe and require early and frequent hemodialysis. There is no specific antidote available.

Obstetrical Acute Renal Failure (ARF)

Obstetrical Acute Renal Failure (ARF) has become a rare complication of the pregnancy in the developed world, but is still rather frequent in the developing countries and responsible for an important maternal fatal morbidity and mortality. Its high incidence is due to the prevalence of unsafe home deliveries and abortions conducted by untrained personal. Additional factors are absence of systematic screening of blood pressure/hypertension, proteinuria, urinary tract infection, and/or incipient renal failure. In Ethiopia, septic abortion is an underlying cause of ARF in 52% of all patients. A recent study by Hachim and colleagues (27), the main etiology of ARF in Morocco is preeclampsia and eclampsia, followed by septic abortion, obstetrical hemorrhages, and in utero fetal death. The recovery of renal function was 87% of the cases. Obstetrical ARF has a bimodal occurrence with the first peak between 8 and 16 weeks of gestation in the context of septic abortions. A second peak seen after 34 weeks is associated mainly with eclampsia, abruptio-placenta post-partum hemorrhages, and puerperal sepsis.

Although the prognosis seems to be favorable, there are a substantial number (~5%) of patients developing chronic kidney failure, mainly due to acute cortical necrosis (28). This severe form of ARF, which has virtually disappeared in the Western world, is still seen in developing countries, particularly in the context of obstetrical ARF. Other causes are snakebites, hemolytic uremic syndrome, and infectious gastroenteritis.

Paraphenylene Diamine (Hair Dye Poisoning)

Paraphenylene diamine (PPD) poisoning has been known for many years (29) and mainly described in Middle Eastern countries (30–33) or Japan (34) in the context of accidental, deliberate, or homicidal ingestion or topical application (especially after a steam bath).

In Sudan, PPD is used by women to color their hair and as a body dye when added to henna (*Lawasonia alba*), a non-toxic substance. Henna on its own needs to be applied two or three times for several hours to give the desired color (dark red or black), which can quickly be achieved with one single application by adding PPD to the henna. PPD in its pure form (90–99%) is available in the local markets and there are no restrictions for its use or trade (29). The major problem of PPD toxicity results from the ingestion of the compound accidentally, in suicidal or homicidal attempts. When added to henna, toxicity may occur through skin absorption.

In Morocco, Takaout beldia indicates a non-toxic vegetable product extracted from the gallnut of Tamaris Orientalis. This non-toxic substance is highly appreciated by woman for its hair-dyeing properties. Its rarefaction resulted in the use of PPD as substitute under the name of Takaout Roumia. Its use for suicidal attempt (ingestion of 3–15 g) in young woman in Morocco and Tunisia become highly prevalent (35). Its ingestion is responsible for a respiratory (cervico-facial edema), muscular (rhabdomyolysis), and ARF due to hypovolemia and myoglobulinuria. The respiratory syndrome mainly determines its prognosis.

A reported series of 171 cases of PPD poisoning was admitted to the medical resuscitation service in Ibn Roshd hospital between January 1994 and October 1997. Twenty-four percent of the patients developed severe ARF and 55 deaths (38.7%) were observed in this study (36). Cases reported with systemic toxicity of PPD had shown various clinical manifestations as well as biochemical histological changes (Table 3).

Deamination has been suggested as a mode of action of PPD, which results in the production of aniline, which may contribute in part to the toxic effects of the compounds (37). PPD induces one of the most striking experimental edema. PPD toxicity is due to altered vascular permeability and

Table 3 Frequency of Clinical Symptoms Observed in 171 Patients with PPD Intoxication in Morocco between 1991 and 2000

Edema	94%
Acute respiratory insufficiency	56%
• Tracheal intubation (72%)	
• Tracheotomy (21%)	
Signs of rhabdomyolysis	88%
Gastrointestinal symptoms (abdominal pain)	53%
Oliguric acute renal failure	32%

Department of Nephrology, Intensive Care Unit, University Hospital Averroes, Casablanca, Morocco. *Source*: From Ref. 29.

involvement of the parasympathetic nervous system (38). Deamination and formation of aniline is claimed to be responsible in part for the toxic symptoms (37). At high concentrations and after a long period of exposure PPD produces cell death. This effect together with lipid peroxidation can be the cause of the production of superoxide and hydrogen peroxide by the auto-oxidation of PPD (39).

In a prospective study performed in the Khartoum Kidney Dialysis Centre and the Sheffield Kidney Institute, 19 renal biopsies out of a series of 23 patients with severe (39%), moderate (35%), and mild intoxication (26%) were studied under light microscopy. Glomerular injury observed in 94% of the biopsies in the form of hypercellularity, membranous proliferation, glomerular swelling, capsular droop and accentuated lobular architecture (40). Tubular lesions were found in 78.9% of the studied samples. Different epithelial necrosis is the most common lesion observed (78.9%) while tubular atrophy had been found in [15.8%] of the studied samples.

There is no specific antidote for the PPD. The early challenge threatening the patient's life is asphyxia due to edema of the upper respiratory tract and the airways. Tracheostomy is a life-saving measurement in this condition (35). Nasotracheal intubation was also proven to be effective (31).

ARF was found to be the second life-threatening effect. Hemo- and peritoneal dialysis had been used as a method of treatment with variable success (31,32,36,41).

Chinese Herbs

In 1991, physicians in Belgium noted an increasing number of women who presented with acute, often near end-stage renal disease following exposure to Chinese herbs at a weight reduction clinic (42,43). An initial survey of seven nephrology centers in Brussels identified 14 women under the age of 50 who had presented with advanced renal failure due to biopsy-proven chronic tubulointerstitial nephritis over a 3-year period. Nine of these patients had been exposed to the same slimming regimen delivered by the same medical clinic, consisting in a mixture of many substances such as appetite suppressants, a diuretic, and Chinese herbs (42). The prescribed Chinese herb, *Stephania tetranda*, had been inadvertently replaced by other herbs containing *Aristolochia* species. As of early 1999, a total of more than 100 cases have been identified, a third of whom have already undergone renal transplantation.

The pathogenesis of Chinese herbal nephropathy is incompletely understood. The plant nephrotoxin, aristolochic acid found in the prescribed mixture, has been proposed as a possible etiologic agent. Support for this hypothesis is provided by findings in animal models of disease (44–46). In one study, rabbits were given intraperitoneal injections of aristolochic acid (0.1 mg AA/kg 5 days a week for 17–21 months) (44). Histologic examination of the kidneys and genitourinary tract revealed renal hypocellular interstitial fibrosis, and atypical and malignant uroepithelial cells. In salt depleted rats, aristolochic acid induced chronic renal failure with interstitial fibrosis (45).

However, in addition to aristolochic acid, patients with Chinese herb nephropathy also received the appetite suppressants, fenfluramine and diethylpropion; these agents have vasoconstrictive properties (47).

Together, these observations suggest that the fast-developing chronic tubulointerstitial renal disease may have been caused by combined exposure to both a potent nephrotoxic substance, aristolochic acid, and to renal vasoconstrictors, fenfluramine/diethylpropion.

In one of the two studies showing a link between Chinese herbal nephropathy and carcinogenesis, an increased dose of aristolochic acid was associated with an enhanced risk of carcinoma (48). Tissue samples revealed aristolochic acid-related DNA adducts, indicating a possible mechanism underlying the development of malignancy. The presence of these adducts was noted in another report of two patients with urolithelial malignancy and Chinese herbal nephropathy (49).

Another possible factor is the abnormal function of p53, a known tumor-suppressor gene. In the second study showing a link between the nephropathy and carcinogenesis, all atypical cells were found to overexpress this protein, thereby suggesting the presence of a mutation in the gene (50).

Affected patients typically present with renal insufficiency with other findings that are typical of a primary tubulointerstitial disease. The blood pressure is either normal or only mildly elevated, protein excretion is only moderately increased (less than 1.5 g/day), and the urine sediment reveals only a few red and white cells. The elevation in protein excretion consists of both albumin and low molecular weight proteins that are normally filtered and then reabsorbed (51). Thus, tubular dysfunction contributes to the proteinuria.

The plasma creatinine concentration at presentation has ranged from 1.4 to 12.7 mg/dL (123–1122 µmol/L) (43). Follow-up studies have revealed relatively stable renal function in most patients with an initial plasma creatinine concentration below 2 mg/dL (176 µmol/L) (52). However, progressive renal failure resulting in eventual dialysis or transplantation may ensue in patients with more severe disease even if further exposure to Chinese herbs is prevented. The risk for progressive disease increases with the duration of exposure (52).

There is no proven effective therapy for this disorder, which typically presents with marked interstitial fibrosis but not prominent inflammation. An uncontrolled study suggested that corticosteroids might slow the rate of loss of renal function (53).

Since this group of investigators in Brussels published their experience (42,43,45,50,54,55), reports from many parts of the developed and developing world describe identical/analogous clinical cases (56–59). Of particular interest is the paper by Yang et al. (60) describing a number of patients with rapidly progressive renal failure and developing urothelial carcinoma associated with regular use of traditional Chinese herbs. Although the authors could not conclusively rule out the presence of aristolochic acid in the herbal medicines in question, their report strongly support the view that phytotoxins are responsible for interstitial renal fibrosis.

Herbal nephropathy deserves greater attention on the part of health authorities. Alternative "natural products" should be subjected to scientific testing that is no less rigorous than that required for conventional treatments. The recent experience of antemisinin (ginghaosu) is very relevant in this context (61). Indeed, after passing the necessary toxicological and pharmacological tests of the active ingredient, a herb used for over 1500 years in the traditional Chinese medicine for fever, turned out to be an excellent antimalarial drug. This is an outstanding example where traditional and modern medicines merge into a powerful medication for the treatment of an important disease worldwide.

REFERENCES

1. Seedat YK, Nathoo BC. Acute renal failure in Blacks and Indians in South Africa: comparison after 10 years. Nephron 1993; 64(2):198–201.
2. Sakuja V, Sud K. Acute renal failure in the tropics. Saudi J Kidney Dis Transplant 1998; 9(3):247–260.
3. Isnard Bagnis C, Deray G, Baumelou A, Le Quintrec M, Vanherweghem JL. Herbs and the kidney. Am J Kidney Dis 2004; 44(1):1–11.
4. De Smet PA. Herbal remedies. N Engl J Med 2002; 347(25):2046–2056.
5. Prakash J. Acute renal failure in epidemic dropsy. Ren Fail 1999; 21(6):707–711.

6. Pasricha CL, Lal S, Malik KS, Biswas PK. An outbreak of epidemic dropsy in a close community. Ind Med Gaz 1939; 74:133–136.

7. Sood NN, Sachdev MS, Mohan M, Gupta SK, Sachdev HP. Epidemic dropsy following transcutaneous absorption of *Argemone mexicana* oil. Trans R Soc Trop Med Hyg 1985; 79(4):510–512.

8. Bhende YM. Vascular changes produced by Argemone oil II-changes in rats given injection of the oil. J Post Grad Med 1956; 2:185.

9. Segasothy M, Swaminathan M, Kong NC, Bennett WM. Djenkol bean poisoning (djenkolism): an unusual cause of acute renal failure. Am J Kidney Dis 1995; 25(1):63–66.

10. Areekul S, Kirdudom P, Chaovanapricha K. Studies on djenkol bean poisoning (djenkolism) in experimental animals. Southeast Asian J Trop Med Pub Health 1976; 7(4):551–558.

11. Burdmann EA, Ando TH, Bennett WM. Personal observation, June 1993.

12. Stewart MJ, Steenkamp V, Zuckerman M. The toxicology of African herbal remedies. Ther Drug Monit 1998; 20(5):510–516.

13. Thomson S. Traditional African medicine: genocide and ethnopiracy against African people. Report to the South African Medicine Control Council, Gaia Research Institute, March 13, 2000 (pdf-copy: www.gaiaresearch.co.za/ tramed.pdf).

14. Venter CP, Joubert PH. Aspects of poisoning with traditional medicines in southern Africa. Biomed Environ Sci 1988; 1(4):388–391.

15. Stewart MJ, Moar JJ, Steenkamp P, Kokot M. Findings in fatal cases of poisoning attributed to traditional remedies in South Africa. Forensic Sci Int 1999; 101(3):177–183.

16. Popat A, Shear NH, Malkiewicz I, Stewart MJ, Steenkamp V, Thomson S, Neuman MG. The toxicity of *Callilepis laureola*, a South African traditional herbal medicine. Clin Biochem 2001; 34(3):229–236.

17. Zoratti M, Szabo I. The mitochondrial permeability transition. Biochem Biophys Acta 1995; 1241(2):139–176.

18. Vancompernolle K, Van Herreweghe F, Pynaert G, Van de Craen M, De Vos K, Totty N, Sterling A, Fiers W, Vandenabeele P, Grooten J. Atractyloside-induced release of cathepsin B, a protease with caspase-processing activity. FEBS Lett 1998; 438(3):150–158.

19. No authors listed. Hepatic and renal toxicity among patients ingesting sheep bile as an unconventional remedy for diabetes mellitus—Saudi Arabia, 1995. MMWR Morb Mortal Wkly Rep 1996; 45(43):941–943 (www.cdc.gov/mmwr/ PDF/wk/mm4543.pdf).

20. Park SK, Kim DG, Kang SK, Han JS, Kim SG, Lee JS, Kim MC. Toxic acute renal failure and hepatitis after ingestion of raw carp bile. Nephron 1990; 56(2):188–193.

21. Choi K, Park SW, Lee KJ, Lee HB, Han HJ, Park SK, Park HS. Grass carp (*Ctenopharyngodon idellus*) bile may inhibit the release of renal dipeptidase from the proximal tubules by nitric oxide generation. Kidney Blood Press Res 2000; 23(2):113–118.

22. Chugh KS, Sakhuja V, Malhotra HS, Pereira BJ. Changing trends in acute renal failure in third-world countries—Chandigarh study. Q J Med 1989; 73(272):1117–1123.

23. Sontz E, Schwieger J. The "green water" syndrome: copper-induced haemolysis and subsequent acute renal failure as consequence of a religious ritual. Am J Med 1995; 98(3):311–315.

24. Akintonwa A, Mabadeje AF, Odutola TA. Fatal poisonings by copper sulfate ingested from "spiritual water". Vet Hum Toxicol 1989; 31(5):453–454.

25. Manzler AD, Schreiner AW. Copper-induced acute hemolytic anaemia. A new complication of hemodialysis. Ann Intern Med 1970; 73(3):409–412.

26. Sarrel PM, Lindsay DC, Poole-Wilson PA, Collins P. Hypothesis: inhibition of endothelium-derived relaxing factor by haemoglobin in the pathogenesis of pre-eclampsia. Lancet 1990; 336(8722):1030–1032.

27. Hachim K, Badahi K, Benghanem M, Fatihi EM, Zahiri K, Ramdani B, Zaid D. Obstetrical acute renal failure. Experience of the nephrology department, Central University Hospital ibn Rochd, Casablanca. Néphrologie 2001; 22(1): 29–31.

28. Chugh KS, Jha V, Sakhuja V, Joshi K. Acute renal cortical necrosis—a study of 113 patients. Ren Fail 1994; 16(1):37–47.

29. Hamdouk MI, Suleiman SM, Kallel H, Bouaziz M, Moutaouakkil S, De Broe ME, Zaid D. Paraphenylene diamine hair dye poisoning. De Broe ME, Porter GA, Bennett WM, Verpooten GA, eds. Clinical Nephrotoxins—Renal Injury from Drugs and Chemicals. 2nd ed. Dordrecht: Kluwer Academic Publ, 2003:611–618.

30. Sir Hashim M, Hamza YO, Yahia B, Khogali FM, Sulieman GI. Poisoning from henna dye and para-phenylenediamine mixtures in children in Khartoum. Ann Trop Paediatr 1992; 12(1):3–6.

31. Bourquia A, Jabrane AJ, Ramdani B, Zaid D. Systemic toxicity of paraphenylenediamine. 4 cases. Presse Med 1988; 17(35):1798–1800.

32. Averbukh Z, Modai D, Leonov Y, Weissgarten J, Lewinsohn G, Fucs L, Golik A, Rosenmann E. Rhabdomyolysis and acute renal failure induced by paraphenylenediamine. Hum Toxicol 1989; 8(5):345–348.

33. Shemesh IY, Mishal Y, Baruchin AM, Bourvin A, Viskoper R, Azuri M. Rhabdomyolysis in paraphenylenediamine intoxication. Vet Hum Toxicol 1995; 37(3):244–245.

34. Saito K, Murai T, Yabe K, Hara M, Watanabe H, Hurukawa T. Rhabdomyolysis due to paraphenylenediamine (hair dye)—report of an autopsy case. Nippon Hoigaku Zasshi 1990; 44(5–6):469–474.

35. Yagi H, el Hind AM, Khalil SI. Acute poisoning from hair dye. East Afr Med J 1991; 68(6):404–411.

36. Charra B, Menebhil L, Bensalama A, Mottaoukkil S. Systemic toxicity of paraphenylene diamine. Works of the 6th Congress of the Arab Society of Nephrology and Renal Transplantation, Marrakech, Morocco, February 21–24, 2000.

37. Nott HW. Systemic poisoning by hair dye. Br Med J 1924; 1:421–422.

38. Tainter ML. The mechanism of oedema production by paraphenylene diamine. J Pharmacol Exp Ther 1924; 24:179–211.

39. Mathur AK, Gupta BN, Narang S, Singh S, Mathur N, Singh A, Shukla LJ, Shanker R. Biochemical and histopathological changes following dermal exposure to paraphenylene diamine in guinea pigs. J Appl Toxicol 1990; 10(5):383–386.

40. Hamdouk M. PPD nephrotoxicity. Paraphenylene Diamine (Hair Dye) Acute Systemic Toxicity. Thesis for Mmed Sci in nephrology. UK: Sheffield Kidney Institute, 2001:34–37.

41. Suliman SM, Homeida M, Aboud OI. Paraphenylenediamine induced acute tubular necrosis following hair dye ingestion. Hum Toxicol 1983; 2(4):633–635.

42. Vanherweghem JL, Depierreux M, Tielemans C, Abramowicz D, Dratwa M, Jadoul M, Richard C, Vandervelde D, Verbeelen D, Vanhaelen-Fastre R, et al. Rapidly progressive interstitial renal fibrosis in young women: association with slimming regimen including Chinese herbs. Lancet 1993; 341(8842):387–391.

43. Depierreux M, Van Damme B, Vanden Houte K, Vanherweghem JL. Pathologic aspects of a newly described nephropathy related to the prolonged use of Chinese herbs. Am J Kidney Dis 1994; 24(2):172–180.

44. Cosyns JP, Dehoux JP, Guiot Y, Goebbels RM, Robert A, Bernard AM, van Ypersele de Strihou C. Chronic aristolochic acid toxicity in rabbits: a model of Chinese herbs nephropathy? Kidney Int 2001; 59(6):2164–2173.

45. Debelle FD, Nortier JL, De Prez EG, Garbar CH, Vienne AR, Salmon IJ, Deschodt-Lanckman MM, Vanherweghem JL. Aristolochic acids induce chronic renal failure with interstitial fibrosis in salt-depleted rats. J Am Soc Nephrol 2002; 13(2):431–436.

46. Van Vleet TR, Schnellmann RG. Toxic nephropathy: environmental chemicals. Semin Nephrol 2003; 23:500.

47. De Broe ME. On a nephrotoxic and carcinogenic slimming regiment. Am J Kidney Dis 1999; 33(6):1171–1173.

48. Nortier JL, Martinez M-C, Schmeiser HH, et al. Urothelial carcinoma associated with the use of a Chinese herb (*Aristolochia fangchi*). N Engl J Med 2000; 342(23):1686–1692.

49. Lord GM, Cook T, Arlt VM, et al. Urothelial malignant disease and Chinese herbal nephropathy. Lancet 2001; 358:1515–1516.

50. Cosyns JP, Jadoul M, Squifflet JP, Wese FX, van Ypersele de Strihou C. Urothelial lesions in Chinese-herb nephropathy. Am J Kidney Dis 1999; 33(6): 1011–1017.

51. Kabanda A, Jadoul M, Lauwerys R, et al. Low molecular weight proteinuria in Chinese herbs nephropathy. Kidney Int 1995; 48:1571–1576.

52. Reginster F, Jadoul M, van Ypersele de Strihou C. Chinese herbs nephropathy presentation, natural history and fate after transplantation. Nephrol Dial Transplant 1997; 12:81–86.

53. Vanherweghem JL, Abramowicz D, Tielemans C, Depierreux M. Effects of steroids on the progression of renal failure in chronic interstitial renal fibrosis: a pilot study in Chinese herbs nephropathy. Am J Kidney Dis 1996; 27:209–215.

54. Cosyns JP, Jadoul M, Squifflet JP, De Plaen JF, Ferluga D, van Ypersele de Strihou C. Chinese herbs nephropathy: aclue to Balkan endemic nephropathy? Kidney Int 1994; 45(6):1680–1688.

55. Vanherweghem JL. Nephropathy and herbal medicine. Am J Kidney Dis 2000; 35(2):330–332.

56. Pourrat J, Montastruc JL, Lacombe JL, Cisterne JM, Rascol O, Dumazer P. Nephropathy associated with Chinese herbal drugs. 2 cases. Presse Med 1994; 23:1669.

57. Pena JM, Borras M, Ramos J, Montoliu J. Rapidly progressive interstitial renal fibrosis due to a chronic intake of a herb (*Aristolochia pistolochia*) infusion. Nephrol Dial Transplant 1996; 11:1359–1360.
58. Ono T, Eri M, Honda G, Kuwahara T. Valvular heart disease and Chinese herb nephropathy. Lancet 1998; 351:991–992.
59. Lord G, Tagore R, Cook T, Gower P, Pusey CD. Nephropathy caused by Chinese herbs in the UK. Lancet 1999; 354:481–482.
60. Yang CS, Lin CH, Chang SH, Hsu HC. Rapidly progressive fibrosing interstitial nephritis associated with Chinese herbal drugs. Am J Kidney Dis 2000; 35:313–316.
61. Vennerstrom JL, Arbe-Barnes S, Brun R, Charman SA, Chiu FC, Chollet J, Dong Y, Dorn A, Hunziker D, Matile H, McIntosh K, Padmanilayam M, Santo Tomas J, Scheurer C, Scorneaux B, Tang Y, Urwyler H, Wittlin S, Charman WN. Identification of an antimalarial synthetic trioxolane drug development candidate. Nature 2004; 430(7002):900–904.

7

Chronic Kidney Disease: Focus on Africa

Saraladevi Naicker
Division of Nephrology, University of the Witwatersrand, Johannesburg, South Africa
Aminu K. Bello and Meguid El Nahas
Sheffield Kidney Institute, University of Sheffield, Sheffield, U.K.

THE GLOBAL CHRONIC KIDNEY DISEASE PROBLEM

The global rise in the number of patients with end-stage renal failure (ESRF) requiring renal replacement therapy (RRT) constitutes a major medical, social, and economic challenge. There are currently more than a million patients on RRT worldwide. This prevalence is expected to double by 2010. Of note, 90% of patients currently treated by dialysis reside in high-income countries. This depicts a clear and direct association between gross national product (GNP) and availability of RRT (1,2). This is coupled with the attendant consequences of increasing cardiovascular morbidity in patients with ESRF; premature mortality associated with chronic kidney disease (CKD) makes it an alarmingly growing public health problem.

The global burden of CKD is heightened by the fact that patients suffering from ESRF (0.1–0.2% of the population of developed countries) are merely the tip of the CKD iceberg. In developed nations, enormous resources are spent on the provision of the increasing demand for RRT; in the United States alone around $18 billion annually with an expected 50% increase by 2010. By contrast, in the developing world, only a few countries can afford a comprehensive RRT program. Thus, in such countries as in most of sub-Saharan Africa, the diagnosis of ESRF amounts to a death sentence. This makes it imperative to develop and adopt preventive strategies towards curtailing the global ravages of CKD.

CLASSIFICATION OF CKD

The Kidney Disease Outcomes Quality Initiative (K/DOQI) of the National Kidney Foundation in the United States (U.S.) has released guidelines for the diagnosis and classification of CKD (3). CKD has been defined as structural or functional abnormalities of the kidney of at least 3 months duration, manifested by either kidney damage (most frequently detected as persistent albuminuria) with or without a decreased glomerular filtration rate (GFR) to a value less than $60\,mL/min/1.73\,m^2$ or a decreased GFR with or without other evidence of kidney damage (3).

K/DOQI stages of CKD:

- Stage 1: Patients with normal GFR, but some evidence of kidney disease as manifested by microalbuminuria/proteinuria, hematuria or histological changes.
- Stage 2: Mild CKD characterized by GFR of $89\text{–}60\,mL/min/1.73\,m^2$ with some evidence of kidney disease as manifested by microalbuminuria/proteinuria, hematuria, or histological changes.
- Stage 3: Moderate CKD with GFR $59\text{–}30\,mL/min/1.73\,m^2$.
- Stage 4: Severe CKD with GFR $29\text{–}15\,mL/min/1.73\,m^2$.
- Stage 5: Also known as renal failure (ESRF) with GFR $<15\,mL/min/1.73\,m^2$, where patient survival depends on a provision of RRT in the form of dialysis or transplantation.

EPIDEMIOLOGY OF ESRF IN SUB-SAHARAN AFRICA

The magnitude of the burden of CKD in sub-Saharan Africa is not accurately known; the vastness and diversity of the region, wars and unrest, the migration of millions of refugees from one country to another, inadequate numbers of trained medical personnel and the lack of regional and national registries are some of the factors that are pivotal in this region.

It is known that there is an increased incidence of CKD in Afro-Americans (4–7). Studies in Egypt (8) and East Africa (9,10) have suggested that CKD is at least 3 to 4 times more frequent in Africa than in more developed countries, with 1–5% of deaths in Egypt annually being due to uremia. Calculations from autopsy studies suggest that death from renal disease must be in the range of 200 per million of the population (pmp) (11). It is estimated that 2–3% of medical admissions in tropical countries are due to kidney disease (12). The annual new patient load for ESRF in North Africa ranges between 34 and 200 pmp (13), figures that are probably an underestimate for sub-Saharan Africa.

CAUSES OF CKD IN AFRICA

Most of the information available is based on hospital-based data. Publications and surveys acknowledge hypertension and glomerular diseases as the two major causes of CKD throughout the region.

Hypertensive Kidney Disease

Hypertension is common in the Black population in Africa (14–16), occurring in 21–25% of the adult Black population of South Africa as reported in two large surveys in the past two decades (15,16). Hypertension was reported as the principal cause of CKD in Nigeria, accounting for 61% of CKD in those patients where the etiology was known in a 10-year study (14). Hypertension was a major cause of CKD in Ghana (17), tropical Africa (18), East Africa (19), and in South Africa, accounting for ESRF in 32% of Blacks in an 8-year study (20) and 34.6% of Blacks in a 6-year study from the South African Dialysis and Transplant Registry (SADTR) involving 3632 patients (21).

Glomerular Disease

The milieu of chronic parasitic, bacterial, and viral infections results in an increased prevalence of glomerulonephritis (GN) and hospital admissions (0.5% in South Africa, 2% in Uganda, and 2.4% in Nigeria) for renal disease and nephrotic syndrome (22). Minimal change disease is uncommon in Blacks, with a preponderance of focal segmental glomerulosclerosis and membrano-proliferative lesions in Black children (23,24) and adults (25); chronic glomer-ulonephritis is therefore a major cause of ESRF in sub-Saharan Africa.

Diabetic Nephropathy

The prevalence of diabetic nephropathy is estimated to be 14–16% in South Africa, 23.8% in Zambia, 12.4% in Egypt, 9% in Sudan, and 6.1% in Ethiopia (26), and it is anticipated to increase. Diabetes mellitus accounted for 11% of patients with ESRF in Nigeria (14) and 9–15% in Kenya (19). Diabetes is listed as the third major cause of ESRF in sub-Saharan Africa in various surveys.

Others

Other renal disorders that are important causes of ESRF in sub-Saharan Africa are lupus nephritis, renal calculi, chronic interstitial nephritis, sickle cell nephropathy, renal tuberculosis, malarial, and HIV-associated nephro-pathy. In North Africa, and Egypt in particular, the nephropathies asso-ciated with hepatitis C virus (HCV) infection are a growing threat in view of the endemic nature of the infection in this country.

RISK FACTORS AND CKD

Susceptibility Factors

The susceptibility, initiation, and progression of CKD are all associated with risk factors. CKD including diabetic nephropathy often clusters within families suggestive of a genetic or familial predisposition. Genetic studies have suggested possible links between CKD and a variety of alterations/polymorphisms of candidate genes including those coding for the renin–angiotensin system (RAS) (27). Racial factors also play a role in the susceptibility to CKD as reflected by the high prevalence of hypertension- and diabetes-related CKD amongst African- and native-Americans in the United States (28) as well as Afro-Caribbeans and Asians in the U.K. (29). Males and the elderly may also be more susceptible to CKD. This would explain their higher prevalence in RRT programs.

Initiation of CKD Factors

In those susceptible individuals, triggering factors would initiate CKD. In the Western world, initiation factors include systemic hypertension, diabetes, obesity, albuminuria, dyslipidemia, and smoking. It is expected that many of these factors will affect an increasing number of individuals in the increasingly westernized societies of the emerging world including Africa.

Traditional Western Risk Factors

In the United States, the Multiple Risk Factors Intervention Study (MRFIT) studying over 300,000 males identified hypertension, obesity, and hyperlipidemia as major risk factors for the development of CKD (28). The Framingham Offspring Study studied 2585 individuals and noted that 9.4% developed CKD (30). Identifiable risk factors included increasing age [odds ratio (OR) = 2.36 per 10-year increment], GFR of less than $90 \, mL/min/1.73 \, m^2$ (OR = 3.01), increased body mass index (OR = 2.60), diabetes (OR = 2.38), smoking (OR = 1.42), and hypertension (OR = 1.57) (30). In Japan, the Okinawa study of over 100,000 individuals identified obesity, smoking and hypertriglyceridemia as predictors of the development of proteinuria (31). In this city, proteinuria (32) as well as obesity (33) also predicted the development of ESRF. The Washington County survey in Maryland, United States, prospectively followed 23,534 men and women over a 20-year period (34). Baseline blood pressure, cigarette smoking [hazard ratio (HR): 2.4 in men and 2.9 in women] and treated diabetes (HR: men: 5 and women: 10.7) were risk factors for the development of CKD (34).

Clearly, common risk factors appear to predispose to both renal and cardiovascular diseases in the developed countries. Early detection and prevention may impact on the outcome of both renal and cardiovascular morbidity and mortality. In developing countries, the risk factor profile for CKD may be determined by the extent of the westernization of the society. Westernized societies may be acquiring a similar risk profile to that of the developed world, with diabetes and hypertension leading the risk factors for CKD.

Infections

Additional risk factors are likely to affect individuals in developing countries. Among these, infections and poverty are two major factors. Developing countries continue to suffer from the burden of infectious diseases and infestations with associated renal insufficiency. The global burden of HIV with 40 million infected individuals (35), HCV (170 millions) (36), malaria (300 million cases/annum) (37), schistosomiasis (200 millions) (38) as well as tuberculosis (200 millions) (39) is compounded by the high incidence of CKD in affected individuals. CKD increases the morbidity and mortality associated with these infections worldwide. The growth in the number of CKD patients attributable to these infections and infestations may parallel the rising number of affected patients with these diseases worldwide. Detection and prevention of CKD programs in the emerging world have to bear the infectious disease burden in mind.

Drugs and Herbs

Many people in Africa consult a traditional healer/herbalist instead of/ before a Western-trained medical practitioner. Herbal ingestion accounts for many instances of acute renal failure in Africa. Mercuric chloride in skin lightening creams has been implicated in the pathogenesis of minimal change and membranous nephropathy in South Africa, Kenya, and Malawi (40). Currently in South Africa, traditional healers and herbalists are to be licensed and registered by the Health Professions Council; this should encourage only trained and skilled practitioners and thus minimize the problem of nephrotoxicity of herbs. In addition, university departments of pharmacy and pharmacology are collaborating with traditional healers and herbalists to identify the therapeutic ingredients in the herbal remedies.

Social Deprivation

Overcrowding, inadequate sanitation, poor nutrition, and chronic infections are considered to be factors in the high prevalence of chronic GN in developing countries. Low socioeconomic status entails a degree of poverty and deprivation levels often associated with limited access to health care among the population. This may constitute an additional and independent risk factor for the initiation and progression of CKD. In the various National Health and Nutrition Examination (NHANES) surveys (41), it has been pointed out that those who are socioeconomically deprived are disproportionately afflicted with a higher burden of CKD. This may reflect delays in diagnosis of conditions predisposing to CKD such as hypertension and diabetes and/or limited access to healthcare leading to poor management. There is little doubt that the socioeconomic conditions of many in Africa and most of the emerging world remain below those of better off individuals in the West. These individuals are likely to share the increased risk of CKD with deprived individuals in the West.

Progression of CKD Factors

Genetic and Racial Factors

CKD progression rate is variable and may depend on a range of factors. These consist of modifiable and non-modifiable factors. The non-modifiable factors involve genetic, racial, age- and gender-related influences. Genetic polymorphisms of a variety of candidate genes thought to be implicated in the progression of CKD have been reported. Racial factors may also influence progression, as for instance in the United States, African Americans are believed to have a faster rate of progressive CKD when compared to Whites. This may clearly impact on the nature of CKD in Africa. In many nephropathies, males have a faster rate of progression than females.

Blacks in South Africa have more severe renal disease: a study of 327 adults with primary GN showed membranoproliferative glomerulonephritis (MPGN) in 35.7%, membranous GN in 21.3%, IgA nephropathy in 0.8%, and minimal change disease in 10.7% of adults (25). The low prevalence of minimal change disease in Blacks was confirmed in a study of 74 Black and 56 Indian children with nephrotic syndrome (42): minimal change disease occurred in 13.5% of Black children and 75% of Indian children; membranous nephropathy occurred in 29.8% of Black and 3.6% of Indian children. A more recent study of 636 children showed an increase in the prevalence of focal and segmental glomerulosclerosis (FSGS) in Black children from 5% to 28.4% and from 1.8% to 20.6% in Indian children (43).

In a study of 394 patients from 1974 to 1981 in Natal, hypertension was reported as the cause of end-stage renal disease (ESRD) in 32% of Blacks, 24% of Indians, and 29% of Mixed race patients; glomerulonephritis in 25% Blacks, White, and Indians and 33% of Mixed race patients; analgesic nephropathy occurred predominantly in Whites, causing ESRF in 33% (20). In contrast, a study of ESRD predominantly in White patients in Johannesburg showed that glomerulonephritis occurred in 32%, analgesic nephropathy in 21%, and hypertension in 2% (44).

In a 6-year study of 3632 patients with ESRD, based on SADTR statistics, hypertension was reported to be the cause of ESRF in 4.3% of Whites, 34.6% of Blacks, 20.9% Mixed race group, and 13.8% of Indians, with 15.9% of essential hypertensives resulting in ESRD and 57% of these undergoing malignant change (21).

Hypertension is common in the urban Black population in Africa (14). Prevalence studies in the adult Black population of Natal showed that hypertension was present in 25% of urban Zulus, 17.2% of Whites, and 14% of Indians (15). The clinical pattern of hypertension in hospitalized patients takes a rapid course with uremia and death, frequently from cerebral hemorrhage. Malignant hypertension is an important cause of morbidity and mortality among urban Black South Africans with hypertension accounting for 16% of all hospital admissions.

Hypertension and Proteinuria

Most notable amongst the modifiable progression factors are systemic hypertension and proteinuria. It has long been established that systemic hypertension is the single most important risk factor for the progression of CKD (45). Studies have identified systolic, diastolic as well as mean arterial blood pressure as putative risks. A wide pulse pressure has also been implicated.

Proteinuria is often considered a reliable predictor of the rate of decline of renal function and a marker of the severity of CKD (3). Patients with persistently high levels of urinary protein excretion (>3–$5\,g/24\,hr$) have in general a much faster rate of progression of CKD when compared to those with mild or moderate proteinuria ($<3\,g/24\,hr$). Proteinuria may in fact be a risk factor for the progression of CKD as it has been implicated in the pathogenesis of tubulointerstitial scarring, inflammation, and fibrosis (46).

The Significance of Albuminuria and Proteinuria in CKD

Albuminuria is not only an early marker of CKD (3) and a predictor of its progression (47) but also a marker of increasing cardiovascular disease (CVD) in those with CKD, hypertension, and diabetes as well as among the general population (48). Considerable interest is now focused on the predictive value of albuminuria as a marker of CVD.

The Prevention of End-Stage Renal and Vascular End-points (PREVEND) study group in the Netherlands has shown that urinary albumin excretion is associated with the risk of significant renal abnormalities in a non-diabetic population (48). In addition, and perhaps of utmost importance, the study established a link between microalbuminuria and cardiovascular as well as all-cause mortality in the general population (48).

Albuminuria is well known to predict cardiovascular morbidity and mortality in diabetics (49). The overall mortality of some diabetic patients may be comparable to that of the general population in the absence of kidney involvement. On the other hand, in the presence of microalbuminuria, it increases by 6 to 8 fold.

In essential hypertension, the rate of decline in kidney function is shown to be proportional to the degree of microalbuminuria with a loss of GFR in microalbuminuric patients twice as fast as in its absence (50).

Metabolic Factors

Dyslipidemia is often a consequence of CKD, but a large body of experimental data suggests a role for hypercholesterolemia in the progression of CKD in diabetic and non-diabetic nephropathies (51). Clinical data also show an association between elevated serum levels of LDL-cholesterol and apolipoprotein B and a faster rate of decline of GFR (51).

Experimental data suggest a link between uric acid concentrations and the progression of hypertensive and toxic nephropathies. In humans, a link between hyperuricemia and the development of systemic hypertension, cardiovascular and renal diseases has been postulated (52).

Obesity

Obesity has been linked in a few studies to a faster rate of progression of CKD. This is particularly true of patients with IgA glomerulonephritis where increased body mass index is associated with a three-fold increased rate of ESRF (53).

Smoking, Caffeine, and Alcohol

Over the last decade, a number of studies have underlined the potentially harmful effect of cigarette smoking on the initiation and progression of diabetic nephropathy (54). Similar observations made in patients with non-diabetic nephropathies suggest a six-fold increase of progression to ESRF in heavy smokers (>15 cigarettes pack year) (55).

Experimental data have suggested a link between caffeine consumption and albuminuria (56). Alcohol intake, in excess of two drinks a day,

Table 1 Risk Factors for Chronic Kidney Disease

Non-modifiable factors	Modifiable factors
Older age	Systemic hypertension (I & P)
Gender (male > female)	Diabetes mellitus (I & P)
Race/ethnicity (African Americans, native Americans, Hispanics > Whites)	Proteinuria (P)
Genetics/familial	Dyslipidemia (I & P)
	Smoking (I & P)
	Obesity (I & P)
	Alcohol consumption (I)
	Infections (I)
	Drugs and herbs/analgesic abuse (I)
	Stones/obstructive uropathy (I)
	Low socioeconomic class (I & P)

Abbreviations: I, initiation; P, progression.

may also increase the risk of ESRF in patients according to a survey undertaken in the United States (57) (Table 1).

ADDRESSING THE PROBLEM

The infrastructure for health is inadequate or non-existent in many parts of sub-Saharan Africa. The challenge is to devise innovative solutions towards prevention and to train and retain its healthcare workers.

The Role of Screening Programs

Screening programs are integral components of CKD prevention programs in all parts of the globe. In order to identify patients at risk of progressive CKD, a number of screening strategies have been implemented over the years; some addressing whole populations, others focussing on those at risk of CKD.

General population screening approaches were carried out in Japan (the Okinawa Screening Program) (31), the United States (U.S.) (National Health and Nutrition Evaluation Survey—NHANES III) (41), the Netherlands (PREVEND Study) (48), and Australia [Australian Diabetes, Obesity and Lifestyle Study (AusDiab Study)] (58). This approach was also adopted in some emerging countries such as Singapore (59), India (Chennai screening program) (60), and Bolivia (61). The latter is an example of a collaborative initiative between a Western nephrologist (Professor G. Remuzzi) and colleagues in South America.

In Japan, the Okinawa screening program (31) was carried out in 1983–1984 and investigated over 106,000 adults who were subsequently followed up for 17 years. The study identified obesity, dyslipidemia, and smoking as significant risk factors for the development of albuminuria. It also identified proteinuria and obesity as major risk factors for the development of CKD.

The U.S.-based NHANES III was a nationally based health survey that recruited 15,626 adult participants. It determined the overall prevalence of CKD among the U.S. population at 11% (representing about 19 million U.S. adults). Of these, 3.3% had stage 1 CKD, 3.0% stage 2, 4.3% stage 3, 0.2% stage 4, and 0.2% stage 5 (41).

In Europe, the PREVEND study in the Netherlands involved about half the population of Groningen, comprising ~40,000 individuals in a cross-sectional survey. The main objective of this study was to determine the prevalence of microalbuminuria in the general population, especially in non-diabetic, non-hypertensive subjects (48). Seven percent of those evaluated were found to have albuminuria. Over a follow-up period of 3 years, individuals with the highest level of albuminuria were found to have the highest incidence of cardiovascular death (48).

In Australia, the Australian Diabetes, Obesity and Lifestyle (AusDiab) study investigated 11,247 participants from May 1999 to December 2000. The survey showed 11% to have significant renal impairment (GFR <60 mL/min) and about 3% were proteinuric (58).

In emerging countries, where whole population screening programs have been undertaken, a similar prevalence of CKD was revealed. The National Kidney Foundation of Singapore is carrying out a comprehensive program for CKD prevention, which was started in the year 2000 and currently involving over 450,000 Singaporeans (59). They have reported significant urinary abnormalities (ranging from 5% to 8% proteinuria and/or hematuria) among the general population (59).

In India, the Chennai community-screening program screened around 25,000 people and found 6% of them to be previously undiagnosed hypertensives and another 4% were found with diabetes mellitus (60). Intensive management of hypertensive and diabetic patients with readily available and cheap drugs in this community achieved target values of control in the majority of screened subjects (60).

In Bolivia, a 16% prevalence rate of asymptomatic urinary abnormalities (proteinuria, hematuria, leucocyturia) was found among the population studied for the early markers of CKD (61).

Other screening programs have targeted those at risk of CKD within the community. This is the case with Australian Aborigines (62) and the Zuni Indians in Southwestern United States (63). The inhabitants of the Tiwi islands are Australian Aborigines with a quarter of all deaths attributed to end-stage renal disease (ESRD). The Tiwi islanders' annual incidence of ESRF is around 2760 pmp (15 times the incidence in the general Australian population). In the Tiwi screening program, the overall prevalence of albuminuria was a staggering 55% (62). When followed up longitudinally, those with albuminuria had a heightened incidence of renal and cardiovascular deaths. Of note, intervention in this high-risk group with an angiotensin converting enzyme inhibitor reduced blood pressure, proteinuria, and the overall mortality (62).

The Zuni Indians have a very high rate of CKD predominantly due to mesangioproliferative glomerulonephritides and diabetic nephropathy, and 2% of the population has ESRF (a prevalence rate of 17,400 pmp) (63).

In 1997, the National Kidney Foundation (United States) initiated the Kidney Early Evaluation Program (KEEP) to identify individuals at risk of CKD and also to determine the prevalence of early stages of CKD among the at-risk population (elderly, diabetics, hypertensives and relatives of CKD patients) (65). So far, the KEEP study showed an overall prevalence of the different stages of CKD (albuminuria, hematuria, decreased GFR) of around 50% (65). Of these numbers, 26% had albuminuria and around 16% had been found with elevated serum creatinine concentrations and other asymtomatic urinary abnormalities represented just 3%.

The Primary Prevention Program at the Soweto Clinics in Johannesburg screened 795 high-risk patients (with hypertension and diabetes mellitus) for the presence of kidney disease; 35% were proteinuric (including 10% of patients with microalbuminuria). At the 6-month review, 60% showed benefit from ACEI and educational intervention, with improvement in systolic and diastolic blood pressure and glycemic control (66).

It is most likely that a targeted approach to identify those with CKD is most effective and would be most suitable for developing nations with limited resources. On the other hand, whole population-based screening programs for hypertension and diabetes are likely to be justifiable by the impact undiagnosed hypertension and diabetes are likely to have in the future on the incidence of CKD in these countries. Early detection followed by primary or secondary prevention would undoubtedly have major impact on the burden of CKD in these countries.

PRIMARY PREVENTION

Infections

Malaria

Chronic malarial infection, amongst other infections, is believed to play an important role in nephrotic syndrome and CKD in the tropics; a 12-year study of 272 children with nephrotic syndrome in Nigeria reported the presence of malarial parasitemia in 38.7% (67). Malaria is also one of the major causes of kidney diseases in Sudan. Much research is directed towards eradication of malaria globally, as well as public education directed at preventing the acquisition of infection.

Hepatitis B Virus (HBV)

Membranous nephropathy due to hepatitis B virus (HBV) was most common in children in endemic areas in Africa. In KwaZulu Natal, South Africa, the prevalence of HBsAg in urban, rural, and institutionalized children was reported to be 6.3%, 18.5%, and 35.4%, respectively (68). HBV-associated nephropathy is the commonest cause of nephrotic syndrome among Black children in KwaZulu Natal; membranous nephropathy is the commonest histological type, present in 43% of 306 Black children with nephrotic syndrome; 86.2% were associated with HBV antigens (69). In Cape Town, 46 of 63 children (86.7%) with membranous nephropathy were HBsAg positive and 80% were HBeAg positive (70); the prevalence of HBsAg in patients with GN other than membranous nephropathy was 10%. In a 14-year study of 70 Black children with nephrotic syndrome from Namibia, 29 (41.4%) were HBV carriers and 26 of them had membranous GN (71).

The HBV vaccine was introduced into the South African Expanded Program on Immunization in 1995; a recent survey showed that there was a significant decline in HBV-related renal disease, with no disease in children <4 years from 2001 and a significant decrease in incidence in children aged 5 to 10 years (72).

Hepatitis C Virus (HCV)

The prevalence of HCV is variable in Africa, with high prevalence rates reported in Egypt; 46% of hemodialysis patients, 47% of patients with chronic liver disease, and 41% of rural adults were HCV positive (73). Blood donors in Mansoura, Egypt, had a HCV infection rate of 16%; 50 of 303 patients with GN were HCV positive; MPGN was present in 54% and cryoglobulinemia was present in 54%, with HCV RNA demonstrated in 66% of these (74). HCV infection was not present in a study of 55 patients with primary GN in Natal, where 45% had type 1 MPGN (75). HCV antibodies were present in 4.8% of 84 hemodialysis and continuous ambulatory peritoneal dialysis (CAPD) patients in Natal, against a 0.2–0.7% prevalence rate in the blood donor population of Natal (76). This is in contrast with a prevalence rate of 21% in 103 hemodialysis patients in the Western Cape, with a blood donor HCV antibody prevalence rate of 0.6–1.2% in the different racial groups (77); HCV antibodies were present in 7.4% of 108 renal allograft recipients in the Western Cape (78). Blood donors in Kenya had an HCV prevalence rate of 0.9%, with 6.3% of transplant patients and 2.6% of patients with chronic hepatitis testing positive (79).

Human Immunodeficiency Virus (HIV)

HIV-associated nephropathy (HIVAN) has been reported as the third major cause of ESRD in Black males aged 24 to 60 in the USRDS (80). A prospective study of 617 patients in Durban in South Africa showed that proteinuria occurred in 6% with HIVAN in 86% of proteinuric subjects, including 85% of those with microalbuminuria (81). Renal disease was present in 51.8% of patients with acquired immunodeficiency syndrome (AIDS) in a study of 79 patients in Nigeria (82). Much effort in Africa and elsewhere is directed at preventing the acquisition of HIV infection by massive public education campaigns, with a reported decline in HIV infection rates in some regions; in addition, antiretrovirals are becoming available at low cost for those who have acquired HIV infections and is anticipated to impact on HIV-related renal disease.

Systemic Hypertension

Systemic hypertension is one of the most important risk factors in the development and progression of CKD. Hypertension is increasing in an epidemic fashion in the population. A growing body of evidence strongly supports the application of lifestyle modification measures in blood pressure (BP) reduction (83). Some of the common lifestyle measures include increased physical activity (exercise) that is associated with lowering of BP independent of other factors. A meta-analysis of 27 randomized trials showed a 4-mmHg net reduction in systolic BP among the subjects exposed to aerobic exercise interventions (84). Another potential benefit of increased physical activity is towards preventing obesity and thus further prevention of hypertension.

A reduced salt consumption is also a key strategy in preventing high BP. This has been shown in a large body of experimental, epidemiological, and clinical evidence. The Trials of Hypertension Prevention Collaborative study has documented the beneficial effects of reduced salt intake in preventing hypertension by about 20% (85). Similarly, it has also been pointed out in the Trials of Non-Pharmacologic Interventions in the Elderly (TONE) that a reduced salt intake independent of weight loss was effective in lowering BP among the elderly subjects studied (86). In the two trials, the total salt (sodium chloride) intake was 6 g/day and thus provided the evidence-base for recommending about 100 mmol/day of salt intake (an equivalent of 6 g/day). But in the dietary approaches to stop hypertension (DASH) study (87), a further reduction in salt intake to 60 mmol/day produced a marked reduction in BP in both hypertensive and non-hypertensive subjects. Further, the DASH study has also shown these effects of salt reduction to be more effective in Blacks than Whites. This may be of significant application among the dwellers of sub-Saharan Africa. The strategies in this direction will involve a marked determination amongst individuals and the food-manufacturing sector to reduce the amount of salt added to cooked and manufactured food substances.

All major studies linking obesity and high BP have shown unequivocally that weight reduction lowers BP (88,89). Moderate alcohol intake and increasing potassium intake has also been shown to be effective in this direction.

Diabetes Mellitus

By the end of the last century, about 151 million persons were estimated to be affected with diabetes mellitus, and it is a leading cause of ESRF worldwide (90,91). The prevention of diabetes will therefore go a long way to reduce the incidence of ESRF due to diabetes.

In South Africa, it is currently estimated that there are 4 million diabetics; however, the burden of diabetic nephropathy is not known. Microvascular complications were studied in 219 patients who had long-standing diabetes mellitus. Persistent proteinuria was present in 25% of Blacks and 18.2% of Indians and almost 40% had a fall in GFR (92).

Increasing evidence suggest that lifestyle modification such as weight reduction, exercise and dietary manipulations can be effective and protective. Findings from the Diabetes Prevention Program (DPP) study demonstrated that diabetes could be prevented or delayed substantially in those at risk by appropriate lifestyle intervention and/or drug treatment (93). In this study, the incidence of diabetes was reduced by 58% through lifestyle interventions and by 31% by treatment with biguanide–metformin in comparison with placebo (93). Most interesting in this study is the generalizabilty of their findings to all racial and ethnic groups, and therefore applicable to sub-Saharan Africa.

The Finnish Diabetes Prevention Study (94) was the first randomized controlled trial to show that lifestyle intervention (weight reduction, decreased fat intake, moderate exercise) could decrease the onset of type 2 diabetes significantly in individuals with abnormal glucose tolerance. From the foregoing, it can be inferred that primary prevention of diabetes by lifestyle modifications is feasible and affordable and can even be carried out in primary care settings with the most basic of facilities.

SECONDARY PREVENTION

There are a lot of established and evidence-based measures of intervention to guard against the progression of established chronic nephropathies as discussed below (Table 2).

Systemic Hypertension and Proteinuria Control

The control of hypertension is the single most important intervention to reduce both albuminuria/proteinuria and to prevent the subsequent development of CKD in both diabetic and non-diabetic nephropathies. It is therefore imperative to aim at early and aggressive reduction of blood pressure in hypertensive patients with CKD. In those, the target blood pressure levels should be less than 130/80 mmHg in the absence of diabetes or proteinuria and <125/75 mmHg in diabetic patients and those with proteinuria in excess of 1 g/24 hour.

These recommendations are based on the Modification of Diet in Renal Disease (MDRD) trial, where it has been shown that strict control of blood pressure could delay time to ESRF by about 1.24 years over a period of 9.4 years (95). In this study, it was confirmed that the rate of progression of CKD was proportional to the severity of proteinuria. This study also showed that the target blood pressure values of those with heavy proteinuria (>3 g/24 hr) should be much lower (MAP ~92 mmHg) than that of those with lower levels of proteinuria (MAP <97 mmHg) in order to achieve a comparable, and slower, rate of decline of GFR.

It has been suggested that in addition to controlling hypertension, the inhibition of the renin angiotensin system (RAS) was essential to the prevention of progressive CKD (96). This may due to the impact angiotensin II has on proteinuria but also on the many other putative actions of these autacoids, including renal pro-inflammatory and pro-fibrotic influences (46). Consequently, numerous studies undertaken in the developed nations have stressed the superiority of ACE inhibitors/ARBs over other antihypertensive

Table 2 Management of CKD: Targets and Interventions

Parameter	Target	Intervention
Blood pressure control		
Proteinuria: none or <1 g/day	<130/80 mmHg (MAP—92 mmHg)	1st step: initially with an ACE inhibitor
>1 g/day	<125/75 mmHg (MAP—90 mmHg)	2nd step: DSR/diuretic
		3rd step: ARB
		4th step: NDHCA
		5th step: alpha-blocker
Proteinuria	<1 g/day	As above using ACE inhibitors
Dyslipidemia	Total cholesterol < 200 mg/dL (5 mmol/L)	Statin (HMG-CoA reductase inhibitor)
	LDL cholesterol < 120 mg/dL (2.2 mmol/L)	
Diet	Moderate protein restriction	0.6–0.75 g/kg/day
	Low salt	4–6 g sodium chloride intake
	Low phosphate	600–800 mmol of phosphate/day
Glycaemic control in diabetes mellitus	HbA1c < 8%	Effective control with diet, oral hypoglycemic agents and/or insulin as appropriate
Smoking	STOP	
Alcohol consumption	Moderate	Restriction to less than 2 drinks/day

Abbreviations: ACE, angiotensin-converting enzyme; ARB, angiotensin-receptor blocker; DSR, dietary salt restriction; NDHCA, non-dihydropyidine calcium antagonist; MAP, mean arterial blood pressure; LDL, low-density lipoprotein; HbA$_1$C, glycated hemoglobin; HMG-CoA, Hydroxymethyl glutaryl CoA.

agents regarding their antiproteinuric and reno-protective effects (45). It could be argued that the majority of these studies were conducted in the Western world with different population characteristics from those of sub-Saharan Africa. However, the African-American Study of Kidney Disease and Hypertension (AASK) confirmed the reno-protective effects of ACEi in Blacks with hypertensive nephropathy, a group previously considered poor responders (97).

Dyslipidemia

Lipid reduction with HMG CoA reductase inhibitors (statins) and other agents has been shown to be protective in experimental models of CKD.

Recent experimental data showed that the statin's effect may be synergistic with the reno-protection provided by ACEi and ARBs (98). Statins have additional effects including anti-inflammatory and antifibrotic influences. In patients with CKD, a systematic review showed that lipid lowering might have a beneficial impact on the rate of progression of CKD (99). Statins are also well established in reducing cardiovascular morbidity and mortality beyond reduction in serum cholesterol.

Smoking

Whilst the effect of cigarette smoking on progressive CKD is becoming increasingly acknowledged, randomized clinical trials supporting such assumptions are still lacking (100). However, it is expected that cessation of smoking will have favorable effects on blood pressure control and benefit individuals at risk of renal as well as cardiovascular diseases. Thus, stopping smoking should be an integral component of retarding CKD progression strategies.

Multiple Therapy Strategy

In the current perspective, the concept of multiple drug therapy is receiving attention after a meta-analysis of over 750 trials involving around 400,000 participants suggested that up to 80% reduction in CVD events can be achieved by a combination treatment with a polypill containing ACE inhibitors, statins, and other cardio-protective agents such as aspirin and vitamins (101). This therapeutic approach can be adopted in the future in some patients with progressive CKD. This may turn out to be a pragmatic and cost-effective approach to reduce the global burden of CKD and the associated CVDs.

MANAGING ESTABLISHED CKD/ESRF

The reality is that there is not enough money for health care in the developing world, especially for expensive and chronic treatment such as renal replacement therapy (RRT). The recently published National Kidney Foundation—Kidney/Dialysis Outcomes Quality Initiative (NKF/K/DOQI) guidelines provide a clear definition, classification, and risk stratification for chronic kidney disease (3). This provides an important framework that should be adopted in management protocols to better identify patients at risk for ESRD and to enable the timeous initiation of intervention strategies aimed at prevention of kidney failure. This is particularly important in developing countries, where limited resources preclude access to RRT in the majority of ESRD patients. Adequate anemia management is important in the CKD patient to prevent cardiovascular morbidity and mortality. Recombinant erythropoietin is an expensive agent and unaffordable for the prevention of anemia in the pre-ESRF patient in many parts of sub-Saharan

Africa. A similar situation exists with the availability and affordability of vitamin D agents and analogues.

Renal Replacement Therapy Options and Availability

Poverty and the high cost of dialysis and transplantation are a problem for the majority of the population of sub-Saharan Africa. The availability of renal replacement therapy is very limited in much of sub-Saharan Africa; in the absence of state funding, therapy is available to patients with medical insurance, employment, or independent financial means. In addition, dialysis facilities are available only in the capital cities in those countries. The exception is South Africa, where the state funds RRT for patients without financial means, if they are eligible for renal transplantation. The majority of African countries offer hemodialysis only; peritoneal dialysis is available in South Africa (about 40% of the dialysis population), Nigeria, Kenya, Cote d'Ivoire, the Democratic Republic of Congo, Congo Republic, Senegal, Zimbabwe, Sudan, Namibia, and Botswana, as well as the countries of North Africa.

Transplantation

Renal transplantation is even more limited in sub-Saharan Africa. Living donor and cadaveric renal transplantation is available in South Africa and Tunisia; living donor transplantation is available in Nigeria, Kenya, and Sudan, and the North African countries. Limited numbers of patients from other countries go abroad for a transplant, with the follow-up and immunosuppression then being carried out in the home country.

RECOMMENDATIONS

The challenge of prevention of progressive CKD in Africa and other developing regions requires a multipronged approach.

1. A priority is a registry to accurately define the magnitude of the problem posed by CKD, requiring governmental, institutional, and global support.
2. Efforts should be made to optimize therapy of hypertension, diabetes mellitus, renal disease, and renal failure; partnerships with pharmaceutical companies are essential to make the reno-protective agents affordable for developing countries.
3. In areas where there are insufficient numbers of physicians and nurses, other allied health workers and members of the public (as in Chennai, India) (60) could be trained to manage these conditions at a local level, with clearly defined criteria for referral of patients.

4. Screen for hypertension and diabetes mellitus at primary health-care level; screening and follow-up of hypertensive and diabetic patients for proteinuria; implementation of recommended targets for control of hypertension and diabetes.
5. Education of patients and healthcare workers with regards to hypertension, diabetes, obesity, and proteinuria.
6. *Public health measures*: Stop/ban smoking in public places, as in South Africa. Promote prudent diet and exercise. Promote a healthy lifestyle from an early age, beginning at primary school.
7. HBV vaccine to be administered widely in endemic areas and to high-risk populations.
8. Governmental support of prevention programs, together with global and other partners.
9. Patients with renal disease should be referred to a nephrologist at an early stage so as to institute measures to retard progression and plan timely transplantation and/or dialysis; this is particularly important where related donors may be available, as a cost-effective strategy.

REFERENCES

1. Lysaght MJ. Maintenance dialysis population dynamics: current trends and long-term implications. J Am Soc Nephrol 2002; 13:37–40.
2. Xue JL, Ma JZ, Louis TA, Collins AJ. Forecast of the number of patients with end-stage renal disease in United States to the year 2010. J Am Soc Nephrol 2001; 12:2753–2758.
3. Anonymous. K/DOQI clinical practice guidelines for chronic kidney disease, evaluation classification and stratification. Kidney disease outcome quality initiative. Am J Kidney Dis 2002; 39(suppl 2):S1–S266.
4. Easterling RE. Racial factors in the evidence and causation of end-stage renal disease. Trans Am Soc Artif Internal Organs 1977; 23:28–33.
5. Mausner JS, Clark JK, Coles BI, Menduke H. An area wide survey of treated end-stage renal disease. Am J Pub Health 1978; 68:166–169.
6. Rostand SG, Kirk KA, Rutsky E, Pate BA. Racial differences in the incidence and treatment of end stage renal disease. N Engl J Med 1982; 306:1276–1279.
7. Trivedi HS, Pang MM. Discrepancy in the epidemiology of nondiabetic chronic renal insufficiency and end stage renal disease in black and white Americans: the Third National Health and Nutrition Examination Survey and United States Renal Data System. Am J Nephrol 2003; 23(6):448–457.
8. Barsoum RS, Rihan ZE, Ibrahim AS, Lebstein A. Long term intermittent haemodialysis in Egypt. Bull World Health Org 1974; 51:647–654.
9. Abdulla K. Chronic renal failure in Northern Iraq. Iraqi Med J 1979; 27:43–46.
10. Abdullah MS. Development of renal services in Kenya. East Afr Med J 1981; 30:9–10.

11. Barsoum RS. Ethical problems in dialysis and transplantation: Africa. Kjellstrand CM, Dosseter JB, eds. Ethical Problems in Dialysis and Transplantation. Dordrecht, The Netherlands: Kluwer Academic Publishers, 1992:169–182.

12. Naicker S. End stage renal disease in sub-Saharan and South Africa. Kidney Int 2003; 63(suppl 83):S119–S122.

13. Barsoum RS. Renal disease in indigenous populations: North Africa. Nephrology 1998; 4:S29–S32.

14. Mabayoje MO, Bamgboye EL, Odutola TA, Mabadeje AF. Chronic renal failure at the Lagos University Teaching Hospital: a 10 year review. Transplant Proc 1992; 24:1851–1852.

15. Seedat YK. Race, environment and blood pressure: the South African experience. J Hypertens 1998; 1:7–12.

16. Steyn K, Gaziano TA, Bradshaw D, Laubscher R, Fourie J. Hypertension in South African adults: results from the Demographic and Health Survey, 1998. J Hypertens 2001; 19:1717–1725.

17. Plange-Rhule J, Phillips R, Acheampong JW, Saggar-Mallik AK, Cappucio FB, Eastwood JB. Hypertension and renal failure in Kumasi, Ghana. J Hum Hypertens 1999; 13(1):37–40.

18. Nseka M, Tshiani KA. Chronic renal failure in tropical Africa. East Afr Med J 1989; 66:109–114.

19. McLigeyo SO, Kayima JK. Evolution of nephrology in East Africa in the last seventy years—studies and practice. East Afr Med J 1993; 70:362–368.

20. Seedat YK, Naicker S, Rawat R, Parsoo I. Racial differences in the causes of end stage renal failure in Natal. South Afr Med J 1984; 65:956–958.

21. Veriawa Y, du Toit E, Lawley CG, Milne FJ, Reinach SG. Hypertension as a cause of end stage renal failure in South Africa. J Hypertens 1990; 4:379–383.

22. Seedat YK. Ethnicity, hypertension, coronary artery disease and renal diseases in South Africa. Ethnicity Health 1996; 1:349–357.

23. Abdurrahman MB, Babaoye FA, Aikhionbare HA. Childhood renal disorders in Nigeria. Pediatr Nephrol 1990; 4(1):88–93.

24. Adhikari M, Bhimma R, Coovadia HM. Focal segmental glomerulosclerosis in children from KwaZulu/Natal, South Africa. Clin Nephrol 2001; 55:16–24.

25. Seedat YK, Nathoo BC, Parag KB, Naiker IP, Ramsaroop R. IgA nephropathy in Blacks and Indians of Natal. Nephron 1988; 50:137–141.

26. Amos AF, McCarty DJ, Zimmet P. The rising global burden of diabetes and its complications. Estimates and projections to the year 2010. Diabet Med 1997; 14:S7–S85.

27. Locatelli F, Del Vecchio L. Natural history and factors affecting the progression of chronic renal failure. El Nahas AM, Anderson S, Harris KPG, eds. Mechanism and Management of Progressive Renal Failure. London: Oxford University Press, 2000:20–79.

28. Klag MJ, Whelton PK, Randall BL, et al. End-stage renal disease in African-Americans and White men: 16-year MRFIT findings. J Am Med Assoc 1997; 277:1293–1298.

29. Buck K, Feehally J. Diabetes and renal failure in Indo-Asians in the UK—a paradigm for the study of disease susceptibility. Nephrol Dial Transplant 1997; 12:1555–1557.

30. Fox CS, Larson MG, Leip EP, Culleton B, Wilson PW, Levy D. Predictors of new-onset kidney disease in a community-based population. JAMA 2004; 18:844–850.

31. Iseki K. The Okinawa Screening Program. J Am Soc Nephrol 2003; 7(suppl 2): S127–S130.

32. Iseki K, Ikemiya Y, Iseki C, Takishita S. Proteinuria and the risk of developing end stage renal disease. Kidney Int 2003; 63(4):1468–1473.

33. Iseki K, Ikemiya Y, Kinjo K, Inoue T, Iseki C, Takishita S. Body mass index and the risk of development of end-stage renal disease in a screened cohort. Kidney Int 2004; 65:1870–1876.

34. Haroun MK, Jaar BG, Hoffman SC, Comstack GW, Klag MJ, Coresh J. Risk factors for chronic kidney disease: a prospective study of 23,534 men and women in Washington County, Maryland. J Am Soc Nephrol 2003; 14: 2934–2941.

35. Joint United Nations Program on HIV/AIDS/World Health Organisation. UNAIDS/WHO Annual Report: AIDS Epidemic Update, Dec. 2003.

36. World Health Organisation. WHO/United Nation Global Population Hepatitis C Prevalence Report, 2000.

37. Wellems TE, Miller LH. Two worlds of malaria. N Engl J Med 2003; 349:1496–1498.

38. Chitsulo L, Engels D, Montresor A, Savioli L. The global status of schistosomiasis and its control. Acta Trop 2000; 77(1):41–51.

39. Drobniewski FA, Caws M, Gibson A, Young D. Modern laboratory diagnosis of tuberculosis. Lancet Infect Dis 2003; 3:142–147.

40. Swanepoel CR, Naicker S, Moosa R, Katz I, Suleiman SM, Twahir M. Nephrotoxins in Africa. De Broe, Porter, Bennett, Verpooten, eds. Clinical Nephrotoxins. 2nd ed. Dordrecht, Boston, London: Kluwer Academic Publishers, 2003:603–610.

41. Coresh J, Astor BC, Greene T, Eknoyan G, Levey AS. Prevalence of chronic kidney disease and decreased kidney function in the adult US population: third National Health and Nutrition Examination Survey. Am J Kidney Dis 2003; 41:1–12.

42. Coovadia HM, Adhikari M, Morel-Maroger L. Clinico-pathological features of the nephrotic syndrome in South African children. Q J Med 1979; 48:77–91.

43. Bhimma R, Coovadia HM, Adhikari M. Nephrotic syndrome in South African children: changing perspectives over 20 years. Pediatr Nephrol 1997; 11(4): 429–434.

44. Meyers AM, Furman KI, Botha JR, Milne FJ, Thomson PD, Louridas G, et al. The treatment of end stage renal disease at the Johannesburg Hospital: a 17 year experience. Part 1. The role of dialysis. South Afr Med J 1983; 64: 515–521.

45. Coles GA, El Nahas AM. Clinical interventions in chronic renal failure. El Nahas AM, Anderson S, Harris KPG, eds. Mechanisms and Management of Progressive Renal Failure. London: Oxford Univeristy Press, 2000:401–423.

46. El Nahas AM. Mechanisms of experimental and clinical renal scarring. In: Davison AM, Cameron JS, Grunfeld J-P, et al., eds. Oxford Textbook of Clinical Nephrology. London: Oxford University Press, 1998:1749–1788.
47. Jafar TH, Stark PC, Schmid CH, et al. Proteinuria as a modifiable risk factor for the progression of non-diabetic renal disease. Kidney Int 2001; 60: 1131–1140.
48. Hillege HL, Fidler V, Diercks GF, van Gilst WH, de Zeeuw D, et al. Prevention of Renal and Vascular End Stage Disease (PREVEND) Study Group. Urinary albumin excretion predicts cardiovascular and non-cardiovascular mortality in general population. Circulation 2002; 106:1777–1782.
49. Mogensen CE. Microalbuminuria predicts clinical proteinuria and early mortality in maturity onset diabetes. New Engl J Med 1984; 310:356–366.
50. Bigazzi R, Bianchi S, Baldari D, Campese VM. Microalbuminuria predicts cardiovascular events and renal insufficiency in essential hypertensives. J Hypertens 1998; 16:1325–1333.
51. Attman P-O. Progression of renal failure and lipids—is there evidence of a link in humans? Nephrol Dial Transplant 1998; 13:545–547.
52. Johnson RJ, Kivlighn SD, Kim YG, Fogo AB. Reappraisal of the pathogenesis and consequence of hyperuricaemia in hypertension, cardiovascular disease and renal disease. Am J Kidney Dis 1999; 33:225–234.
53. Bonnet F, Defrele C, Sassolas A, et al. Excessive body weight as a new independent risk factor for clinical and pathological progression in primary IgA nephropathy. Am J Kidney Dis 2001; 37:720–727.
54. Orth SR, Ritz E, Schrier RW. The renal risks of smoking. Kidney Int 1997; 51:1669–1677.
55. Remuzzi G. Cigarrete smoking and renal function impairment. Am J Kidney Dis 1993; 33:807–813.
56. Tofovic SP, Jackson EK. Effects of long-term caffeine consumption on renal function in spontaneously hypertensive heart failure prone rats. J Cardiovasc Pharmacol 1999; 33:360–366.
57. Parekh RS, Klag MJ. Alcohol: role in the development of hypertension and end-stage renal disease. Curr Opin Nephrol Hypertens 2001; 10:385–390.
58. Chadban SJ, Briganti EM, Kerr PG, Dunstan DW, Welborn TA, Zimmet PZ, Atkins RC. Prevalence of kidney damage in Australian adults: the AusDiab Kidney Study. J Am Soc Nephrol 2003; 14:S131–S138.
59. Ramirez SP, Hsu SI, McClellan W. Taking a public health approach to the prevention of end-stage renal disease: the NKF Singapore Program. Kidney Int 2003; 63(suppl 83):S61–S65.
60. Mani MK. Prevention of chronic renal failure at the community level. Kidney Int 2003; 63(suppl 83):S86–S89.
61. Plata R, Silva C, Yahuita J, Perez L, Schieppati A, Remuzzi G. The first clinical and epidemiological programme on renal disease in Bolivia: a model for prevention and early diagnosis of renal diseases in the developing countries. Nephrol Dial Transplant 1998; 13(12):3034–3036.
62. McDonald SP, Maguire GP, Hoy WE. Renal function and cardiovascular risk markers in a remote Australian Aboriginal community. Nephrol Dial Transplant 2003; 18:1555–1561.

63. Stidley CA, Shah VO, Narva AS, et al. A population-based, cross-sectional survey of the Zuni Pueblo: a collaborative approach to an epidemic of kidney disease. Am J Kidney Dis 2002; 39:358–368.

64. Maschio G, Alberti D, Janin G, Locatelli F, Mann JFE, Motolese M, Ponticelli C, Ritz E, Zucchelli P. The angiotensin-converting-enzyme inhibition in Progressive Renal Insufficency Study Group. Effect of the angiotensin-converting-enzyme inhibitor Benazepril on the progression of chronic renal insufficiency. N Engl J Med 1996; 334:939–945.

65. Brown WW, Peters RM, Ohmit SE, Keane WF, et al. Early detection of kidney disease in community settings. The Kidney Early Evaluation Program (KEEP). Am J Kidney Dis 2003; 42:22–35.

66. Katz I. Kidney and kidney related chronic diseases in South Africa and chronic disease intervention program experiences. Adv Chronic Kidney Dis 2005; 12(1):14–21.

67. Okoro BA, Okafor HU, Nnoli LU. Childhood nephrotic syndrome in Enugu, Nigeria. West Afr J Med 2000; 19:137–141.

68. Kew MC. Progress towards the comprehensive control of hepatitis B in Africa: a view from South Africa. Gut Suppl 1996; 38(2):S31–S36.

69. Bhimma R, Coovadia HM, Adhikari M. Hepatitis B virus-associated nephropathy in black South African children. Pediatr Nephrol 1998; 11:429–434.

70. Wiggelinkhuizen J, Sinclair-Smith C. Membranous glomerulopathy in childhood. S Afr Med J 1987; 72:184–187.

71. van Buuren AJ, Bates WD, Muller N. Nephrotic syndrome in Namibian children. S Afr Med J 1999; 89(10):1088–1091.

72. Bhimma R, Coovadia HM, Adhikari M, Connolly CA. Impact of HBV vaccine on HBV-associated membranous nephropathy. Arch Pediatr Adolesc Med 2003; 157:1025–1030.

73. Abdel-Wahab MF, Zakaria S, Kamel M, Abdel-Khaliq MK, Mabrouk MA, Salama H, Esmat G, Thomas DL, Strickland GT. High seroprevalence of hepatitis C infection among risk groups in Egypt. Am J Trop Med Hyg 1994; 51(5):563–567.

74. Sabry AA, Sobh MA, Irving WL, Grabowska A, Wagner BE, Fox S, Kudesia G, El Nahas AM. A comprehensive study of the association between hepatitis C virus and glomerulopathy. Nephrol Dial Transplant 2002; 17(2): 239–245.

75. Madala ND, Naicker S, Singh B, Naidoo M, Smith AN, Rughubar K. The pathogenesis of membranoproliferative glomerulonephritis in KwaZulu-Natal, South Africa is unrelated to hepatitis C virus infection. Clin Nephrol 2003; 60(2):69–73.

76. Soni PN, Tait DR, Kenoyer DG, Fernandes-Costa F, Naicker S, Gopaul W, Simjee AE. Hepatitis C virus antibodies among risk groups in a South African area endemic for hepatitis B virus. J Med Virol 1993; 40(1):65–68.

77. Cassidy MJ, Jankelson D, Becker M, Dunne T, Walzl G, Moosa MR. The prevalence of antibodies to hepatitis C virus in 2 haemodialysis units in South Africa. S Afr Med J 1995; 85(10):996–998.

78. Moosa MR, Becker M, Cassidy MJD. Hepatitis C virus antibodies in renal allograft recipients. Saudi J Kidney Dis 1996; 7(suppl 1):S141–S144.

79. Ilako FM, McLigeyo SO, Riyat MS, Lile GN, Okoth FA, Kaptich D. The prevalence of hepatitis C virus in renal patients, blood donors and patients with chronic liver disease in Kenya. East Afr Med J 1995; 72(6):362–364.

80. Szczech LA, Kalayjian R, Rodriguez R, Gupta S, Coladonato J, Winston J. Adult AIDS Clinical Trial Group Renal Complications Committee. The clinical complications and antiretroviral dosing patterns of HIV-infected patients receiving dialysis. Kidney Int 2003; 63:2295–2301.

81. Han TM, Naicker S, Ramdial PK, Assounga AGH. Microalbuminuria is a manifestation of HIV-associated nephropathy in South African HIV seropositive patients. Abstracts of the EDTA/ERA Congress, May 2004.

82. Agaba EI, Agaba PA, Sirisena ND, Anteyi EA, Idoko JA. Renal disease in the acquired immunodeficiency syndrome in north central Nigeria. Niger J Med 2003; 12(3):120–125.

83. Appel LJ. Lifestyle modification as a means to prevent and treat high blood pressure. J Am Soc Nephrol 2003; 14:S99–S102.

84. Whelton SP, Chin A, Xin X, He J. Effect of aerobic exercise on blood pressure: a meta-analysis of randomised, controlled trials. Ann Int Med 2002; 136:493–503.

85. The Trials of Hypertension Prevention Collaborative Research Group. Effects of weight loss and sodium reduction intervention on blood pressure and hypertension incidence in overweight people with high-normal blood pressure. The Trials of Hypertension Prevention, Phase II. Arch Intern Med 1997; 157: 657–667.

86. Whelton PK, Appel LJ, Espeland MA, et al. for the TONE Collaborative Research Group. Efficacy of sodium reduction and weight loss in the treatment of hypertension in older persons: main results of the randomised, controlled trial of nonpharmacologic interventions in the elderly (TONE). JAMA 1998; 279:839–846.

87. Obarzanek E, Proschan MA, Vollmer WM. Individual blood pressure responses to changes in salt intake: results from the DASH-Sodium trial. Hypertension 2003; 42(4):456–459.

88. Diaz ME. Hypertension and obesity. J Hum Hypertens 2002; 16(suppl 1): S18–S22.

89. Redon J. Hypertension in obesity. Nutr Metab Hypertens 2002; 11:S18–S22.

90. Zimmet P, Alberti KGMM, Shaw J. Global and societal implications of the diabetes epidemic. Nature 2001; 414:782–787.

91. King H, Auber RE, Herman WH. Global burden of diabetes, 1995–2025: prevalence, numerical estimates, and projections. Diabetes Care 1998; 21: 1414–1431.

92. Motala AA, Pirie FJ, Gouws E, Amod A, Omar MA. Microvascular complications in South African patients with long-duration diabetes mellitus. S Afr Med J 2001; 91(11):987–992.

93. The Diabetes Prevention Program Research Group. Reduction in the incidence of type 2 diabetes with lifestyle intervention or metformin. N Engl J Med 2002; 346:393–403.

94. Lindstrom J, Eriksson JG, Valle TT, et al. Prevention of diabetes mellitus in subjects with impaired glucose tolerance in the Finnish Diabetes Prevention

Study: results from a randomised clinical trial. J Am Soc Nephrol 2003; 14:S108–S113.

95. Peterson JC, Adler S, Burkart JM, et al. Blood pressure control, proteinuria, and the progression of renal disease. The Modification of Diet in Renal Disease Study. Ann Intern Med 1995; 123:754–762.

96. Remuzzi G, Bertani T. Pathophysiology of progressive nephropathies. N Engl J Med 1998; 339:1448–1456.

97. Hsu CY, Lin F, Vittinghof E, Schlipak MG. Racial differences in the progression from chronic renal insufficiency to end-stage renal disease in the United States. J Am Soc Nephrol 2003; 14(11):2902–2907.

98. Zoja C, Corna D, Camozzi D, Cattaneo D, et al. How to fully protect the kidney in a severe model of progressive nephropathy: a multidrug approach. J Am Soc Nephrol 2002; 13:2898–2908.

99. Fried LF, Orchard TJ, Kasiske BL, et al. Effects of lipid reduction on the progression of renal disease: a meta-analysis. Kidney Int 2001; 59:260–269.

100. Orth SR, Stockmann A, Conradt C, et al. Smoking as a risk factor for end-stage renal failure in men with primary renal disease. Kidney Int 1998; 54:926–931.

101. Wald NJ, Law MR. A strategy to reduce cardiovascular disease by more than 80%. BMJ 2003; 326:1419–1422.

8

Diabetic Nephropathy: Present and Future Challenges

Arrigo Schieppati and Piero Ruggenenti
Division of Nephrology and Dialysis, Azienda Ospedaliera Ospedali Riuniti di Bergamo—'Mario Negri' Institute for Pharmacological Research, Bergamo, Italy

Giuseppe Remuzzi
Department of Medicine and Transplantation, Asienda Ospedaliera Ospedali Riuniti di Bergamo—'Mario Negri' Institute for Pharmacological Research, Bergamo, Italy

THE GROWING BURDEN OF DIABETES MELLITUS

Diabetes is rapidly becoming a major global health problem. According to WHO estimates, the prevalence of diabetes will grow from the actual 177 million people to more than 300 million by year 2025 (1). Much of this increase will occur in developing countries and will be due to population growth, aging, unhealthy diets, obesity, and sedentary lifestyles.

By 2025, while most people with diabetes in developed countries will be aged 65 years or more, in developing countries most will be in the 45 to 64 year age bracket and affected in their most productive years (2). In many countries, even in developed countries, there are a large number of undiagnosed and improperly controlled patients with diabetes. People with diabetes are prone to both short- and long-term complications, which will be a tremendous increasing burden for healthcare systems of all countries.

Table 1 reports the estimates of the prevalence of diabetes mellitus in the world by regions. Data are made available by the International Diabetes

Table 1 Estimated Prevalence of Diabetes Mellitus by WHO Regions

Region	Number of patients with diabetes	Estimated prevalence (million people) (%)
Africa	2.5	1.1
Southeast Asia	49	7.5
Western Pacific	46	3.8
Europe	32	5.5
North America	21	7.8
East Mediterranean, Middle East	14	6.4
South a Central America	11	4.8

Source: From Ref. 3.

Federation's "Diabete Atlas" which reports either data by WHO regions and by individual countries (3). Diabetes affects some 49 million people in the Southeast Asian region, making it the largest region in terms of diabetic population, although the disease is not yet considered a problem with high priority in almost all the countries of the region. In the Western Pacific region lives 25% of the global population, 20% in China alone. The region also includes Indonesia with a population exceeding 200 million. The region has the second highest number of people with diabetes in the world with an estimated 46 million in the adult population. In the last three decades, the Eastern Mediterranean and Middle East have experienced significant social and economic changes, progressive urbanization, decreasing infant mortality, and an increasing life expectancy. In addition, the traditional ways of life in most countries have given way to adoption of Western behavior and lifestyle, reflected by the changes in nutritional pattern, increasing rates of obesity, and diabetes. There are an estimated 11 million people with diabetes in the South and Central American region. Type 2 diabetes is among the first 10 causes of mortality in the adult population. Africa has currently approximately 2.5 million diabetic patients, but this number is probably underestimated. Estimates from some countries suggest that the African diabetic population is bound to increase dramatically over the next few decades.

The global rise of diabetes prevalence is associated with the rising epidemic of obesity (4).

More than 80% of cases of type 2 diabetes can be attributed to obesity, which may also account for many diabetes-related deaths. The risk of type 2 diabetes increases with the degree and duration of obesity, diet, and the central distribution of body fat (5,6). Type 2 diabetes mellitus is strongly associated with obesity in all ethnic groups (7).

Weight gain precedes the onset of diabetes (8). Weight gain after age 18 years in women and after age 20 years in men also increases the risk of type 2 diabetes, and the excess risk for diabetes with even modest weight gain is substantial (9,10). Conversely, weight loss is associated with a decreased risk of type 2 diabetes (9). WHO estimates that there are more than 1 billion overweight adults, and at least 300 million obese people (4). The rising epidemic reflects the profound changes in society and in behavioral patterns of communities over recent decades. There has been a worldwide nutrition transition characterized by increased consumption of more energy-dense, nutrient-poor foods with high levels of sugar and saturated fats, combined with reduced physical activity (11).

These are the driving forces behind the increase of obesity rates that have risen three-fold or more since 1980. The obesity epidemic is not confined to industrialized societies, but is evident also in developing countries, where it coexists with malnutrition. In summary, the rise of obesity and diabetes prevalence are two different but closely linked aspects of a global epidemiological transition from communicable to noncommunicable diseases that is taking place worldwide.

DIABETIC NEPHROPATHY

Diabetic nephropathy is a chronic complication that develops in approximately one-third of all patients with diabetes. The cumulative risk of proteinuria, as a marker of renal damage, after 20 years of diabetes mellitus is approximately 30% in type 1 and type 2 diabetes (12,13).

The cumulative risk of renal failure, as defined as serum creatinine greater than 1.4 mg/dL, after 3 years of persisting proteinuria in approximately 40% in both types of diabetes and after 5 years of proteinuria is close to 60%.

It is the most frequent cause of end-stage renal disease in the United States, Europe, and Japan. In the United States, the incidence of diabetic nephropathy has increased by 150% in the past 10 years, a trend also seen in Europe (14,15). In North America, 40% of prevalent patients on dialysis in 2001 had diabetic nephropathy (14). Projection of the U.S. population shows that in the year 2030, the prevalent diabetic population under treatment for ESRD may be as large as 1.3 million patients (14). Actual costs for treating diabetic patients with ESRD in dialysis are 30% higher than for patients with a primary diagnosis of glomerulonephritis and 13% higher than for patients with hypertension or other diseases (14). There are limited data on the prevalence of diabetic nephropathy in developing countries. In Latin America, a renal registry that collects data from 20 countries with a population of more than 500 million people reports that the prevalence of diabetic nephropathy among ESRD patients is 33%, varying from 19% of Brazil to 49% of Mexico (16). In India, data suggest that diabetic nephropathy may be the cause of up to 41% of ESRD cases (17). Other Asian countries may have similar figures (14). It seems therefore reasonable, by extrapolating data from developed countries, to predict that diabetic nephropathy is going to be a major health problem of worldwide dimension. Parallel with the rise in the prevalence of diabetes mellitus, there will be a rise of diabetic nephropathy.

Diabetic patients on dialysis fare worse than nondiabetic patients. They have a 22% higher mortality at 1 year and a 15% higher mortality at 5 years than patients without diabetes (14). About half of this excess mortality can be attributed to cardiovascular causes. In a Canadian study, clinical and echocardiographic data were collected from a cohort of 433 patients with ESRD who survived for an average of 41 months (18). At inception of dialysis, diabetic patients ($n = 116$) had more left ventricular hypertrophy, ischemic hart disease, and cardiac failure than nondiabetics. After starting dialysis, diabetic patients had similar rates of progression of echocardiographic changes and new cardiac failure as nondiabetics, but higher rates of new ischemic heart disease, overall mortality, and cardiovascular mortality. This study confirms the impression that the burden of clinically manifest cardiac disease in diabetic patients starting ESRD treatment is huge. Indeed, in a random sample of 4025 patients with ESRD entering dialysis, the prevalence of coronary heart disease was 46.4% in diabetic patients and 32.2% in nondiabetics, a highly statistical difference on multivariate analysis (19). In patients undergoing coronary angiography in preparation for renal transplantation, the prevalence of coronary lesions is as high as 30–40% (20).

In diabetic patients, renal transplantation reduced the risk of acute coronary syndromes in comparison to dialysis treatment, although the risk is substantially higher than the risk of the nondiabetic population (21). In summary, diabetic nephropathy is a high-risk condition for cardiovascular and non-cardiovascular morbidity and mortality. Indeed, renal insufficiency by any cause has a significant impact on cardiovascular disease outcome. Among many others, it is worth mentioning two recently published papers. Investigators of the Valsartan in Acute Myoscardial Infarction Trial (VALIANT) identified 14,527 patients with complicated myocardial infarction who had a measured serum creatinine (22). They calculated the glomerular filtration rate (GFR) with the modification of diet in renal disease (MDRD) formula, and patients were grouped according to their estimated GFR. In these patients, the risk of death from cardiovascular causes increased with declining GFR. The authors concluded that even mild renal disease should be considered a major risk factor for cardiovascular complication after a myocardial infarction. The study of Go and co-workers (23) was conducted in a large population of more than 1 million adults within an integrated system of health care. In these people, serum creatinine had been measured, and GFR could be estimated by MDRD formula. After adjustment, the risk of death increased as GFR declined below $60 \, \text{mL/min}/1.73 \, \text{m}^2$. A similar independent graded association was noted between reduced GFR and cardiovascular events. The concern that kidney disease could be underestimated as

Table 2 Stages of Diabetic Nephropathy

Definition	Features
Normoalbuminuria	Albuminuria: $<30 \, mg/24 \, hr$, or $<20 \, \mu g/min$
	Normal or increased GFR
Microalbuminuria	Albuminuria: $30–300 \, mg/24 \, hr$, or $20–200 \, \mu g/min$
	Normal GFR
Macroalbuminuria	Albuminuria: $>300 \, mg/24 \, hr$, or $>300 \, \mu g/min$
	Declining GFR
End-stage renal disease	Kidney failure, need of renal replacement therapy

a risk factor for development of cardiovascular disease has been voiced by the American Heart Association, which has issued a scientific statement to recommend that patients with chronic kidney diseases are considered at the highest risk group for cardiovascular disease (24).

CLINICAL MANIFESTATIONS OF DIABETIC NEPHROPATHY

The first sign of renal involvement in patients with type 2 diabetes is most often microalbuminuria (urinary albumin excretion, $30–300 \, mg/24 \, hours$, or $20–200 \, \mu g/min$), which is classified as incipient nephropathy (25) (Table 2). Microalbuminuria affects 20–40% of patients 10 to 15 years after the onset of diabetes. Progression to Macroalbuminuria (urinary albumin excretion $>300 \, mg/24 \, hr$, or $>200 \, \mu g/min$), or overt nephropathy, occurs in 20–40% of patients over a period of 15 to 20 years after the onset of diabetes. Once macroalbuminuria is present, creatinine clearance declines at a rate that varies widely from patient to patient; the average reduction is $10–12 \, mL/min/year$ in untreated patients (13).

Blood pressure is usually normal in type 1 diabetes at the stage of normoalbuminuria, and increases only after the onset of microalbuminuria and with the progression of nephropathy (26). Most of type 2 diabetic patients with normoalbuminuria are hypertensive and blood pressure increases with the development of diabetic nephropathy (27).

FACTORS ASSOCIATED WITH DEVELOPMENT OF DIABETIC NEPHROPATHY

Clinical studies have found a link between a number of clinical or laboratory features and the risk of developing diabetic nephropathy. It is important to detect the factors since some of them are remediable and can direct preventive interventions. However, it should also be noted that none of these potential factors is as yet sufficiently predictive in the individual patient (Table 3).

Table 3   Risk Factors for Diabetic Nephropathy

- Duration of diabetes
- Familial and genetic factors
- Race
- Hyperglycemia
- High blood pressure
- Dyslipidemia
- Proteinuria
- Smoking

Duration

Diabetic nephropathy develops 10 to 15 years after the onset of the disease both in type 1 and type 2 diabetes. There are few studies showing that the incidence of albuminuria in patients with diabetes is below 10% during the first 10 years of disease, and then rises to 20% and 30% in the following 10 years (28,29). Duration of the diabetes is strongly associated with development of proteinuria in Pima Indians in whom the duration of diabetes is known with accuracy because they are systematically monitored for glucose tolerance (30). Sometimes, albuminuria is already present in patients with type 2 diabetes at the time when diabetes is found. In most patients, diabetes precedes the diagnosis of nephropathy by several years. In others, however, the development of microalbuminuria is close to the onset of type 2 diabetes, and in some cases it may even precede the disease (31). There are subjects with preclinical diabetes, in whom microalbuminuria is a feature of the metabolic syndrome secondary to decreased insulin sensitivity (insulin resistance) (32,33). Insulin resistance per se is at least in part genetically determined (34), and may predispose to the development of renal disease in diabetic people (35).

Familial and Genetic Factors

There are some studies suggesting that a predisposition to develop diabetic nephropathy may be inherited (36). An elegant study in Pima Indians showed that the chance of developing diabetic nephropathy was more than double in people whose parents were both affected by diabetic nephropathy as compared to people whose parents did not have nephropathy (37). Those patients with only one parent with diabetic nephropathy were somewhere in between. Other studies have shown that there is a definite greater risk for diabetic nephropathy in some families. Also, a family history of hypertension has been associated with an increased risk of diabetic nephropathy (38).

At the present time, the gene(s) responsible for determining diabetic nephropathy have not been identified, although several candidate genes have been proposed. In particular, attention has been focused on the renin–angiotensin system.

There is a growing body of evidence that maternal diabetes during pregnancy is associated with obesity in childhood and development of diabetes mellitus later in life (39). The association between low birth weight and increase lifetime risk of insulin resistance, or type 2 diabetes later in life, has been found (40,41). The disadvantaged people belonging to racial minority of developed countries, and the large population of poor of developing countries are particularly exposed to the risk of intrauterine growth retardation (42).

Race

The U.S. Renal Data System (14) and population-based studies (43,44) as well as intervention trials (45) found that compared with Caucasian, racial minorities in the United States are disproportionately affected by diabetes and have excessive risk of complication such as end-stage renal disease. Studies have shown that in African Americans and Hispanics microvascular complications occur more frequently, while macrovascular complications may be more frequent in Caucasians (46). In 2003, Young and colleagues (47) conducted a longitudinal cohort study, in 429,919 veterans with diabetes, to determine racial differences in the prevalence of diabetic nephropathy. After adjustment for age, sex, and economic status, African Americans, Asians, Hispanics, and Native Americans were also more likely to have diabetic end-stage renal disease than Caucasians. African Americans and Native Americans were also more likely to have early diabetic nephropathy than Caucasians (adjusted odd ratio: 1.3 for African Americans, and 1.5 for Native vs. Caucasians).

Burden and coworkers (48) noted that Asians in the United Kingdom had 14 times the incidence of diabetic end-stage renal disease as the Caucasians in the same region. In Australia, Aborigines in some remote areas have an incidence of end-stage renal disease (ESRD) of more than 500 per million or more and the proportion of people with diabetes as a cause of ESRD is 47% as compared to 17% of non-indigenous people (49). The observation that the risk of diabetic nephropathy is increased in such genetically disparate populations suggests that there could be primary role for socioeconomic factors, such as diet, poor control of hyperglycemia, hypertension, and obesity. However, the importance of genetic influences in the racial risk to diabetic nephropathy cannot be excluded. In the study mentioned before (47), even after adjustments to the increased incidence of hypertension and lower socioeconomic status in African Americans, there still appears to be a greater risk of end-stage renal disease due to diabetic nephropathy in African Americans than in Caucasians.

Hyperglycemia

An association between hyperglycemia and the development and progression of the microvascular complications of diabetes (retinopathy, nephropathy, and neuropathy) has been suggested from several studies. Originally suggested by a study in 18 patients with type 1 diabetes by Nyberg and colleagues (50), the association between high levels of hemoglobin A1c (HbA1c) and diabetic nephropathy was confirmed in a number of studies involving a large number of patients (51,52). The association has been confirmed in the prospective Diabetes Control and Complications Trial (DCCT) (53), in which patients with type 1 diabetes were randomly assigned to receive either conventional therapy or intensive insulin therapy. The mean HbA1c values during the 9-year study were 7.2% with intensive therapy as opposed to 9.1% with conventional therapy. The study showed that strict glycemic control could both delay the onset of microvascular complications (primary prevention) and slow the rate of progression of already present complications (secondary intervention). Intensive insulin therapy is also effective at a somewhat later stage, after microalbuminuria develops (54).

A meta-analysis of 226 patients with type 1 diabetes found similar results: in patients with no albuminuria or microalbuminuria, the odds ratio for increasing albumin excretion was 0.34 in patients receiving intensive therapy as compared with those receiving conventional therapy (i.e., the risk was reduced by approximately 66%) (55).

The role of hyperglycemia in the development of microalbuminuria in type 2 diabetes has been suggested by some studies (56–58). A retrospective study from Minnesota showed that hyperglycemia is a strong predictor of proteinuria in type 2 diabetes (56). The United Kingdom Prospective Diabetes Study (UKPDS) of patients with type 2 diabetes found that fewer patients treated with intensive versus conventional therapy had progression of microalbuminuria and proteinuria over 15 years of follow-up (57). The STENO group study compared two groups of type 2 diabetes, and showed that intensified multifactorial intervention in patients with type 2 diabetes and microalbuminuria slowed progression to overt nephropathy, and progression of retinopathy and autonomic neuropathy (58).

Hypertension

High blood pressure is closely related with kidney damage in diabetes. While patients with type 1 diabetes develop hypertension later in the course of the disease, a very large proportion of patients with type 2 diabetes (up to 50%) have high blood pressure even before they develop diabetes (59). Hypertension may be present for years at the time of diagnosis and precedes the development of diabetic nephropathy. In a study performed in Germany, blood pressure was measured in 92 patients with recent onset diabetes using ambulatory blood pressure monitoring; 57% of these patients had high blood pressure, according to WHO definition, while only 23% had a completely normal blood pressure (60).

High blood pressure significantly increases the risk of subsequent albuminuria. In a retrospective analysis, it was found that diabetic patients who subsequently developed albuminuria had more frequent and more severe high blood pressure in the pre-albuminuric period than patients who did not develop albuminuria (61).

Once kidney damage is established, hypertension is a strong risk factor for deterioration of kidney function. A close correlation between hypertension and rate of loss of kidney function has been documented both in type 1 and type 2 diabetes: patient who have high blood pressure experience a more rapid loss of glomerular filtration rate than patients with normal blood pressure (62,63). The experience of the Steno Diabetes Center in Denmark, with 301 type 1 diabetes patients followed for 7 years with yearly assessment of kidney function, showed that the loss of kidney function was directly associated with hypertension: those patients with higher blood pressure and also faster decline of kidney function (51).

Dyslipidemia

Abnormalities of lipid profile are often present in patients with kidney disease and are usually considered the consequence of kidney dysfunction. However, they can also play a role in causing and aggravating glomerular damage. Several studies in type 1 and type 2 diabetes have observed a correlation between hypercholesterolemia and the progression of diabetic nephropathy (56,59,63,64). In a small study, it was shown that patients with serum cholesterol levels higher than 7 mmol/L had a faster decline of glomerular filtration rate than patients with cholesterol below that threshold (the two groups of patients had similar blood pressure, albuminuria, and HbA1c) (65). The Steno Diabetes Center's study, mentioned above (51), showed that elevated serum cholesterol acts as an independent progression promoter in diabetic nephropathy.

In addition, it is important to remember that dyslipidemia remains a strong risk factor for cardiovascular complications of diabetes.

Proteinuria

Excretion of the proteins in the urine is a hallmark of kidney damage. Diseased glomerular capillaries let protein pass through their walls and spill into the urine. Recent animal and human studies have suggested that excessive urinary protein excretion is not only a marker of damage, but is also a promoter of progression (66). Increased glomerular permeability of proteins results in the accumulation of proteins in proximal tubular cells and may trigger the activation of vasoactive and inflammatory substances, which contributes to cellular proliferation and interstitial inflammation, ultimately leading to accelerated renal scarring and fibrosis (67). Indeed, patients with severe proteinuria have a faster rate of loss of kidney function (68). Proteinuria is also a powerful predictor, and a risk factor per se, of cardiovascular mortality in type 2 diabetes (69).

Smoking

Smoking is a strong predictor of kidney disease in type 1 diabetes (70). Also, heavy smoking increases the risk of developing type 2 diabetes by a factor of 1.9, and in diabetics who smoke more than 25 cigarettes a day, the risk of developing proteinuria is two times greater than in nonsmokers (71,72). Some studies have also suggested that heavy smoking can accelerate progression of diabetic nephropathy to ESRD (72). The mechanisms are not well understood; smoking increases blood pressure acutely and this rise in blood pressure may be responsible of some damage to glomerular capillaries.

THE ASSOCIATION OF NEPHROPATHY AND OTHER DIABETIC COMPLICATIONS

The presence of diabetic nephropathy is a bad prognostic sign in patients with type 1 and type 2 diabetes. Not only because they are at risk of ESRF and they may end up with chronic dialysis, but also because the other complications are exacerbated by the presence of kidney involvement.

Diabetic complications are often designed as microvascular and macrovascular in nature, since they are caused by alterations of small or medium or large arterial vessels of vital organs such as the retina, peripheral nerves, heart, brain, aorta, arteries of the limbs, etc. The relationship between diabetic nephropathy and other complications has been object of intense scrutiny by several investigators, and it has been concluded that diabetic nephropathy makes all those complications worse. Here they will be briefly reviewed.

Cardiovascular Complications

Microalbuminuria is associated with increased risk of cardiovascular complications in diabetic patients (73). The WHO Multinational Study of Vascular Disease in Diabetes (74) involved 1188 patients with type 1 diabetes and 3234 patients with type 2 diabetes, aged 35 to 55. Compared with patients with no proteinuria, all-cause mortality ratios were 1.5 and 2.9 for type 1 patients with light and heavy proteinuria, respectively, and 1.5 (1.2–1.8) and 2.8 (2.3–3.4) for type 2 patients in the WHO Multinational Study of Vascular Disease in Diabetes. Proteinuria was associated with significantly increased mortality from renal failure, cardiovascular disease, and all other causes of death.

The EURODIAB Prospective Complication Study (75) examined risks factors for coronary heart disease in 2329 type 1 diabetic patients and found a strong predictive value of baseline albuminuria. In the multivariate Cox proportional hazard models, the standardized hazards ratio for albuminuria was 1.64 in men and 1.33 in women. The Heart Outcome Prevention Evaluation (HOPE) (76) study involved more than 9000 patients. Albuminuria predicted an increased risk of cardiovascular endpoints in patients with or without diabetes, and the relative risk was higher for diabetic persons than non-diabetic (RR 1.97 and 1.61, respectively). A meta-analysis of 11 cohort studies representing a total of 2138 patients with type 2 diabetes confirmed a significant association between microalbuminuria and total and cardiovascular mortality, the overall odds ratio for death being 2.4 and for cardiovascular morbidity and mortality 2.0 (69).

A retrospective analysis on patients undergoing percutaneous coronary intervention (77) showed that on average diabetic patients were older, had more cardiovascular morbidity, and were more likely to have multivessel disease as compared to nondiabetic patients. Diabetics had also a higher chance of having another myocardial infarction or a need of additional revascularization at 5 years (77).

The Thrombolysis and Angioplasty in Myocardial Infarction (TAMI) trial included 148 diabetics and 923 nondiabetic patients in whom cardiac catheterization was performed at 90 minutes and 7 to 10 days after thrombolytic therapy (78). Compared to nondiabetics, the diabetic patients had a significantly higher incidence of coronary multivessel disease (66% versus 46%) and a greater number of diseased vessels.

Several risk factors for cardiovascular disease cluster in subjects with type 2 diabetes and microalbuminuria, including insulin resistance, hypertension, obesity, dyslipidemia, hyperuricemia, chronic inflammation, oxidative stress. All of them may be a manifestation of increased insulin resistance and independently contribute to the excess of cardiovascular morbidity and mortality in diabetic patients with microalbuminuria as compared with those with normoalbuminuria (79). In these patients, insulin resistance may be per se an independent risk factor for cardiovascular disease, and microalbuminuria may reflect a marker of widespread endothelial dysfunction that independently contributes to the development of micro- and macrovascular disease (80).

The risk of cardiovascular events is further increased in people with overt nephropathy. In these patients, the systemic abnormalities associated with overt proteinuria and decreased renal function, including more severe hypertension and dyslipidemia, coagulation abnormalities, hyperhomocysteinemia, anemia, deranged calcium–phosphate homeostasis, and hyperparathyroidism with secondary vascular calcifications, dramatically contribute to promote and accelerate macrovascular disease (81).

Patients with diabetes have an abnormal lipid profile. Serum low-density lipoprotein (LDL) and tryglycerides are increased while high-density lipoprotein (HDL) is reduced in diabetic patients (82,83). This lipid pattern is associated with increased cardiovascular morbidity and mortality. The presence of incipient diabetic nephropathy worsens the abnormal lipid profile, thereby increasing the risk of cardiovascular complications. As diabetic nephropathy progress to overt proteinuria and kidney insufficiency, changes in the lipid profile are exacerbated.

Retinopathy

Retinopathy is a severely invalidating complication of diabetes causing blindness in a large number of patients (84). Retinal lesions are divided into two large categories: background or nonproliferative, and proliferative retinopathy. Background diabetic retinopathy is a less severe form characterized by microvascular changes restricted to the retina that seldom influence visual acuity, and can ultimately be identified in virtually all people with type 1 and in a high proportion of those with type 2 diabetes mellitus (85). Proliferative diabetic retinopathy is a more severe disease characterized by ischemia-induced proliferation of new retinal vessels, affects up to 25% of type 1 and type 2 diabetic patients over 15 to 25 years of disease duration, and is a major cause of blindness (84). Diabetes duration (85), poor metabolic control (86), and high blood pressure (87) are risk factors for both forms of retinopathy and promote their progression over time. The association of retinopathy with nephropathy is particularly strong in type 1 (88), while is less well documented in type 2 diabetes (89). Some ethnic groups seem to be exposed to greater risk than others. In a clinical study that involved 815 type 2 diabetic patients, 144 of whom where Hispanics, Estacio and coworkers (90) found that, after controlling for severity and duration of diabetes, Hispanics had significantly more risk of retinopathy than non-Hispanic Whites (odd ratio 2.13). The presence of albuminuria, defined as urinary albumin excretion $>200\,\mu g/min$, was a predictor for retinopathy among the Hispanic (odds ratio 11.1, $p = 0.03$) but not the White patients.

Proliferative and nonproliferative retinopathies are characterized by abnormalities of the retinal microvasculature. The similarities between retinal capillaries and glomerular vessels, together with the close link between retinopathy and nephropathy, suggest that a common mechanism is responsible for both conditions.

Neuropathy

Diabetic patients may suffer from diabetic neuropathies. Chronic hyperglycemia is a major determinant of diabetic neuropathy (91), although microvascular disease and secondary ischemia and hypoperfusion also contribute to the development of this complication (92).

Peripheral neuropathy leads to numbness and sometimes pain and weakness in the limbs. Autonomic neuropathy causes problems in every organ including the digestive tract, heart, and sexual organs. There is a close relation between the duration of the diabetes and the onset of neuropathy. On the other hand, the relationship between diabetic neuropathy and nephropathy is less well established. One study has suggested, however, that neuropathy may play a role in damaging the kidney (93). In type 1 diabetes patients, the continuous monitoring of blood pressure for 24 hours showed that nocturnal drop of blood pressure observed in healthy individuals is attenuated, and on the average blood pressure remains higher than normal during the sleep (94). This loss of blood pressure regulation may be due to autonomic neuropathy, which may in turn contribute to the development of diabetic nephropathy. Symptoms of diabetic neuropathy may worsen with the progression of renal insufficiency and uremia may contribute.

PREVENTION AND TREATMENT OF DIABETIC NEPHROPATHY

During the last years, a great deal of knowledge has been gathered from clinical studies to indicate that it is possible to reduce the incidence and the rate of progression of diabetic nephropathy. In this chapter, we will summarize the available evidences and will provide a concise set of recommendation for prevention and management of diabetic nephropathy (Table 4).

Glycemic Control

Several studies have indicated that control of glycemia retards the development of diabetic nephropathy. The Diabetes Control and Complication Trial (DCCT) was conducted in type 1 diabetic patients under the aegis of the National Institute of Diabetes and Digestive and Kidney Diseases (NIDDK) from 1983 to 1993 and involved 1441 patients (53). A group of them was treated with a so-called intensive regimen for controlling blood glucose, which was kept around 150 mg/dL on the average, while a group of patients followed what was then the conventional therapy. There was a 50% reduction of diabetic nephropathy among patients in the intensive treatment group with normal albuminuria. However, this study showed that there was no advantage from intensive glycemic control in patients who were already albuminuric at the beginning of the study.

The United Kingdom Prospective Diabetes Study (UKPDS) was undertaken in type 2 diabetic patients and showed that intensive control of blood glucose with oral hypoglycemic agents or insulin reduces the risk of diabetic nephropathy and other microvascular complications, but not macrovascular complications (57).

In the subgroup of participants in the UKPDS who were overweight (defined as >120% of ideal body weight), the effect of the metformin in reducing the risk of kidney failure was similar to that of other hypoglycemic agents, but metformin resulted in a significantly lower risk of myocardial infarction than did the other agents (95). In another study conducted in Japan in type 2 diabetes, intensive glucose control with three or more insulin injections per day led to a lower rate of new or progressive nephropathy

Table 4 Management of Risk Factor in Diabetic Nephropathy

Risk factor	Treatment	Result of treatment
Hyperglycemia	Tight glycemic control with insulin, oral hypoglycemic agents, lifestyle modification	Prevent appearance of albuminuria, may delay progression of nephropathy
High blood pressure	Drugs: ACE inhibitors, angiotensin receptor antagonists, diuretics, non-dyhydropiridinic, calcium blockers, beta blockers Lifestyle modification: salt restriction, exercise, loss of weight in excess	Prevent albuminuria, delay progression
Dyslipidemia	Lifestyle modification Drugs: statins, fibrates (caution if renal failure)	May delay progression of nephropathy
Smoking	Stop smoking	May prevent nephropathy and delay progression

over a period of 6 years compared to conventional therapy (7.7% vs. 28%) (96). These studies have not established a threshold for glycemic control. However, the current practice guidelines of the most important scientific societies suggest that glycemic control should achieve an HbA1c level of less than 7% (97,98).

The impact of intensive metabolic control on the progression of renal insufficiency in patients with macroalbuminuria and declining renal function has been disappointing (99,100). In these small nonrandomized trials, the rate of decline of GFR and rise of proteinuria were not ameliorated by intensive blood glucose control. At this stage of diabetic renal damage, blood pressure control has probably greater potential of reno-protection than intensive metabolic control. Moreover, a cautionary note is needed for intensive metabolic control in people with advanced diabetic nephropathy. The half-life of insulin is prolonged in patients with decreased renal function (101), exposing them to the risk of developing hypoglycemia. Sulfonylurea compounds also accumulate in renal failure (102), and metformin should be avoided in patients with serum creatinine greater than 1.5 mg/dL (103).

Blood Pressure Control

High blood pressure accelerates the progressive increase in albumin levels in patients with type 2 diabetes who have initially normal albumin levels and accelerates the loss of kidney function in those with overt nephropathy (104). Renal insufficiency further increases blood pressure, thereby establishing a vicious circle that accelerates progression to end-stage renal disease and increase cardiovascular complications. Both effects are prevented or limited by drugs that lower blood pressure.

Choice of Drugs

The earliest descriptions of a beneficial effect of antihypertensive therapy on diabetic nephropathy date back to the early 1980s (104). At the end of that decade, studies described the beneficial effects of a new class of antihypertensive drugs, the angiotensin converting enzyme (ACE) inhibitors. In 1993, a clinical study demonstrated that the ACE inhibitor captopril significantly reduced the risk of progression of overt diabetic nephropathy in type 1 diabetics with macroalbuminuria (105). More recently, two studies examined the effect of blockade of the renin–angiotensin system with angiotensin receptor blocker on the progression of renal disease in patients with type 2 diabetes and macroalbuminuria.

The Reduction of Endpoints in NIDDM with the Angiotensin II Antagonist Losartan (RENAAL) study showed that, as compared with conventional treatment alone, losartan decreased the level of urinary protein excretion by 35% and reduced the risk of end-stage kidney disease by 28% (106). In the Irbesartan Diabetic Nephropathy Trial (IDNT), the risk of a doubling of the base-line serum creatinine level, the onset of ESRF, or death from any cause was 20% lower in patients treated with irbesartan than in those treated with conventional therapy and 23% lower than in those treated with amlodipine (107).

Studies have also examined the possibility to prevent the progression from microalbuminuria to overt nephropathy in both type 1 and type diabetes. In 1994, Viberti and colleagues (108) showed that captopril therapy significantly impeded progression to clinical proteinuria and prevented the increase in albumin excretion rate in normotensive, type 1 diabetic patients with persistent microalbuminuria. A meta-analysis of 12 studies in type 1 diabetic patients with microalbuminuria showed that ACE inhibitors reduced the risk of progression to macroalbuminuria by 62% as compared to placebo (109). The beneficial effect of ACE inhibition is long lasting and is associated with GFR preservation (110). The role of ACE inhibition in type 2 diabetic patients was studied by Ravid et al. (111), who showed that enalapril offered long-term protection (7 years follow-up) against the development of nephropathy in normotensive patients with type 2 diabetes mellitus who have microalbuminuria.

In a subgroup of patients with type 2 diabetes of the Heart Outcomes Prevention Evaluation (HOPE) study, at similar blood pressures, an ACE inhibitor resulted in a 24% greater decrease in the rate of progression to overt nephropathy than did placebo in patients with type 2 diabetes and normoalbuminuria or microalbuminuria (112).

In the Irbesartan in Patients with Type 2 Diabetes and Microalbuminuria (IRMA) study, treatment of type 2 diabetes patients with irbesartan (an angiotensin receptor antagonist) at a dose of 300 mg/day decreased the level of urinary albumin excretion by 38% from base line, and reduced the risk of progression to macroalbuminuria by 70% as compared with placebo (113).

In term of primary prevention, while there are no studies that examine the role of ACE inhibition in type 1 patients, very recently published data showed that ACE inhibitors are capable to prevent the development of microalbuminuria in hypertensive, normoalbuminuric type 2 diabetic patients. In the Bergamo Nephrologic Diabetes Complications Trial (BENEDICT), 1204 patients were randomly assigned to receive at least 3 years of treatment with trandolapril plus verapamil, trandolapril alone, verapamil alone, or placebo (114). The primary endpoint was the development of persistent microalbuminuria (overnight albumin excretion 20 μg/min at two consecutive visits). The primary outcome was reached in 5.7% of the subjects receiving trandolapril plus verapamil, 6.0% of the subjects receiving trandolapril, 11.9% of the subjects receiving verapamil, and 10.0% of control subjects receiving placebo. Trandolapril plus verapamil and trandolapril alone delayed the onset of microalbuminuria by factors of 2.6 and 2.1, respectively. In summary, a large body of evidence has been gathered in the last 10 years to support the recommendation that patients with type 1 and type 2 diabetes with hypertension should be treated with an ACE inhibitor or an angiotensin receptor blocker in order to prevent microalbuminuria, macroalbuminuria, and progression of overt nephropathy (115).

This treatment is to be considered safe and cost-effective. Hyperkalemia is a recognized risk of antagonists of the renin–angiotensin system, but pooled data from large clinical trials suggest that the risk is low (106,107). Only 1.5% of patients treated with ACE inhibitors or angiotensin II-receptor antagonists were withdrawn from trials because of hyperkalemia, and no deaths were reported in association with hyperkalemia in any treatment group.

Other Drugs

Dihydropyridine calcium-channel blockers (e.g., nifedipine and amlodipine) may worsen proteinuria and accelerate the progression of disease in patients with nondiabetic or diabetic nephropathy (116). At any level of blood pressure control, patients with diabetes who were treated with dihydropyridine calcium-channel blockers had more severe proteinuria and a more rapid decline in the glomerular filtration rate than those treated with other antihypertensive agents (117). In the IDNT study, patients on amlodipine had an outcome comparable or even worse than those on placebo (107). However, in the RENAAL study, the effect of losartan in reducing the risk of kidney events was not diminished by concomitant use of dihydropyridine calcium-channel blockers (108).

The Appropriate Blood Pressure Control in Diabetes (ABCD) Trial compared the effects of intensive vs. moderate blood pressure control on the incidence and progression of type 2 diabetic complications, using a calcium-channel blocker, nisoldipine vs. an ACE inhibitor, enalapril (118). The mean blood pressure achieved was 132/78 mmHg in the intensive group and 138/86 mmHg in the moderate control group. During the 5-year follow-up period, no difference was observed between intensive vs. moderate blood pressure control and those randomized to nisoldipine vs. enalapril with regard to the change in creatinine clearance. After the first year of antihypertensive treatment, creatinine clearance stabilized in both the intensive and moderate blood pressure control groups in those patients with baseline normo- or microalbuminuria. In contrast, patients starting with overt albuminuria demonstrated a steady decline in creatinine clearance of 5 to 6 mL/min/1.73 m^2/year throughout the follow-up period whether they were on intensive or moderate therapy. There was also no difference between the interventions with regard to individuals progressing from normoalbuminuria to microalbuminuria or microalbuminuria to overt albuminuria.

Beta-blockers may also be beneficial in the treatment of diabetic nephropathy. In the United Kingdom Prospective Diabetes Study, beta-blockers and ACE inhibitors were equally effective in lowering the incidence of microalbuminuria and macroalbuminuria in patients with type 2 diabetes (119). A small study involving patients with overt nephropathy also found that beta-blockers and ACE inhibitors had similar protective effects on kidney function (120).

The question of whether beta-blockers offer as much kidney protection as angiotensin II-receptor antagonists needs to be answered by a direct comparison of the two classes of drugs. No large studies have compared the effects of diuretics, beta-blockers, or calcium-channel blockers with the effects of ACE inhibitors or angiotensin receptor antagonists in patients with diabetes who have overt nephropathy.

Combination of Antihypertensive Drugs

Most often more than one drug is required to obtain an ideal blood pressure control in diabetic patients, a clinical observation confirmed by IDNT and RENAAL studies, raising the question of which is the best combination of drugs. The favorable effects of inhibitors of the renin–angiotensin system on proteinuria are increased by sodium restriction and by concomitant administration of diuretics or non-dihydropyridine calcium-channel blockers. In patients with type 2 diabetes who have microalbuminuria, the combined treatment with lisinopril and candesartan was more effective in reducing blood pressure and albuminuria than either drug alone (121).

Blood Pressure Goals

The optimal range of blood pressure in patients with type 2 diabetes is unclear. In the Hypertension Optimal Treatment (HOT) Trial involving patients with type 2 diabetes, there were no more cardiovascular events when diastolic blood pressure was 70–84 mmHg than when it was 85 mmHg or higher (122). However, if diastolic blood pressure was less than 70 mmHg, the rates of cardiovascular events increased by 11% for each additional reduction of 5 mmHg, with an attendant increase in mortality. In accordance with the "standards of medical care in diabetes mellitus," the position statement on "hypertension management in adults with diabetes," and other recommendations issued by the American Diabetes Association (123), the primary goal of therapy for non-pregnant diabetic patients of more than 18 years of age is to decrease blood pressure to and maintain it at <130 mmHg mmHg systolic and <80 mmHg diastolic. The seventh report of the Joint National Committee on Prevention, Detection, Evaluation, and Treatment of High Blood Pressure (JNC 7) recommendations (124) include prompt initiation of pharmacological therapy simultaneously with lifestyle modification, a lower blood pressure goal (<130/80 mmHg), and antihypertensive medications specific to the comorbid conditions. In particular, ACE inhibitors and ARBs are recommended for patients with heart failure, diabetes, and CKD. Guidelines proposed by the NKF-K/DOQI Work Group on Hypertension and Antihypertensive Agents (125) are largely consistent with recommendations by JNC 7 and ADA.

Treatment of Dyslipidemia

An analysis of 13 controlled trials (involving a total of 362 subjects, 253 of whom had diabetes) showed that statins decreased proteinuria and preserved the glomerular filtration rate in patients with chronic kidney disease—effects that are not entirely explained by a reduction in blood cholesterol (126).

Dietary Protein Restriction

It has been suggested from experimental studies that the reduced dietary protein intake may protect the kidney against loss of function. Indeed, a study involving patients with type 1 diabetes and nephropathy showed that, as compared with a high intake of protein and phosphorus, restriction of protein and phosphorus (0.6 g of protein per kilogram of body weight per day and 500–1000 mg of phosphorus per day) reduced the loss of the glomerular filtration rate, lowered blood pressure, and stabilized kidney function in some patients (127). Restriction of protein intake to 0.8 g/kg/day, which is consistent with the recommended daily allowance, also reduces the rate of progression to end-stage kidney disease in patients with type 1 diabetes (128). There have been no large randomized trials of protein restriction in patients with type 2 diabetes mellitus.

Lifestyle Modification

Lifestyle modifications are difficult to assess in a controlled fashion. There are to be considered with attention two well-designed studies, which showed that lifestyle interventions, which achieved only modest changes in weight, were sufficient to obtain an important reduction in the incidence of diabetes. The Finnish Diabetes Prevention study (129) enrolled 522 middle-aged overweight subjects, who were randomized to an intervention program, consisting in counseling aimed to reduce weight, to reduce fat intake, to increase fiber intake and physical exercise; or to a control group. Subjects in the intervention group lost an average of 4.2 kg of body weight, while the control group did not lose weight. During the trial, the risk to develop diabetes was reduced by 58% in the intervention group.

The Diabetes Prevention Program study was conducted in the United States (130). Overweight subjects were randomized to placebo, metformin, or lyfestyle changes. Lyfestyle changes were more effective than metformin and placebo in reducing the incidence of diabetes in this high-risk population. The role of weight loss with lifestyle modifications has not yet been formally assessed in diabetic nephropathy. Both the mentioned studies showed that, although effective, the intervention required a considerable effort from well-trained staff, and the long-term maintenance of lifestyle changes are difficult to assess. On the other hand, physical activity and weight loss are of medical benefit, not just for preventing diabetes but also for improving
cardiovascular health and quality of life, and should be encouraged.

Smoking Cessation

Smoking, besides increasing the risk of cardiovascular events, is an independent risk factor for the development of nephropathy in patients with type 2 diabetes and is associated with an accelerated loss of kidney function (131,132). Smoking cessation alone may reduce the risk of disease progression by 30%, which meant that smoking cessation might be the most effective measure than any other pharmacological intervention to date (133).

PREVENTION OF DIABETIC NEPHROPATHY IN DEVELOPING COUNTRIES

The World Health Organization is strongly committed to fighting diabetes and its complications, which are posing a tremendous threat to health globally. WHO interventions are particularly aimed to prevent and treat diabetes in developing countries, which are going to carry the heaviest burden of the rising epidemic of diabetes. It is a tremendously complex task, but we can learn from pilot experiences, which show that simple and inexpensive screening programs could be feasible at low cost even in poor countries, and also simple and inexpensive treatments are plausible and possibly effective. As an example, the Kidney Help Trust rural project in India, which was able to screen for high blood pressure, diabetes, and chronic kidney disease in a rural population of 25,000 people with the help of six health social workers, at a cost of less than $6000 per year, a mere 25 cents per capita. An excellent blood pressure control was achieved among hypertensive patients, while blood glucose control in diabetics was considered good (134).

RECOMMENDATIONS

In summary, there is a great deal of information from clinical studies that allows to provide a set of recommendations aimed to prevent the development of diabetic nephropathy, reduce the risk of disease progression, and prevent cardiovascular complications. This is a tremendously important task, with extremely relevant implication from a public health point of view, as documented by the emphasis that national and international agencies, such as WHO, put on the subject. Treatment should include (Tables 4 and 5):

> smoking cessation;
> lifestyle modifications such as weight loss, exercise reduction alcohol
> intake;
> control of high blood pressure;
> tight glucose control;
> treatment of dislypidemia;
> moderate restriction of dietary protein intake.

The first choice for antihypertensive treatment should be an ACE inhibitor or angiotensin II-receptor antagonist because each decreases both blood pressure and albuminuria; the dose should be titrated upward to the moderate or high range, as tolerated, to achieve a systolic pressure below 130 mmHg and a diastolic pressure below 80 mmHg.

Serum potassium and creatinine should be checked in all patients 7 days after the initiation of treatment with drugs that block the renin–angiotensin system and after any increase in the dose of such drugs. A beta-blocker or diuretic—or if these agents are inadequate, a non-dihydropyridine calcium-channel blocker—should be added if ACE inhibitors or angiotensin II-receptor antagonists are insufficient to maintain blood pressure in the desired range. We consider adding dihydropyridine calcium-channel blockers or alpha-blockers only when the target for blood pressure is not met with the use of these other approaches.

The same approach is advisable in hypertensive patients with normo-albuminuria, in order to delay or prevent nephropathy. If tolerated, drugs

Table 5 Goals of Intervention for Prevention and Management of Diabetic Nephropathy

Variable	Target
Blood glucose	HbA1c $<7\%$
Systolic blood pressure	$<130\,\text{mmHg}$
Diastolic blood pressure	$<80\,\text{mmHg}$
LDL Cholesterol	$<115\,\text{mg/dL}$
Dietary protein	$<0.8\,\text{g/kg}$ body weight
Other measures	Stop smoking, weight loss, physical exercise, moderate alcohol intake

Current practice guidelines for patients with incipient and overt diabetic nephropathy.
Source: From Ref. 135.

that inhibit the renin–angiotensin system are also recommended for normotensive patients with microalbuminuria or macroalbuminuria; reduction of the albumin level is the main goal in such patients.

Restriction of dietary protein (a maximum of 0.8 g per kilogram of body weight per day, corresponding to about 10% of total daily caloric intake) has been rigorously studied only in patients with type 1 diabetes, but it may also be beneficial in those with type 2 diabetes.

Although studies of statins have not been designed specifically to examine their use in patients with kidney disease, available data suggest that these medications may not only reduce the risk of cardiovascular disease but also slow the loss of kidney function.

REFERENCES

1. King H, Aubert RE, Herman WH. Global burden of diabetes, 1995–2025: prevalence, numerical estimates, and projections. Diabetes Care 1998; 21: 1414–1431.
2. Wild S, Roglic G, Green A, Sicree R, King H. Global prevalence of diabetes: estimates for the year 2000 and projections for 2030. Diabetes Care 2004; 27:1047–1053.
3. International Diabetes Federation e-Atlas. Available at http://www.idf.org/e-atlas/home/ accessed October 2004.
4. World Health Organization. Obesity and overweight. Fact sheet available at http://www.who.int/dietphysicalactivity/media/en/gsfs_obesity.pdf as accessed October 2004.
5. Felber JP. From obesity to diabetes. Pathophysiological considerations. Int J Obes Relat Metab Disord 1992; 16:937–952.
6. Chan JM, Rimm EB, Colditz GA, Stampfer MJ, Willett WC. Obesity, fat distribution, and weight gain as risk factors for clinical diabetes in men. Diabetes Care 1994; 1:961–969.

7. van Dam RM, Rimm EB, Willett WC, Stampfer MJ, Hu FB. Dietary patterns and risk for type 2 diabetes mellitus in U.S. men. Ann Intern Med 2002; 136:201–209.

8. Mokdad AH, Ford ES, Bowman BA, et al. Prevalence of obesity, diabetes, and obesity-related health risk factors, 2001. JAMA 2003; 289:76–79.

9. Colditz GA, Willett WC, Rotnitzky A, Manson JE. Weight gain as a risk factor for clinical diabetes mellitus in women. Ann Intern Med 1995; 122: 481–486.

10. Willett WC, Dietz WH, Colditz GA. Guidelines for healthy weight. N Engl J Med 1999; 341:427–434.

11. Report of the Joint WHO/FAO Expert Consultation on Diet, Nutrition and the Prevention of Chronic Diseases (Geneva, 28 January–1 February 2002)— WHO Technical Report Series No. 916). Available at http://www.who.int/ nut/documents/trs_916.pdf. Accessed October 2004.

12. Parving HH, Hommel E, Mathiesen E, et al. Prevalence of microalbuminuria, arterial hypertension, retinopathy and neuropathy in patients with insulin dependent diabetes. Br Med J 1988; 296:156–160.

13. Ritz E, Orth SR. Nephropathy in patients with type 2 diabetes mellitus. N Engl J Med 1999; 341:1127–1133.

14. U.S. Renal Data System. USRDS 2003 Annual Data Report: Atlas of End-Stage Renal Disease in the United States. Bethesda, MD: National Institutes of Health, National Institute of Diabetes and Digestive and Kidney Diseases, 2003.

15. European Dialysis and Transplant Association. Report on management of renal failure in Europe, XXVI, 1995. Nephrol Dial Transplant 1996; 11(suppl 7):1–32.

16. Zatz R, Romão JE, Noronha IL. Nephrology in Latin America, with special emphasis on Brazil. Kidney Int 2003; 63(s83):S131–S134.

17. Sakhuja V, Sud K. End-stage renal disease in India and Pakistan: burden of disease and management issues. Kidney Int 2003; 63(s83):S115–S118.

18. Foley RN, Culleton BF, Parfrey PS, et al. Cardiac disease in diabetic end-stage renal disease. Diabetologia 1997; 40:1307–1312.

19. Stack AG, Bloembergen WE. A cross-sectional study of the prevalence and clinical correlates of congestive heart failure among incident US dialysis patients. Am J Kidney Dis 2001; 38:992–1000.

20. Dikow R, Ritz E. Cardiovascular complications in the diabetic patient with renal disease: an update in 2003. Nephrol Dial Transplant 2003; 18:1993–1998.

21. Hypolite IO, Bucci J, Hshieh P, et al. Acute coronary syndromes after renal transplantation in patients with end-stage renal disease resulting from diabetes. Am J Transplant 2002; 2:274–281.

22. Anavekar NS, McMurray JJ, Velazquez EJ, et al. Relation between renal dysfunction and cardiovascular outcomes after myocardial infarction. N Engl J Med 2004; 351:1285–1295.

23. Go AS, Chertow GM, Fan D, McCulloch CE, Hsu CY. Chronic kidney disease and the risks of death, cardiovascular events, and hospitalization. N Engl J Med 2004; 351:1296–1305.

24. Sarnak MJ, Levey AS, Schoolwerth AC, et al. Kidney disease as a risk factor for development of cardiovascular disease: a statement from the American

Heart Association Councils on Kidney in Cardiovascular Disease, High Blood Pressure Research, Clinical Cardiology, and Epidemiology and Prevention. Hypertension 2003; 42:1050–1065.

25. Ruggenenti P, Remuzzi G. The diagnosis of renal involvement in non-insulin-dependent diabetes mellitus. Curr Opin Nephrol Hypertens 1997; 6:141–145.

26. Mogensen CE, Hansen KW, Pedersen MM, Christensen CK. Renal factors influencing blood pressure threshold and choice of treatment for hypertension in IDDM. Diabetes Care 1991; 14(suppl 4):13–26.

27. Hypertension in Diabetes Study (HDS): I. Prevalence of hypertension in newly presenting type 2 diabetic patients and the association with risk factors for cardiovascular and diabetic complications. J Hypertens 1993; 11:309–317.

28. Andersen AR, Christiansen JS, Andersen JK, Kreiner S, Deckert T. Diabetic nephropathy in Type 1 (insulin-dependent) diabetes: an epidemiological study. Diabetologia 1983; 25:496–501.

29. Pugh JA, Medina R, Ramirez M. Comparison of the course to end-stage renal disease of type 1 (insulin-dependent) and type 2 (non-insulin-dependent) diabetic nephropathy. Diabetologia 1993; 36:1094–1098.

30. Nelson RG, Kunzelman CL, Pettitt DJ, Saad MF, Bennett PH, Knowler WC. Albuminuria in type 2 (non-insulin-dependent) diabetes mellitus and impaired glucose tolerance in Pima Indians. Diabetologia 1989; 32:870–876.

31. Tapp Rj, Dip G, Shaw JE, et al. Albuminuria is evident in the early stages of diabetes onset: results from the Austrialian Diabetes, Obesity and Lifestyle Study (AusDiab). Am J Kidney Dis 2004; 44:792–798.

32. Reaven GM. Banting Lecture 1988: role of insulin resistance in human disease. Diabetes 1988; 37:1595–1607.

33. DeFronzo RA, Ferrannini E. Insulin resistance. A multifaceted syndrome responsible for NIDDM, obesity, hypertension, dyslipidemia, and atherosclerotic cardiovascular disease. Diabetes Care 1991; 14:173–194.

34. Cameron AJ, Shaw JE, Zimmet PZ. The metabolic syndrome: prevalence in worldwide populations. Endocrinol Metab Clin North Am 2004; 33:351–375.

35. Chen J, Muntner P, Hamm LL, et al. The metabolic syndrome and chronic kidney disease in U.S. adults. Ann Intern Med 2004; 140:167–174.

36. Seaquist ER, Goetz FC, Rich S, Barbosa J. Familial clustering of diabetic kidney disease. Evidence for genetic susceptibility to diabetic nephropathy. N Engl J Med 1989; 320:1161–1165.

37. Pettitt DJ, Saad MF, Bennett PH, Nelson RG, Knowler WC. Familial predisposition to renal disease in two generations of Pima Indians with type 2 (non-insulin-dependent) diabetes mellitus. Diabetologia 1990; 33:438–443.

38. Viberti GC, Keen H, Wiseman MJ. Raised arterial pressure in parents of proteinuric insulin dependent diabetics. Br Med J 1987; 295:515–517.

39. Martorell R, Stein AD, Schroeder DG. Early nutrition and later adiposity. J Nutr 2001; 131:S874–S880.

40. Nelson RG, Morgenstern H, Bennett PH. Intrauterine diabetes exposure and the risk of renal disease in diabetic Pima Indians. Diabetes 1998; 47:1489–1493.

41. Nelson RG, Morgenstern H, Bennett PH. Birth weight and renal disease in Pima Indians with type 2 diabetes mellitus. Am J Epidemiol 1998; 148:650–656.

42. Nelson RG. Intrauterine determinants of diabetic kidney disease in disadvantaged populations. Kidney Int 2003; 63(suppl 83):S13–S16.
43. Brancati FL, Whittle JC, Whelton PK, et al. The excess incidence of diabetic end-stage renal disease among blacks. A population-based study of potential explanatory factors. JAMA 1992; 268:3079–3084.
44. Smith SR, Svetkey LP, Dennis VW. Racial differences in the incidence and progression of renal diseases. Kidney Int 1991; 40:815–822.
45. Brancati FL, Whelton PK, Randall BL, Neaton JD, Stamler J, Klag MJ. Risk of end-stage renal disease in diabetes mellitus: a prospective cohort study of men screened for MRFIT. Multiple Risk Factor Intervention Trial. JAMA 1997; 278:2069–2074.
46. Karter AJ, Ferrara A, Liu JY, Moffet HH, Ackerson LM, Selby JV. Ethnic disparities in diabetic complications in an insured population. JAMA 2002; 287:2519–2527.
47. Young BA, Maynard C, Boyko EJ. Racial differences in diabetic nephropathy, cardiovascular disease, and mortality in a national population of veterans. Diabetes Care 2003; 26:2392–2399.
48. Burden ML, Woghiren O, Burden AC. Diabetes in African Caribbean, and Indo-Asian ethnic minority people. J R Coll Phys Lond 2000; 34:343–346.
49. McDonald SP, Russ GR. Current incidence, treatment patterns and outcome of end-stage renal disease among indigenous groups in Australia and New Zealand. Nephrology 2003; 8:42–48.
50. Nyberg G, Blohme G, Norden G. Impact of metabolic control in progression of clinical diabetic nephropathy. Diabetologia 1987; 30:82–86.
51. Breyer JA, Bain RP, Evans JK, et al. Predictors of the progression of renal insufficiency in patients with insulin-dependent diabetes and overt diabetic nephropathy. The Collaborative Study Group. Kidney Int 1996; 50:1651–1658.
52. Hovind P, Rossing P, Tarnow L, Smidt UM, Parving HH. Progression of diabetic nephropathy. Kidney Int 2001; 59:702–709.
53. The Diabetes Control and Complications Trial Research Group. The effect of intensive treatment on the development and progression of long-term complications in insulin dependent diabetes mellitus. N Engl J Med 1993; 329: 977–986.
54. Feldt-Rasmussen B, Mathiesen ER, Deckert T. Effect of two years of strict metabolic control on progression of incipient nephropathy in insulin-dependent diabetes. Lancet 1986; 2:1300–1304.
55. Wang PH, Lau J, Chalmers TC. Meta-analysis of effects of intensive blood-glucose control on late complications of type I diabetes. Lancet 1993; 341: 1306–1309.
56. Ballard DJ, Humphrey LL, Melton LJ III, Frohnert PP, Chu PC, O'Fallon WM, Palumbo PJ. Epidemiology of persistent proteinuria in type II diabetes mellitus. Population-based study in Rochester, Minnesota. Diabetes 1988; 37:405–412.
57. UK Prospective Diabetes Study (UKPDS) Group. Intensive blood-glucose control with sulphonylureas or insulin compared with conventional treatment and risk of complications in patients with type 2 diabetes (UKPDS 33). Lancet 1998; 352:837.

58. Gaede P, Vedel P, Parving HH, Pedersen O. Intensified multifactorial intervention in patients with type 2 diabetes mellitus and microalbuminuria: the Steno type 2 randomized study. Lancet 1999; 353:617–622.
59. Ritz E, Stefanski A. Diabetic nephropathy in type II diabetes. Am J Kidney Dis 1996; 27:167–194.
60. Keller CK, Bergis KH, Fliser D, Ritz E. Renal findings in patients with short-term type 2 diabetes. J Am Soc Nephrol 1996; 7:2627–2635.
61. Hasslacher C, Wolfrum M, Stech G, Wahl P, Ritz E. Diabetic nephropathy in type II diabetes: effect of metabolic control and blood pressure on its development and course. Dtsch Med Wochenschr 1987; 112:1445–1449.
62. Rossing P, Hommel E, Smidt UM, Parving HH. Impact of arterial blood pressure and albuminuria on the progression of diabetic nephropathy in IDDM patients. Diabetes 1993; 42:715–719.
63. Gall MA, Nielsen FS, Smidt UM, Parving HH. The course of kidney function in type 2 (non-insulin-dependent) diabetic patients with diabetic nephropathy. Diabetologia 1993; 36:1071–1078.
64. Yokoyama H, Tomonaga O, Hirayama M, et al. Predictors of the progression of diabetic nephropathy and the beneficial effect of angiotensin-converting enzyme inhibitors in NIDDM patients. Diabetologia 1997; 40:405–411.
65. Mulec H, Johnson SA, Bjorck S. Relation between serum cholesterol and diabetic nephropathy. Lancet 1990; 335:1537–1538.
66. Remuzzi G. Nephropathic nature of proteinuria. Curr Opin Nephrol Hypertens 1999; 8:655–663.
67. Abbate M, Remuzzi G. Proteinuria as a mediator of tubulointerstitial injury. Kidney Blood Press Res 1999; 22:37–46.
68. Jafar TH, Stark PC, Schmid CH, et al. AIPRD Study Group. Angiotensin-converting enzymne inhibition and progression of renal disease. Proteinuria as a modifiable risk factor for the progression of non-diabetic renal disease. Kidney Int 2001; 60:1131–1140.
69. Dinneen SF, Gerstein HC. The association of microalbuminuria and mortality in non-insulin-dependent diabetes mellitus. A systematic overview of the literature. Arch Intern Med 1997; 157:1413–1418.
70. Muhlhauser I, Sawicki P, Berger M. Cigarette-smoking as a risk factor for macroproteinuria and proliferative retinopathy in type 1 (insulin-dependent) diabetes. Diabetologia 1986; 29:500–502.
71. Orth SR, Ritz E, Schrier RW. The renal risks of smoking. Kidney Int 1997; 51:1669–1677.
72. Sawicki PT, Didjurgeit U, Muhlhauser I, Bender R, Heinemann L, Berger M. Smoking is associated with progression of diabetic nephropathy. Diabetes Care 1994; 17:126–131.
73. Deckert T, Yokoyama H, Mathiesen E, et al. Cohort study of predictive value of urinary albumin excretion for atherosclerotic vascular disease in patients with insulin dependent diabetes. BMJ 1996; 312:871–874.
74. Stephenson JM, Kenny S, Stevens LK, Fuller JH, Lee E. Proteinuria and mortality in diabetes: the WHO Multinational Study of Vascular Disease in Diabetes. Diabet Med 1995; 12:149–155.

75. Soedamah-Muthu SS, Chaturvedi N, Toeller M, et al. For the EURODIAB Prospective Complications Study Group. Risk factors for coronary heart disease in type 1 diabetic patients in Europe: the EURODIAB Prospective Complications Study. Diabetes Care 2004; 27:530–537.

76. Gerstein HC, Mann JF, Yi Q, et al. HOPE Study Investigators. Albuminuria and risk of cardiovascular events, death, and heart failure in diabetic and non-diabetic individuals. JAMA 2001; 286:421–426.

77. Stein B, Weintraub WS, Gebhart SP, et al. Influence of diabetes mellitus on early and late outcome after percutaneous transluminal coronary angioplasty. Circulation 1995; 91:979–989.

78. Granger CB, Califf RM, Young S, et al. Outcome of patients with diabetes mellitus and acute myocardial infarction treated with thrombolytic agents. The Thrombolysis and Angioplasty in Myocardial Infarction (TAMI) Study Group. J Am Coll Cardiol 1993; 21:920–925.

79. Haffner SM, Mykkanen L, Festa A, Burke JP, Stern MP. Insulin-resistant pre-diabetic subjects have more atherogenic risk factors than insulin-sensitive pre-diabetic subjects: implications for preventing coronary heart disease during the prediabetic state. Circulation 2000; 101:975–980.

80. Stehouwer CD, Nauta JJ, Zeldenrust GC, Hackeng WH, Donker AJ, den Ottolander GJ. Urinary albumin excretion, cardiovascular disease, and endo-thelial dysfunction in non-insulin-dependent diabetes mellitus. Lancet 1992; 340:319–323.

81. Ishimura E, Shoji T, Emoto M, et al. Renal insufficiency accelerates athero-sclerosis in patients with type 2 diabetes mellitus. Am J Kidney Dis 2001; 38(4 suppl 1):S186–S190.

82. Garg A, Grundy SM. Management of dyslipidemia in NIDDM. Diabetes Care 1990; 13:153–169.

83. O'Brien T, Nguyen TT, Zimmerman BR. Hyperlipidemia and diabetes melli-tus. Mayo Clin Proc 1998; 73:969–976.

84. Klein R, Klein BE. Vision disorders in diabetes. In: National Diabetes Data Group. Diabetes in America. 2nd ed. Bethesda, MD: NIH Publication No. 95–1468. National Institutes of Health, National Institute of Diabetes and Digestive and Kidney Diseases, 1995:293.

85. Klein R, Klein BE, Moss SE, Davis MD, DeMets DL. The Wisconsin epi-demiologic study of diabetic retinopathy. III. Prevalence and risk of diabetic retinopathy when age at diagnosis is 30 or more years. Arch Ophthalmol 1984; 102:527–532.

86. Klein R, Klein BE, Moss SE, Cruickshanks KJ. Relationship of hyperglyce-mia to the long-term incidence and progression of diabetic retinopathy. Arch Intern Med 1994; 154:2169–2178.

87. Cignarelli M, De Cicco ML, Damato A, et al. High systolic blood pressure increases prevalence and severity of retinopathy in NIDDM patients. Diabetes Care 1992; 15:1002–1008.

88. Chavers BM, Mauer SM, Ramsay RC, Steffes MW. Relationship between reti-nal and glomerular lesions in IDDM patients. Diabetes 1994; 43:441–446.

89. Christensen PK, Larsen S, Horn T, Olsen S, Parving HH. Causes of albuminuria in patients with type 2 diabetes without diabetic retinopathy. Kidney Int 2000; 58:1719–1731.

90. Estacio RO, McFarling E, Biggerstaff S, et al. Overt albuminuria predicts diabetic retinopathy in Hispanics with NIDDM. Am J Kidney Dis 1998; 31:947–953.

91. Stevens MJ, Feldman EL, Greene DA. The aetiology of diabetic neuropathy: the combined roles of metabolic and vascular defects. Diabet Med 1995; 12:566–579.

92. Kilo S, Berghoff M, Hilz M. Freeman RTI—neural and endothelial control of the microcirculation in diabetic peripheral neuropathy. Neurology 2000; 54(6):1246–1252.

93. Sundkvist G, Lilja B. Autonomic neuropathy predicts deterioration in glomerular filtration rate in patients with IDDM. Diabetes Care 1993; 16:773–779.

94. Lurbe E, Redon J, Kesani A, et al. Increase in nocturnal blood pressure and progression to microalbuminuria in type 1 diabetes. N Engl J Med 2002; 347:797–805.

95. UK Prospective Diabetes study (UKPDS) Group. Effect of intensive blood glucose control with metformin on complications in overweight patients with type 2 diabetes (UKPDS 34). Lancet 1998; 352:854–865.

96. Ohkubo Y, Kishikawa H, Araki E, et al. Intensive insulin therapy prevents the progression of diabetic microvascular complications in Japanese patients with non-insulin-dependent diabetes mellitus: a randomized prospective 6-year study. Diabet Res Clin Pract 1995; 28:103–117.

97. American Diabetes Association. Standards of medical care in diabetes. Diabetes Care 2004; 27(suppl 1):S15–S35.

98. Meltzer S, Leiter L, Daneman D, et al. 1998 Clinical practice guidelines for the management of diabetes in Canada. CMAJ 1998; 159(suppl 8):S1–S29.

99. Viberti GC, Bilous RW, Mackintosh D, Bending JJ, Keen H. Long term correction of hyperglycaemia and progression of renal failure in insulin dependent diabetes. Br Med J (Clin Res Ed) 1983; 286:598–602.

100. Tamborlane WV, Puklin JE, Bergman M, et al. Long-term improvement of metabolic control with the insulin pump does not reverse diabetic microangiopathy. Diabetes Care 1982; 5(suppl 1):58–64.

101. Mak RH, DeFronzo RA. Glucose and insulin metabolism in uremia. Nephron 1992; 61:377–382.

102. Charpentier G, Riveline JP, Varroud-Vial M. Management of drugs affecting blood glucose in diabetic patients with renal failure. Diabetes Metab 2000; 26(suppl 4):73–85.

103. Bailey CJ, Turner RC. Metformin. N Engl J Med 1996; 334:574–579.

104. Mogensen CE. Microalbuminuria, blood pressure and diabetic renal disease: origin and development of ideas. In: Mogensen CE, ed. The Kidney and Hypertension in Diabetes Mellitus. 5th ed. Boston: Kluwer, 2000:655–706.

105. Lewis EJ, Hunsicker LG, Bain RP, Rohde RD. The effect of angiotensin-converting-enzyme inhibition on diabetic nephropathy. N Engl J Med 1993; 329:1456–1462.

106. Brenner BM, Cooper ME, de Zeeuw D, et al. Effects of losartan on renal and cardiovascular outcomes in patients with type 2 diabetes and nephropathy. N Engl J Med 2001; 345:861–869.

107. Lewis EJ, Hunsicker LG, Clarke WR, et al. Renoprotective effect of the angiotensin-receptor antagonist irbesartan in patients with nephropathy due to type 2 diabetes. N Engl J Med 2001; 345:851–860.

108. Viberti G, Mogensen CE, Groop LC, Pauls JF. Effect of captopril on progression to clinical proteinuria in patients with insulin-dependent diabetes mellitus and microalbuminuria. European Microalbuminuria Captopril Study Group. JAMA 1994; 271:275–279.

109. The ACE Inhibitors in Diabetic Nephropathy Trialist Group. Should all type 1 diabetic microalbuminuric patients receive ACE inhibitors? A meta-regression analysis. Ann Intern Med 2001; 134:370–379.

110. Mathiesen ER, Hommel E, Hansen HP, et al. Randomized controlled trial of long term efficacy of captopril on preservation of kidney function in normotensive patients with insulin dependent diabetes and microalbuminuria. Br Med J 1999; 319:24–25.

111. Ravid M, Lang R, Rachmani R, Lishner M. Long-term renoprotective effect of angiotensin-converting enzyme inhibition in non-insulin-dependent diabetes mellitus. Arch Intern Med 1996; 156:286–289.

112. Heart Outcomes Prevention Evaluation Study Investigators. Effects of ramipril on cardiovascular and microvascular outcomes in people with diabetes mellitus: results of the HOPE study and MICRO-HOPE substudy. Lancet 2000; 355:253–259.

113. Parving H-H, Lehnert H, Bröchner-Mortensen J, Gomis R, Andersen S, Arner P. The effect of irbesartan on the development of diabetic nephropathy in patients with type 2 diabetes. N Engl J Med 2001; 345:870–878.

114. Ruggenenti P, Fassi A, Ilieva AP, et al. Bergamo Nephrologic Diabetes Complications Trial (BENEDICT) Investigators. Preventing microalbuminuria in type 2 diabetes. N Engl J Med 2004; 351:1941–1951.

115. Bakris GL, Williams M, Dworkin L, et al. Preserving renal function in adults with hypertension and diabetes: a consensus approach. Am J Kid Dis 2000; 36:646–661.

116. Bakris GL. Renal effects of calcium antagonists in diabetes mellitus: an overview of studies in animal models and in humans. Am J Hypertens 1991; 4(suppl): S487–S493.

117. Weidmann P, Schneider M, Bohlen L. Therapeutic efficacy of different antihypertensive drugs in human diabetic nephropathy: an updated meta-analysis. Nephrol Dial Transplant 1995; 10(suppl 9):39–45.

118. Estacio RO, Jeffers BW, Gifford N, Schrier RW. Effect of blood pressure control on diabetic microvascular complications in patients with hypertension and type 2 diabetes. Diabetes Care 2000; 23(suppl 2):S54–S64.

119. UK Prospective Diabetes Study Group. Efficacy of atenolol and captopril in reducing risk of macrovascular and microvascular complications in type 2 diabetes: UKPDS 39. BMJ 1998; 317:713–720.

120. Nielsen FS, Rossing P, Gall MA, Skott P, Smidt UM, Parving H-H. Long-term effect of lisinopril and atenolol on kidney function in hypertensive NIDDM subjects with diabetic nephropathy. Diabetes 1997; 46: 1182–1188.

121. Mogensen CE, Neldam S, Tikkenen I, et al. Randomized controlled trial of dual blockade of renin–angiotensin system in patients with hypertension, microalbuminuria, and non-insulin dependent diabetes: the Candesartan and Lisinopril Microalbuminuria (CALM) study. BMJ 2000; 321:1440–1444.

122. Hansson L, Zanchetti A, Carruthers SG, et al. Effects of intensive blood-pressure lowering and low-dose aspirin in patients with hypertension: principal results of the Hypertension Optimal Treatment (HOT) randomised trial. Lancet 1998; 351:1755–1762.

123. Arauz-Pacheco C, Parrott MA, Raskin P, American Diabetes Association. Hypertension management in adults with diabetes. Diabetes Care 2004; 27(suppl 1):S65–S67.

124. Chobanian AV, Bakris GL, Black HR, et al. National Heart, Lung, and Blood Institute Joint National Committee on Prevention, Detection, Evaluation, and Treatment of High Blood Pressure; National High Blood Pressure Education Program Coordinating Committee. The seventh report of the Joint National Committee on Prevention, Detection, Evaluation, and Treatment of High Blood Pressure: the JNC 7 report. JAMA 2003; 289:2560–2572.

125. Kidney Disease Outcomes Quality Initiative (K/DOQI). K/DOQI clinical practice guidelines on hypertension and antihypertensive agents in chronic kidney disease. Am J Kidney Dis 2004; 43(suppl 5):S65–S73.

126. Fried LF, Orchard TJ, Kasiske BL. Effect of lipid reduction on the progression of renal disease: a meta-analysis. Kidney Int 2001; 59:260–269.

127. Zeller K, Whittaker E, Sullivan L, Raskin P, Jacobson HR. Effect of restricting dietary protein on the progression of renal failure in patients with insulin-dependent diabetes mellitus. N Engl J Med 1991; 324:78–84.

128. Hansen HP, Tauber-Lassen E, Jensen BR, Parving H-H. Effect of dietary protein restriction on prognosis in type 1 diabetic patients with diabetic nephropathy [abstr]. Presented at the European Diabetic Nephropathy Study Group 14th Annual Meeting, County Durham, United Kingdom, May 2001.

129. Tuomilehto J, Lindstrom J, Eriksson JG, et al. Finnish Diabetes Prevention Study Group. Prevention of type 2 diabetes mellitus by changes in lifestyle among subjects with impaired glucose tolerance. N Engl J Med 2001; 344:1343–1350.

130. Knowler WC, Barrett-Connor E, Fowler SE, et al. Diabetes Prevention Program Research Group. Reduction in the incidence of type 2 diabetes with lifestyle intervention or metformin. N Engl J Med 2002; 346:393–403.

131. Hovind P, Rossing P, Tarnow L, Parving HH. Smoking and progression of diabetic nephropathy in type 1 diabetes. Diabetes Care 2003; 26:911–916.

132. Ritz E, Ogata H, Orth SR. Smoking: a factor promoting onset and progression of diabetic nephropathy. Diabetes Metab 2000; 26(suppl 4):54–63.

133. Chuahirun T, Simoni J, Hudson C, Seipel T, Khanna A, Harrist RB, Wesson DE. Cigarette smoking exacerbates and its cessation ameliorates renal injury in type 2 diabetes. Am J Med Sci 2004; 327:57–67.

134. Mani MK. Prevention of chronic renal failure at the community level. Kidney Int 2003: 63(s83):86–89.

135. Remuzzi et al. N Engl J Med 2002; 346:1145.

9

Albuminuria: A New Target for Therapy? Treat the Kidney to Protect the Heart

Dick de Zeeuw

Department of Clinical Pharmacology Groningen, University Medical Center, Groningen, The Netherlands

Meguid El Nahas

Sheffield Kidney Institute, University of Sheffield, Sheffield, U.K.

INTRODUCTION

Chronic diseases (kidney, diabetes, heart disease) constitute about 50% of the total disease burden in the general population, but carry about 80–90% of healthcare budgets in the Westernized world. In particular, the number of those suffering from type 2 diabetes is dramatically growing and is expected to have doubled within the next 20 years. In fact, while the global burden may double in the next 20 years, that of the developing countries is more likely to treble. Such a health threat is hanging over the populations in the developing World where already major increases in the prevalence of type 2 diabetes have been reported and where causes for morbidity and mortality are shifting from infectious towards cardiovascular. Both in the Westernized as well as in the developing World, healthcare resources will be unable to face such growing demands. Therefore, emphasis has to shift from secondary to primary prevention, meaning that we need to detect those that are at risk of diabetes as well as its complications chronic kidney (CKD) and CV (CVD) diseases and treat them before CKD and CVD initiation.

Patients with mild renal dysfunction run an increased risk of the so-called end-organ failure and subsequently death. This is particularly evident in patients with type 2 diabetes mellitus, in which mild renal dysfunction heralds diabetic nephropathy, vascular disease, and most notably cardiovascular death. Thus, although patients with renal dysfunction are often treated with the intention of protecting them against further kidney damage, one should realize that the most frequent morbidity and mortality is of cardiovascular origin.

The initial and usually mild dysfunction of the kidney is called stage I or stage II chronic kidney disease (CKD) according to the US National Kidney Foundation (NKF) K/DOQI guidelines (1). This is evidenced by a more than normal loss of proteins in the urine, particularly albumin, and/or a decreased glomerular filtration rate. An abnormal urinary loss of albumin is called microalbuminuria when it ranges between 30 and 300 mg/day (20–200 µg/min), when higher it is called macroalbuminuria or proteinuria.

The classical cardiovascular risk profiling of patients at risk for cardiovascular and or renal disease is based on classical parameters derived from the Framingham study: age, sex, and modifiable factors such as blood pressure, cholesterol, body weight, diabetes, and smoking. These parameters not only allow us to classify the risk profile of a given patient when first seen, but they also allow to define our therapeutic strategies aiming to minimize these risk factors/markers. For instance, blood pressure control in those with hypertension decreases renal and cardiovascular risk. Similarly, control of plasma lipid abnormalities affords both cardiovascular and renal protection, although the latter awaits confirmation in large hard-endpoint trials. Optimization of diabetes control has been a major step in preventing life-threatening end-organ damage in type 2 diabetes, reducing renal as well as cardiovascular risks.

By far, the biggest added therapeutic step has been the introduction of interventions able to manipulate the renin-angiotensin-aldosterone system (RAAS), such as angiotensin converting enzyme inhibitors (ACEi) and AII receptor blockers (ARB). A large body of evidence suggests that these drugs add to renal and cardiovascular protection beyond blood pressure control (2–10). It remains uncertain as to why the blockade of the RAAS has such potent cardio- and reno-protective effects. This was initially thought to be due to their reduction of circulating and/or organ angiotensin-II levels. However, increasing doubts on whether that is the sole protective mechanism has stimulated search for alternatives. Both ACEi and ARB, as well as the forthcoming rennin inhibitors, share a clear antiproteinuric effect beyond their antihypertensive effects. Since albuminuria has been associated to cardiovascular and renal risk, one could only speculate as to the possibility that the effect of ACEi and ARB on albuminuria might explain the end-organ protection of inhibition of the RAAS. Even if this relationship is not directly causal, albuminuria and its reduction could be used as surrogate (intermediate) marker for effectiveness of therapy.

The following paragraphs will try to define albuminuria as the (renal) risk marker for cardiovascular and renal end-organ damage, and more importantly to mark it as the novel target for therapy of the 21st century protecting both the kidney and the cardiovascular system, thus arguing that monitoring the therapeutic effect on the kidneys in order to protect the heart and blood vessels. The emphasis of the review will be on patients and studies relating to type 2 diabetes.

ALBUMINURIA: A MARKER OF END-ORGAN DAMAGE

Renal

Albuminuria has been considered a marker of renal damage for decades. The classical hypothesis is that albuminuria or proteinuria is a consequence of renal damage, and as such marks the degree of severity of renal damage/ disease. However, with the work of Williams et al. (11) a turning point was established in this thought process. Williams observed a relationship between the degree of proteinuria and the rate of decline in renal function. This could on the one hand confirm the classical hypothesis, on the other hand it could also be interpreted that proteinuria is associated or even contributing to renal dysfunction. Later clinical work from Groningen in the Netherlands (12) provided clinical evidence that proteinuria is associated with renal dysfunction and that therapy leading to a reduction of proteinuria is associated with protection of the kidneys against further fall in GFR.

Remuzzi and Bertani (13) wrote a landmark review and hypothesis in which they identified albuminuria as a cause, and not just the consequence, of kidney damage in several experimental models. They argued that when albumin is filtered in too high quantities, the proximal tubule becomes overloaded with tubular reabsorption. This, in turn, triggers the release by tubules cells of inflammatory chemokines and cytokines that may contribute to interstitial inflammation. Whether the damage is caused by the native albumin protein itself or by a modified albumin, or by molecules attached to the protein, remains still to be clarified. The relevance of this hypothesis to the clinical situation has been subject of controversy and ongoing debates.

Despite this ongoing cause–effect debate, the predictive power of albumin excretion for progressive renal functional loss is very strong. Clinical studies consistently show that in diabetic and nondiabetic renal disease, despite treatment of all risk factors, albuminuria remains the dictating parameter that predicts the risk for ESRD (4,14). This predictive power appears to be present at all levels of albumin excretion; even high normal albumin excretion rates (15–30 mg/day) predict subsequent risk for renal functional loss in the general population (Fig. 1) (15,16) as has been previously well

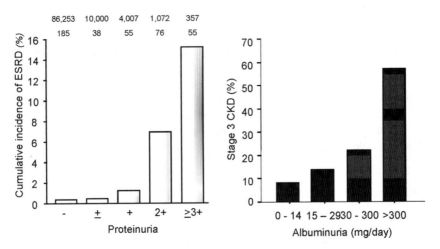

Figure 1 The predictive power of urinary albumin excretion for loss of renal function in the general population. The more proteinuria/albuminuria is excreted, the higher the chance of reaching end-stage renal disease in the next 17 years (15), and the higher the chance of reaching stage 3 (K/DOQI guidelines) renal function loss, (GFR <60 mL/min) during 4-year follow-up (16).

established in the diabetic population (17). Thus, excess albumin excretion in the urine predicts the risk for excessive loss of renal function. Whether it is a marker or maker of renal damage and functional loss is still debatable.

Cardiovascular

The most intriguing part of the above story on albuminuria is that it not only predicts renal outcome, but it also predicts cardiovascular morbidity and mortality. This was already known for quite some years, since the Framingham study (the same study that established the classical CV risk factors) established already in 1984 that proteinuria is an important risk marker of CV mortality (18). The fact that it was never added to the risk profiling is quite intriguing, but may have to do with the fact that it was not as accurately measurable or that it was thought that it was not a modifiable factor. Hillege et al. (19) recently showed that, like for the kidney, albuminuria is at all levels from normal to micro- and macroalbuminuria, predictive of CV events (Fig. 2). Indeed, many studies have shown without any doubt that elevated levels of albuminuria, be it at the low (microalbuminuria) or high (macroalbuminuria) end of the spectrum, are highly predictive for CV morbidity and mortality in many studies both for brain, heart, and peripheral vessels. This holds true in the general

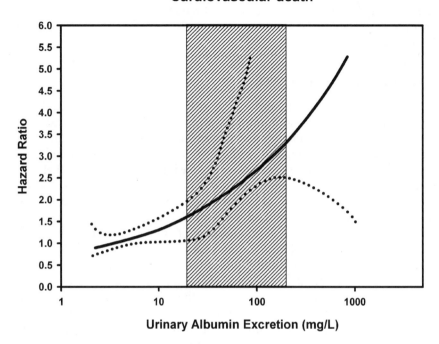

Figure 2 The predictive power of urinary albumin excretion for cardiovascular mortality in the general population (19).

population (19–22), as well as in diabetes (23,24), in hypertension (25), or in subjects with already increased CV risk (26).

The exact mechanism of this albuminuria-associated CV risk is not known. However, there is accumulating evidence that microalbuminuria is associated with endothelial dysfunction (27). This endothelial dysfunction by itself is then preconditioning the vessels for more atherosclerotic risk with all its consequences. Thus, endothelial dysfunction may be the common mechanism of damage both to the kidney and to the cardiovascular system. In the kidney, this may initiate a vicious cycle as endothelial dysfunction would lead to increased albuminuria/proteinuria, which may in turn lead to further glomerular and tubulointerstitial damage. Also, the adaptive changes taking place within the kidney due to endothelial dysfunction including changes in the RAAS may contribute to CV damage. Albuminuria may also reflect the severity of kidney damage; renal insufficiency is associated with increased CV risk (28). Thus, excess renal albumin leakage is associated with increased risk for cardiovascular morbidity and mortality. Albuminuria remains therefore a potent predictor and marker of not only renal but CV risk. Whether it is a risk factor as such awaits confirmation through selective interventions capable of reducing albuminuria in isolation in order to establish whether they would also reduce CV morbidity and mortality.

RAAS-INTERVENTION LOWERS ALBUMINURIA

The importance of albuminuria as a risk predictor for renal and CV disease became much more relevant when drugs were discovered that actually lower albuminuria. Michielsen et al. and Arisz et al. found that non-steroidal antiinflammatory drugs (NSAIDs) are capable of lowering the proteinuria. This effect was associated with a reduction in GFR and appeared to disappear directly after the drug was discontinued (29,30). In 1986, Vriesendorp et al. (12) and Lagrue et al. (31) were the first to show (albeit in non-randomized retrospective clinical trials involving a small number of patients) that lowering of albuminuria with NSAIDs resulted in renal protection. The big disadvantage of such interventions was the fact that high doses of NSAIDs were needed to obtain this anti-proteinuric effect and this was associated with significant side effects. In 1985, Heeg et al. (32), published on the antiproteinuric effect of ACE inhibitors in nondiabetics, while Taguma et al. (33) and Hommel et al. (34) confirmed such effect in patients with diabetic nephropathy. These early observations have since been followed by numerous confirmatory reports (35,36). The fact that both AII-antagonists, renin inhibitors, and more recently aldosterone antagonists have similar antiproteinuric effects (37–39) makes it clear that interventions on all components of the RAAS lead in general to a reduction of albuminuria/proteinuria. Such antiproteinuric effect seems to be in addition to the blood pressure lowering capacity of these agents (37); in fact, one can separate the dose response of proteinuria from that of the blood pressure (40).

RAAS-INTERVENTION OFFERS ORGAN PROTECTION BEYOND BLOOD PRESSURE EFFECTS

Blockade of the RAAS is not only an attractive way to lower a high blood pressure, but animal experimentation suggested it has additional organ-protective effects. These effects are attributed to many different characteristics of RAAS-interventions mainly focusing on inhibiting the numerous potentially detrimental effects of angiotensin II. Several classical trials have consistently shown that both renal and cardiovascular protection can be achieved beyond blood pressure control. The design of such studies was usually comparing two or three treatment arms of which one was containing the RAAS-intervention. Initially, many such clinical trials failed to dissoci-ate the beneficial effects of manipulation of the RAAS from better blood pressure control. But more, recently, better-designed trials were more convincing.

Renal Protection Trials

For the renal protections trials, we will use type 2 diabetes as an example. Renal damage in diabetes is characterized by: (1) the transition from normal urine albumin excretion to microalbuminuria, (2) the transition from micro-albuminuria to macroalbuminuria (the latter phase is called diabetic nephropathy), and finally the stage from macro to end-stage renal disease (ESRD) and/or death. Figure 3 shows that several different landmark trials have successfully targeted the RAAS to prevent the risk of transition from one stage to the next. In the BENDEDICT trial, transition from normal to microalbuminuria was prevented by the ACEi trandolapril compared to the CCB verapamil that had little impact (10). In the IRMA2 trial, patients

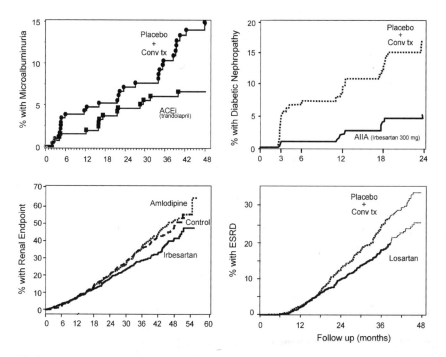

Figure 3 Reno-protective effect of RAAS-intervention in different stages of renal diabetic "disease": transition from normoalbuminuria to microalbuminuria (*top left panel*; BENEDICT); transition from microalbuminuria to macroalbuminuria (*top right panel*; IRMA-2); transition from macroalbuminuria to renal endpoint (*bottom left panel*; IDNT); transition from macroalbuminuria to ESRD (*bottom right panel*; RENAAL).

were protected by the ARB irbesartan from progression from microalbuminuria to overt proteinuria, diabetic nephropathy (5). In the HOPE study,
ramipril protected high CV risk patients from progressing from normo- to
micro- or from micro- to macroalbuminuria (41). Finally, in the Captopril
Collaborative Trial in type 1 diabetes (3), the IDNT (irbesartan) trial (8)
and RENAAL (losartan) (7) trials in type 2 diabetes, patients were protected
from progressive renal insufficiency or ESRD. All these trials confirmed that
the reno-protective effects of RAAS-intervention are due to more than only
blood pressure lowering as in most of these trials blood pressure control was
comparable in the experimental groups. However, the Captopril Collaborative Trial showed significantly lower blood pressure levels in captopril-
treated diabetics and randomization was flawed as the control group had
significantly higher baseline proteinuria (3).

The reno-protective effect of RAAS-intervention is not only present in
different stages of diabetes but is also shown in nondiabetics renal disease.
In particular, the AASK trial showed renal protection in African-American
patients with nephrosclerosis (42), and the REIN trial showed renal protection in nondiabetics proteinuric renal disease (4). Thus, RAAS-intervention
is associated with renal protection, which appears to be present beyond the
blood pressure lowering effect of the drugs. Interestingly, in all these trials
the RAAS-intervention arms showed relatively more lowering of albuminuria when compared to controls.

Cardiovascular

There are a large number of studies showing that RAAS-intervention is
cardioprotective in a range of cardiovascular diseases including those affecting diabetic patients. An in-depth review of these studies is beyond the scope
of this chapter. The HOPE study showed that the ACEi ramipril offers cardiovascular protection in hypertensive patients with one or more additional
CV risk factors (6). This study tested against placebo, and since there was a
marked difference in blood pressure in favor of the ACEi arm, one may
wonder whether this cardiovascular protection is actually to be ascribed
to a special effect of the ACEi ramipril or merely to a better blood pressure
control. However, the LIFE study later showed, in hypertensive patients
with left-ventricular hypertrophy, that the ARB losartan offered better
cardiovascular protection compared the beta-blocker atenolol, with comparable blood pressure control suggesting protection over and above good
blood pressure control (9). Interestingly, in both studies, the most notable
cardiovascular protection was observed in the diabetic sub-groups of
patients. Recently, Asselbergs et al. (43) showed that even in the general
population with only microalbuminuria, if one compares the effect of the
ACEi fosinopril to placebo treatment, one sees a "tendency towards"
cardiac protection. Again in all of the above studies showing more

cardioprotection in the RAAS-intervention arm, there was a higher fall in albumin excretion rate compared to controls.

ALBUMINURIA REDUCTION PREDICTS THE END-ORGAN PROTECTION

Albuminuria has been associated with increased risk for end-organ damage. Interventions affecting the RAAS have been associated with decrease in urinary albumin/protein excretion as well as with end-organ protection. Thus, is the organ protective effect of RAAS-intervention directly associated with its antialbuminuric effect or is the reduction in albuminuria merely a paraphenomenon of the overall end-organ protection afforded by these agents?

Several other therapies are associated with reduction of albuminuria or proteinuria apart from RAAS-intervention. NSAIDs reduce albuminuria as does the switch from high or normal dietary protein intake to a low protein intake (LPD). The reduction in albuminuria by NSAIDs, LPD, or RAAS-intervention follows within weeks after start of the therapies or diet. Is the degree of this initial reduction in albuminuria predictive of the long-term organ protection? In general, one can say that 100% reduction of urinary albumin excretion means full organ protection for years to come, whereas no reduction in albuminuria means little or no organ protection.

Renal

El Nahas et al. (44) were the first to show in 1984, albeit in a very small group of patients, that LPD induced a variable degree of reduction in proteinuria. Interestingly, when they followed the evaluated renal functional response to LPD, they noted that the patients who benefited most were those whose proteinuria fell the most significantly on a protein-restricted diet (44). Similar data were later found by Gansevoort et al. (45) in a retrospective study using an ACE inhibitor therapy. Later Apperloo et al. (46) and Rossing et al. (47) confirmed in nondiabetic as well as in diabetic cohorts, respectively, that the degree of antiproteinuric or antialbuminuric effect of therapy determines for the individual patient, the degree of renal protection (46,47) (Fig. 4).

Similar findings were later observed in large trials such as REIN (ramipril) (4), IRMA-2 (irbesartan) (5), RENAAL (losartan) (14), and IDNT (irbesartan) (48). These trials showed in several stages of diabetic and nondiabetic renal disease that the extent of reduction of albuminuria/ proteinuria upon instituting a RAAS-intervention predicts the renal outcome, in hard endpoints such as transition to diabetic nephropathy, doubling of serum creatinine, or even ESRD. IRMA-2 showed in diabetic microalbuminurics that increasing doses of irbesartan was paralleled by albuminuria

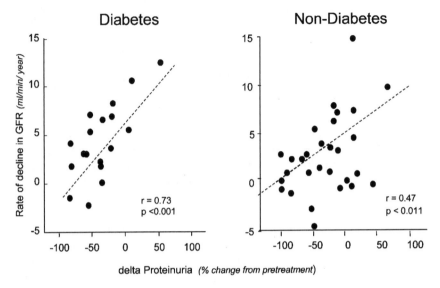

Figure 4 The initial proteinuria/albuminuria lowering response to therapy predicts the renal outcome (decline in GFR during follow-up) both in individual diabetic (*left panel*) and nondiabetic patients. *Source*: Adapted from Refs. 46, 47.

reduction followed by enhanced renal protection. Both IDNT and RENAAL showed in diabetic nephropathy that the more albuminuria is reduced early during the course of treatment, the more significant the prevention of doubling of serum creatinine and/or ESRD (Fig. 5, *left panel*). The RENAAL trial even showed that if one corrected the outcome of the trial for the albuminuria-lowering effect of losartan, the ARB has no additional advantage compared to the control group. In other words, in the RENAAL trial, the extra renal protection provided by the ARB treatment is directly linked to the drug's antiproteinuric effect.

The mechanism of this renal protection linked to albuminuria reduction remains unclear. It would be tempting to interpret the data implying that reduction of albuminuria results in less filtered and reabsorbed proteins, thus leading to less renal inflammation, interstitial fibrosis and functional decline. Whilst, experimental data would support such contention, there are considerable difficulties in extrapolation of this hypothesis to the clinical situation. Also, interstitial inflammation is not a feature of early diabetic nephropathy (microalbuminuria nor even early macroalbuminuria), it appears late in the course of the disease when scarring is prominent. Clearly, other mechanisms may come into play to link albuminuria/proteinuria and its reduction to progressive renal scarring and dysfunction.

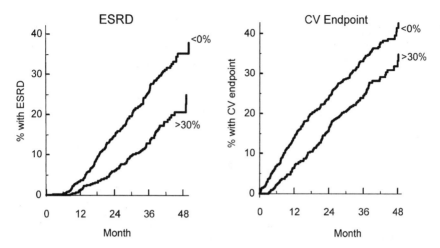

Figure 5 The initial albuminuria lowering response to therapy predicts both the renal (*left panel*) and cardiovascular (*right-hand panel*) outcome during 4 yr continued therapy. Those with more than 30% albuminuria reduction are better protected than those with no change or a rise in albuminuria upon therapy. *Source*: Adapted from Ref. 14.

Cardiovascular

The effect of albuminuria reduction as a predictor for cardiovascular outcome has been first described by de Zeeuw et al. (24) in a post hoc study of the RENAAL trial (24). Indeed, the more significant the reduction of albuminuria with losartan during the first couple of months, the more extensive the protection against cardiovascular events in these diabetics nephropathy patients (Fig. 5, *right panel*). Similar data have been obtained in the LIFE trial in hypertensives with LVH and with varying degree of albuminuria at baseline of which most (70%) were normoalbuminuria (<30 mg/day). Nevertheless, the change in albuminuria occurring upon therapy, appeared to be predictive of the cardiovascular outcome; rise in albuminuria was associated with more CV events, whereas a reduction in albuminuria was associated with cardioprotection (H. Ibsen, personal communication).

Whether the reduction of albuminuria and cardioprotection are causally linked remains to be established, as it is difficult to explain how a reduction in albuminuria would lead to cardiovascular risk reduction. The current explanation would be that the predictive effect of albuminuria for CV events is related to the associated vascular (endothelial) dysfunction (27). Therapies that restore endothelial functional integrity may lead to less glomerular albumin leak and therefore a reduction in albuminuria along with an improved vascular outcome. Whether a reduction of vascular albumin leak is itself protective to vessels and restores endothelial function is more difficult to envisage, but will undoubtedly warrant further investigation. For instance, albumin and associated fatty acids may be taken up by endothelial cells through albumin binding proteins acting as receptors and cause injury. Also, excessive transit of albumin and bound lipids through the vascular wall and their uptake by smooth muscle cells may affect vascular function and integrity. It is interesting in that respect that cellular uptake of albumin stimulates the release of a wide range of pro-inflammatory and pro-fibrotic mediators including the possible generation of angiotensin II.

ALBUMINURIA, A TARGET FOR THERAPY TITRATION

Whatever the mechanism of the renal and cardioprotective effect of RAAS-interventions, the reduction in albuminuria is a good marker for the organ-protective effectiveness of such therapies. Despite the relative success of using RAAS-interventions, the absolute remaining renal (and cardiovascular) risk is still incredibly high. It is important to realize that the prediction of that remaining risk is again highly predicted by the residual level of albuminuria. Despite the fact that therapy may reduce albuminuria substantially (thereby reducing renal risk substantially), if the remaining albuminuria level remains elevated, the patient still runs a considerable risk of both ESRD and CV morbidity and mortality. In fact, it appears that the absolute level of albuminuria is the risk-determining factor regardless of whether this level is at baseline or after treatment (14). This argues for aggressive anti-albuminuric/proteinuric interventions to minimize risks.

There are several ways to enhance the antialbuminuric efficacy of RAAS-intervention. Most important is to optimize the effect of ACEi by combining the therapy with low sodium intake or a diuretic (49). This strategy will result in a further lowering of the blood pressure as well as a further lowering of albuminuria or proteinuria. Secondly, increasing the dose of ACEi or ARB will increase the antialbuminuric effect (50,51). Most importantly, titrating the intervention to albuminuria reduction should be done independently from blood pressure lowering titration; Laverman et al. (40) showed that individual may respond differently to RAAS-intervention dose increase in terms of blood pressure and proteinuria. Lastly, combining an ACEi with an ARB has been shown to have additive effects. The COOP-ERATE trial in nondiabetic renal disease showed that combining an ACEi with an ARB will not only enhance the antiproteinuric effect but also enhance the renal protective effect compared to single-drug regimen (52).

SECONDARY TO PRIMARY PREVENTION, PARTICULARLY IN DEVELOPING COUNTRIES

It is imperative to develop reliable and affordable tools to detect those at risk of CKD and CVD. This is all the more urgent in the developing countries where early detection may lead to effective interventions aimed at primary prevention. The growing epidemic of diabetes and its complications is most likely to devastate health care in the developing world unless early interventions to detect and prevent complications are in place. Measurement and detection of increased urinary albumin excretion are such strategies. It predicts in the general population (even at levels below the currently defined abnormal range of microalbuminuria: 30–300 mg/day) the risk for both renal and cardiovascular disease, as well as interestingly the risk for developing new-onset diabetes (19–22,53).

In fact, albuminuria is easy and cheap to measure. Standard techniques for measuring albumin in urine are nearly all based on antibody interaction with albumin. There are several ways of detecting this complex varying from radiolabels, coloring of the complex, to precipitation techniques such as nephelometry or turbidometry. All these techniques have in common the detection of immunoreactive albumin. The antibodies to detect urinary albumin, are raised against serum albumin.

Although this is still considered a sound approach, it was recently found that albumin could also appear in urine in a so-called non-immunoreactive form. This can be measured by a novel HPLC technique (Accumin®, AusAm Biotechnologies Inc). Several authors have found that this new technique may pick up microalbuminuria in earlier stages of the disease, and may be even more sensitive in its relation with CV disease (54,55). Thus, development of new antibodies that detect all forms of albumin in the urine may be a way forward in the future for more accurate prediction of renal and CV risk.

All these techniques have in common the fact that they need to be carried out in a standardized laboratory environment. Particularly for developing countries, one should be able to measure albumin at a point of care. Although albuminuria can be semi-quantitatively measured with a urine dipstick technique (Micral®, Roche Laboratories), accurate measurements in the field may be extremely valuable both in a setting of the future practicing physician needing to titrate his medication to albuminuria, and also in the current setting for the developing countries. Fortunately, new devices are available that can accurately and rapidly measure albumin with "desktop" machines (Hemocue Urine Albumin®, Bayer DCA 2000®).

When should we test urine for albumin? Certainly in case of diabetes, urine albumin testing is obligatory according to most national and international guidelines. In case of hypertension, it is certainly advisable (and according to some guidelines more than recommendable) that one measures urinary albumin, since it enhances the risk profiling of the individual. In the future, it may become standard to test for albuminuria in the obese and even the general population visiting the general physician/primary care setting. An exception may be the use of such urine albumin measurements in the developing countries. As one may appreciate from the work of Correa-Rotter et al. (56), the need for simple and inexpensive predictors for CV/renal morbidity and mortality is raising dramatically in the developing countries. Next to blood pressure, albuminuria and renal function evaluation by serum creatinine measurement may be such "easy" markers for risk. In these countries, this may well lead to early (primary) intervention strategies, certainly given the fact that treatment in advanced stages is cost-effective, but that more early-stage treatment is even more cost-saving (57). The cost-effectiveness of albuminuria detection in diabetics has been well established. Doubts persist regarding the wisdom and cost-effectiveness of whole population screening for proteinuria; some have found them not to be cost-effective unless it targeted those at higher risk such as the elderly (58). However, such analysis did not take into consideration the potential cost-effectiveness of reducing cardiovascular risk linked to proteinuria, they focused exclusively on the renal protection benefit (58). Whether, albuminuria screening in the general population is cost-effective remains to be established. Whilst, the advantage of albuminuria detection are increasingly recognized, cost implications and effectiveness has to be established before embarking on potentially costing screening exercises in the general population of developing countries.

Finally, having a measurement of albumin in the urine should lead to action in case the result is "abnormal." The definition of normal is now still based on historical findings in diabetes, in which microalbuminuria is defined as "abnormal", ranging from 30 to 300 mg of albumin in the urine per day. Since daily collection of urine is very cumbersome, timed overnight collected urine, or even spot urines are often preferred. Normal ranges for timed overnight urinary albumin samples are defined as between 20 to 200 µg/min. For spot urine samples, the normal range is between 20 to 200 mg/L. Since this latter urine may be diluted or concentrated, correction of albumin concentration values using urinary creatinine is often practiced. The normal range for this urinary albumin creatinine ratio (ACR) is 3 to 30 mg/mmol. However, gender differences in urinary creatinine excretion may further complicate this issue. Until proven different, the standard for normal urinary albumin levels should thus be <30 mg/day or <20 mg/L. This allows correct interpretation of all of the data from the past. Changing borders will only lead to more confusion. Certainly, just like with the definition of normal blood pressure, boundaries for normal albuminuria will shift in the future.

SUMMARY

There is ample evidence that risk-stratification for end-organ damage should include excreted proteins in the urine (albuminuria/proteinuria), along with blood pressure levels, cholesterol levels, presence of diabetes and/or obesity, and smoking. Given the high residual cardiovascular and renal risk under conventional risk reduction strategies, the enormous additional impact of albuminuria on patient morbidity and mortality, and the marked predictive value of albuminuria lowering on cardiovascular and renal protection, one should use the current drug armamentarium to specifically target albuminuria and reduce it as effectively as possible independently of other risk factors.

The fact that reduced renal function, be it albuminuria or decreased filtration power, enhances the vulnerability of the cardiovascular system for progressive failure, as well as the fact that reno-protective strategies are directly related to cardiovascular protection, suggest that the way to a better heart is through a better kidney. This opens the door for multiorgan disease management and therapy in a disease with multiorgan involvement and failure like diabetes. The predictive power of albuminuria for renal and CV disease risk, above and beyond traditional risk profiling, provides us with a tool to detect and take preventive measures even before the diseases are present. Given the threat of growing chronic renal and CV diseases in both the Westernized and particularly the developing world, albuminuria measurement may become a very important vehicle to improve health care and control the healthcare budget. Research is urgently needed to establish the cost-effectiveness of such approaches in order to convince Government agencies to support widespread detection and prevention programs.

REFERENCES

1. National Kidney Foundation. K/DOQI clinical practice guidelines for chronic kidney disease: evaluation, classification, and stratification. Am J Kidney Dis 2002; 39:S1–S266.
2. Maschio G, Alberti D, Janin G, et al. Effect of the angiotensin-converting-enzyme inhibitor benazepril on the progression of chronic renal insufficiency. N Engl J Med 1996; 334:939–945.
3. Lewis EJ, Hunsicker LG, Bain RP, Rohde RD. The effect of angiotensin-converting-enzyme inhibition on diabetic nephropathy. N Engl J Med 1993; 329:1456–1462.
4. No authors listed. Randomised placebo-controlled trial of effect of ramipril on decline in glomerular filtration rate and risk of terminal renal failure in proteinuric, nondiabetic nephropathy. The GISEN Group (Gruppo Italiano di Studi Epidemiologici in Nefrologia). Lancet 1997; 349(9069):1857–1863.
5. Parving H-H, Lehnert H, Brochner-Mortensen J, et al, for the Irbesartan in Patients with Type 2 Diabetes and Microalbuminuria Study Group. The effect of irbesartan on the development of diabetic nephropathy in patients with type 2 diabetes. N Engl J Med 2001; 345:870–878.
6. Yusuf S, Sleight P, Pogue J, Bosch J, Davies R, Dagenais G. Effects of an angiotensin-converting-enzyme inhibitor, ramipril, on cardiovascular events in high-risk patients. The Heart Outcomes Prevention Evaluation Study Investigators. N Engl J Med 2000; 342(3):145–153.

7. Brenner BM, Cooper ME, de Zeeuw D, et al., for the RENAAL Study Investigators. Effects of losartan on renal and cardiovascular outcomes in patients with type 2 diabetes and nephropathy. N Engl J Med 2001; 345: 861–869.
8. Lewis EJ, Hunsicker LG, Clarke WR, et al., for the Collaborative Study Group. Renoprotective effect of the angiotensin-receptor antagonist irbesartan in patients with nephropathy due to type 2 diabetes. N Engl J Med 2001; 345: 851–860.
9. Dahlöf B, Devereux RB, Kjeldsen SE, et al., for the LIFE study group. Cardiovascular morbidity and mortality in the Losartan Intervention for Endpoint Reduction In Hypertension Study (LIFE): a randomised trial against atenolol. Lancet 2002; 359:995–1003.
10. Ruggenenti P, Fassi A, Ilieva AP, et al. Bergamo Nephrologic Diabetes Complications Trial (BENEDICT) Investigators. Preventing microalbuminuria in type 2 diabetes. N Engl J Med 2004; 351(19):1941–1951.
11. Williams PS, Fass G, Bone JM. Renal pathology and proteinuria determine progression in untreated mild/moderate chronic renal failure. Q J Med 1988; 67(252):343–354.
12. Vriesendorp R, Donker AJ, et al. Effects of nonsteroidal anti-inflammatory drugs on proteinuria. Am J Med 1986; 81(2B):84–94.
13. Remuzzi G, Bertani T. Is glomerulosclerosis a consequence of altered glomerular permeability to macromolecules? Kidney Int 1990; 38(3):384–394
14. De Zeeuw D, Remuzzi G, Parving H-H, et al. Proteinuria, a target for renoprotection in patients with type 2 diabetic nephropathy: lessons from RENAAL. Kidney Int 2004; 65:2309–2320.
15. Iseki K, Ikemiya Y, Iseki C, Takishita S. Proteinuria and the risk of developing end-stage renal disease. Kidney Int 2003; 63(4):1468–1474.
16. Verhave JC, Gansevoort RT, et al. An elevated urinary albumin excretion predicts de novo development of renal function impairment in the general population. Kidney Int 2004; 92:S18–S21.
17. Mogensen CE. Microalbuminuria as a predictor of clinical diabetic nephropathy. Kidney Int 1987; 31(2):673–689.
18. Kannel WB, Stampfer MJ, et al. The prognostic significance of proteinuria: the Framingham study. Am Heart J 1984; 108:1347–1352.
19. Hillege HL, Fidler V, et al. Urinary albumin excretion predicts cardiovascular and noncardiovascular mortality in the general population. Circulation 2002; 106:1777–1782.
20. Borch-Johnsen K, Feldt-Rasmussen B, Strandgaard S, Schroll M, Jensen JS. Urinary albumin excretion. An independent predictor of ischemic heart disease. Arterioscler Thromb Vasc Biol 1999; 19(8):1992–1997.
21. Klausen K, Borch-Johnsen K, et al. Very low levels of microalbuminuria are associated with increased risk of coronary heart disease and death independently of renal function, hypertension, and diabetes. Circulation 2004; 110: 32–35.
22. Romundstad S, Holmen J, et al. Microalbuminuria and all-cause mortality in 2,089 apparently healthy individuals: a 4.4-year follow-up study. The Nord-Trøndelag Health Study (HUNT), Norway. Am J Kidney Dis 2003; 42:466–473.

23. Mogensen CE. Microalbuminuria predicts clinical proteinuria and early mortality in maturity-onset diabetes. N Engl J Med 1984; 310(6):356–360.

24. De Zeeuw D, Remuzzi G, Parving H-H, et al. Albuminuria, a therapeutic target for cardiovascular protection in type 2 diabetic patients with nephropathy. Circulation 2004; 110:921–927.

25. Wachtell K, Ibsen H, et al. Albuminuria and cardiovascular risk in hypertensive patients with left ventricular hypertrophy: the LIFE study. Ann Intern Med 2003; 139:901–906.

26. Gerstein HC, Mann JF, Yi Q, et al. Albuminuria and risk of cardiovascular events, death, and heart failure in diabetic and nondiabetic individuals. JAMA 2001; 286(4):421–426.

27. Stehouwer CDA, Henry RMA, et al. Microalbuminuria is associated with impaired brachial artery flow-mediated vasodilation in elderly individuals without and with diabetes: further evidence for a link between microalbuminuria and endothelial dysfunction. The Hoorn Study. Kidney Int 2004; 92:S42–S44.

28. Hillege HL, Girbes AR, de Kam PJ, Boomsma F, de Zeeuw D, Charlesworth A, Hampton JR, van Veldhuisen DJ. Renal function, neurohormonal activation, and survival in patients with chronic heart failure. Circulation 2000; 102(2): 203–210.

29. Michielsen P, Lambert PP. Effects of corticosteroid and indomethacin treatment on proteinurai. Bull Mem Soc Med Hop paris 1967; 118:217–232.

30. Arisz L, Donker AJ, Brentjens JR, van der Hem GK. The effect of indomethacin on proteinuria and kidney function in the nephrotic syndrome. Acta Med Scand 1976; 199:121–125.

31. Lagrue G, Laurent J, Belghiti D. Renal survival in membranoproliferative glomerulonephritis (MPGN): role of long-term treatment with non-steroid anti-inflammatory drugs (NSAID). Int Urol Nephrol 1988; 20:669–677.

32. Heeg JE, de Jong PE, van der Hem GK, de Zeeuw D. Reduction of proteinuria by angiotensin converting enzyme inhibition. Kidney Int 1987; 32:78–83.

33. Taguma Y, Kitamoto Y, Futaki G, Ueda H, Monma H, Ishizaki M, Takahashi H, Sekino H, Sasaki Y. Effect of captopril on heavy proteinuria in azotemic diabetics. N Engl J Med 1985; 313:1617–1620.

34. Hommel E, Parving HH, Mathiesen E, Edsberg B, Damkjaer Nielsen M, Giese J. Effect of captopril on kidney function in insulin-dependent diabetic patients with nephropathy. Br Med J (Clin Res Ed) 1986; 293:467–470.

35. Gansevoort RT, Sluiter WJ, et al. Antiproteinuric effect of blood-pressure-lowering agents: a meta-analysis of comparative trials. Nephrol Dial Transplant 1995; 10(11):1963–1974.

36. Kasiske BL, Kalil RS, Ma JZ, Liao M, Keane WF. Effect of antihypertensive therapy on the kidney in patients with diabetes: a meta-regression analysis. Ann Intern Med. 1993; 118:129–138.

37. Gansevoort RT, de Zeeuw D, et al. Is the antiproteinuric effect of ACE inhibition mediated by interference in the renin–angiotensin system? Kidney Int 1994; 45(3):861–867.

38. Andersen S, Tarnow L, Rossing P, Hansen BV, Parving H-H. Renoprotective effects of angiotensin II receptor blockade in type 1 diabetic patients with diabetic nephropathy. Kidney Int 2000; 57:601–606.

39. van Paassen P, de Zeeuw D, Navis G, de Jong PE. Renal and systemic effects of continued treatment with renin inhibitor remikiren in hypertensive patients with normal and impaired renal function. Nephrol Dial Transplant 2000; 15(5): 637–643.

40. Laverman GD, Andersen S, Rossing P, Navis G, de Zeeuw D, Parving HH. Renoprotection with and without blood pressure reduction. Kidney Int Suppl. 2005; (94): S54–S59 .

41. Mann JF, Gerstein HC, Yi QL, Lonn EM, Hoogwerf BJ, Rashkow A, Yusuf S. Development of renal disease in people at high cardiovascular risk: results of the HOPE randomized study. J Am Soc Nephrol 2003; 14:641–647.

42. Agodoa LY, Appel L, Bakris GL, et al. African American Study of Kidney Disease and Hypertension (AASK) Study Group. Effect of ramipril vs amlodipine on renal outcomes in hypertensive nephrosclerosis: a randomized controlled trial. JAMA 2001; 285:2719–2728.

43. Asselbergs FW, Diercks FH, et al. Effects of fosinopril and pravastatin on cardiovascular events in microalbuminuric subjects; results of the PREVEND IT. Circulation 2004; 110(18):2809–2816.

44. El Nahas AM, Masters-Thomas A, et al. Selective effect of low protein diets in chronic renal diseases. Br Med J (Clin Res Ed) 1984; 289(6455):1337–1341.

45. Gansevoort RT, de Zeeuw D, de Jong PE. Long-term benefits of the antiproteinuric effect of angiotensin-converting enzyme inhibition in nondiabetic renal disease. Am J Kidney Dis 1993; 22:202–206.

46. Apperloo AJ, De Zeeuw D, et al. Short-term antiproteinuric response to antihypertensive treatment predicts long-term GFR decline in patients with nondiabetic renal disease. Kidney Int 1994; 45:S174–S178.

47. Rossing P, Hommel E, et al. Reduction in albuminuria predicts a beneficial effect on diminishing the progression of human diabetic nephropathy during antihypertensive treatment. Diabetologia 1994; 37:511–516.

48. Hunsicker LG, Atkins RC. Impact of Irbesartan, blood pressure control, and proteinuria on renal outcomes in the Irbesartan Diabetic Nephropathy Trial. Kidney Int 2004; 92:S99–S101.

49. Buter H, Hemmelder MH, et al. The blunting of the antiproteinuric efficacy of ACE inhibition by high sodium intake can be restored by hydrochlorothiazide. Nephrol Dial Transplant 1998; 13:1682–1685.

50. Laverman GD, Henning RH, de Jong PE, Navis G, de Zeeuw D. Optimal antiproteinuric dose of losartan in nondiabetic patients with nephrotic range proteinuria. Am J Kidney Dis 2001; 38:1381–1384.

51. Andersen S, Rossing P, Juhl TR, Deinum J, Parving HH. Optimal dose of losartan for renoprotection in diabetic nephropathy. Nephrol Dial Transplant 2002; 17:1413–1418.

52. Nakao N, Yoshimura A, Morita H, Takada M, Kayano T, Ideura T. Combination treatment of angiotensin-II receptor blocker and angiotensin-converting-enzyme inhibitor in nondiabetic renal disease (COOPERATE): a randomised controlled trial. Lancet 2003; 361:117–124.

53. Brantsma AH, Bakker SJL, Hillege HL, de Zeeuw D, de Jong PE, Gansevoort RT. Urinary albumin excretion is an independent predictor of development of type 2 diabetes mellitus [abstr]. ASN 2004.

54. Comper WD, Osicka TM. Albumin-like material in urine. Kidney Int 2004; 92:S67–S68.
55. Brinkman JW, Bakker SJL, et al. Which method for quantifying urinary albumin excretion gives what outcome? A comparison of immunonephelometry with high-performance liquid chromatography. Kidney Int 2004; 92:S69–S75.
56. Correa-Rotter R, Naicker S, et al. Demographic and epidemiologic transition in the developing world: role of albuminuria in the early diagnosis and prevention of renal and cardiovascular disease. Kidney Int 2004; 92:S32–S37.
57. Palmer AJ, Rodby RA. Health economics studies assessing irbesartan use in patients with hypertension, Type 2 diabetes and microalbuminuria. Kidney Int 2004; 92:S118–S120.
58. Boulware LE, Jaar BG, Tarver-Car ME, Brancati FL, Powe NR. Screening for proteinuria in US adults: a cost-effectiveness analysis. JAMA 2003; 290: 3101–3114.

10

Renal Transplantation in Developing Countries

S. Adibul Hasan Rizvi, S. A. Anwar Naqvi, and Ejaz Ahmed

*Sindh Institute of Urology and Transplantation,
Dow Medical College, Karachi, Pakistan*

INTRODUCTION

The developing countries are a heterogeneous collection of countries geographically spanning most of Asia, Africa, Latin America, and Middle East (Fig. 1). Historically, these regions have been the birthplace of many civilizations, but unfortunately most have lagged behind in progress even after the end of colonial period; some being reduced to utter poverty. The World Bank defines them economically according to GNP per capita into low-income countries where the average gross income is less than $785 per capita and low-mid-income countries where the income is between $786 and $3125 per capita (1). Some countries in these regions have GNP exceeding $3125 per capita but share similar problems with the strictly defined developing countries and are therefore included in this category. Eighty percent of the world population lives in these countries; however, they only have access to 15% of world resources. The healthcare budget as percentage of GNP in these countries ranges from 0.8% to 2% compared to 10–15% in the developed world. In addition to economic deprivation, most of the countries in the developing world have unstable governments, inconsistent health priorities and policies, civic unrest, and rapid population growth. Under these economic constraints and an inadequate infrastructure, the government

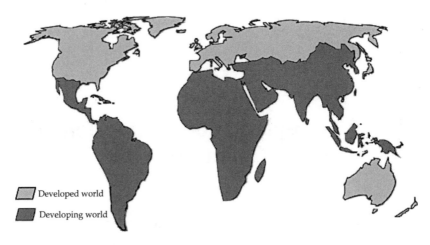

Figure 1 The developing world.

and medical communities in the region have struggled to develop successful transplant programs.

BURDEN OF ESRF IN THE DEVELOPING WORLD

Few countries in the developing world have organized registry of end-stage renal disease (ESRD) patients and data from most of rest are estimates based on dialysis centers in larger metropolitan cities. With half of the population living in rural areas, these figures underestimate the actual burden. On a worldwide basis, there is a direct relationship between GNP and patients receiving renal replacement therapy (RRT). The GNP per capita and prevalence of RRT in less developed Eastern European countries are less than half of Western Europe (2). The contrast becomes more striking when we move to developing countries. In India, where it is estimated that 100,000 patients develop ESRD each year, 90% never see a nephrologist (3). Though the estimated incidence of ESRD in developing countries is similar to the developed world, there is a huge difference in prevalence of patients receiving RRT (Fig. 2).

In addition to the underestimated burden of ESRD patients, another problem is late presentation, which may be detrimental to the prospect of subsequent renal transplantation (4). Late presentation is almost the norm in developing countries. A large proportion is critically ill on first presentation with advanced uremia and pulmonary edema leading to a high early mortality (5). In a study from Sao Paulo, Brazil, 58% (106/184) of the patients with chronic kidney failure (CKF) were diagnosed less than a month prior to the start of maintenance dialysis; 6-month survival of

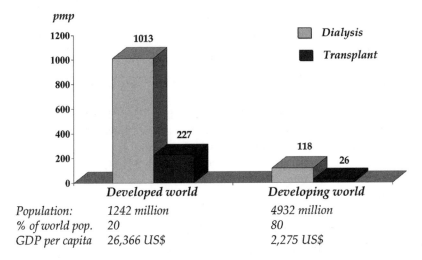

Figure 2 Prevalence of renal replacement therapy at end of 2001, developed versus developing world (120,121).

patients presenting late was 18% lower than those diagnosed early (6). Inadequate dialysis and delay in creation of permanent vascular access leads to frequent infection and malnutrition, while exposure to hepatitis viruses further decreases the prospect of transplantation.

ETIOLOGY OF ESRF AND IMPLICATIONS FOR TRANSPLANT

There are significant regional differences in the causes of ESRD; nevertheless, chronic glomerular disease, diabetes mellitus, hypertensive nephrosclerosis, and chronic interstitial nephritis remain the leading causes of ESRF (Table 1) (7–10). A disproportionately high number of patients present with small smooth kidneys and preceding history is non-contributory to identify the cause (5,11). Considering the fact that majority of transplants in developing countries are from living donors, recurrence of undiagnosed

Table 1 Proportion of Known Causes of ESRD in Different Regions

	Latin America (7)	India (8)	N. Africa (9)	China (10)
Chronic glomerular disease (%)	12.1	23.6	11.24	60.6
Diabetes (%)	24.5	23.2	5–20	4.3
Hypertension (%)	19.5	4.1	5–21	3.9
Chronic interstitial nephritis (%)	—	16.5	14–32	—

original disease and subsequent graft failure reflects loss of a kidney and waste of precious resources. This holds true for certain glomerular disease like focal and segmental glomerulosclerosis (FSGS), sporadic hemolytic uremic syndrome (HUS), and oxalosis (12).

There are some renal diseases concentrated in distinct geographic regions of the developing world. This includes nephrolithiasis in the so-called Afro-Asian stone belt stretching from rim of North Africa, Middle East across to South Asia. Familial Mediterranean Fever in the Mediterranean basin causes recurrent amyloid deposition in transplanted kidney (13). In Africa, schistosomiasis frequently affects urinary tract, bladder fibrosis and active chronic pyelonephritis complicates the management of transplant recipients (14).

RENAL TRANSPLANTATION IN DEVELOPING COUNTRIES—THE PROBLEMS

The progress of renal transplantation in developing countries has been patchy. In some African countries it has yet to start; for most countries, the overall provision of health care and its standard determines the transplant activities; however, there are exceptions. Impediments to, and hindrances in evolution of a successful transplant program can be broadly classified into following groups:

    a. Cost and economics
    b. Donor issues
    c. Religious aspects
    d. Socio-cultural aspects
    e. Awareness and education
    f. Organisational aspects
    g. Ethics and commercialism
    h. Immunosuppression
    i. Infections

Cost and Economics

In developing countries, due to the lower cost of transplantation, to have a functioning transplant becomes less expensive compared to dialysis 1 to 2 years after operation (15); successful rehabilitation and gainful employment are other advantages. Pre-emptive transplantation can further reduce the overall cost, but this is only possible in a minority due to late presentation (16). Despite these distinct advantages, allocating the operational cost of transplantation and that of subsequent immunosuppression from the healthcare budget may not be possible, as it is already strained by expenditure made on debt payment, political stability, and purchase of weapons. Yearly cost of maintaining a transplant can be 5 to 10 times the GNP in many developing countries and on a nationwide scale can theoretically consume quarter of healthcare budget. For these reasons, transplantation activity runs parallel with GNP in most countries (Fig. 3).

The cost of the transplant operation varies widely among different countries, depending on whether a public or private facility is used as well as local economic norms. In general, public care hospital costs are less than half of private care facilities. In countries where initial transplant cost is not supported by the government or reimbursed by employer or health insurance, transplantation is limited to a wealthy few or to those who can obtain the loans. Similarly, maintenance immunosuppression cost is not supported by state or insurance in many countries, and self-financed patients are forced to decrease or discontinue costly immunosuppressants (17).

Donor Issues

Donor source in different parts of developing countries is shown in Figure 4.

Living Donors

Living donors account for nearly half of overall transplant activity, and in some countries it is the predominant type of transplantation. Living-related transplant activity is helped by extended families and strong intra-familial ties. However, finding a suitable donor from within the family may not always be easy. Experience from an exclusive live-related transplant center showed that from an average of six potential donors per recipient in each family at initial work-up, the final outcome is 1.6 donors per recipient. Fear of surgery and refusal by family members were the main reasons for unwillingness to donate, accounting for 36% of dropout. For willing

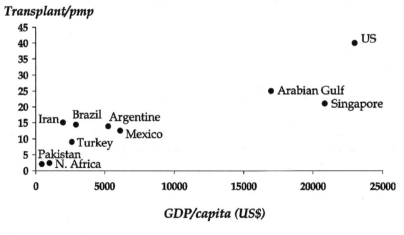

Figure 3 Relation of GDP and transplant activity in selected regions.

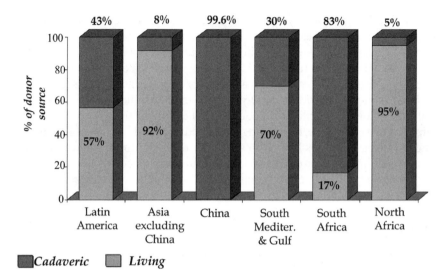

Figure 4 Donor source in different regions.

donors, blood group incompatibility and unidentified medical problems, including diabetes mellitus and hypertension emerged as main factors preventing donation (18). In regions with high prevalence of hepatitis B and hepatitis C asymptomatic carriers are identified during donor work-up, and centers vary in accepting them as donors.

Living-unrelated transplant activity has progressively increased in all regions of the developing world; in Asia 40% of all living donor transplants are from unrelated donors with spousal transplant making 22% of all unrelated activity (19). *Issues related to live-unrelated transplantation including financial and ethical aspects are discussed separately.*

Cadaveric Donors

Experience from Latin American countries suggests that successful cadaveric programs are possible in developing countries. Even among countries in the same geographical regions with equal health expenditure there is wide variation. Economics and organization of cadaveric transplant are certainly more complex and it is the society understanding and motivation, which determines cadaveric transplant activity. The reasons for relatively low cadaver transplant activity in these regions are multiple and are discussed in following sections.

Religion

Most religions practiced in these regions have a progressive and supportive view about organ donation. Culture, traditional values, and beliefs are often mixed up with religious norms and it is difficult to analyze religious impediments to transplantation in developing countries.

There is a large Muslim population in Asia, Middle East, and North Africa, and Islam views life as a gift from God and places great importance on hygiene, health, and prevention of diseases (20). Islamic ethicists allow living donation and removal of organs from the deceased provided there is goodwill and unconditional consent. Islamic scholars and the general population of Middle Eastern Muslims have played an active role in encouraging cadaveric transplantation and have enacted laws supporting it. This is not the case in South Asia where Muslim jurists though agreeing with its potential benefits have not actively supported organ donation (21).

Historically, Christian scholars have been the earliest supporters of transplantation. In both Catholics and Protestant faiths, organ donation from live donors is widely encouraged as a charitable act; organ removal from a deceased person is not considered a hindrance for successful resurrection. As in Muslim population socio-cultural beliefs explain the wide variation regarding organ transplantation in different regions.

In Hinduism, practiced by a large population of South Asia, donation of organs is an individual decision. Traditionally, Hindu texts associate death with respiratory failure and there seems no resistance to death defined on basis of brain-function criteria (21). Failure of transplant act in India to encourage cadaveric transplantation is again down to organizational and socio-cultural reasons.

Buddhism in Asian countries honor those people who donate their bodies and organs for the advancement of medical science and saving lives although there is ambivalence about brain-death criteria (22). Chinese traditional religious thoughts influenced by Confucianism and Taoism are not explicit about organ transplantation, but brain-death criteria are not accepted easily in China (23).

Sociocultural Issues

Living donation is easily accepted in most populations of diverse socio-cultural background, but this is not the case with cadaveric donations. Reverence for the dead is extremely deep-rooted and intactness of the body at the time of burial is considered essential in some cultures; organ removal is considered to be a mutilation of the body. Deceased family members often refuse permission for organ removal, even if explicitly consented by person during their life. It has taken decades in some countries to get cadaveric transplant law to be enacted; however, transplantation rates are poor; this holds true for Asia and is not confined to a particular religion. Japan though a highly developed country only implemented a cadaveric transplantation law in 1997; in Korea a brain-death law was enforced in 2002, whereas in the Philippines, which has a predominantly Christian population, there is negligible cadaveric transplant activity. Cadaveric transplantation law in Pakistan, a Muslim state, has yet to be passed.

Public Awareness and Education

Knowledge about successful renal transplantation as a therapy for ESRF and its potential benefits may not be known to the common man and even the non-specialist medical community in developing countries. The fact that organs can be removed from a "dead person" for the benefit of someone with organ failure is a new concept for the uneducated masses.

Nothing generates greater apprehension and reservation in the minds of people, than the concept of brain death; illiteracy is only partly responsible in generating such feelings. Nationwide programs to improve public awareness and education are seldom undertaken; even for educated people, brain death equates with premature death pronouncement. Mistrust of the medical community and emotional distress to family members have been cited as reasons for unwillingness to become a donor, despite agreeing in principle with cadaveric donation.

The concept unfortunately is not clear either among doctors and paramedical staff who are unaware of procedural details of brain-death confirmation and organ retrieval (24).

Organization and Infrastructure

Implementing laws of organ transplantation to facilitate cadaveric transplant activity runs into practical problems. In most countries, trained surgical teams and transplant physicians are available; however, specially trained paramedical and nursing staff are less easy to find. Overall intensive care facilities are not evenly distributed throughout the country and are limited in number. Transporting accident victims is difficult, especially over long distances and the intensive care unit (ICU) may not accept cases with little hope of survival. In general, ICUs are poorly equipped and are often forced to ration ventilators. Once in the ICU, a potential donor may be missed if the medical team is not especially trained or motivated. Efforts to sustain a potential donor with maximum support are prematurely terminated. Paucity of regional transplant coordinators and social workers especially trained in family counseling decreases the chances of consent (25,26).

Transplant units often work in isolation as nationwide coordination for organ allocation only exists in few countries. The rate of cadaveric transplantation doubled in Turkey after the establishment of a National Coordination Center and organizational improvement (27). Tissue typing laboratories are sparse and wanting in equipment and technically trained staff. In the absence of an organized waiting list of ESRD patients and organ sharing network, allocation is either local and therefore decreases the probability of best match or less commonly cross-match based.

Ethical Issues and Commercialism in Developing Countries

As living kidney donation still accounts for most transplant activity, ethical issues dominate not only in the setting of unrelated transplantation but also for related donors. One can argue about emotional exploitation of a reluctant donor by family members, which may not be apparent to the transplant team; however, for most related donors organ donation is a gratifying experience after a successful transplantation (28,29).

Of the unrelated donors, one category is emotionally related donors which include either spouse or close friends. This has certainly expanded the donor pool with results equivalent to, or better than, cadaveric kidneys (30). Though it is ethically accepted, almost everywhere women are more often the donors and less often the recipients of kidney (31). A "friend" motive to donate his kidney in socioeconomic deprived countries may not be truly altruistic. It is the emotionally unrelated living kidney transplantation involving the sale of kidneys that has been the subject of intensive ethical debate, and has raised concerns about the safety of such practice in developing countries.

The experience from South Asia casts serious doubts about the justification of paid unrelated living transplantation. Poverty, lack of an organized cadaveric program, and availability of trained transplant personnel encouraged commercial transplantation in India in 1980. Despite an organ transplant act in 1994, these have continued (32); it is estimated that 50–60% of transplantation being performed in India are from paid unrelated donors (33). The absence of organ donation law in Pakistan has encouraged paid unrelated renal transplant, which has progressively increased and accounted for 45% transplants performed in 2001 (34); recipients of such transplant are affluent people and foreigners. Small private hospitals with little ancillary facilities can be the setting for transplants and early discharge is encouraged. Post-transplant follow-up is non-existent or inadequate. Though large-scale follow-up is not available, a higher mortality due to transmission of communicable disease has been observed (35).

Donor safety is ignored and there are well-documented cases of transplantation of diseased kidneys and even half of horseshoe kidneys (36). Even in donors a high rate of morbidity and mortality has been reported (37). Though extreme poverty makes this option attractive to many, they fall prey to middlemen who siphon off half of the promised money. In a survey of paid Indian kidney donors, 75% of participants whose motive for donating kidneys was payment of debts, continued to be in debt; 90% reported significant deterioration in health and over 80% said they would not recommend such a step to others (38).

Ethicists have argued that by removing the middlemen and profiteering motive, and implementation of some form of regulation, a fair system can be evolved. Others have argued that banning sale of organs may remove the best option these poor people have (39). The Iranian experience, where the state agrees to act as a third party to regulate a system of organ purchase from voluntary kidney donors in exchange for monetary gain does not support such an assumption. In an interview with 300 kidney vendors, Zargooshi (40) found poverty (79%), negative impact on employment (65%), isolation from society (70%), depressive anxiety (60%), and other negative impact, which deteriorated the previous economical and health status.

Paid donor renal transplantation exerts a negative impact on live-related renal transplantation, as it allows wealthy patients and their families to opt for it as happened in Iran. Societal motivation to develop cadaveric transplant progression damps down (41).

Another type of unrelated transplant is the use of kidneys from executed prisoners. The practice is prevalent in some regions though its exact extent is not known. It has been condemned by all transplant societies; however, individuals have argued that execution itself and not the removal of kidneys after legal process is undignified. There are strong arguments against this practice, including promotion and modification of execution process to facilitate organ retrieval (42).

There are instances of removal of kidneys without consent from people who went to hospitals for other reasons and were unaware of the nature of operation (33). The worst incidence was the killing of patients of a mental hospital to obtain kidneys (43).

Immunosuppression

Cyclosprin in combination with steroid and azathioprine remains the cornerstone of immunosuppression in developing countries. Usual initial dose and target levels of cyclosporin are lower than that recommended and practiced in developed countries. The reasons are partly economical, but there are some suggestions that higher dose is unnecessary and potentially nephrotoxic due to racial and genetic differences in drug handling (44,45). Diltiazem and ketoconazole are often used to reduce cyclosprin dosage for financial reasons; 30–60% reduction in cyclosporin dosage has been reported without significant long-term effects (46,47). Significant reduction or complete withdrawal of cyclosporin after varying period of stable graft function is practiced in some centers; however, this cost-saving measure can be potentially counterproductive if the graft is lost (48).

Mycophenolate mofetil use is limited by cost to high-risk patients. At doses used in developed countries gastro-intestinal side effects are more frequent. There is overall increase in its usage and that of tacrolimus in more prosperous regions consequent to trials conducted in developed countries (49,50). Sirolimus is either not available or infrequently used.

Generic versions of cyclosprin and more recently mycophenolate mofetil are available. For some preparation, well-conducted trials of bio-equivalence have been reported (51). In some countries, these are the predominant preparations prescribed as cost saving is enormous and experience from individual centers regarding their efficacy and safely justifies it. Induction with biological agents is practiced less frequently due to high cost and fear of over immunosuppression with its attendant risk of prevalent and opportunistic infections. Use of biological agents to treat rejection varies among centers.

Infections

In developing countries, post-transplantation infections are the major cause of morbidity, and compared to developed countries is the most common cause of patient loss after successful renal transplantation (52,53). Many factors contribute to it:

- poor hygienic conditions and health education;
- high prevalence of communicable disease;
- lack of clean potable water and sewage disposal;
- limited diagnostic facilities;
- malnutrition.

Infection complicates the course of as many as 75% of transplant recipients; in general, they reflect the endemicity in that population. Common diarrheal illness and respiratory tract infection occur with the same or higher frequency as is prevalent in the community. Of 35 patients hospitalized due to infection at a transplant center in Turkey during 1 year, 42.8% had upper respiratory tract infection and 28.6% had acute gastroenteritis (54). A report from Brazil found that transplant recipient in lower socioeconomic group had more infections (55). Infections of particular relevance for developing countries are briefly discussed here.

Bacterial Infections

Bacterial infections involving the lungs and urinary tract are the commonest source of sepsis. Causative organisms in pneumonic illness have ranged from usual community-acquired organisms like streptococcus pneumonia and *Hemophilus influenzae* to multidrug-resistant gram-negative organisms (56). The etiologic agent may remain unidentified due to the common practice of empiric wide spectrum antibiotic, as isolation techniques are limited.

Epidemiology and the clinical course of urinary tract infections in developing regions exhibit unusual features. Frequency of infection is higher than expected; organisms resistant to commonly used antibiotics are very prevalent due to indiscriminate use of antibiotics in community and hospital. Acute graft dysfunction with overt or occult pyelonephritis is not uncommon and it is not rare to see unsuspected pyelonephritis in graft biopsy. Coexistent infection and rejection on biopsy have been reported and infection can follow antirejection treatment (57,58). Cases of graft loss solely due to recurrent or persistent urinary tract infection have been observed. Management is problematic; prophylaxis with co-trimoxazole or ciprofloxacin may be ineffective (59). The organism may be sensitive to only a few injectable antibiotics and their administration for 4 to 6 weeks as recommended in early post-transplant period, becomes impractical.

Parasitic and Helminthic Infections

Transplanted patients in regions with endemic parasitic infection have the same risks of developing disease as the general population but the clinical course may be more aggressive.

In tropical regions, malaria is the most common parasitic infection affecting transplant recipients. It is not clear if mortality is higher than local non-immunosuppressed patients developing the disease; however, response to standard anti-malarial drug seems adequate (60).

Trypanosomiasis (Chaga's disease), is endemic in South America; new infection after transplantation and reactivation have been reported (61). As with malaria, response to treatment is not blunted but prophylactic treatment for those receiving heavy immunosuppression is suggested.

Of the helminthic infection, strongyloidiasis in tropical regions can follow a very aggressive course after transplantation. Severe disease confined to the intestine or lungs, as well as a disseminated disease has been reported. The presence of eosinophilia in appropriate setting should alert and a search for larva in the stool and other body fluids be made. Ameobiasis which on occasion may become invasive can lead to colonic perforation (Fig. 5A–C).

Fungal Infections

Both superficial and systemic fungal infections are more prevalent in developing countries after transplantation with deep infections carrying a high mortality. Environmental factors have an important bearing. The overall incidence of systemic fungal infection in tropics is 4.7% (62).

Invasive aspergillosis involves the lung and early diagnosis using bronchoalveolar lavage (BAL) and transbronchial biopsy can be life saving as amphotericin can be started without undue delay. Mortality can be as high as 50–90% (63). Rare cases of aspergillosis involving transplanted kidney with rupture of graft vessel have been reported. The same is true for mucormycosis, which in addition to the rhinocerebral form and pneumonic illness can affect transplanted kidney (Fig. 6A, B).

Viral Infections

The herpes group of viruses and those causing hepatitis cause considerable morbidity and mortality in transplant recipients especially in developing region.

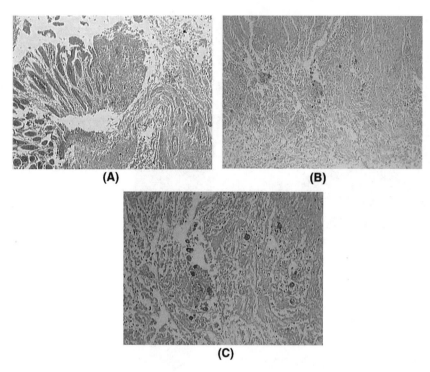

Figure 5 (A) Ameobic ulcer (B) *Entaneoba histolytica* in muscle layer of colonic wall. (C) High-power view showing individual parasites.

Herpes virus group: Among the herpes viruses, Cytomegalovirus is the most commonly encountered infection and many have detrimental effect on graft function and survival. In the adult population of the developing world, a very high seropositivity for CMV has been observed at time of transplantation (64). This combined with lower intensity of immunosuppression may well account for its comparatively lower incidence in some series (65). It may go unrecognized due to lack of available diagnostic tests including quantitative polymerase chain reaction (PCR) and antigenemia-based tests. Prophylactic strategies as practiced in developed countries may not be necessary for reasons mentioned above and are too expensive. Pre-emptive treatment with intravenous gancyclovir at time of treatment with antilymphocyte antibodies has been shown to be cost effective (66).

Cytomegalovirus detection test based on pp-65 antigen has a high sensitivity and if available can be used to detect early CMV disease. Selective treatment of these patients with intravenous gancyclovir is a safe and economically viable option (67). Oral formulation of gancyclovir and the recently introduced valacyclovir and valgancyclovir are yet to be used in

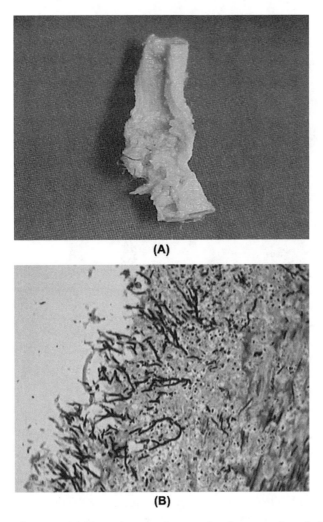

Figure 6 (A) Transplant renal artery showing necrosis and sloughing (B) Histology of arterial wall showing aspergillus invading intima.

developing countries on large scale and may be prohibitively expensive; even intra-venous gancyclovir is not easily available, costly, and death due to invasive CMV disease has been reported due to non-affordability (68).

Hepatitis viruses: Current prevalence of hepatitis C and hepatitis B virus infections in dialysis patients of developing countries range from 10% to 68% and 10% to 45%, respectively; this causes considerable problems in pre- and post-transplant period (69).

Hepatitis C virus infection: Short- and medium-term patient and graft survival does not seem to be affected by HCV infection (70,71). However, longer follow-up studies show a negative impact on patients' survival in the second decade after transplantation (72).

Screening and selection of HCV-positive patients in high prevalent areas for transplantation puts tremendous strain on already meager resources. It is suggested that screening should be done with a third-generation anti-HCV ELISA, which has a high sensitivity (73,74). Even if the test is available, it may not detect all patients harboring HCV and tests for HCV RNA may be necessary (75). HCV RNA detection tests are labor-intensive, prohibitively expensive, and only selected laboratories in developing countries have them.

Liver biopsy is usually necessary for diagnosis and staging of chronic liver disease in HCV patients awaiting transplant (76). The risk of post-biopsy bleeding is high in under-dialyzed patients typical of developing country and equipments for the transjugular approach carry its own cost when available.

Established cirrhosis is a relative contraindication for subsequent transplantation. Patients with chronic hepatitis without cirrhosis are by far the largest group and perhaps the biggest dilemma for subsequent transplantation. Interferon treatment in dialysis patients can achieve a sustained response in as many as 30–70% after 12 months of therapy (77). This response is maintained post-transplantation with no detrimental effect on subsequent graft survival (78). Interferon therapy post-renal transplant is less effective and can precipitate rejection. Ideally all patients, especially those with active chronic hepatitis, should be treated with interferon before transplantation. The cost of interferon therapy and its duration prevents its widespread application in developing countries where more resources should be saved for subsequent transplant operation and cost of immunosuppression. In these patients, the use of ribavarine is contraindicated in view of severe renal insufficiency and the associated high-risk profile of the drug.

There are insufficient data about the antiviral effects of mycophenolate mofetil to recommend its preferential use in HCV-positive patients. In addition, it makes the immunosuppressive regime more costly compared to azathioprine, which is still widely used in developing countries.

Donors with Positive Hepatitis Serology

Anti-HCV-positive donors are more likely to transmit infection if they are HCV RNA-positive (79,80). Those who are HCV RNA-negative can be considered for anti-HCV-negative recipients if choice is limited. Recipients who are anti-HCV-positive with HCV RNA positively can be grafted with anti-HCV-positive kidney, as adverse effect of superinfection with a different genotype is small (81). Among 17 participant countries in Asian transplant registry, HCV antibody-positive donors to anti-HCV-positive recipient is allowed in 10 countries; however, for HCV antibody-negative recipients such donors are accepted in two countries (19).

Hepatitis B infection: Chronic hepatitis B virus infection is highly prevalent in Asia. In Taiwan, the prevalence of HBV infection in the general population is 15% and a much higher prevalence of 19.2% and 20.9% in dialysis and transplant patients, respectively (82). Poor outcome in earlier reports led to the exclusion of HBsAg-positive patients from transplant list in some centers till they become HBsAg negative (83). More recent reports suggest that bad outcome is limited to patients with pre-existing cirrhosis (71).

Pre-transplant ALT levels are poor predictors of severity of liver disease before and after transplantation. High pre-transplant viral load (HBeAg positive or DNA$>10^5$ copies mL) has been associated with reduced 10-year survival after renal transplantation (84). Liver histology before transplant may be a very useful guide in selecting patients and it is suggested that all HBV-positive transplant candidates, like their HCV-positive counterparts, without clinical or radiological features of cirrhosis should undergo liver biopsy, but this is not practiced routinely in developing countries. For those with chronic hepatitis pre-transplant, treatment with lamivudine or interferon is suggested. With or without pre-treatment, subsequent transplant policy in this group is variable among centers.

Lamivudine post-transplantation has been shown to be effective and a meta-analysis of its use, which included five studies from Asia, showed a mean overall estimate for HBV DNA and HBeAg clearance of 91% and 27%, respectively, but loss of HBsAg was infrequent. The mean overall estimate of ALT normalization was 81% (85). In patients with varying severity of chronic hepatitis on biopsy and HBV DNA greater than 10^5 copies/mL, it is prudent to start treatment before transplant. Emergence of lamivudine resistance in general and its cost become a limiting factor with prolonged treatment. Interferon therapy is only safe before transplant as previously discussed.

Tuberculosis after renal transplantation: The reported incidence of tuberculosis after renal transplantation has been as high as 15.2% in developing world compared to 0.36% in the developed countries (86,87). Though tuberculosis can develop at any time post transplantation, the majority of cases occur within the first year of transplantation. Presentation can be atypical being masked by immunosuppression. A relatively higher frequency of extra-pulmonary lesion and disseminated disease is encountered (Figs. 6 and 7) (88).

Bacteriological diagnosis by smear and culture of body secretion and fluids have limitations and take time. PCR-based tests are not available in every center and more importantly their specificity in endemic areas has shown wide variation (89).

Radiological changes in the organ involved though by no means pathognomic, sometime suggest the diagnosis in the right setting. The classic apical cavitation on chest X-ray in cases of documented pulmonary involvement is seldom seen in immunosuppressed patients (90). In cases with pulmonary involvement and scanty sputum production, BAL may be helpful.

Histological examination of the accessible biopsy site is another way of confirming diagnosis, which may show typical granuloma with or without caseation. It may not be easy to confirm the diagnosis of TB and a therapeutic trial in appropriate setting is justified (91).

The well-known interaction of cyclosporin with rifampicin necessitates 150–200% increment in cyclosprin dosage with considerable cost burden. A regimen that excludes rifampicin can be employed but the duration of treatment is prolonged (90). The emergence of TB resistant to conventional

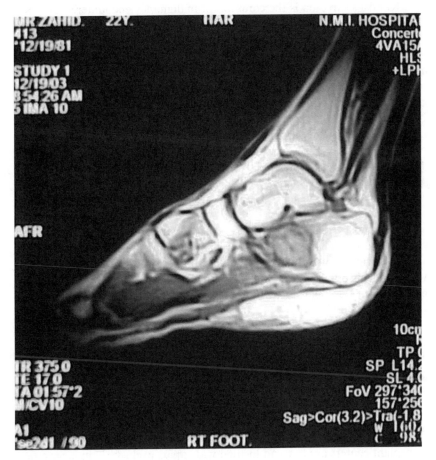

Figure 7 MRI showing tuberculous osteomyelitis of calcaneus.

drugs requires administration of second-line drugs, which are expensive and not easily available. Despite these limitations, successful treatment of post-renal transplant tuberculosis is possible, though the risk of death may be increased by 20–25% (92). Relapse after successful treatment is uncommon.

Whether or not isoniazid (INH) prophylaxis should be given in endemic areas is a debatable issue. Preliminary results from an ongoing randomized trial at our own center have shown a trend of lower incidence in the INH-treated group (93).

POST-TRANSPLANTATION MALIGNANCY

Geographical area, genetic predisposition and type of immunosuppression account for a slightly different pattern of malignancy following renal transplantation in developing countries.

Kaposi's sarcoma is the commonest malignancy encountered in Saudi Arabia, Egypt, Pakistan, and the non-White population of South Africa (94,95); the average time of appearance is 21 months post-transplantation (96). Therapeutic approaches include reduction or complete withdrawal of immunosuppression depending on the extent of disease with or without surgery and radiation. Visceral involvement carries a poor prognosis for patients' survival (Fig. 8) (97). Human herpes virus 8 also known as Kaposi's sarcoma herpes virus (KSHV) is causally associated with Kaposi's sarcoma as its incidence in renal transplant recipient parallels the geographic seroprevalence of KSHV in these regions (98).

Non-Hodgkin's extranodal lymphoma can involve unusual sites; gastrointestinal involvement was considerably higher (88%) in a series reported from Mexico, which contrasts with the 12–24% reported in larger series from developed countries (99).

Early post-transplant lymphoproliferative disease is strongly associated with EBV, especially in children. In the non-immunosuppressed population, latent EBV infection is linked to the development of Burkit's lymphoma in Africa and nasopharyngeal carcinoma in Southeast Asia. Data from these regions about these particular tumors in the setting of renal transplantation is lacking.

Bladder cancer comprised 14% of all malignancies reported from Egypt, which is six times more than that reported in the Cincinnati Transplant Registry (94). Concomitant presence of schistosomial infection explains the high incidence in this region. Routine cystoscopy at regular intervals in those who had schistosomiasis before transplantation is necessary.

MONITORING AND OUTCOME

Transplant centers are few and located wide apart exclusively in large cities. Frequency of patients' follow-up is partly limited by long-distance travel,

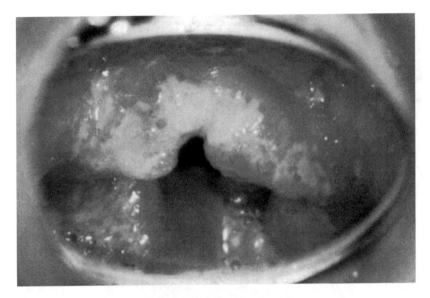

Figure 8 Laryngeal tuberculosis in a transplant recipient.

which is costly, inconvenient, consumes valuable time and working hours. Coordination among centers and an organized primary healthcare system is lacking, forcing patients to always attend the same unit even for trivial medical problems.

Compliance is reportedly better in those who receive immunosuppressants free of charge (100). It is not surprising that self-financed patient don't comply well with costly immunosuppressant for long periods, in addition lower socioeconomic group on its own has been shown to correlate with poor compliance (101,102). In a study from India, non-compliance to drugs and follow-up was found in 21.7% of 152 recipients. Low income, residence long distance away from hospital, female sex, and low level of education were factors more frequent in non-compliant group. There was higher incidence of chronic infection and death in non-compliant group (103). Non-compliance was the third most common cause of graft loss in a study from Taiwan and 82% of non-compliant patients lost their grafts (104).

There is a wide variation regarding drug level monitoring and practice of performing biopsy for graft dysfunction. Availability and center preference determine the frequency of cyclosporin monitoring, cost is an important issue restricting its use to first few weeks or in cases with acute dysfunction.

Acute rejection is often diagnosed on clinical grounds, as graft biopsy adds to the cost of subsequent management and histopathologists familiar with transplant biopsy interpretation are hard to find. Laboratories well equipped to process biopsy tissue in a standard way are far and few.

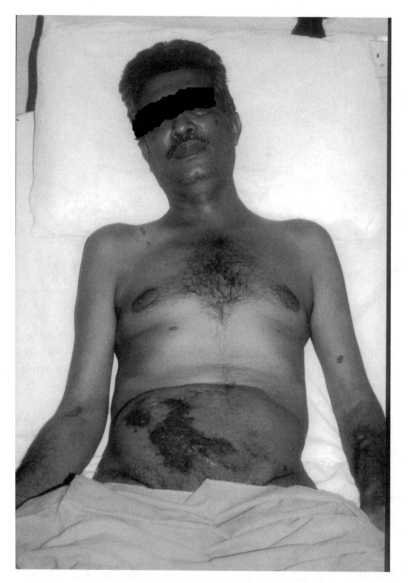

Figure 9 Extensive cutaneous lesion of Kaposi sarcoma in a transplant recipient.

Despite these limitations, 1-year graft survival has reached 90% in some centers of developing countries. Overall graft survival at 1 and 5 years are inferior to those reported from developed countries. Center effect, lack of appropriate diagnostic facilities, tailoring immunosuppression to curtail cost, frequency and accuracy of follow-up are all contributory. Chronic rejection is the most common cause of long-term graft loss.

Infection-related mortality is the main cause of patient loss reported from most centers. Cardiovascular diseases ranked second to infection compared to developed countries, where it is the leading cause of patient loss (34,105,106).

PEDIATRIC TRANSPLANTATION

Late diagnosed anomalies of kidney and urinary tract make a significant proportion of known cases of ESRD in children in developing countries. Due to consanguineous marriages, hereditary diseases are common. Underlying disease remains obscure in 40–50% of cases. The care of children with ESRD is more complex and demanding. Dedicated units staffed with pediatric nephrologists do not exist in developing countries. Identification of renal disease is late and by the time they reach a renal care facility, which usually caters for adult population, considerable growth retardation has already occurred. Often they are considered too small and technically demanding for a transplant operation and not offered this modality. Those who are accepted face enormous problems in getting a permanent vascular access, which in itself requires expertise. Frequent infection with temporary access decreases their transplant prospect, as CAPD is not well organized in developing countries (107).

Early live-related transplantation is the best option for children with ESRD, but parents who have to look after other siblings in a usual large family are often reluctant to donate, having reservations about its potential benefit (108). Children with abnormalities of lower urinary tract are usually considered difficult or impossible to transplant. A cadaveric program if exists is more likely to allocate a kidney to an adult.

For these reasons, pediatric transplantation accounts for less than 5% of all transplants and 80–90% are from living donors. The mean age of children is high as those under 5 years are seldom transplanted (109). Detection of early post-transplant complications in children requires high index of suspicion and ancillary diagnostic facilities, which are not uniformly available in developing countries. Monitoring of immunosuppression, which sometimes requires frequent drug levels, adds to cost and complexity in managing children post transplant (110). Despite these problems, individual centers 1- and 5-year graft survival of live-related pediatric transplants have ranged from 85% to 90% and 65% to 72%, respectively (111,112). Results of cadaveric transplantation in children are even more sparse, out of the 217 pediatric transplants in Brazil at a single center, 64 (29.5%) received a cadaveric kidney. Combined 1- and 5-year patient and graft survival rates were 97%, 95%, 90%, and 72%, respectively (105). As in the adult population, infections cause considerable morbidity and mortality in the post-transplant period in children.

RENAL TRANSPLANT IN SPECIFIC REGIONS

Asia

The average annual transplant rate remains below 10 per million population and living donor transplantation forms the bulk of transplant activity. It is only in China, where almost all renal transplantations are from cadaveric donors; however, the relative proportion of cadaveric transplants using kidneys from executed prisoners is unknown. Renal transplantation units are not run by government, and those with medical insurance get reimbursement for 1 year of transplant cost (112). In sharp contrast, in neighboring South Korea, transplantation activity predominantly uses living donors with one-third being unrelated. Korea has also developed a swap (donor exchange) program for patients with willing but incompatible donors (106).

Southeast Asia has a generally low transplant rate though some of the economies are fairly prosperous. Singapore has the highest transplant rate of 21 pmp, half of them being cadaveric. The same proportion of cadaveric transplants are performed in Thailand. Indonesia, the most populous country in the region, has very low transplantation activity.

The Indian sub-continent relies heavily on living donation. The menace of commercial unrelated transplant has been discussed earlier. Following the approval of cadaveric transplantation law in India in 1995, 523 cadaveric transplants have been performed till the end of 2003 (G. Abraham, personal communication, 2004).

In Iran, state-sponsored and -controlled paid living unrelated transplant has flourished and now accounts for most transplants performed there. This has happened at the expense of live-related transplant. Waiting lists have shrunken as transplantation activity has reached 27 cases per million per year (113).

Middle East and South Mediterranean

In Turkey and Saudi Arabia, where financial constraints are low and cadaveric laws have existed for a while, organizational aspects of renal transplantation are much better. In these countries, cadaveric transplant activity is about 20–30% of total transplants (27). Patients transplanted abroad from live-unrelated donors now outnumber locally transplanted patients in Saudi Arabia (F. A. M. Shaheen and A. A. Khedr, personal communication, 2004).

In Lebanon, cadaveric transplantation was established in 1990, but it makes only 10% of yearly transplant activity and living-unrelated transplants accounts for the majority of patients. Israel has a very well-developed transplant program. Combined living and cadaveric transplant activity is equal to developed countries transplant rates.

Africa

For Africa as a whole, transplant activity is the lowest compared to other developing regions, averaging below 5 pmp/year. Transplantation is limited to North African countries and South Africa. Only few countries in sub-Saharan and West Africa have renal transplantation programs.

Egypt accounts for majority of transplant among North African nations. Between 1993 and 2002, 3000 renal transplants were performed, with almost all using live donors (114). Unrelated transplantation makes a large proportion. Cadaveric transplant activity has picked up in Tunisia. Twenty-five percent of transplants are cadaveric and a presumed consent type of law has existed since 1991.

South Africa has a well-established cadaveric transplant program, where cadaveric transplantation law has existed since 1984. Of the 300 yearly transplants performed, 250 are from cadaveric donors. There is a low rate of organ donation by Muslim families and the Black population (115).

Latin America

Average transplant rate in Latin America now exceeds 10 per million population (pmp) and nearly half are living donors. As in other regions, there are differences among countries.

Renal transplantation rate in Brazil reached 22 pmp in 2001, which is more than double the Latin American average. Organizational improvement had a positive effect in increasing cadaveric transplantation activity (119). Argentine, Chile, and Colombia have two-third of transplants from cadaveric donors. Mexico has a predominant living donor transplant program.

Overall renal transplantation is better organized in Latin American countries with nine of 18 countries surveyed having some type of registry. Use of newer immunosuppressive drugs including MMF and tacrolimus (FK506) has increased and the same holds true for polyclonal and monoclonal antibodies with over 50% of countries and reporting their use in variable proportion (117).

THE WAY FORWARD

The hallmark of the developing world is poverty. Between one-third and one-half of the population in these countries lives on less than a dollar a day. The economies in these countries are predominantly agrarian and crop failures are not uncommon. Borrowing from international donor agencies, which show little compassion for the poor makes them vulnerable when debt servicing is being negotiated. Moreover, inefficiency and lack of transparency allow very little of the funds trickling down to the sick. As a result, whereas the industrialized nations spend 10–15% GDP on health care, most poorer countries can only spare less then 1%. The fragile economies preclude health insurance to be a viable option. Under such difficult circumstances, expectations from the government to sponsor a comprehensive renal rehabilitation program are unrealistic. Ways to organize and improve the current situation of renal transplantation in developing countries are discussed below.

Prevention of Renal Disease

The goal of prevention of renal disease will remain elusive, but diseases such as diabetes mellitus and hypertension could be targeted across the countries in urban and rural government clinics and hospitals. Blood pressure monitoring and basic clinical laboratory together with the use of ultrasound would help improve better detection and monitoring of patients. Measures to slow the progression of renal disease would be a small but important measure. However, many would continue to reach ESRF and there is no substitute for transplantation for reasons of cost, quality of life, and rehabilitation.

Government Community Partnership

Any meaningful dialysis and transplantation program will have to seek funding sources other than that of the State. Involvement of community through participation of the affluent is one workable option. To create a viable and sustainable model, it should be supported jointly by community and the government. Dialysis and transplantation centers should be encouraged in public sector hospitals not only to make it cost effective but also to provide access to the poor population who form the vast majority. SIUT has tried to create one such model.

History of SIUT

SIUT had its beginning in 1972 as an eight-bedded Urology ward within the premises of a large public sector hospital in Karachi, Pakistan. The hospital caters for low-income city dwellers and poor rural population. To begin with, neglected stone cases formed the bulk of workload in the ward and many had renal impairment. Shear necessity forced the beginning of peritoneal dialysis in 1975 and in-house modified physiological saline was the only solution available for this purpose. This therapy was not suitable in many patients and hemodialysis facility was acquired in 1977. Hemodialysis machine with coil dialyzer was the earliest. It was soon realized that Urology ward had to establish a dialysis unit not only to cater for its own patient but also for all those coming to other medical wards with renal failure. Donation was sought from community who realized and appreciated free and dedicated services being offered to the poor. They responded generously once their confidence was gained. A fully functional hemodialysis unit with four machines became operational in 1981. General urology services continued expanding and so was the number of patients on maintenance dialysis. After getting sponsorship by a charity foundation, which contributed to the cost of surgery and maintenance immunosuppression, live-related renal transplantation was started in November 1985. Until 1990, annual transplantation rate was 20 and post-transplant management was done by urologist as there was no trained nephrologists available. Ancillary test like tissue typing and drug level used to be done abroad. All investigation facilities for transplantation were gradually established under one roof, decreasing dependence on costly private facilities. A team concept was evolved with emphasis on early and coordinated effort by different specialists for complex medical problems. Good outcome at no cost to the poor patient motivated the community whose participation increased from individual to corporate donors. To ensure transparency, SIUT is supervised by Board of Governors comprising members of government, community representatives from different walks of life, and philanthropists. The government contributes 40% of budget and rests comes from community as donation. From year 2000 onwards, 100 to 120 live-related renal transplantation are being performed annually and all are getting free maintenance immunosuppressive drugs from this institute.

Donor Source

In developing countries, large family size is common and intrafamilial donor can support a modest transplantation program. Unrelated donors should be discouraged because the financial inducements will push the program towards unbridled commercialism, witnessed in India in the 1990s. Only the rich will be able to afford to pay for the unrelated donor transplantation, whereas the donors invariably will be the poor who would be induced to donate without due informed consent. If unchecked, this will result in mushrooming into transplant tourism, e.g., patients from Middle East and Europe are traveling to Pakistan for living unrelated donors. In fact, liberalizing of visas may see wandering donors from developing countries in the garb of laborers at the door step of richer nations. But most importantly, donor safety and follow-up would be almost impossible under such circumstances.

Education

The next step would be to educate the society of the benefits of cadaver donation. Transplantologist will have to motivate the society especially journalist and writers in print and electronic media about the benefits of transplantation. Acceptance of brain-death criteria will pave the way for increasing renal transplantation as well as initiating non-renal transplantation. Given the resistance to cadaver donor transplantation due to socio-cultural reasons, non-heart beating donor may be the most feasible option in the beginning.

Immunosuppression

Under economic constraints, it is difficult to formulate guidelines for maintenance immunosuppression. In patients with three or fewer mismatches, it is safe to start treatment with calcineurin inhibitors in dosage, which are non-nephrotoxic for local population along with prednisolone and azathioprine. Use of generic preparation of cyclosporin and concomitant administration of diltiazem can make the regime more affordable without compromising safety. It is preferable to continue lower and economically affordable dose of cyclosporine than its complete discontinuation (48). Withdrawal of cyclosporine after 12 months of stable graft function can be attempted in very good matched kidneys that never had acute rejection episode (118). Slow tapering of cyclosporine over 2 to 3 months before discontinuation decreases the chances of acute rejection. A higher dose of azathioprine on stopping cyclosporin may afford some protection in combination with prednisolone.

Mycophenolate is advisable in cases with more mismatches or in those who develop early acute rejection while on azathioprin; however, this makes immunosuppression very costly. Use of mycophenolate for first few months after transplant is a more economically viable option in such situation with later substitution by azathioprine (119).

Induction treatment with biological agents should best be limited to high-risk patients and IL2 receptor blockers are preferable as risk of subsequent infection is lower.

Infection Control

It is difficult to balance immunosuppression and risk of infection in developing countries. Measures to prevent infection should start from pre-transplant period. Correction of anatomical abnormalities of urinary tract and ensuring that tract is sterile is a must. Identification and treatment of active TB before transplant is necessary. Immunization status against common infectious diseases especially HBV and tetanus must be ensured. In the peri-operative and early hospital stay, universal precautions are often ignored and emphasis shifts on wide spectrum prophylactic antibiotics for long periods. Hand washing and targeted short-term prophylactic antibiotic offer good protection at low cost. Minimizing blood transfusion and early removal of drains and catheters are other protective measures.

At discharge, patients should be advised to consume clean water and avoid commercially cooked food. Cotrimoxazole prophylaxis against PCP is recommended. Topical oral antifungal may offer some protection against candida. INH prophylaxis against TB remains a contentious issue. Patients should be encouraged to contact the transplant center during all febrile illness and provision of isolation for potentially contagious or undiagnosed infectious patients must be ensured.

Regional Cooperation

Regional countries, i.e., South Asian block could explore the possibility of manufacturing dialysis machines and consumables. Dialysis concentrate can be produced indigenously in most countries with some help from the industry, resulting in cost saving of up to 40%. Local pharmaceutical industry should be encouraged to manufacture generic immunosuppressants of comparable efficacy.

Regional training centers for physicians and surgeons, nurses, and technicians could organize courses and workshops to promote collaboration and understanding. Registry for dialysis and transplantation could focus on outcomes and regional issues, e.g., immunosuppression and infections. The use of Internet would further augment registry and organ sharing in the future. The above measures can enhance the present dismal transplantation rate of less than 10 per million population to double in the foreseeable future.

ACKNOWLEDGMENTS

We are grateful to Prof. Fazal Akhtar, Dr. Zahid Anwar Khan, Dr. Javed Kazi, Dr. Rubina Naqvi, Dr. Rahel Aziz, Dr. Kashif Manzoor, Dr. Farhana Amanullah, Dr. Tahir Aziz, Dr. Seema Hashmi, and Dr. Salman Imtiaz, who participated in this study. The authors also thank the library and secretarial staff of SIUT.

REFERENCES

1. World Bank Research World Development Reports. http://econ.worldbank.org/wdr.
2. De Vecchi AF, Dratwa M, Wiedemann ME. Healthcare systems and end stage renal disease (ESRD) therapies—an international review: costs and reimbursement/ funding of ESRD therapies. Nephrol Dial Transplant 1999; 14(suppl 6):31–41.
3. Kher V. End stage renal disease in developing countries. Kidney Int 2002; 62:350–362.
4. Lameire N, Van Biesen W. The pattern of referral of patients with end stage renal disease to the nephrologist—a European survey. Nephrol Dial Transplant 1999; 14(suppl 6):16–23.
5. Rao M, Juneja RB, Shirly M, Jacob CK. Hemodialysis for end stage renal disease in Southern India—a perspective from a tertiary referral care centre. Nephrol Dial Transplant 1998; 13:2492–2500.
6. Sesso R, Belasco AG. Late diagnosis of chronic renal failure and mortality on maintenance dialysis. Nephrol Dial Transplant 1996; 11:2417–2420.

7. Fernandez-Cean J. Renal replacement therapy in Latin America. Kidney Int 2000; 57(suppl 74):S55–S59.
8. Mittal S, Kher V, Gulati S, Agarwal LK, Arora P. Chronic renal failure in India. Ren Fail 1997; 19:763–770.
9. Barsoum RS. End stage renal disease in North Africa. Kidney Int 2003; 63(suppl 83):S111–S114.
10. Guanyu W, Nan C, Jiaqi Q, Shanyan L, Qinjun X, Dechang D. Nephrology, dialysis and transplantation in Shanghai, 1999. Nephrol Dial Transplant 2000; 15:961–963.
11. Ball S, Lloyd J, Cairns T, Cook T, Palmer A, Cattell V, Taube D. Why is there so much end stage renal failure of undetermined cause in UK Indo-Asians? Q J Med 2001; 94:187–193.
12. Cameron JS. Recurrent renal disease after renal transplantation. Curr Opin Nephrol Hypertens 1994; 3:602–607.
13. Karakayali H, Demirag A, Moray G, Ersoy E, Turan M, Bilgin N, Haberal M. Impact of amyloidosis on long-term survival in kidney transplantation. Transplant Proc 1999; 31:3221–3223.
14. Sobh MA, el-Agroudy AE, Moustafa FE, Shokeir AA, el-Shazly A, Ghoneim MA. Impact of schistosomiasis on patient and graft outcome after kidney transplantation. Nephrol Dial Transplant 1992; 7:858–864.
15. Hu RH, Lee PH, Tsai MK, Lee CY. Medical cost difference between renal transplantation and hemodialysis. Transplant Proc 1998; 30:3617–3620.
16. el-Agroudy AE, Donia AF, Bakr MA, Foda MA, Ghoneim MA. Preemptive living-donor kidney transplantation: clinical course and outcome. Transplantation 2004; 77:1366–1370.
17. Isaacs RB. Optimal transplant immunosuppression: a case of the haves and have nots? Am J Kidney Dis 2001; 37:160–163.
18. Jawad F, Hussain Z, Ahmed E, Akhtar F, Hussain M, Sheikh R, Aziz T, Ahmed S, Naqvi A, Rizvi A. Problems of donor selection in a living related renal transplant program. Transplant Proc 1998; 30:3643.
19. Ota K. Current status of organ transplantations in Asian countries. Transplant Proc 2003; 35:8–11.
20. Gatrad AR. Muslim customs surrounding death, bereavement, postmortem examinations, and organ transplants. BMJ 1994; 309:521–523.
21. Veatch RM. Introduction: religious and cultural perspectives in organ transplantation. Transplantation Ethics. Georgetown University PressWashington, DC20001–39.
22. Nolan K. Buddhism, Zen and bioethics. In: Lustig BA, Brody BA, Engelhardt HT Jr, McCullough LB, eds. Bioethics Yearbook: Theological Developments in Bioethics, 1990–1992. Vol. 3. Boston: Kluwer Academic, 1993:204–205.
23. Qiu RZ. Ethical problems in dialysis and transplantation. Chinese perspectives. Kjellstrand CM, Dosseter JB, eds. Ethical Problems in Dialysis and Transplantation. Boston: Kluwer Academic, 1992:227–228.
24. Erdogan O, Yucetin L, Tuncer M, Boston: Kececioglu N, Gurkan A, Akaydin M, Yakupoglu G. Attitudes and knowledge of Turkish physicians about organ donation and transplantation. Transplant Proc 2002; 34:2007–2008.

25. Shaheen FA, Souqiyyeh MZ, Ramprassad K, Attar MB. Current issues and problems of transplantation in the Middle East: the Arabian Gulf. Transplant Proc 2001; 33:2621–2622.

26. Shroff S, Navin S, Abraham G, Rajan PS, Suresh S, Rao S, Thomas P. Cadaver organ donation and transplantation—an Indian perspective. Transplant Proc 2003; 35:15–17.

27. Haberal M, Emiroglu R, Karakayali H, Moray G, Arslan G, Bilgin N. Cadaver kidney transplantation and the nation wide donor organ coordination system in Turkey. Cecka MJ, Terasaki PI, eds. Clinical Transplants 2001. Los Angeles: UCLA Tissue Typing Laboratory, 2002:201–206.

28. Campbell A, Gillett C, Jones C. Organ and tissue transplantation. Medical Ethics. 3rd ed. Oxford: Oxford University Press, 2001:129–146.

29. Johnson EM, Anderson JK, Jacobs C, Suh G, Humar A, Suhr BD, Kerr SR, Matas AJ. Long-term follow-up of living kidney donors: quality of life after donation. Transplantation 1999; 67:717–721.

30. Sesso R, Klag MJ, Ancao MS, Whelton PK, Seidler A, Sigulem D, Ramos OL. Kidney transplantation from living unrelated donors. Ann Intern Med 1992; 117:983–989.

31. Singh P, Kumar A, Bhandari M, Sharma RK, Gupta A. Kidney donation from wives, an exploitation or social compulsion. The XIIth International Congress on Psychonephrology, Yokohama, Japan, 2000.

32. Jha V. Paid transplants in India: the grim reality. Nephrol Dial Transplant 2004; 19:541–543.

33. Chugh KS, Jha V. Commerce in transplantation in Third World countries. Kidney Int 1996; 49:1181–1186.

34. Rizvi SAH, Naqvi SAA, Zafar MN. Renal transplantation in Pakistan. Cecka MJ, Terasaki PI, eds. Clinical Transplants 2001. Los Angeles: UCLA Tissue Typing Laboratory, 2002:191–200.

35. Salahudeen AK, Woods HF, Pingle A, Nur-El-Huda Suleyman M, Shakuntala K, Nandakumar M, Yahya TM, Daar AS. High mortality among recipients of bought living-unrelated donor kidneys. Lancet 1990; 336: 725–728.

36. Higgins R, West N, Fletcher S, Stein A, Lam F, Kashi H. Kidney transplantation in patients travelling from the UK to India or Pakistan. Nephrol Dial Transplant 2003; 18:851–852.

37. Call to legalise live organ trade. http://news.bbc.co.uk/2/hi/health/3041363.htm. (19th May 2003).

38. Goyal M, Mehta RL, Schneiderman LJ, Sehgal AR. Economic and health consequences of selling a kidney in India. JAMA 2002; 288:1589–1593.

39. Radcliffe-Richards J, Daar AS, Guttmann RD, Hoffenberg R, Kennedy I, Lock M, Sells RA, Tilney N. The case for allowing kidney sales. International Forum for Transplant Ethics. Lancet 1998; 351:1950–1952.

40. Zargooshi J. Quality of life of Iranian kidney "donors". J Urol 2001; 166: 1790–1799.

41. Mani MK. Development of cadaver renal transplantation in India. Nephrology 2002; 7:177–182.

42. Cameron JS, Hoffenberg R. The ethics of organ transplantation reconsidered: paid organ donation and the use of executed prisoners as donors. Kidney Int 1999; 55:724–732.
43. Chaudhary V. Argentina uncovers patients killed for organs. BMJ 1992; 304:1073–1074.
44. Wong HS, Morad Z. Neoral (cyclosporine) C2 monitoring in renal transplant recipients: a single-center experience in Asia. Transplant Proc 2003; 35: 230–231.
45. Tan J, Tang X. A retrospective analysis of Neoral C2 monitoring in Chinese renal transplantation recipients. Transplant Proc 2003; 35:232–233.
46. Abraham MA, Thomas PP, John GT, Job V, Shankar V, Jacob CK. Efficacy and safety of low-dose ketoconazole (50 mg) to reduce the cost of cyclosporine in renal allograft recipients. Transplant Proc 2003; 35:215–216.
47. El-Agroudy AE, Sobh MA, Hamdy AF, Ghoneim MA. A prospective, randomized study of coadministration of ketoconazole and cyclosporine A in kidney transplant recipients: ten-year follow-up. Transplantation 2004; 77:1371–1376.
48. Jha V, Muthukumar T, Kohli HS, Sud K, Gupta KL, Sakhuja V. Impact of cyclosporine withdrawal on living related renal transplants: a single-center experience. Am J Kidney Dis 2001; 37:119–124.
49. Suleymanlar G, Tuncer M, Sarikaya M, Ersoy F, Aktan S, Yakupoglu G, Karpuzoglu T. The cost effectiveness of mycophenolate mofetil in the first year after living related renal transplantation. Transplant Proc 2001; 33:2780–2781.
50. Kim HC, Park SB, Han SY, Whang EA, Jeon DS, Kim HT, Cho WH, Park CH. Primary immunosuppression with tacrolimus in renal transplantation: a single center experience. Transplant Proc 2003; 35:217–218.
51. Masri MA, Haberal M, Rizvi A, Stephan A, Bilgin N, Naqvi A, Barbari A, Kamel G, Zafar N, Emiroglu R, Colak T, Manzoor K, Matha V, Kamarad V, Rizk S, Itany AR, Shehedeh I. The pharmacokinetics of equoral versus neoral in stable renal transplant patients: a multinational multicenter study. Transplant Proc 2004; 36:80–83.
52. Rizvi A, Naqvi A, Hussain Z, Hafiz S, Hashmi A, Zafar N, Akhtar F, Ahmed E, Hussain M, Askari A. Factors influencing graft survival in living-related donor kidney transplantation at a single center. Transplant Proc 1998; 30:712–716.
53. Barsoum RS. Renal transplantation in a developing country: the Egyptian 17 year experience. Afr J Health Sci 1994; 1:30–36.
54. Tokalak I, Basaran O, Emiroglu R, Karakayali H, Bilgin N, Haberal M. Problems in postoperative renal transplant recipients who present to the emergency unit: experience at one center. Transplant Proc 2004; 36:184–186.
55. Ianhez LE, Sampaio M, Fonseca JA, Sabbaga E. The influence of socioeconomic conditions in renal posttransplant infection. Transplant Proc 1992; 24:3100.
56. Jha V, Sakhuja V, Gupta D, Krishna VS, Chakrabarti A, Joshi K, Sud K, Kohli HS, Gupta KL. Successful management of pulmonary tuberculosis in renal allograft recipients in a single center. Kidney Int 1999; 56:1944–1950.
57. Ahmed E, Akhtar F, Hashmi A, Imtiaz S, Hussain Z, Hafeez S, Naqvi A, Rizvi A. Acute graft dysfunction due to pyelonephritis: value and safety of graft biopsy. Ren Fail 2003; 25:509–512.

58. Chan PC, Cheng IK, Wong KK, Li MK, Chan MK. Urinary tract infections in post-renal transplant patients. Int Urol Nephrol 1990; 22:389–396.
59. Ergin F, Arslan H, Yapar G, Karakayali H, Haberal M. Urinary tract infections in renal transplant recipients. Transplant Proc 2003; 35:2685–2686.
60. Gueco I, Saniel M, Mendoza M, Alano F, Ona E. Tropical infections after renal transplantation. Transplant Proc 1989; 21:2105–2107.
61. Cantarovich F, Vazquez M, Garcia WD, Abbud FM, Herrera C, Villegas HA. Special infections in organ transplantation in South America. Transplant Proc 1992; 24:1902–1908.
62. Chugh KS, Sakhuja V, Jain S, Talwar P, Minz M, Joshi K, Indudhara R. High mortality in systemic fungal infections following renal transplantation in third-world countries. Nephrol Dial Transplant 1993; 8:168–172.
63. Oner-Eyuboglu F, Karacan O, Akcay S, Arslan H, Demirhan B, Haberal M. Invasive pulmonary fungal infections in solid organ transplant recipients: a four-year review. Transplant Proc 2003; 35:2689–2691.
64. Rao M, Finny GJ, Abraham P, Juneja R, Thomas PP, Jacob CK, Sridharan G. Cytomegalovirus infection in a seroendemic renal transplant population: a longitudinal study of virological markers. Nephron 2000; 84:367–373.
65. Tsai MK, Lee PH, Hu RH, Lee CJ. Infectious complications in renal transplant recipients: a 10-year review of cyclosporine-based immunosuppression. Transplant Proc 1998; 30:3125–3126.
66. Chak WL, Choi KS, Wong KM, Chan YH, Chau KF, Li CS. Pharmaco-economic analysis of preemptive gancyclovir therapy in the prevention of cytomegalovirus infections in high-risk renal graft recipients. Transplant Proc 2003; 35:280–281.
67. Said T, Nampoory MR, Pacsa AS, Johny KV, Nair MP, Abdel-Haleem M, Samhan M, Al-Mousawi M. Cytomegalovirus infection in kidney transplant recipients: early diagnosis and monitoring of antiviral therapy by the antigenemia assay. Transplant Proc 2001; 33:2799–2801.
68. Jha R, Narayen G, Sinha S, Kadeer K, Prasad KN. Symptomatic herpes virus infections in post renal transplant. Transplant Proc 2003; 35:284–285.
69. Fehr T, Ambuhl PM. Chronic hepatitis virus infection in patients on renal replacement therapy. Nephrol Dial Transplant 2004; 19:1049–1053.
70. Pereira BJ, Natov SN, Bouthot BA, Murthy BV, Ruthazer R, Schmid CH, Levey AS. Effects of hepatitis C infection and renal transplantation on survival in end-stage renal disease. The New England Organ Bank Hepatitis C Study Group. Kidney Int 1998; 53:1374–1381.
71. Naqvi A, Aziz T, Hussain M, Zafar N, Muzaffar R, Kazi J, Akhtar F, Ahmad E, Hashmi A, Hussain Z, Rizvi A. Outcome of living-related donor renal allografts in hepatitis C antibody-positive recipients. Transplant Proc 1998; 30:793.
72. Mathurin P, Mouquet C, Poynard T, Sylla C, Benalia H, Fretz C, Thibault V, Cadranel JF, Bernard B, Opolon P, Coriat P, Bitker MO. Impact of hepatitis B and C virus on kidney transplantation outcome. Hepatology 1999; 29: 257–263.
73. Fabrizi F, Lunghi G, Raffaele L, Guarnori I, Bacchini G, Corti M, Pagano A, Erba G, Locatelli F. Serologic survey for control of hepatitis C in

haemodialysis patients: third-generation assays and analysis of costs. Nephrol Dial Transplant 1997; 12:298–303.

74. Abdel-Hamid M, El-Daly M, El-Kafrawy S, Mikhail N, Strickland GT, Fix AD. Comparison of second- and third-generation enzyme immunoassays for detecting antibodies to hepatitis C virus. J Clin Microbiol 2002; 40:1656–1659.

75. al Meshari K, al Ahdal M, Alfurayh O, Ali A, De Vol E, Kessie G. New insights into hepatitis C virus infection of hemodialysis patients: the implications. Am J Kidney Dis 1995; 25:572–578.

76. Boyacioglu S, Gur G, Yilmaz U, Korkmaz M, Demirhan B, Bilezikci B, Ozdemir N. Investigation of possible clinical and laboratory predictors of liver fibrosis in hemodialysis patients infected with hepatitis C virus. Transplant Proc 2004; 36:50–52.

77. Huraib S, Tanimu D, Romeh SA, Quadri K, Al Ghamdi G, Iqbal A, Abdulla A. Interferon-alpha in chronic hepatitis C infection in dialysis patients. Am J Kidney Dis 1999; 34:55–60.

78. Gursoy M, Bilezikci B, Colak T, Koksal R, Demirhan B, Karavelioglu D, Boyacioglu S, Bilgin N, Arslan G. Histologic outcome of hepatitis C virus infection in renal transplant recipients and the effect of pretransplantation interferon treatment. Transplant Proc 2000; 32:558–560.

79. Kirk AD, Heisey DM, D'Alessandro AM, Knechtle SJ, Odorico JS, Rayhill SC, Sollinger HW, Pirsch JD. Clinical hepatitis after transplantation of hepatitis C virus-positive kidneys: HLA-DR3 as a risk factor for the development of posttransplant hepatitis. Transplantation 1996; 62(12):1758–1762.

80. Tokumoto T, Tanabe K, Simizu T, Shimmura H, Iizuka J, Ishikawa N, Oshima T, Yagisawa T, Goya N, Nakazawa H, Toma H. Kidney transplantation from a donor who is HCV antibody positive and HCV-RNA negative. Transplant Proc 2000; 32(7):1597–1599.

81. Widell A, Mansson S, Persson NH, Thysell H, Hermodsson S, Blohme I. Hepatitis C superinfection in hepatitis C virus (HCV)-infected patients transplanted with an HCV-infected kidney. Transplantation 1995; 60(7):642–647.

82. Hu RH, Lee PH, Chung YC, Huang MT, Lee CS. Hepatitis B and C in renal transplantation in Taiwan. Transplant Proc 1994; 26:2059–2061.

83. Roy DM, Thomas PP, Dakshinamurthy KV, Jacob CK, Shastry JC. Long term survival in living related donor renal allograft recipients with hepatitis B infection. Transplantation 1994; 58:118–119.

84. Fairley CK, Mijch A, Gust ID, Nichilson S, Dimitrakakis M, Lucas CR. The increased risk of fatal liver disease in renal transplant patients who are hepatitis Be antigen and/or HBV DNA positive. Transplantation 1991; 52:497–500.

85. Fabrizi F, Dulai G, Dixit V, Bunnapradist S, Martin P. Lamivudine for the treatment of hepatitis B virus-related liver disease after renal transplantation: meta-analysis of clinical trials. Transplantation 2004; 77:859–864.

86. Naqvi A, Rizvi A, Hussain Z, Hafeez S, Hashmi A, Akhtar F, Hussain M, Ahmed E, Akhtar S, Muzaffar R, Naqvi R. Developing world perspective of posttransplant tuberculosis: morbidity, mortality, and cost implications. Transplant Proc 2001; 33:1787–1788.

87. Vandermarliere A, Van Audenhove A, Peetermans WE, Vanrenterghem Y, Maes B. Mycobacterial infection after renal transplantation in a Western population. Transplant Infect Dis 2003; 5:9–15.

88. Yildiz A, Sever MS, Turkmen A, Ecder T, Besisik F, Tabak L, Ece T, Kilicarslan I, Ark E. Tuberculosis after renal transplantation: experience of one Turkish centre. Nephrol Dial Transplant 1998; 13:1872–1875.

89. Cavusoglu C, Cicek-Saydam C, Karasu Z, Karaca Y, Ozkahya M, Toz H, Tokat Y, Bilgic A. Mycobacterium tuberculosis infection and laboratory diagnosis in solid-organ transplant recipients. Clin Transplant 2002; 16:257–261.

90. Mossa MR, Bouwens C. Tuberculosis in renal allograft recipients: the South African experience. Transplant Rev 1997; 11:84.

91. Sakhuja V, Jha V, Varma PP, Joshi K, Chugh KS. The high incidence of tuberculosis among renal transplant recipients in India. Transplantation 1996; 61:211–215.

92. Qunibi WY, al-Sibai MB, Taher S, Harder EJ, de Vol E, al-Furayh O, Ginn HE. Mycobacterial infection after renal transplantation—report of 14 cases and review of the literature. Q J Med 1990; 77:1039–1060.

93. Naqvi R, Akhtar S, Ahmed E, Akhtar F, Naqvi A, Rizvi A. Randomized trial of isoniazid prophylaxis in renal transplant recipients in a highly prevalent region for tuberculosis [abstr]. J Am Soc Nephrol 2003; 14:661A.

94. Bakr MA, Sobh M, el-Agroudy A, Sally S, Fouda MA, el-Mekresh M, Moustafa F, el-Baz M, Wafa E, Ghoneim MA. Study of malignancy among Egyptian kidney transplant recipients. Transplant Proc 1997; 29:3067–3070.

95. Margolius LP. Kaposi's sarcoma and other malignancies in renal transplant recipients. Transplant Rev 1996; 10:129.

96. Qunibi W, Akhtar M, Sheth K, Ginn HE, Al-Furayh O, DeVol EB, Taher S. Kaposi's sarcoma: the most common tumor after renal transplantation in Saudi Arabia. Am J Med 1988; 84:225–232.

97. Woodle ES, Hanaway M, Buell J, Gross T, First MR, Trofe J, Beebe T. Israel Penn International Transplant Tumor Registry. Kaposi sarcoma: an analysis of the US and international experiences from the Israel Penn. International Transplant Tumor Registry. Transplant Proc 2001; 33:3660–3661.

98. Singh N. Infections with human herpes virus 6,7 and 8. In: Bowden RA, Jungman PL, Paya CV, eds. Transplant Infection. 2nd ed. Chapter 23. Lippincott William & Wilkinspp, Philadelphia 2003; 367–374.

99. Nalesnik MA. Involvement of the gastrointestinal tract by Epstein–Barr virus-associated posttransplant lymphoproliferative disorders. Am J Surg Pathol 1990; 14(suppl 1):92–100.

100. Chisholm MA, Vollenweider LJ, Mulloy LL, Jagadeesan M, Wade WE, DiPiro JT. Direct patient care services provided by a pharmacist on a multidisciplinary renal transplant team. Am J Health Syst Pharm 2000; 57: 1994–1996.

101. Rodriguez A, Diaz M, Colon A, Santiago-Delpin EA. Psychosocial profile of noncompliant transplant patients. Transplant Proc 1991; 23:1807–1809.

102. Meyers KE, Thomson PD, Weiland H. Noncompliance in children and adolescents after renal transplantation. Transplantation 1996; 62:186–189.

103. Sharma AK, Gupta R, Tolani SL, Rathi GL, Gupta HP. Evaluation of socio-economic factors in noncompliance in renal transplantation. Transplant Proc 2000; 32:1864.

104. Lee CJ. Organ transplantation practices in Taiwan. Transplant Proc 1992; 24:1824–1827.

105. Keitel Ferreira Dos Santos, Garcia, et al. Twenty five year experience with renal transplantation at Santa Casa Hospital, Porto Alegve. In: Cecka MJ, Terasaki PI, eds. Clinical Transplants 2001. Los Angeles: UCLA Tissue Typing Laboratory, 2002:163–170.

106. Kim SI, Kwon KH, Huh KH, Lee JH, Kim YS, Park K. Experience with cyclosporine in adult living donor kidney transplantation: from 1984 to 2002 at Yonsei University. Transplant Proc 2004; 36(suppl 2):S186–S192.

107. Haberal M, Bereket G, Karakayali H, Arslan G, Moray G, Bilgin N. Pediatric renal transplantation in Turkey: a review of 56 cases from a single center. Pediatr Transplant 2000; 4:293–299.

108. Phadke K, Ballal S, Venkatesh K, Sundar S. Pediatric renal transplantation—Indian experience. Indian Pediatr 1998; 35:231–235.

109. al Baba MA, Shaheen FA, Sheikh IA, Nivien K, Alkhader A, Fallatah A. Experience of Jeddah Kidney Center in pediatric renal transplantation. Transplant Proc 1998; 30:3679–3680.

110. Rizvi SA, Naqvi SA, Hussain Z, Hashmi A, Akhtar F, Zafar MN, Hussain M, Ahmed E, Kazi JI, Hasan AS, Khalid R, Aziz S, Sultan S. Living-related pediatric renal transplants: a single-center experience from a developing country. Pediatr Transplant 2002; 6:101–110.

111. Ojeda Duran S, Ochoa Ponce C, Ortiz Lopez H, et al. Experience de 10 anos de transplante renal en ninos en el occidente de Mexico. Arch Venez Pediatr 1999; 62 (suppl 2):179.

112. Lin S. Nephrology in China. A great mission and momentous challenge. Kidney Int 2003; 63(suppl 83):S108–S111.

113. Ghods AJ. Changing ethics in renal transplantation: presentation of Iran model. Transplant Proc 2004; 36:11–13.

114. Barsoum R, Bakr MA. The Egyptian renal transplant experience. Cecka MJ, Terasaki PI, eds. Clinical Transplants 2000. Los Angeles: UCLA Tissue Typing Laboratory, 2001:359–360.

115. Kahn D, Botha JR, Naicker S, Karrusseitt VOL, Haffejee A, Pascoe. Renal transplantation in South Africa. Cecka MJ, Terasaki PI, eds. Clinical Transplants 2000. Los Angeles: UCLA Tissue Typing Laboratory, 2001: 394–395.

116. Zatz R, Romao JE Jr, Noronha IL. Nephrology in Latin America, with special emphasis on Brazil. Kidney Int Suppl 2003; 83:S131–S134.

117. Santiago Delpin EA, Duro Garcia V. The 11th report of the Latin American Transplant Registry: 62,000 transplants. Transplant Proc 2001; 33:1986–1988.

118. Kahn D, Ovnat A, Pontin AR, Swanepoel CR, Cassidy MJ. Long-term results with elective cyclosporine withdrawal at three months after renal transplantation—appropriate for living-related transplants. Transplantation 1994; 58: 1410–1412.

119. Wuthrich RP, Cicvara S, Ambuhl PM, Binswanger U. Randomized trial of conversion from mycophenolate mofetil to azathioprine 6 months after renal allograft transplantation. Nephrol Dial Transplant 2000; 15:1228–1231.
120. Moeller S, Gioberge S, Brown G. ESRD patients in 2001: global overview of patients, treatment modalities and development trends. Nephrol Dial Transplant 2002; 17:2071–2076.
121. Collins AJ, Kasiske B, Herzog C, Chen S, et al. 2003 Annual Data Report. International comparisons. Am J Kidney Dis 2003; 42:S174–S180.

11

End-Stage Renal Failure in African Americans

Lawrence Agodoa

National Institute of Diabetes and Digestive and Kidney Diseases
National Institutes of Health, Bethesda, Maryland, U.S.A.

INTRODUCTION

Terminal kidney failure, also referred to as end-stage renal disease (ESRD), is defined as the stage at which RRT must be initiated to sustain life. Chronic kidney disease (CKD), with the subsequent progression to ESRD, imposes a relentless socioeconomic burden on patients, society, and health-care systems. The continued growth of the ESRD population has substantial public policy implications worldwide. Over the last decade, the number of ESRD patients in the United States grew at an exponential rate, doubling from 201,454 in 1991 to 406,081 in 2001. With the continued growth rate, projections to the end of this decade are sobering, with 651,000 patients estimated to be receiving ESRD treatment by 2010 in the United States (1).

The greatest incidence and prevalence of ESRD are reported in the United States and Japan with incidence rates in excess of 300 cases per million population. However, most of the developed nations have experienced staggering increases in both prevalence and incidence rates. More frighteningly and potentially devastating are the reports of alarming increases in renal disease in developing countries whose economies can hardly support the bare necessities. It is imperative, therefore, that preventive measures and early detection and treatment be instituted worldwide.

The greatest burden of kidney disease has been in indigenous peoples worldwide. Although the exact explanation is yet to be found, it has been observed that transition of these populations from their traditional ways of life, including diets, to Western European life style has accelerated development of diseases such as diabetes and hypertension that ultimately lead to damage to the kidneys. In the United States, it has long been recognized that ESRD is more common in certain racial and ethnic groups (2–4). These disparities in renal disease incidence have been shown to be greatest in African Americans (NHANES III, 1988–1994) (5). However, the African-American population is not an exception; these disparities have been noted in other racial and ethnic groups in the United States, such as American Indians, Alaska Natives, Native Hawaiians and Other Pacific Islanders, Asians, and Hispanics. Similar racial and ethnic disparities have been reported in other countries, including United Kingdom, Australia, and New Zealand (6–8).

Racial and ethnic minorities in the United States also exhibit increases in key risk factors for the development of chronic kidney disease, and display disparities and a significant gap with the White population. For example, Hispanic Americans are twice as likely to die from diabetes; American Indians and Alaska Natives have a diabetes rate more than twice that of Whites; more than 65% of African-American and Mexican-American women are overweight as defined by a body mass index (BMI) above 25; more than 10% cent of non-Hispanic Black women in the age group 40 to 60 are severely obese, with BMI over 40; American Indian children have obesity rates more than twice as high as the rest of the population; Hispanic Americans also have higher rates of obesity and high blood pressure than Whites.

The higher rates of diabetes and obesity mean that these populations also suffer from higher rates of the complications, such as the microvascular complications in the eyes, nerves, and kidneys; lower extremity amputations; development of type 2 diabetes and obesity in the children of diabetic mothers; and hypertension and coronary heart disease. Because these racial and ethnic minority groups tend to be the ones with the highest inequalities in income and education, they also tend to have less access to quality health care and to education and information programs to help them manage their disease and disorders.

Some of the risk factors and comorbid conditions may appear early in the course of renal failure, others may occur as renal disease progresses. Therefore, it is essential that patients with chronic kidney disease be identified early, and effective preventive management initiated to slow progression and aborts the development of some of the comorbid conditions. The exact number of patients with chronic renal insufficiency is difficult to ascertain. However, analyzing data from the third National Health and Nutrition Examination Survey (NHANES III), a cross-sectional nationally representative sample of the U.S. civilian non-institutionalized population that uses a stratified, multistage probability cluster design with over-sampling of Mexican Americans, African Americans, and elderly, Jones and colleagues reported that African Americans adults have nearly three times higher prevalence of mild to moderate elevations of serum creatinine levels (≥ 2.0 mg/dL). They also estimated that there might be as many as 10–15 million persons in the United States with various levels of renal dysfunction (5).

The National Institute of Diabetes and Digestive and Kidney Diseases (NIDDK) and the Health Care Financing Administration (HCFA, now the Centers for Medicare and Medicaid, CMS) collaborated in 1988 to develop the United States Renal Data System (USRDS) database with the data reported to the CMS on the Medicare ESRD patients. Additional data are added to the database through special studies carried out by the USRDS. The USRDS currently has information on over 96% of ESRD patients in the United States. Through the data collected and analyzed by the USRDS, the spectrum of kidney disease in the United States has been well characterized. Most of the data reported in this chapter comes from the annual data reports of the USRDS.

INCIDENCE AND PREVALENCE OF ESRD

It was estimated that the total number of beneficiaries in the U.S. ESRD program at its inception in 1973 was approximately 10,000. This number has dramatically increased to a period prevalence of 512,574 treated ESRD patients in 2002 (Fig. 1). The incidence rate has also progressively increased and 100,359 new cases were treated in 2002 (9). Since its inception in 1988, the USRDS has reported data that racial and ethnic minorities in the United States, especially African Americans, are disproportionately afflicted with ESRD. Since the early days of RRT in the United States and the Medicare program, racial and ethnic minorities, especially African Americans, have exhibited disproportionate affliction with renal disease. As shown in Figure 2, in 2002, the incidence rates (adjusted for age, gender, and cause of renal disease), by race, were 256 per million population for Caucasians compared with 982 for African Americans, 514 for American Indians and Alaska Natives, and 344 for Asians and Pacific Islanders (USRDS, 2004). The reported incidence rate of ESRD in Hispanic Americans in 2002 was 481 per million population. Data reporting for Hispanics commenced in 1995, and there is reason to believe that this rate is lower than expected due to under-reporting. The period and point prevalence rates, likewise, confirm the higher rates of affliction of racial and ethnic minorities with ESRD.

CAUSES OF ESRD

Two diseases, namely diabetes mellitus and hypertension cause approximately 70% of all new adult ESRD cases in the United States. Glomerulonephritis

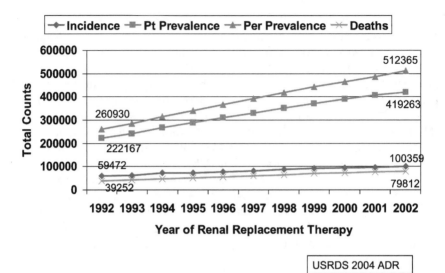

Figure 1 Time trend of end-stage renal disease (ESRD) in the United Stages, 1992–2002. Pt Prevalence = point prevalence; Per Prevalence = period prevalence. *Source:* From Ref. 9.

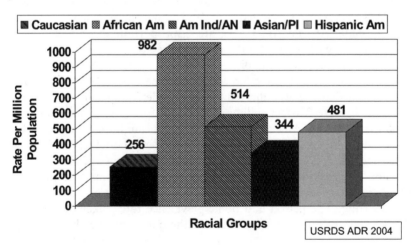

Figure 2 Racial differences in the incidence of ESRD, 2002; adjusted for age, gender, and cause of ESRD. African Am = African Americans, Am In/AN = American Indians and Alaska Natives; Asian/PI = Asians and Pacific Islanders; Hispanic Am = Hispanic Americans. *Source:* From Ref. 1.

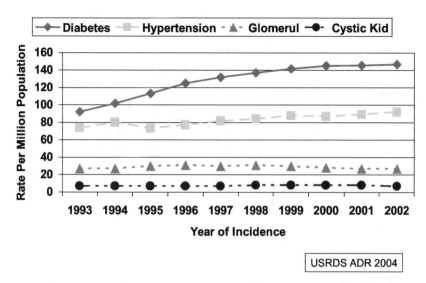

Figure 3 Time trends in the causes of end-stage renal disease in the United States, 1993–2002. Rates are per million population, adjusted for age, gender, and race. ◆ Diabetes = diabetes mellitus; ■ Hypertension; ▲ Glomerul = glomerulonephritis; • Cystic Kid = cystic kidney disease. *Source*: From Ref. 9.

and cystic kidney diseases contribute about 10% (Fig. 3). However, other "rarer" diseases causing ESRD, such as the human immunodeficiency syndrome virus (HIV), are also important contributors, especially in African Americans.

Diabetic Kidney Disease

Since the early 1970s, diabetes mellitus has remained the leading cause of ESRD in the United States. Comparatively, it has been a relatively minor contributor in the causes of ESRD in Europe, Australia, and New Zealand. In the United States, the prevalence rate of diabetes in African American men is nearly 50% greater than that of White men; for African American women the rate is approximately 100% greater than in White women. Diabetes afflicts Hispanics (1.9 times that of non-Hispanic Whites) and Native Americans (2.8 times that of non-Hispanic Whites) at an even higher rate (10). It is the primary cause of ESRD in all racial and ethnic groups, but at a much higher rate in American Indians, Alaska Natives, and African Americans (9) (Fig. 4). In African Americans, especially, it was the second leading cause of ESRD prior to 1995. The age distribution is similar for all races, in that the highest prevalence rates are in the 65 to 79 year age group, except for American Indians and Alaska Natives where the highest incidence rate is in the 60 to 69 year age group. Curiously, however, even

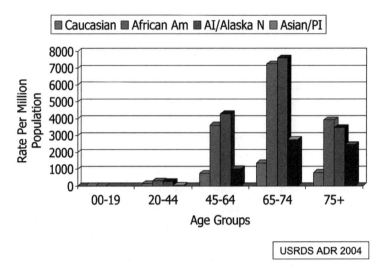

Figure 4 Incidence rates of diabetic end-stage renal disease by age and race; adjusted for gender, 1999–2002. Rates are per million population. African Am = African American; AI/Alaska N = American Indians and Alaska Natives; Asian/PI = Asians and Pacific Islanders. *Source*: From Ref. 9.

though this disease is practically unusual in children primarily because of the time it takes established diabetes to cause sufficient injury to the kidneys and to progress to end stage, there has been increasing frequency of the diagnosis of diabetic ESRD in African American girls, and to a minor extent, in Caucasian children. The gender difference is not the same in all the races. For Caucasians and Asians, men have a higher incidence rate of diabetic ESRD than women. In African Americans, American Indians, and Alaska Natives, women have a higher incidence rate than men.

It has been postulated that the continuing rise in the incidence of diabetic ESRD is due to a combination of increasing incidence rate of diabetes in the United States, as well as ineffective therapy to retard progression of diabetic renal disease in the early stages of development. The early effects of diabetes on the kidneys include microalbuminuria and hyperfiltration. Subsequently, the damage progresses to gross proteinuria and relentless decrease in glomerular filtration rate to end stage. Some investigators suggest that intervening early in the course of the disease would be more effective than after the disease has been established.

Several landmark studies assessed the effect of modulation of the renin–angiotensin–aldosterone axis on the nephropathy of type 2 diabetes. One of the studies in the early phase of type 2 diabetic nephropathy showed that treatment with angiotensin receptor blockers (ARBs) resulted in reduction of microalbuminuria, and/or progression to gross proteinuria (11).

Two other clinical trials were conducted in type 2 diabetic patients with gross proteinuria and reduced glomerular filtration rate. Both studies showed that the use of ARBs in the late stages was effective in reducing, but not preventing, progression of the disease (12,13). From these studies, it can be concluded that diabetic ESRD can be delayed if patients in the advanced stages of the disease are treated with ARBs. There are also indications that treatment in the early stages of the disease with ARBs will reduce the incidence, and eventually the prevalence of the disease.

Hypertension

Although the rate of rise in the incidence rate of hypertensive ESRD has diminished over the past decade, it remains a major cause of ESRD in African Americans. Among the racial and ethnic groups, only African Americans have shown a substantial increase in the prevalence of hypertension (14,15). Mexican Americans, on the other hand, have shown poorer control of hypertension (65% that of African Americans or Whites), and this relatively poorer control may have implications for the future rates of ESRD development in this group (16).

The incidence of hypertensive ESRD is very high among younger African Americans, nearly 20 times the incidence of Caucasians in the 20- to 44-year-old group (9). As illustrated in Figure 3, the incidence rate of hypertensive ESRD has continued to increase, over the past two decades, but less dramatically in the last five. This rate of increase has been greatest in African Americans. Prior to 1995, it was the leading cause of ESRD in African Americans, but currently the second leading cause of ESRD. In 2002, of the 100,359 new cases of ESRD, 27,227 (27%) were reportedly caused by hypertension. In the period 1999–2002, the incidence rates (per million population) of hypertensive ESRD by race, adjusted for age were 60 for Caucasians, 62 for American Indians and Alaska Natives, 98 for Asians and Pacific Islanders, and 337 for African Americans, with a Black/White ratio of approximately 6:1 (Fig. 5); the rate was higher in men than in women, for all races. Patients older than 80 years had the highest incidence rate of hypertensive ESRD.

It is unclear whether the high incidence of hypertensive kidney disease, especially among African Americans, is a result of damage from severe essential hypertension potentiated by environmental nephrotoxins, use of illicit or prescribed drugs, or other factors (17–20). The higher prevalence of hypertension in the African-American population suggests that hypertensive nephrosclerosis is more common in this population. Hypertension in general occurs earlier and is more severe in African Americans. Compared to the Caucasian population, African Americans in the 20- to 44-year age group have a higher incidence and prevalence of hypertensive end-stage

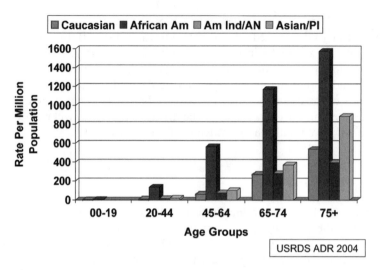

Figure 5 Incidence of hypertensive end-stage renal disease by race and age, 1999–2002; adjusted for gender. African Am = African Americans; Am Ind/AN = American Indians and Alaska Natives; Asian/PI = Asians and Pacific Islanders. *Source*: From Ref. 9.

renal disease. Therefore, the magnitude of this disease entity in the African-American population is due to the combination of a higher prevalence of hypertensive nephrosclerosis and a faster rate of progression.

Until recently, there was no effective way to halt progression to end stage once the disease developed. However, the results of the recently completed African American Study of Kidney Disease and Hypertension (AASK) clinical trial has shown that progression can be slowed even in the advanced stage of the disease by the use of angiotensin converting enzyme inhibitors (ACEI). In that study, patients without significant proteinuria showed no significant worsening of the disease with adequate control of the blood pressure. In the presence of proteinuria, however, even at the level of 300 mg per 24 hours, the disease showed faster progression unless ACEI were used (21,22). There are no reported studies on the effect of intervention in the early phases of the disease. However, some investigators suggest that treatment of hypertension in the early phases of the disease should result in prevention of ESRD. The presence of proteinuria mandates the use of ACEI.

Glomerulonephritis

Primary and secondary glomerulonephritides constitute the third most frequently reported cause of ESRD in the United States. The incidence rate is higher in men than in women. Overall, African Americans have the highest rate of ESRD due to glomerulonephritis. However, racial and ethnic distribution varies by the type of glomerulonephritis. For example, IgA nephropathy and IgM nephropathy are less frequent in African Americans; on the other hand, focal and segmental glomerulosclerosis (FSGS) and nephropathy due to systemic lupus erythematosus (SLE) are more common in African Americans than Caucasians.

The current epidemic of infection with the human immunodeficiency virus (HIV) has resulted in an important cause of ESRD. Although the total number of cases in the U.S. ESRD population is relatively few, it comprises the third leading cause of ESRD in African Americans, and is as much as 10 times the incidence rate in Caucasians (23–26). With increasing use of anti-retroviral drugs, one would expect a positive effect on the incidence of HIV nephropathy in all racial and ethnic groups. However, there is inconsistent reporting of HIV infection in the ESRD population; therefore, the direct effect of increasing use of HAART is difficult to ascertain at this time.

There are currently no consistent effective therapies for the glomerulonephritides. Immunosuppressive therapy was tried in patients with primary and some secondary (such as SLE) glomerulonephritides with inconsistent results. In general, however, these diseases are accompanied by proteinuria. Proteinuric kidney diseases have been shown to respond well to drugs that inhibit the renin–angiotensin–aldosterone axis (27–29). Therefore, it is recommended that therapeutic regimens for glomerular diseases should contain ACEI.

Tubulo-Interstitial and Cystic Kidney Diseases

This is a group of diseases that are non-glomerular and non-vascular in origin, including autosomal dominant polycystic kidney disease (ADPKD), chronic pyelonephritis, hereditary nephritis, analgesics and other drugs, and heavy metals. Most of the individuals in this group have ADPKD. These diseases constitute only about 4% of the total incident ESRD population. Even at this low incident rate, African Americans are afflicted at a higher rate than other racial and ethnic groups. There is approximately 25% higher incidence rate in men in all racial and ethnic groups. The peak incidence is in the 70- to 79-year age group (9).

Treatment is non-uniform; in instances where the causative agent is known, removal from exposure may diminish the rate of progression. ESRD is inevitable when patients are discovered at the stage 4 of the National Kidney Foundation's Kidney Disease Outcomes Quality Initiative (K/DOQI) (30). In the case of autosomal dominant polycystic kidney disease, treatment has been mostly symptomatic, essentially of the hypertension that is frequently associated with this disease. However, it has been demonstrated that the pathogenic mechanisms include clonal expansion of partially differentiated epithelial cells that are dysregulated, undergo apoptosis, and have been

shown to secret several growth factors, chemokines, proinflammatory cytokines, nucleotides, matrix metalloproteinases, lysosomal enzymes, and
vasoactive substances; therefore, there are many potential interventions.
Many of these are in the initial stages of experimentation, and will likely
lead to the development of novel therapies that will prevent progression
of the disease to end stage (31–33).

MODALITIES OF THERAPY FOR ESRD

The kidneys are primarily responsible for maintaining the body's homeostasis,
including removal of metabolic waste products, maintenance of acid–base
homeostasis, control of fluid balance, immunological surveillance, and, very
importantly, endocrine and hormonal regulation, including metabolism and
regulation of insulin levels, erythropoietin synthesis, parathyroid hormone
regulation, and gonadal function. A successful RRT should, therefore,
include all the kidney functions lost when ESRD ensues. Earlier in the development of RRT, investigators focused primarily on correcting acid–base,
fluid, and electrolyte disorders. Dialysis was the outcome of those early considerations. It is, therefore, not surprising that although dialysis has resulted
in saving the life of the patient with ESRD from immediate death, neither
the quality of life nor the expected remaining life years are returned to the
pre-renal failure level. Successful renal transplant, on the other hand,
returns the patient to near normal quality of life and lifespan.

Hemodialysis

Minorities, especially African Americans with the high incidence rate of
ESRD, are referred for specialist care later in the course of their disease than
Caucasians. Therefore, they are more likely to have more advanced disease
and more complications from the renal failure. Compared with Caucasians,
African Americans, by the time they see renal care specialists, are more
likely to have hypoalbuminemia and severe anemia at the initiation of
hemodialysis and are less likely to receive erythropoietin therapy before
dialysis (34). Some investigators also believe that this late referral results
in more urgent placement on hemodialysis (35–37). Furthermore, late referral is associated with an increased chance of dialysis catheter use (38–40).

 The preferred vascular access for chronic hemodialysis is an autologous
arteriovenous fistula rather than a synthetic arteriovenous graft or intravenous catheter due to the lower rates of thrombosis and infection (41,42).
Despite these recommendations and available outcome data, African
Americans more commonly have synthetic grafts compared with Caucasians.
Late referral, which necessitates immediate access placement, may be one of
the causes for this discrepancy (39,40).

In 2002, of the 100,359 incident patients, 98,313 (98%) received hemodialysis as the initial modality of therapy. African Americans comprised 29% of the incident dialysis patient population and 38% of the prevalent dialysis population, compared with Caucasians who comprised 63% of the incident dialysis population and only 54% of the prevalent dialysis population. The decrease in the proportion of Caucasians in the prevalent population is mainly due to their referral for renal transplantation.

The prescribed dose, and hence the delivered dose of dialysis is more likely to be sub-optimal in African-American hemodialysis patients despite clear guidelines for hemodialysis dose and frequent monitoring (43,44). A dialysis dose less than the recommended level is associated with higher mortality; paradoxically, however, the survival of African Americans on hemodialysis is better than Whites (9,45). Interestingly, the relationship between dialysis dose and mortality risk appears to be weakest in African Americans (43). However, there may be a potential for improved survival with the combination of timely referral, optimal angio access, and appropriate dialysis delivery.

Approximately 50% of all deaths in hemodialysis patients is due to cardiovascular causes, defined as acute myocardial infarction, pericarditis, atherosclerotic heart disease, caridomyopathy, cardiac arrhythmia, cardiac arrest, valvular heart disease, and cerebrovascular disease. In spite of poorer pre-ESRD care and higher rate of hypertension in African Americans, morbidity and mortality due to cardiovascular causes is lower in African Americans than Caucasians on hemodialysis.

Peritoneal Dialysis

The two predominant modes of peritoneal dialysis in the United States are chronic ambulatory peritoneal dialysis (CAPD) and continuous cycling peritoneal dialysis (CCPD). In general, there has been a gradual decrease in the use of peritoneal dialysis in the United States. A decade ago, approximately 14% of the incident of ESRD patients was treated with peritoneal dialysis; however, by the 2002, only 6.6% received this modality of treatment.

There are racial differences in peritoneal dialysis use; Caucasians and Asian Americans are more likely to choose peritoneal dialysis compared to African Americans and Native Americans (9,46–48). For example, in the Southeast, one study observed that African Americans were 50% less likely, compared with Caucasians, to select peritoneal dialysis as an initial mode of ESRD treatment. The choice of peritoneal dialysis tends to be a function of education, socioeconomic status, cultural bias related to health behavior and body image, physician bias, and communication barriers (46).

Renal Transplantation

Kidney transplantation is the treatment of choice for ESRD patients (49,50). However, in the past two decades, the growing need for organs has outstripped the supply of kidneys. Therefore, the rate of transplantation has declined. In 1991, the rate of transplantation was approximately 8 per 100 patient years, and in the year 2002 the rate had declined to approximately 4.9 per 100 patient years (9). The waiting time for African Americans to receive organ is longer than that of Caucasians, and is increasing at an even greater rate.

The shortage of organs is contributed to by the lower rate of organ donation among African American, Native American, and Hispanic American communities, compared with Caucasians (51–53), and six antigen matching is less frequent for African Americans than for Caucasians. With the faster rate of growth of ESRD incidence rates among African Americans, their chances of receiving kidney transplants are substantially lower than Whites (54–57).

In the United States, the majority of renal transplants are deceased donor organs. The decline in the rate of deceased donor kidney transplants has been responsible for the overall decline in the transplantation rate. Living organ donor transplantation, on the other hand, has shown improvement, especially in living unrelated organs. In the period 1999–2002, the transplantation rate for first deceased donor kidney transplant by race was 3.5 per 100 patient years on dialysis for Caucasians, compared with 2.2 for African Americans, 2.4 for Native Americans, and 3.3 for Asians. The mean time to first deceased donor renal transplant for African Americans in the year 2002 was 1382 days compared with 817 days for Caucasians and 1197 for Hispanic Americans.

Overall, the first year graft survival probability for deceased donor kidneys has substantially improved over the past decade from 80.2% in 1991 to 89.2% in 2001. However, the dramatic improvement seen in this short-term graft survival has not been maintained in the longer term, i.e., 10 years, graft survival increased from 26.7 in 1987 to 36.7 in 1992. The difference between African Americans and Caucasians is not significant in the short term; one-year graft survival probabilities in 2001 were 90.6 for Caucasians and 87.3 for African Americans. On the other hand, the difference remains large in long-term graft survival; the 10-year graft survival in 1992 was 39.1 for Caucasians, compared with 25.0 in African Americans.

The differential rates of graft failure in African Americans and Caucasians are not entirely clear. However, HLA mismatches may play a significant role. The greater genetic diversity in the African-American community contributes to the difficulty in getting perfect HLA matches for organ transplantation in African Americans, resulting in chronic immunological injury. Also, more severe hypertension and other non-immunological insults may contribute to the greater rate of graft loss.

The patient death rate for deceased donor renal transplants is higher for African Americans than for Caucasians (9).

Living donor transplant rates in the period 1999–2002 were 2.6 per 100 patient years on dialysis for Caucasians, 0.7 for African Americans, 1.2 for Native Americans, and 1.7 for Asians (9). The mean time to first living donor transplant in the year 2002 was 481 days for African Americans, compared with 234 for Caucasians and 418 for Hispanic Americans. There has been noticeable improvement in both the short-term (one year) and the long-term (10 years) graft survival probabilities for living donor organs. However, as in the experience with deceased donor organs, the improvement in the 10-year graft survival is modest, compared with the one-year survival. African Americans have lower graft survival in both the short term and long term compared with Caucasians. Patient death rate is also higher for African Americans (9).

The major racial barriers that contribute to and maintain the large differences in the transplantation rates between African Americans and Caucasians include reluctance to accept transplants, comorbid conditions, limited access, lack of appropriate counseling by healthcare providers, longer waiting times, sociodemographic factors, dialysis facility practice patterns, perceptions of care, and less trust in the healthcare system (58–62).

MORBIDITY AND MORTALITY IN ESRD

Morbidity

Morbidity in patients treated for ESRD is defined in terms of all cause and cause-specific hospitalization. Events such as acute myocardial infarction and problems with vascular access are frequent causes for hospitalization. In general, peritoneal dialysis patients spend more days, and transplant patients spend fewer days in the hospital. Overall, there is not a significant difference between African Americans and Caucasians in the rate of first hospitalization for all ESRD patients. However, in dialysis patients, African Americans have a lower rate of first hospitalization, but spend more time in the hospital when they receive renal transplants (9).

Mortality

Despite advances in dialysis technology and transplantation, long-term survival in ESRD is dreadfully low. Almost half of all deaths are due to cardiovascular disease. The second most common cause of death is sepsis. Hypoalbuminemia at initiation of dialysis is an indicator for poor survival. Severe anemia and low dialysis dose are associated with poor prognosis in ESRD. Despite evidence that non-White patients are more likely to have

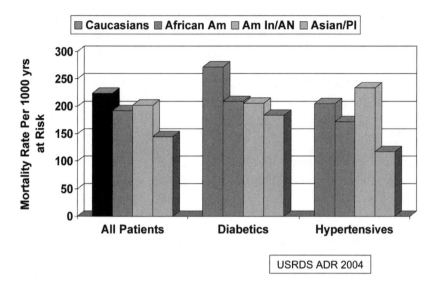

Figure 6 Annual mortality rate per 1000 patient years at risk for hemodialysis patients by race and diagnosis, 2002. African Am = African Americans; Am In/AN = American Indians and Alaska Natives; Asian/PI = Asians and Pacific Islanders. *Source*: From Ref. 9.

these poor survival indicators as well as limited pre-ESRD care, the survival rates in dialysis are higher for racial and ethnic minorities compared with Caucasians. In the year 2002, the annual death rate for all ESRD patients (per 1000 patient years) was 183 for Caucasians, compared with 176 for African Americans, 172 for Native Americans, and 128 for Asians. For hemodialysis patients, the annual death rate was 224 for Caucasians, 192 for African Americans, 202 for Native Americans, and 145 for Asians (9) (Fig. 6). Overall, the better survival of African Americans and other racial and ethnic minority groups than Caucasians is poorly understood, and requires further exploration.

In general, kidney transplantation is associated with better survival and quality of life. Although African Americans have poorer survival than Caucasians, irrespective of graft function, there is a substantial survival benefit when compared with patients on the waiting list or on dialysis (63).

SUMMARY AND DISCUSSION

End-stage renal disease is a major public health problem in the United States. In spite of general improvement in health status of Americans and increased longevity, the incidence rate of ESRD continues to increase. The escalating incidence rate is seen in all racial and ethnic groups, but racial and ethnic minorities, especially African Americans, American Indians, and Alaska Natives have the highest rates. They seem to develop ESRD at a younger age, and suffer a higher burden of disease than Caucasians. Although the two most frequent causes of ESRD, namely type 2 diabetes mellitus and hypertension, are also more common in the minority groups, their higher prevalence does not entirely explain the disproportionate burden of renal disease. It is possible that other factors, including socioeconomic status, exposure to unidentified environmental agents, and genetic pre-disposition play important roles in the development and progression of kidney disease.

The greater burden of chronic kidney disease and end-stage renal disease in racial and ethnic minorities can be reduced through specific educational programs targeted at these communities. The recently initiated National Kidney Disease Education Program (NKDEP) by the National Institute of Diabetes and Digestive and Kidney Diseases of the National Institutes of Health has, as its initial goal, targeted the African-American community. The pilot program was carried out in four communities that were predominantly African American. The expansion of the program nationally still places a greater emphasis in racial and ethnic minority communities.

It is quite intriguing that the racial and ethnic minorities that carry a disproportionate burden of ESRD have better survival than Caucasians. There is no ready explanation for this phenomenon, and requires further research. Finally, in addition to health education, there is need for preventive programs especially in developing countries.

REFERENCES

1. U.S. Renal Data System (USRDS). USRDS 20021 Annual Data Report: Atlas of End-Stage Renal Disease in the United States. Bethesda, MD: National Institutes of Health, National Institute of Diabetes and Digestive and Kidney Diseases, 2002.
2. Easterling RE. Racial factors in the incidence and causation of end-stage renal disease (ESRD). Trans Am Soc Artif Intern Organs 1977; 23:28–33.
3. Rostand SG, Kirk KA, Rutsky EA. Racial differences in the incidence and treatment for end-stage renal disease. N Engl J Med 1982; 306:1276–1279.
4. Ferguson R, Grim CE, Opgenorth TJ. The epidemiology of end-stage renal disease; the six-year South-Central Los Angeles experience, 1980–1985. Am J Pub Health 1987; 77:864–865.
5. Jones CA, McQuillan GM, Kusek JW, Eberhardt MS, Herman WH, et al. Serum creatinine levels in the US population: Third National Health and Nutrition Examination Survey. Am J Kidney Dis 1998; 32:992–999.
6. UK Renal Registry. The Fifth Annual Report of the UK Renal Registry, 2003. Available from http://www.renalreg.com/home.htm.

7. McDonald SP, Russ GR, Kerr PG. ESRD in Australia and New Zealand at the end of the millennium: a report from the ANZDATA registry. Am J Kidney Dis 2002; 40:1122–1131.

8. McDonald SP, Russ GR. Current incidence, treatment patterns and outcome of end-stage renal disease among indigenous groups in Australia and New Zealand. Nephrology 2003; 8:42.

9. U.S. Renal Data System. USRDS 2004 Annual Data Report. Atlas of End Stage Renal Disease in the United States. Bethesda, MD: National Institute of Diabetes and Digestive and Kidney Diseases, 2004.

10. Harris MI, Flegal KM, Cowie CC, Eberhardt MS, Goldstein DE, et al. Prevalence of diabetes, impaired fasting glucose and impaired glucose tolerance in U.S. adults. The Third National Health and Nutrition Examination Survey, 1988–1994. Diabetes Care 1998; 21(4):518–524.

11. Parving HH, Lehnert H, Brochner-Mortensen J, Gomis R, Andersen S, Arner P. The effect of irbesartan on the development of diabetic nephropathy in patients with type 2 diabetes. N Engl J Med 2001; 345:870–878.

12. Lewis EJ, Hunsicker LG, Clarke WR, et al. Renoprotective effect of the angiotensin-receptor antagonist ibesartan in patients with nephropathy due to type 2 diabetes. N Engl J Med 2001; 345:851–860.

13. Brenner BM, Cooper ME, de Zeeuw D, et al. Effects of losartan on renal and cardiovascular outcomes in patients with type 2 diabetes and nephropathy. N Engl J Med 2001; 345:861–869.

14. Klag MJ, Stamler J, Brancati FL, Neaton JD, Randall BL, Whelton PK. End-stage renal disease in African-American and white men: 16-year MRFIT findings. J Am Med Assoc 1977; 277(16):1293–1298.

15. Coresh J, Wei GL, McQuillan G, Brancati FL, Levey AS, et al. Prevalence of high blood pressure and elevated serum creatinine level in the United States: findings from the Third National Health and Nutrition Examination Survey (1988–1994). Arch Intern Med 2001; 161:1207–1216.

16. Burt VL, Whelton P, Roccella EJ, Brown C, et al. Prevalence of hypertension in the US adult population. Results from the Third National Health and Nutrition Examination Survey, 1988–1991. Hypertension 1995; 3:305–313.

17. Perneger TV, Whelton PK, Klag MJ. Risk of kidney failure associated with the use of acetaminophen, aspirin and nonsteroidal anti-inflammatory drugs. N Engl J Med 1994; 331:1675–1679.

18. Sandler DP, Smith JC, Weinberg CR, et al. Analgesic use and chronic renal disease. N Engl J Med 1989; 320:1238–1243.

19. Norris KC, Thornhill-Joynes M, Robinson C, Strickland T, et al. Cocaine use, hypertension and end-stage renal disease. Am J Kidney Dis 2001; 38(3): 523–528.

20. Norris KC, Thornhill-Joynes M, Tareen N. Cocaine use and chronic renal failure. Semin Nephrol 2001; 21(4):362–366.

21. Agodoa LY, Appel L, Bakris GL, Beck G, Bourgoignie J, et al., for the African American Study of Kidney Disease and Hypertension (AASK) Study Group. Effect of ramipril vs amlodipine on renal outcomes in hypertensive nephrosclerosis. A randomized controlled trial. J Am Med Assoc 2001; 285:2719–2728.

22. Wright JT Jr, Bakris G, Greene T, Agodoa LY, et al., for the African American Study of Kidney Disease and Hypertension Study Group. Effect of blood pressure lowering and antihypertensive drug class on progression of hypertensive kidney disease: results of the AASK trial. J Am Med Assoc 2002; 288: 2421–2431.

23. Winston JS, Burns GC, Klotman PE. The human immunodeficiency virus (HIV) epidemic and HIV-associated nephropathy. Semin Nephrol 1998; 18(4): 373–377.

24. Monahan M, Tanji N, Klotman PE. HIV-associated nephropathy: an urban epidemic. Semin Nephrol 2001; 21(4):393–402.

25. Klotman PE. HIV-associated nephropathy. Kidney Int 1999; 56:1161–1176.

26. Maschio G, Alberti D, Janin G, et al. Effect of the angiotensin-converting-enzyme inhibitor benazepril on the progression of chronic renal insufficiency. The Angiotensin-Converting-Enzyme Inhibition in Progressive Renal Insufficiency Study Group. N Engl J Med 1996; 334(15):939–945.

27. GISEN Group. Randomized placebo-controlled trial of effect of ramipril on decline in glomerular filtration rate and risk of terminal renal failure in proteinuric, non-diabetic nephropathy. The GISEN Group (Gruppo Italiano di Studi Epidemiologici in Nefrologia). Lancet 1997; 349:1857–1863.

28. Ruggenenti P, Perna A, Gherardi G, Gaspari F, Benini R, Remuzzi G. Renal function and requirement for dialysis in chronic nephropathy patients on long-term ramipril: REIN follow-up trial. Gruppo Italiano di Studi Epidemiologici in Nefrologia (GISEN). Ramipril efficacy in nephropathy. Lancet 1998; 352:1252–1256.

29. National Kidney Foundation K/DOQI Working Group. Clinical practice guidelines for chronic renal disease evaluation, classification, and stratification. Am J Kidney Dis 2002; 39:S46–S75.

30. Bogdanova N, Markoff A, Horst J. Autosomal dominant polycystic kidney disease—clinical and genetic aspects. Autosomal dominant polycystic kidney disease—clinical and genetic aspects. Kidney Blood Pressure Res 2002; 25(5): 265–283.

31. Davis ID, MacRae, Dell K, Sweeney WE, Avner ED. Can progression of autosomal dominant or autosomal recessive polycystic kidney disease be prevented? Semin Nephrol 2001; 21(5):430–440.

32. Qian Q, Harris PC, Torres VE. Treatment prospects for autosomal-dominant polycystic kidney disease. Kidney Int 2001; 59(6):2005–2022.

33. Ifudu O, Dawood M, Iofel Y, Valcourt JS, Friedman EA. Delayed referral of black, Hispanic, and older patients with chronic renal failure. Am J Kidney Dis 1999; 33:728–733.

34. Schmidt RJ, Domico JR, Sorkin MI, Hobbs G. Early referral and its impact on emergent first dialyses, health care costs, and outcome. Am J Kidney Dis 1998; 32:278–283.

35. Stack AG. Determinants of modality selection among incident US dialysis patients: results from a national study. J Am Soc Nephrol 2002; 13: 1279–1287.

36. Winkelmayer WC, Glynn RJ, Levin R, Owen W Jr, Avorn J. Late referral and modality choice in end-stage renal disease. Kidney Int 2001; 60:1547–1554.

37. Astor BC, Eustace JA, Powe NR, et al. Timing of nephrologist referral and arteriovenous access use: the CHOICE Study. Am J Kidney Dis 2001; 38:494–501.
38. Stehman-Breen CO, Sherrard DJ, Gillen D, Caps M. Determinants of type and timing of initial permanent hemodialysis vascular access. Kidney Int 2000; 57:639–645.
39. Arora P, Obrador GT, Ruthazer R, et al. Prevalence, predictors, and consequences of late nephrology referral at a tertiary care center. J Am Soc Nephrol 1999; 10:1281–1286.
40. NKF-DOQI clinical practice guidelines for vascular access. National Kidney Foundation-Dialysis Outcomes Quality Initiative. Am J Kidney Dis 1997;30: S150–S191.
41. Hoen B, Paul-Dauphin A, Hestin D, Kessler M. EPIBACDIAL: a multicenter prospective study of risk factors for bacteremia in chronic hemodialysis patients. J Am Soc Nephrol 1998; 9:869–876.
42. Owen WF Jr, Chertow GM, Lazarus JM, Lowrie EG. Dose of hemodialysis and survival: differences by race and sex. J Am Med Assoc 1998; 280:1764–1768.
43. Seghal AR. Outcomes of renal replacement therapy among blacks and women. Am J Kidney Dis 1993; 35:S148.
44. Frankenfield DL, Rocco MV, Frederick PR, Pugh J, McClellan WM, Owen WF Jr. Racial/ethnic analysis of selected intermediate outcomes for hemodialysis patients: results from the 1997 ESRD Core Indicators Project. Am J Kidney Dis 1999; 34:721–730.
45. Barker-Cummings C, McClellan W, Soucie JM, Krisher J. Ethnic differences in the use of peritoneal dialysis as initial treatment for end-stage renal disease. J Am Med Assoc 1995; 274:1858–1862.
46. Saade M, Joglar F. Chronic peritoneal dialysis: seven-year experience in a large Hispanic program. Peritoneal Dial Int 1995; 15:37–41.
47. Nolph KD, Cutler SJ, Steinberg SM, Novak JW, Hirschman GH. Factors associated with morbidity and mortality among patients on CAPD. Am Soc Artif Intern Organs Trans 1987; 33:57–65.
48. Port FK, Wolfe RA, Mauger EA, Berling DP, Jiang K. Comparison of survival probabilities for dialysis patients vs. cadaveric renal transplant recipients. J Am Med Assoc 1993; 270:1339–1343.
49. Wolfe RA, Ashby VB, Milford EL, et al. Comparison of mortality in all patients on dialysis, patients on dialysis awaiting transplantation, and recipients of a first cadaveric transplant. N Engl J Med 1999; 341:1725–1730.
50. Danielson BL, LaPree AJ, Odland MD, Steffens EK. Attitudes and beliefs concerning organ donation among Native Americans in the upper Midwest. J Transplant Coord 1998; 8:153–156.
51. Epstein AM, Ayanian JZ, Keogh JH, et al. Racial disparities in access to renal transplantation—clinically appropriate or due to underuse or overuse? N Engl J Med 2000; 343:1537–1544.
52. Bleyer AJ, Tell GS, Evans GW, Ettinger WH Jr, Burkart JM. Survival of patients undergoing renal replacement therapy in one center with special emphasis on racial differences. Am J Kidney Dis 1996; 28:72–81.

53. Alexander GC, Sehgal AR. Barriers to cadaveric renal transplantation among blacks, women, and the poor. J Am Med Assoc 1998; 280:1148–1152.
54. Eggers PW. Racial differences in access to kidney transplantation. Health Care Financing Rev 1995; 17:89–103.
55. Gaylin DS, Held PJ, Port FK, et al. The impact of comorbid and sociodemographic factors on access to renal transplantation. J Am Med Assoc 1993; 269: 603–608.
56. Soucie JM, Neylan JF, McClellan W. Race and sex differences in the identification of candidates for renal transplantation. Am J Kidney Dis 1992; 19:414–419.
57. Ayanian JZ, Cleary PD, Weissman JS, Epstein AM. The effect of patients' preferences on racial differences in access to renal transplantation. N Engl J Med 1999; 341:1661–1669.
58. Ozminkowski RJ, White AJ, Hassol A, Murphy M. Minimizing racial disparity regarding receipt of a cadaver kidney transplant. Am J Kidney Dis 1997; 30:749–759.
59. Sanfilippo FP, Vaughn WK, Peters TG, et al. Factors affecting the waiting time of cadaveric kidney transplant candidates in the United States. J Am Med Assoc 1992; 267:247–252.
60. Hata Y, Cecka JM, Takemoto S, Ozawa M, Cho YW, Terasaki PI. Effects of changes in the criteria for nationally shared kidney transplants for HLA-matched patients. Transplantation 1998; 65:208–212.
61. Ellison MD, Breen T, Cunningham P, Daily O. Blacks and whites on the UNOS renal waiting list: waiting times and patient demographics compared. Transplant Proc 1993; 25:2462–2466.
62. Isaacs RB, Lobo PI, Nock SL, Hanson JA, Ojo AO, Pruett TL. Racial disparities in access to simultaneous pancreas-kidney transplantation in the United States. Am J Kidney Dis 2000; 36:526–533.
63. Isaacs RB, Nock SL, Spencer CE, et al. Racial disparities in renal transplant outcomes. Am J Kidney Dis 1999; 34:706–712.

12

Histopathologic Patterns in Hypertensive Nephrosclerosis in African Americans

Yihan Wang and Agnes B. Fogo

Department of Pathology, Vanderbilt University Medical Center, Nashville, Tennessee, U.S.A.

INTRODUCTION

Hypertensive nephrosclerosis is one of the leading causes of end-stage renal disease (ESRD) as listed in registries throughout the world, and particularly affects African Americans (1,2). In the United States, African Americans constitute approximately 30% of new ESRD patients entering dialysis programs, but only 12.6% of the general U.S. population. In this patient group, 30% of ESRD is attributed to hypertension (3). This overall age- and sex-adjusted incidence is at least five times higher than in non-African Americans in the United States. Hypertension in African Americans also develops 10 years earlier than in Caucasians. Thus, in the age group of 20 to 44 years old, the excess incidence in African Americans is even more striking, with a 20-fold higher incidence of ESRD (4–8). African Americans have a 50–75% higher prevalence of hypertension compared to other Americans, with two to three times greater prevalence of more severe stage 2 and stage 3 hypertension (8).

Multiple likely risk factors for this racial difference in hypertensive nephrosclerosis leading to ESRD in the United States include, but are not limited to, a lack of access to medical care, socioeconomic status, severity and duration of hypertension, education level, alcohol and drug abuse (4,5,7,8). However, these factors alone cannot account for the excess disease burden in African Americans. Additional factors, such as nephron endowment and genetic predisposition have thus been postulated. Genetically and/or environmentally induced amplification of profibrotic mechanisms, such as the renin–angiotensin system (RAS) and transforming growth factor-β (TGF-β) may be more prevalent in African Americans (9–12). Importantly, even with similar blood pressure (BP) control, African Americans with hypertension and renal insufficiency have a more rapid fall in renal function than Caucasians (13,14). However, this disease progression can be modified with aggressive interventions. The recent update on the African American Study of Kidney Disease (AASK) intervention trial showed that BP control with angiotensin I converting enzyme (ACE)-inhibitor and additional antihypertensives could slow progressive loss of GFR in African Americans with hypertensive nephrosclerosis (5). Further understanding of the nature of end organ damage and possible mechanisms could lead to further advances in therapy. This review will describe the histopathology and discuss possible pathogenesis of these lesions in African Americans.

MORPHOLOGY

General

The AASK study was designed to determine if interventions with antihypertensives could affect progressive loss of GFR in African Americans with presumed hypertensive nephrosclerosis. Indeed, ACEI was found to have a greater efficacy than a calcium channel blocker, although patients needed an average of 2.6 drugs to achieve BP goals (5). Entry criteria included Black race, adults with moderate renal insufficiency, and lack of marked proteinuria or other clinical findings to suggest disease other than hypertensive nephrosclerosis. In the pilot phase, an important objective was to determine if the clinical diagnosis of hypertensive nephrosclerosis indeed was accurate. The typical clinical features of hypertensive nephrosclerosis are hypertension, followed by a decrease in glomerular filtration rate, commonly accompanied by proteinuria and hematuria. Histologically, the so-called "hypertensive nephrosclerosis" is defined by sclerosis of vessels with extensive global glomerulosclerosis and proportional tubulointerstitial fibrosis in the absence of other defining lesions. Typical lesions are vascular wall medial thickening with frequent arteriolar hyaline deposition, varying degree of arterial intimal fibrosis, interstitial fibrosis with proportional tubular atrophy, focal glomerular ischemic changes with variable thickening and wrinkling of the basement membrane, and varying foot process effacement. A group of 46 patients consented to undergo protocol biopsy, with adequate tissue obtained in 39. This AASK pilot study importantly confirmed that renal biopsies in African Americans with a clinical diagnosis of hypertensive nephrosclerosis show morphological lesions consistent with this diagnosis. These changes of hypertensive nephrosclerosis were widespread in nearly all cases in the AASK biopsy study (15). Importantly, no evidence of other significant primary underlying renal disease was found in these protocol biopsies, underscoring the accuracy of the clinical diagnosis in these patients. One patient had mesangial deposits, one had GBM thickening (without any clinical evidence of diabetes), and two had cholesterol emboli, without systemic evidence of disease related to these lesions.

Glomeruli

Glomeruli with ischemic injury in hypertensive nephrosclerosis are postulated to eventually progress to global glomerulosclerosis. Global glomerulosclerosis can be classified as either solidified or obsolescent type. Obsolescent glomeruli are defined as glomeruli in which Bowman's space is occupied by collagenous, PAS-positive material, and the tuft is retracted (Fig. 1), as first described by McManus and Lupton (16) in 1960 as "ischemic obsolescence." Solidified glomeruli are defined as glomeruli in which the entire tuft is solidified, in the absence of the collagenous change in the capsular space (Fig. 2), as described first by Fahr (17) in 1925 and subsequently revisited by Bohle and Ratschek (18), using the term "decompensated benign nephrosclerosis."

Glomerulosclerosis may also be segmental in hypertension-associated nephrosclerosis. The differentiation of primary versus secondary segmental sclerotic lesions may be challenging. Our criteria for diagnosis of secondary

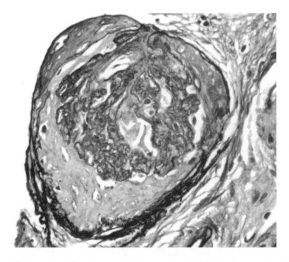

Figure 1   Obsolescent glomerulus. Global glomerulosclerosis with Bowman's space filled by collagenous material and retraction of the tuft as first described by McManus in 1960 as "ischemic obsolescence" (Jones' silver stain, ×400).

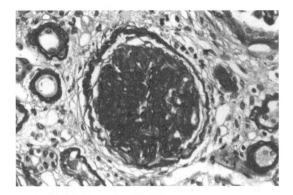

Figure 2 Solidified glomerulus. Globally sclerosed glomerulus with solidification of the entire tuft, in the absence of accumulated collagenous material in the capsular space, the so-called "decompensated benign nephrosclerosis" as described first by Fahr in 1925 (periodic acid Schiff stain, ×400).

focal segmental glomerulosclerosis (FSGS) associated with hypertensive nephrosclerosis include, in addition to the segmental sclerosis, the predominance of small, shrunken, globally sclerotic glomeruli, the presence of periglomerular fibrosis, glomerular basement membrane corrugation, increased lucency of the lamina rara interna, and sub-total foot process effacement by EM, and disproportionately severe vascular lesions relative to sclerosis (Fig. 3) (15,19). Of course, the clinical history is of utmost importance in delineating the time sequence of hypertension, renal insufficiency, and

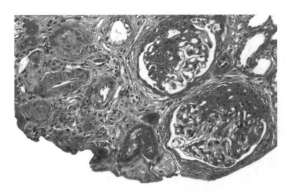

Figure 3 Secondary segmental sclerosis. Glomeruli show segmental sclerosis with adhesions to Bowman's capsule and surrounding tubulointerstitial fibrosis. Features suggesting arterionephrosclerosis as the underlying etiology include periglomerular fibrosis, glomerular basement membrane corrugation, and interlobular arteries with medial thickening and intimal fibrosis and tortuosity (periodic acid Schiff stain, ×200).

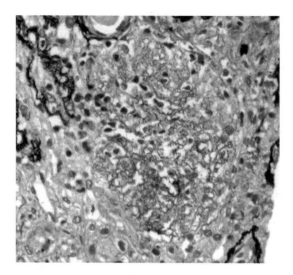

Figure 4 "Disappearing" glomerulus. This resorbing globally sclerotic glomerulus still shows remaining recognizable corrugated glomerular basement membranes, but with dissolution of Bowman's capsule, becoming continuous with the fibrotic interstitium. This process ultimately leads to apparent disappearance of sclerotic glomeruli (Jones' silver stain, ×400).

proteinuria. Of note, the extent of global glomerulosclerosis may be under-estimated based on hematoxylin and eosin stain examination, as resorbing globally sclerosed glomeruli may not be evident. These disappearing glomeruli show partial disappearance or absence of Bowman's capsule, which in some cases extends to partial dissolution of the globally sclerotic glomeruli, which then become continuous with the fibrotic interstitium (Fig. 4).

Vasculature

The so-called "benign hypertensive nephrosclerosis" vascular lesions vary depending on the size of the vessels involved. Arcuate and larger arteries show intimal fibrosis and sometimes splitting of the internal elastic lamina. Interlobular arteries show fibroelastic intimal expansion with reduplication of the internal elastic lamina. Small arteries and arterioles show medial thickening with multilayered smooth muscle cells and intimal proliferation. Arteriolar hyalinosis of afferent arterioles, typically eccentric, is common. In contrast, accelerated hypertensive nephrosclerosis shows lesions in interlobular arteries with marked intimal edema, proliferation of myointimal cells with mucoid matrix, which later organizes to a characteristic concentric "onionskin" pattern of intimal fibrosis. These alterations may also affect the arcuate arteries and extend into arterioles. Sometimes blood constituents in the vascular wall in the subendothelial space, such as red blood cell fragments and intraluminal fibrin thrombi, may be seen. Malignant hypertensive nephrosclerosis is diagnosed morphologically when fibrinoid necrosis of the vessel wall is present. Malignant hypertension as a presenting finding is now rare in the United States. However, in a large series reported in Brazil of 81 biopsied patients who presented with primary hypertensive nephrosclerosis underlying their moderate renal insufficiency, 43% showed lesions indicative of malignant nephrosclerosis (20).

Tubulointerstitium

Tubular changes in hypertensive nephrosclerosis generally are non-specific and most often are secondary to vascular and glomerular lesions. Tubulointerstitial fibrosis in hypertensive nephrosclerosis is proportional to glomerulosclerosis. Tubular lesions are proportional to interstitial fibrosis and consist of atrophic epithelium, thickened basement membrane, and occasional proteinaceous casts.

Possible pathophysiologic mechanisms are as follows:

1. *Hemodynamic injury*: Hypertension can result in renal vascular injury. Vasoconstriction or vasodilation of afferent arterioles in different nephrons might both contribute to lesions. Afferent arteriolar vasoconstriction might cause glomerular ischemic injury that leads to glomerular simplification, followed by tubular injury that leads to tubular atrophy, tubulointerstitial infiltrate and fibrosis, and ultimate loss of GFR. Conversely, afferent arteriolar vasodilation in remnant nephrons can contribute to glomerular hypertension, glomerular hypertrophy, and associated glomerulosclerosis, proteinuria, and progressive renal failure (21).

Correlation and extent of lesions were investigated further in biopsies from patients enrolled in the pilot phase of the AASK trial. Importantly, these biopsies confirmed that African American patients with this clinical diagnosis had lesions of hypertensive nephrosclerosis. The extent of global glomerulosclerosis in this population was extraordinary, involving on average $43 \pm 26\%$ of glomeruli in this population with average age of 53 ± 11 years old. Interestingly, the extensive global glomerulosclerosis did not correlate with vascular thickening, nor did the vascular lesions correlate with degree of hypertension. Vascular and glomerular sclerosis and interstitial fibrosis did correlate with the reciprocal of serum creatinine (18). These results suggest the possibility that a primary microvascular disease could contribute to both hypertension and renal lesions (see below).

For obvious ethical reasons, a control population was not included in the AASK study. We therefore also studied our clinical renal biopsies to compare hypertensive nephrosclerosis lesions in biopsied African Americans and Caucasians (22). Clearly, in this retrospective study, clinical criteria for renal biopsy determined the study population. Perneger et al. (23) have elegantly demonstrated that the presumptive, clinical diagnosis of hypertensive nephrosclerosis is made much more commonly in African Americans than in Caucasians. Therefore, it is expected that especially in African Americans with hypertension and renal insufficiency, a renal biopsy would only be done when the clinical situation was atypical for hypertensive nephrosclerosis or was more severe. All cases from our renal biopsy files from both African Americans and Caucasians with a clinicopathologic diagnosis of hypertensive nephrosclerosis, in the absence of other disease as verified by IF and/or EM, were reviewed.

As expected, in this study, biopsied African Americans were younger than Caucasians, and had higher serum creatinine and proteinuria. Total global glomerulosclerosis was extensive in both African Americans and Caucasians (all patients $42 \pm 3\%$; African Americans $50 \pm 5\%$ vs. Caucasians $39 \pm 4\%$), as also seen in the AASK trial. Surprisingly, solidified glomeruli were significantly increased in African Americans vs. Caucasians ($25 \pm 6\%$ vs. $8 \pm 2\%$). These solidified glomeruli were associated with segmental glomerulosclerosis, and with clinically worse disease. In contrast, the extent of obsolescent glomeruli was similar in African Americans and Caucasians ($24 \pm 5\%$ vs. $31 \pm 4\%$). Solidified glomeruli did not increase with aging, while obsolescent glomeruli did, suggesting different pathogenesis of these two types of global sclerosis.

A multiple linear regression analysis was performed to examine if the clinical parameters of proteinuria, mean arterial pressure (MAP), serum creatinine, and age could predict the severity of structural injury observed. Of note, total global sclerosis and vascular sclerosis were poorly predicted by this model ($R^2 = 0.16$). MAP did not contribute to the prediction by the model of any morphologic lesions, and proteinuria accounted only minimally for the variability of global glomerulosclerosis. In summary, in this study, neither age, nor blood pressure or proteinuria was good predictor of severity of structural injuries. Thus, both our retrospective biopsy study and the AASK renal biopsy data do not support a simple linear relationship between hypertension, vascular sclerosis, and ultimately global glomerulosclerosis.

2. *Vasoreactivity*: What then could account for the extensive global glomerulosclerosis in African American patients with hypertensive nephrosclerosis? We speculate that the coexistence of solidified glomeruli with segmental glomerulosclerosis in our biopsy study could reflect an increased vasoreactivity in susceptible populations (22). African Americans tend to show a larger increase in blood pressure level than Caucasians during stress, particularly to stimuli that elicit a vasoconstrictor response (24–26). Autoregulatory response to hypertension, resulting in vasospasm, could be excessive in patients susceptible to develop hypertension, like in some African Americans (27). Thus, we speculate that global vasoconstrictive ischemia could result in complete collapse and solidification of the glomerulus.

Further, we hypothesize that adaptation and segmental resistance to collapse and/or reflow, with possible attendant segmental hypertension/hyperfiltration, could give rise to segmental sclerotic lesions associated with solidification in those patients. Thus, vasospasm could reflect primary microvascular injury and endothelial dysfunction that then caused hypertension, or occurred in response to hypertension, in susceptible patients. It is thus possible that a primary renal microvascular disease results in hypertension, glomerulosclerosis, and interstitial fibrosis (28).

In 1989, Muirhead and Pitcock described different characteristics of malignant nephrosclerosis in African Americans versus Caucasians (29,30). In this study, they examined renal biopsy or nephrectomy specimens from African Americans and Caucasians with previous very severe hypertension (group average BP, 255/171 mmHg) and varying degree of renal functional impairment, with tissue obtained after BP was controlled. Both populations showed onionskin intimal thickening with intramural deposition of acid mucopolysaccharides and thickening of the media. However, the renal biopsies from African Americans with malignant hypertension failed to show fibrinoid necrosis of the small arteries and afferent arterioles and proliferative glomerulitis, unlike those of Caucasian patients. Instead, African Americans showed prominent glomerular collapse and ischemic changes, and more marked myointimal fibroplasia and arteriolar hyalinosis. These findings further support differences in vasoactive responses and injury mechanisms, with resulting differences in both severity and phenotype of lesions in African Americans vs. Caucasians.

Population-based studies of African Africans with hypertension and chronic kidney disease (CKD) are limited. Data from a single center from South Africa of its Black patients with ESRD presenting for dialysis from 1972 to 1976 showed that essential malignant hypertension was the commonest single cause of ESRD, accounting for about half of ESRD cases (31). These patients were on average 39.9 years old for the males vs. 33.4 years for the females. No patients under age 30 had malignant hypertension. In two more recent studies reported in the early 1990s from Nigeria, hypertensive nephrosclerosis accounted for 23% and 43%, respectively, of chronic renal failure cases (32,33). The authors of the largest of these two studies of 1980 CKD patients, observed that the frequency and severity of apparent essential hypertension in this Black Nigerian population with associated renal failure, were similar to that observed in African Americans (32). Whether similar genetic and environmental risk factors for hypertension-associated sclerosis, as we discuss in the latter population, are also relevant for the African Africans remains to be proven.

Marked myointimal fibroplasia with mucoid changes and fibrinoid necrosis were observed as prominent features in renal biopsies in these African Blacks in South Africa and Nigeria with essential malignant hypertension (34,35). Histological findings did not change in tissue from

1956 versus 1989, despite better antihypertensive drug availability (34). Of note, fibrinoid necrosis was insignificant or absent in African Americans with malignant hypertension as described by Muirhead and Pitcock (30). In the above two series of South African and Nigerian Blacks with malignant hypertension, fibrinoid necrosis was present in 44% of renal biopsies (34), and 76% of renal biopsies and autopsies (35). Autopsied South African Black patients with malignant hypertension from the 1956–1961 era showed fibrinoid necrosis in 92% (34). Of note, the above patients had very severe hypertension, 227/145 and 206/137 mmHg, respectively, for these two studies (34,35). The lesser fibrinoid necrosis in African Americans with similarly severe malignant hypertension suggests possible differences in susceptibility to pressure-associated end organ damage vs. African Africans. Additional possibilities include differences in antihypertensive treatment and time of presentation.

3. *Accelerated aging*: Vascular sclerosis and glomerulosclerosis increase in normal populations with aging, but the rate varies widely in different populations. The extent of global sclerosis in the overall normal adult U.S. population under age 50 years is estimated to be 1–3%, increasing up to 30% by age 80 years in the United States, based on the formula [(age/ 2 − 10) = %sclerosis] (36,37). Elegant studies by Tracy et al. (38) have shown less aortic fibroplasia and renal sclerosis at all ages in the native Mexican population in Mexico compared to the U.S. population. Interestingly, first- and second-generation Hispanic immigrants to the United States had increasing renal vascular sclerosis to levels intermediate between Mexico City natives and other U.S. residents (39). These findings support an interplay of genetic and environmental factors in determination of vascular sclerosis. In a similar morphologic study of Bolivian Indians, only minimal vessel wall changes occurred with aging (40). In this population-based autopsy study of 27 people of La Paz, Bolivia, an age range of 15–78 years was studied. Only minimal intimal fibroplasia was observed at all ages, even in the most elderly subjects, compared to populations of the United States. Elderly Japanese hypertensive patients also showed only minimal glomerulosclerosis, even less than expected for age in the normal, non-hypertensive U.S. Caucasian population (41,42). These 30 subjects with hypertension, ranging from 71 to 84 years, had only minimal or no glomerulosclerosis, with obsolescent glomeruli present in 21 of 30 patients (41). In comparison, only half of the 10 aging patients without hypertension examined showed glomerular obsolescence. Arteriolar sclerosis with medial hypertrophy, proliferation, and hyalinosis was present in all those with hypertension. Only two of these 30 hypertensive patients showed additional malignant hypertensive changes of fibrinoid necrosis.

Within the United States, the vessel wall thickening increase with age in normal African Americans was shown to be even more severe than in the Caucasian population (43). These worse vascular lesions in population-based autopsies coexisted with higher screening clinic blood pressures measured in the African American population compared to the Caucasians in the same New Orleans region. However, even these blood pressure differences, if extrapolated to the autopsied patients in that area, would not completely account for the greater vascular wall thickening in the African American population. These observations point to possible differences in injury set point, rates, and mechanisms of vascular lesions between populations, both in "normal" aging and in response to injury. Of note, in our study of African Americans and Caucasians, we observed an increase of obsolescent, but not solidified glomeruli with increasing age (22). These observations point to different mechanisms leading to the varying phenotypes of sclerosis.

4. *Decreased nephron number*: Low birth weight, defined as birth weight less than 2.5 kg at term birth, may be due to both environmental and genetic factors. Low birth weight is more common in African Americans than in Caucasians. This low birth weight, possibly due to its association with fewer nephrons present at birth, is also postulated by Barker and Brenner (44,45) to be linked to increased risk of cardiovascular disease and renal disease. Lower nephron number is postulated to further increase hemodynamic stress on the remaining nephrons (44,46). However, in neither the AASK nor in our retrospective biopsy study was there a direct correlation of blood pressure with sclerosis, supporting other or additional mechanisms of sclerosis.

Glomerular hypertrophy is another abnormality, which has been a marker of glomerulosclerosis in a variety of settings. We have postulated that abnormal glomerular growth could be linked to activation of profibrotic mechanisms, ultimately resulting in sclerosis. We therefore examined whether glomerular size differed in normal African American and Caucasian populations (47). Data were gathered from age- and body mass index-matched sudden/traumatic deaths in patients without cardiovascular disease. Glomerular volume was significantly greater in African Americans vs. Caucasians. Interestingly, the distribution pattern was different in the two groups. The African American population showed an apparent Gaussian distribution of glomerular size. In contrast, the Caucasian population had a bi-modal distribution, with a sub-group with enlarged glomerular size comparable to that in the African American population (47). Studies from transplant donors have confirmed larger glomerular size in apparently normal African American donors versus Whites (48). Several studies have linked larger glomerular size at baseline to worse long-term outcome after transplant (49,50). These larger nephrons could possibly reflect lower nephron number, and increased susceptibility to injury with less organ reserve. Of interest in this regard are Dr. Hoy's findings in the African American and Australian Aboriginal populations (51). Autopsy study of 37 African Americans and 19 Caucasians showed a strong correlation of birth weight and glomerular number. The data predict an increase of 257,426 glomeruli for each kilogram increase in birth weight (52). Studies from Australian Aborigines and non-Aborigines, African Americans and U.S. Caucasians revealed large variability in glomerular number, with inverse correlation to glomerular corpuscular volume (53). Studies in Aboriginal patients with renal insufficiency have revealed varied histopathology, with frequent lesions related to previous infection. However, of note, marked glomerular enlargement is present in those biopsies that show only sclerotic lesions, perhaps reflecting fewer nephrons at birth (54). We postulate that environmental and genetic influences leading to fewer nephrons at birth may also promote injury in adults, in addition to the possible increased hemodynamic injury when fewer nephrons are present. Maturation and number of glomeruli could be influenced by functional polymorphisms of genes involved not only in renal/glomerular development but also in scarring mechanisms. Augmented fibrotic responses to injury and subsequent renal and vascular sclerosis in adulthood could thus be linked to polymorphisms that also result in a developmental environment that affects glomerular development and growth. The renin–angiotensin–aldosterone system (RAS) is one of several such candidate mediators with effects on both embryonic and maturational development of the kidney, and subsequent response to injury.

5. *Genetics*: Specific polymorphisms in ACE, angiotensinogen and the angiotensin type 1 receptor genes have been linked with cardiovascular disorders, including hypertension, myocardial infarction and cardiac hypertrophy in both African American and other population (55). Familial clustering of chronic renal failure has been especially noted in African Americans (4,56), and angiotensinogen gene mutations were increased in African Americans with essential hypertension, compared to Caucasian hypertensive populations (11). The insertion/deletion (I/D) polymorphism of the ACE gene has also been studied extensively. The D polymorphism has been associated with higher RAS activity, augmented response to angiotensin II, and progression (57). This D allele is significantly more frequent in African American populations compared to Caucasians (12,58). Interestingly, a study from Spain showed that hypertensive patients with impaired GFR more frequently were homozygous for DD, compared to normal ACE genotype distribution in hypertensive patients with preserved renal function (59). This small study suggests the possibility of a contributing role for DD genotype to progressive GFR loss in hypertensive patients. Conversely, patients with II or I/D genotypes could be more resistant to renal sclerosing injuries.

Pharmacological inhibition of the RAS inhibits maturational glomerular growth in animal models (60). Angiotensinogen knockout mice have increased mesangial matrix and arteriosclerosis, despite low blood pressures, and also have decreased glomerular maturation and hypoplastic papilla, pointing to a crucial role of the RAS in development (61). Excess RAS is equally deleterious to the kidney as its absence, pointing to a crucial role for a finely balanced local RAS in kidney development and injury. In transgenic mice with increased copy number of the ACE gene, and thus increased RAS activity, abnormal structural development, with small glomeruli and vascular sclerosis, was also present (62). The RAS also modulates the sclerosis that occurs in association with aging in experimental models: chronic angiotensin inhibition treatment even regressed age-related sclerosis in rats in glomeruli and blood vessels (63).

The prevalence of "salt sensitivity" in African Americans paralleling the incidence of hypertension is higher than in Caucasians throughout the first six decades of life. The cause of the racial disparities remains elusive. Studies suggest that African Americans have a heightened response to a sodium load (64) and may also have an intrinsic impairment in overall ability to excrete a sodium load (65). Aviv and his colleagues propose that habitual consumption of high salt in African Americans causes chronic intermittent tubular hyperperfusion of the macula densa, resulting in a rightward and upward resetting of the operating point for tubuloglomerular feedback. The resetting of the operating point is postulated to cause an imbalance between the vascular tones of the afferent/efferent arterioles, a rise in the glomerular capillary hydraulic pressure, and consequent hyperfiltration. Increased susceptibility to glomerular hypertension/hyperfiltration of African Americans on a high salt intake may explain their proclivity to progressive renal injury associated with essential hypertension (66,67). High salt intake in African Americans may be an independent factor causing renal damage regardless of blood pressure. Rats infused with angiotensin II causing transient hypertension developed mild tubulointerstitial fibrosis and afferent arteriolosclerosis, with subsequent recurrent hypertension following a high salt diet. These studies demonstrate that experimentally induced microvascular and interstitial injury can result in salt-sensitive hypertension. Further, the development of even subtle renal injury may alter the renal ability to excrete salt (68). Genetic and/or environmental elevation of serum uric acid has been proposed as an initial factor in development of endothelial dysfunction and subsequent tubulointerstitial fibrosis and hypertension (69,70). Preliminary studies from the group of Johnson show an intriguing link of elevated serum uric acid and essential hypertension in children with reduced birth weight and endothelial dysfunction. The authors postulate that maternal hyperuricemia could inhibit nephron development in utero (70). Experimental data from rats support that increased uric acid could initiate subtle tubulointerstitial lesions and thus cause hypertension (68,69). Whether these factors are indeed causal in human hypertension, and particularly the hypertension-associated nephrosclerosis in African Americans, remains to be determined.

Transforming growth factor beta (TGF-βl) is a fibrogenic cytokine with manifold actions, including cell proliferation and differentiation, development, matrix turnover, tissue repair, apoptosis, and immune response. TGF-β1 promotes the accumulation of extracellular matrix by increasing expression of extracellular matrix genes and by inhibiting production of proteins mediating proteolysis (71). Thus, increased TGF-β1 is often, but not invariably, linked to increased extracellular matrix and glomerulosclerosis. Higher circulating levels of TGF-β1 in the normal African American population in African Americans with ESRD or hypertension compared to Caucasian counterparts was demonstrated by August and Suthanthiran (72). A polymorphism of TGF-β1 with homozygosity for the arginine allele at codon 25 has been postulated to contribute to heightened TGF-β1 actions (10). Increased expression of TGF-β1 even at normal baseline in African Americans could thus promote imbalanced matrix metabolism and augmented tubulointerstitial fibrosis and glomerulosclerosis, yet another potential mechanism contributing to the racial differences in hypertension-associated lesions. Numerous additional vasoactive and/or fibrogenic molecules have been postulated to contribute to hypertension-associated lesions in African Americans. For example, circulating levels of endothelin-1, another profibrotic vasoconstrictor, are elevated in African Americans with essential hypertension compared to that in Caucasians (73). However, specific proof of a causal link for any of these factors to lesions in humans is not available. The observed link of obesity and FSGS, and the recent surge in incidence of obesity and dysmetabolic syndrome coinciding with the increase of hypertension-associated renal sclerosis, have led to an interesting hypothesis by Kincaid-Smith (74) that these may be causally linked. Direct data in African Americans with hypertensive nephrosclerosis to investigate this intriguing possibility are lacking.

SUMMARY

In summary, renal biopsy data suggest that there may be differing phenotypes of glomerulosclerosis in African Americans versus Caucasians. The precise mechanisms underlying the severe global glomerulosclerosis characteristic of hypertension-associated lesions have not been established. The AASK study and additional human data do not support a direct linear relationship between hypertension and the associated lesions. Additional potential mechanisms underlying the renal injury include decreased nephron number possibly related to polymorphisms of factors that could also influence fibrotic responses in adulthood, abnormal acceleration of aging, abnormal vasoreactivity or other primary microvascular diseases. Whether altered genotypes for the renin–angiotensin system affect vascular/glomerular structure from the earliest stages in utero to aging in the hypertensive African American population remains to be elucidated.

REFERENCES

1. Valderrabano F, Gomez-Campdera F, Jones EH. Hypertension as cause of end-stage renal disease: lessons from international registries. Kidney Int 1998; 54(suppl 68):S60–S66.
2. U.S. RENAL DATA SYSTEM. USRDS 1999 Annual Data Report. Am J Kidney Dis 1999; 34(suppl l):S40–S151.
3. U.S. Data System. USRDS 2002 Annual Data Report: Atlas of End Stage Renal Disease in the United States, Bethesda, National Institutes of Health, National Institutes of Diabetes and Digestive and Kidney Diseases, 2002.
4. Freedman BI, Spray BJ, Tuttle AB, Buckalew VM. The familial risk of end-stage renal disease in African-Americans. Am J Kidney Dis 1993; 21:387–393.
5. Agodoa LY, Appel L, Bakris GL, Beck G, Bourgoignie J, Briggs JP, Charleston J, Cheek D, Cleveland W, Douglas JG, Douglas M, Dowie D, Faulkner M, Gabriel A, Gassman J, Greene T, Hall Y, Hebert L, Hiremath L, Jamerson K, Johnson CJ, Kopple J, Kusek J, Lash J, Lca J, Lewis JB, Lipkowitz M, Massry S, Middleton J, Miller ER III, Norris K, O'Connor D, Ojo A, Phillips RA, Pogue V, Rahman M, Randall OS, Rostand S, Schulman G, Smith W, Thornley-Brown D, Tisher CC, Toto RD, Wright JT Jr, Xu S. African American Study of Kidney Disease and Hypertension (AASK) Study Group: effect of ramipril vs amlodipnie on renal outcomes in hypertensive nephrosclerosis: a randomized controlled trial. JAMA 2001; 285:2719–2728.
6. Shulman NB, Hall WD. Renal vascular disease in African-Americans and other racial minorities. Circulation 1931; 83:1477–1479.
7. Martins D, Tareen N, Norris KC. The epidemiology of end-stage renal disease among African Americans. Am J Med Sci 2002; 323:65–71.
8. Freedman BL. End-stage renal failure in African-Americans: insights in kidney disease susceptibility. Nephrol Dial Transplant 2002; 17:138–200.
9. Suthanthiran M, Khanna A, Cukran D, Adhikarla R, Sharma VK, Singh T, August P. Transforming growth factor-beta 1 hyperexpression in African American end-stage renal disease patients. Kidney Int 1998; 53:639–644.
10. Li B, Khanna A, Sharma V, Singh T, Suthanthiran M, August P. TGF-beta1 DNA polymorphisms, protein levels, and blood pressure. Hypertension 1999; 33:271–275.
11. Bloem LJ, Manatunga AK, Tewksbury DA, Pratt JH. The serum angiotensinogen concentration and variants of the angiotensinogen gene in white and black children. J Clin Invest 1995; 95:948–953.
12. Duru K, Farrow S, Wang J-M, Lockette W, Kurtz T. Frequency of a deletion polymorphism in the gene for angiotensin converting enzyme is increased in African Americans with hypertension. Am J Hypertens 1994; 7:759–762.
13. Shulman NB, Ford CE, Hall WD, Blaufox MD, Simon D, Langford HG, Schneider KA. Prognostic value of serum creatinine and effect of treatment of hypertension on renal function. Results from the hypertension detection and follow-up program. The Hypertension Detection and Follow-up Program Cooperative Group. Hypertension 1989; 13(suppl 5):180–193.
14. Klag MJ, Whelton PK, Randall BL, Neaton JD, Brancati FL, Stamler J. End-stage renal disease in African-American and white men. 16-year MRFIT findings. JAMA 1997; 277:1293–1298.

15. Fogo A, Breyer JA, Smith MC, Cleveland WH, Agodoa L, Kirk KA, Glassock R. Accuracy of the diagnosis of hypertensive nephrosclerosis in African Americans: a report from the African American Study of Kidney Disease (AASK) Trial. AASK Pilot Study Investigators. Kidney Int 1997; 51:244–252.
16. McManus JFA, Lupton CH Jr. Ischemic obsolescence of renal glomeruli: the natural history of the lesions and their relation to hypertension. Lab Invest 1960; 9:413–434.
17. Fahr T. Pathologische Anatomie des Morbus Brightii. In: Henke F, Lubarsch O, eds. Handbuch der Speziellen Pathologischen Anatomie und Histologie. Vol. 6. Part 1. Berlin: Springer, 1925:156.
18. Bohle A, Ratschek M. The compensated and the decompensated form of benign nephrosclerosis. Pathol Pract Res 1982; 174:357–367.
19. Rossini M, Fogo AB. Interpreting segmental glomerular sclerosis. Curr Diag Pathol 2004; 10:1–10.
20. Caetano ER, Zatz R, Saldanha LB, Praxedes JN. Hypertensive nephrosclerosis as a relevant cause of chronic renal failure. Hypertension 2001; 38:171–176.
21. Toto RB. Hypertensive nephrosclerosis in African Americans. Kidney Int 2003; 64:2331–2341.
22. Marcantoni C, Ma L-J, Federspiel C, Fogo AB. Hypertensive nephrosclerosis in African-Americans vs Caucasians. Kidney Int 2002; 62:172–180.
23. Pemeger TV, Whelton PK, Klag MJ, Rossiter KD. Diagnosis of hypertensive end stage renal disease: effect of patients' race. Am J Epidemiol 1995; 141:10–15.
24. Pickering TG. Hypertension in blacks. Curr Opin Nephrol Hypertens 1994; 3:207–212.
25. Walker AJ, Bassett DR Jr, Duey WJ, Howley ET, Bond V, Torok DJ, Mancuso P. Cardiovascular and plasma catecholamine responses to exercise in blacks and whites. Hypertension 1992; 20:542–548.
26. Treiber FA, Musante L, Braden D, Arensman F, Strong WB, Levy M, Leverett S. Racial differences in hemodynamic responses to the cold face stimulus in children and adults. Psychosom Med 1990; 52:256–296.
27. Luke RG. Hypertensive nephrosclerosis: pathogenesis and prevalence. Nephrol Dial Transplant 1999; 14:2271–2278.
28. Freedman BL, Iskandar SS, Appel RG. The link between hypertension and nephrosclerosis. Am J Kidney Dis 1995; 25:207–221.
29. Dustan HP. Does keloid pathogenesis hold the key to understanding black/white differences in hypertension severity? Hypertension 1995; 26:858–862.
30. Muirhead EE, Pitcock JA. Histopathology of severe vascular damage in blacks. Clin Cardiol 1989; 12:58–65.
31. Gold CH, Isaacson C, Levin J. The pathological basis of end-stage renal disease in blacks. S Afr Med J 1982; 61:263–265.
32. Ojogwu LI. The pathological basis of endstage renal disease in Nigerians: experience from Benin City. West Afr J Med 1990; 9:193–196.
33. Adelekun TA, Akinsola A. Hypertension induced chronic renal failure: clinical features, management and prognosis. West Afr J Med 1998; 17:104–108.

34. Isaacson C, Milne FJ, van Niekerk I, Kenyon MR, Mzamane DV. The renal histopathology of essential malignant hypertension in black South Africans. S Afr Med J 1991; 80:173–176.

35. Kadiri S, Thomas JO. Focal segmental glomerulosclerosis in malignant hypertension. S Afr Med J 2002; 92:303–305.

36. Kappel B, Olsen S. Cortical interstitial tissue and sclerosed glomeruli in the normal human kidney, related to age and sex. A quantitative study. Virchows Arch (Pathol Anat) 1980; 387:271–277.

37. Smith SM, Hoy WE, Cobb L. Low incidence of glomerulosclerosis in normal kidneys. Arch Pathol Lab Med 1989; 113:1253–1256.

38. Tracy RE, Berenson GS, Cueto-Garcia L, Wattigney WA, Barrett TJ. Nephrosclerosis and aortic atherosclerosis from age 6 to 70 years in the United States and Mexico. Virchows Arch A Pathol Anat Histopathol 1992; 420:479–488.

39. Tracy RE, Guileyardo JM. Renovasculopathies of hypertension in Hispanic residents of Dallas, Texas. Arch Med Res 1999; 30:40–48.

40. Tracy RE, Rios-Dalenz JL. Rarity of hypertensive stigmata in aging renocortical arteries of Bolivians. Virchows Arch 1994; 424:307–314.

41. Tamura T. Histologic features of renal biopsies from patients with essential hypertension and from the aged. Japanese Circulation J 1966; 30:829–862.

42. Katafuchi R, Takebayashi S. Morphometrical and functional correlations in benign nephrosclerosis. Clin Nephrol 1987; 28:238–243.

43. Tracy RE. Renovasculopathies of hypertension and the rise of blood pressure with age in blacks and whites. Semin Nephrol 1996; 16:126–133.

44. Brenner EM, Chertow GM. Congenital oligonephropathy and the etiology of adult hypertension and progressive renal injury. Am J Kidney Dis 1994; 23: 171–175.

45. Lackland DT, Bendall HE, Osmond C, Egan BM, Barker DJ. Low birth weights contribute to high rates of early-onset chronic renal failure in the Southeastern United States. Arch Intern Med 2000; 160:1472–1476.

46. Keller G, Zimmer G, Mall G, Ritz E, Amann K. Nephron number in patients with primary hypertension. N Engl J Med 2003; 348:101–108.

47. Pesce C, Schmidt K, Fogo A, Okoye MI, Kim R, Striker LJ, Striker GE. Glomerular size and the incidence of renal disease in African Americans and Caucasians. J Nephrol 1994; 7:355–358.

48. Abdi R, Slakey D, Kittur D, Racusen LC. Heterogeneity of glomerular size in normal donor kidneys: impact of race. Am J Kidney Dis 1998; 32:43–46.

49. Abdi R, Slakey D, Kittur D, Burdick J, Racusen L. Baseline glomerular size as a predictor of function in human renal transplantation. Transplantation 1998; 66:329–333.

50. Li M, Nicholls KM, Becker GJ. Risk factors for late renal allograft dysfunction: effects of baseline glomerular size. J Nepbrol 2002; 15:620–625.

51. Spencer J, Wang Z, Hoy W. Low birth weight and reduced renal volume in Aboriginal children. Am J Kidney Dis 2001; 37:915–920.

52. Hughson M, Farris AB III, Douglas-Denton R, Hoy WE, Bertram JF. Glomerular number and size in autopsy kidneys: the relationship to birth weight. Kidney Int 2003; 63:2113–2122.

53. Hoy WE, Douglas-Denton RN, Hughson MD, Cass A, Johnson K, Bertram JF. A stereological study of glomerular number and volume: preliminary findings in a multiracial study of kidneys at autopsy. Kidney Int Suppl 2003; 83:S31–S37.

54. Young RJ, Hoy WE, Kincaid-Smith P, Seymour AE, Bertram JF. Glomerular size and glomerulosclerosis in Australian aborigines. Am J Kidney Dis 2000; 36:481–489.

55. Teio KK. Angiotensin converting enzyme genotypes and disease. Br Med J 1995; 311:76–77.

56. Ferguson R, Grim CE, Opgenorth TJ. A familial risk of chronic renal failure among blacks on dialysis? J Clin Epidemiol 1988; 41:1189–1196.

57. Hunley TE, Julian BA, Phillips JA III, Summar ML, Yoshida H, Horn RG, Brown NJ, Fogo A, Ichikawa I, Kon V. Angiotensin converting enzyme gene polymorphism: potential silencer motif and impact on progression in IgA nephropathy. Kidney Int 1996; 49:571–577.

58. Rutledge DR, Kubilis P, Browe CS, Ross EA. Polymorphism of the angiotensin I converting enzyme gene in essential hypertensive patients. Biochem Mol Biol Int 1995; 35:661–668.

59. Fernandez-Llama P, Poch E, Oriola J, Botey A, Coll E, Darnell A, Rivera F, Revert L. Angiotensin converting enzyme gene I/D polymorphism in essential hypertension and nephroangiosclerosis. Kidney Int 1998; 53:1743–1747.

60. Fogo A, Yoshida Y, Yared A, Ichikawa I. Importance of angiogenic action of angiotensin II in the glomerular growth of maturing kidneys. Kidney Int 1990; 38:1068–1074.

61. Niimura F, Labosky PA, Kakuchi J, Okubo S, Yoshida H, Oikawa T, Ichiki T, Naftilan AJ, Fogo A, Inagami T, Hogan BL, Ichikawa I. Gene targeting in mice reveals a requirement for angiotensin in the development and maintenance of kidney morphology and growth factor regulation. J Clin Invest 1995; 96: 2947–2954.

62. Krege JH, Kim HS, Moyer JS, Jennette JC, Peng L, Hiller SK, Smithies O. Angiotensin-converting enzyme gene mutations, blood pressures, and cardiovascular homeostasis. Hypertension 1997; 29:150–157.

63. Ma LJ, Nakamura S, Whitsirt JS, Marcantoni C, Davidson JM, Fogo AB. Regression of sclerosis in aging by an angiotensin inhibition-induced decrease in PAI-1. Kidney Int 2000; 58:2425–2436.

64. Weir MR, Chrysant SG, McCarron DA, Canossa-Terris M, Cohen JD, Gunter PA, Lewin AJ, Mennella RF, Kirkegaard LW, Hamilton JH, Weinberger MH, Weder AB. Influence of race and dietary salt on the antihypertensive efficacy of an angiotensin converting enzyme inhibitor or a calcium channel antagonist in salt-sensitive hypertensives. Hypertension 1998; 31:1088–1096.

65. Hall JE. Mechanisms of abnormal renal sodium handling in obesity-hypertension. Am J Hypertens 1997; 10:S49–S55.

66. Aviv A, Hollenberg NK, Weder AB. Sodium glomerulopathy: tubuloglomerular feedback and renal injury in African Americans. Kidney Int 2004; 65: 361–368.

67. Aviv A, Hollenberg NK, Weder A. Urinary potassium excretion sodium sensitivity in blacks. Hypertension 2004; 43:707–713.

68. Johnson RJ, Herrera-Acosta J, Schreiner GF, Rodriguez-Iturbe B. Subtle acquired renal injury as a mechanism of salt-sensitive hypertension. N Engl J Med 2002; 346:913–923.
69. Johnson RJ, Rideout BA. Uric acid and diet—insights into the epidemic of cardiovascular disease. N Engl J Med 2004; 350:1071–1073.
70. Feig DI, Nakagawa T, Karumanchi SA, Oliver WJ, Kang DH, Finch J, Johnson RJ. Hypothesis: uric acid, nephron number, and the pathogenesis of essential hypertension. Kidney Int 2004; 66:281–287.
71. Border WA, Noble NA. Transforming growth factor beta in tissue fibrosis. N Engl J Med 1994; 331:1286–1292.
72. August P, Suthanthiran M. Transforming growth factor beta and progression of renal disease. Kidney Int 2003; 64(suppl 87):S99–S104.
73. Ergul S, Parish DC, Puett D, Ergul A. Racial differences in plasma endothelin-1 concentrations in individuals with essential hypertension. Hypertension 1996; 28:652–655.
74. Kincaid-Smith P. Hypothesis: obesity and the insulin resistance syndrome play a major role in end-stage renal failure attributed to hypertension and labelled hypertensive nephrosclerosis. J Hypertens 2004; 22:1051–1055.

13

Kidney Disease in Ethnic Minority Populations of the United Kingdom

John Feehally
The John Walls Renal Unit, Leicester General Hospital, Leicester, U.K.

Liz Lightstone
*Renal Section, Division of Medicine,
Imperial College London, Hammersmith Hospital, London, U.K.*

INTRODUCTION

In this chapter, we discuss kidney disease in the ethnic minority populations of the United Kingdom (UK). The UK is an increasingly multicultural society, with growing numbers of migrant people with differing disease susceptibilities to those of the native North European Caucasian population. There are two major migrant populations. The first is African Caribbean, a migration predominantly from former British colonies in the West Indies, which started in the early 1950s and continued steadily thereafter. The second is a South Asian population, either migrant directly from India, Pakistan, and Bangladesh, or reaching the UK via sub-Saharan Africa; these people having originally migrated from the Indian subcontinent to Africa predominantly in the first half of the 20th century. The South Asian migration to the UK started in the 1960s with a very rapid surge in the early 1970s, when political changes in sub-Saharan Africa resulted in an urgent need to relocate. The South Asian population has markedly varied cultural and religious backgrounds, including substantial populations of Gujarati-speaking Hindus, Punjabi-speaking Sikhs, Urdu-speaking Muslims, and a number of other smaller groups. From the

1990s onwards, a wider range of migrant populations have also begun to move to the UK, particularly from Africa, including some asylum seekers.

Disease variations in the South Asian population include marked increases in susceptibility to type 2 diabetes, coronary heart disease, and kidney disease (1,2). In African Caribbeans, there is an additional susceptibility to hypertension and the subsequent end organ damage.

It is common to emphasize the increased susceptibility to kidney disease in these and other ethnic minority populations, but perhaps it should instead be considered that it is the White European population, which is uniquely at low risk of kidney disease, whether for genetic reasons, or because the environmental changes of urbanization have been imposed so much more slowly.

The increased prevalence of chronic kidney disease (CKD) in minority populations presents a major economic challenge for the delivery of health care in the UK for those in whom end-stage renal disease (ESRD) is established or inevitable. Opportunities must therefore be grasped to detect kidney disease earlier in these populations and intervene to delay or prevent ESRD. Finally, the rapid migration events of the last half century have created a "human laboratory," which offers exciting opportunities to investigate the pathogenesis of this increased susceptibility to kidney disease.

EPIDEMIOLOGY

A high incidence of ESRD has been identified in South Asians and African Caribbeans in the UK compared to Whites of European origin, comparable to the rates seen in minority populations in other developed countries, including African Americans, Native Americans, Australian Aboriginals, and Maoris and Pacific Islanders in New Zealand. How these rates compare to those for similar populations in developing countries remains uncertain since, in the absence of comprehensive nephrology care, there are few robust data on the prevalence of CKD and ESRD in those regions (3).

Several studies have shown 3–5-fold higher rates of ESRD among South Asians and Blacks in the UK. We showed a similar incidence of ESRD [as judged by acceptance onto a renal replacement therapy (RRT) program] between 1982 and 1988 in two very distinct South Asian populations in the UK: 115 per million population per year (pmp/yr) for a predominantly Punjabi population served by the Hammersmith Hospital in West London, and 123 pmp/yr for a Gujarati population in Leicester, four-fold higher than the incidence in the White populations in those units (2). A similar high prevalence of ESRD was reported among South Asians and Blacks in Birmingham, UK (4). Data from Coventry, another city with a large ethnic population, identified an even higher take on rate in 1992–1995. Importantly, there was an exponential rise in rates of ESRD with age and a widening differential between Whites and ethnic minorities, four-fold higher

Table 1 Relative Risk (RR) for End-Stage Renal Disease in Asian & Black Populations Compared with Whites. UK Data Are Shown as Well as Data from the United States, Canada, and Australia

	Indo Asians	Blacks	Indigenous population
Lightstone et al., 1995 (2)	2.86–5.34	—	—
Ball et al., 2001 (6)	3.8	2.81	—
Roderick et al., 1994 (7)			
Age 16–54 years	3.1	3.0	
Age 55–64 years	6.0	5.5	
Age >65 years	8	7.8	
Roderick et al., 1996 (8)			—
Age 16–54 years	3.6–3.8[a]	3.6–2.9	
Age 55–64 years	5.1–8.4	3.6–6.5	
Age >65 years	5.1–8.9	4.8–10.1	
Cass et al., 2001 (9)	—	—	1.39–31.05[b]
Dyck et al. (10,11)	—	—	2.56 (non-DM ESRD) 16.2 (DM ESRD)
USRDS 2004 http:// www.usrds.org/atlas.htm	(SE Asians) 1.34	3.83	Hispanic 1.88 Native American 2.0

[a]RR for males and females, respectively.
[b]Regional RR for Indigenous people versus total adult Australian population.

in those aged 30 to 39 years, but 10-fold higher in those aged 60 to 69 years (5). Table 1 summarizes a number of studies in the UK, demonstrating the relative risk of ESRD among Asian and Black populations compared with Whites. Comparative data from the United States, Canada, and Australia are also shown.

Many studies have shown increased prevalence of diabetes and hypertension in the South Asian (1,12) and Black populations (13,14), and also evidence that diabetic nephropathy and hypertensive nephropathy are more common causes of ESRD (2,6,14–17). Nevertheless, when patients have been evaluated by renal biopsy, it is more common to find glomerular disease, complicated by hypertension, rather than primary hypertension as the cause of ESRD (17). Focal segmental glomerulosclerosis and reflux nephropathy are also more common in both South Asians and Blacks compared to Whites, whilst adult polycystic kidney disease is rare. Our own data also showed an excess among South Asians of ESRD of unknown cause, associated with bland urine sediment and small smooth kidneys on renal imaging. This was particularly common among women, accounting for 50% of the Asian women compared with only 10% of White women(2). It has been suggested this may be a late presentation of interstitial nephritis, possibly due to tuberculosis (18,19).

More recently higher rates of interstitial nephritis have been reported in South Asians compared to Whites (20) although a possible etiological role for tuberculosis has not been established. However, the same authors present anecdotal data, suggesting that treatment with corticosteroids (combined with isoniazid prophylaxis) may improve renal function in those with biopsy-proven idiopathic interstitial nephritis (20). ESRD is also much more common in South Asian children than in Whites, although a high proportion of this excess is due to genetic causes and congenital malformations, possibly associated with the high rates of consanguinity, especially amongst Pakistani Asians (21).

Renal diseases, some of which may not progress to ESRD, are also more common among UK ethnic populations. Lupus nephritis is more common not only in Blacks (as is seen in North America) but also among South Asians (22,23). High rates of minimal change nephrotic syndrome have also been reported in Asian children (24,25).

While this increase in ESRD may represent a true increase in severe renal disease, it is possible that the differing natural history of other comorbidities may influence the size of the population, which requires RRT. For example, a longitudinal study of African Caribbeans and Europeans with type 2 diabetes suggests that the former group is relatively protected from heart disease, which might increase survival to ESRD, even if there were no difference in the rate of diabetic nephropathy per se (26). However, in the South Asian population, there is still an increase in ESRD even though cardiovascular disease is more common in those with type 2 diabetes (1,27,28). Another possibility is that the renal disease is no more common, but there is an increased susceptibility to progression of renal disease to ESRD. In the UK, the limited available data are conflicting on this point: a small retrospective study from Leicester reports no difference in rate of progression to ESRD of diabetic nephropathy in South Asians compared to Whites: median time to ESRD from first referral to a nephrology clinic (when mean serum creatinine was 270 µmol/L) was 20 months in both groups (29). However, a retrospective analysis from North London suggests that there was more rapid progression of diabetic nephropathy in South Asians: median time for doubling of serum creatinine from identification of impaired kidney function (mean serum creatinine > 170 µmol/L) was 30 months in South Asians and 70 months in Whites and African Caribbeans (30).

While it is usually straightforward to establish the incidence of ESRD by ascertaining incident patients starting RRT, it has proven far harder to establish the incidence and prevalence of CKD in ethnic communities. There have been several UK community studies, which have looked at the prevalence of renal impairment defined by serum creatinine (31,32) and have identified similar rates of CKD to those reported in the United States' National Health and Nutrition Examination Survey (NHANES) III study (33). However, none of these studies has so far focused on UK regions with large ethnic populations. A study now being undertaken in a primary care setting in West London will for the first time identify the prevalence of CKD (as judged by reduced estimated GFR and albuminuria) in a predominantly South Asian community. Preliminary data suggest no difference in the prevalence of stage 3 CKD of all causes in South Asians compared to Whites in a district where the incidence of ESRD is known to be four times higher, implying more rapid progression towards ESRD (34). Importantly, the prevalence of 4% of the population studied having an estimated GFR of $<60\,\mathrm{mL/min/1.73\,m^2}$ is very similar to that in African Americans and Whites in the NHANES III survey in the United States (35). As well as establishing the prevalence and causes of CKD in this community, it will also give the opportunity to see if appropriate preventative treatments are being implemented in this population known to have high rates of type 2 diabetes and hypertension.

PATHOGENESIS

Three broad influences may contribute to the increased susceptibility to CKD in ethnic minority populations. They are genetic susceptibility, susceptibility provoked by environmental factors, and susceptibility induced by the previous effects of fetal environment (12). It is improbable that any of these three factors is exclusive, more likely they interact with variable contributions. The particular migration patterns of the UK population afford a special opportunity to investigate the relative contributions of genetic and environmental influences on susceptibility to renal disease.

Genetics

There is substantial indirect evidence to support a genetic basis for susceptibility. However, it is important to emphasize that no specific gene distribution has yet been associated with risk of ESRD in these populations, although plausible candidate genes can be proposed from current understanding of both susceptibility to renal disease and risk of progression to ESRD. Indirect evidence strongly suggests a genetic susceptibility to progressive renal disease regardless of etiological factors. This is based on the broad susceptibility to ESRD in these populations whether due to diabetic nephropathy, hypertensive nephrosclerosis, or a range of other parenchymal renal diseases. There is also an increased risk of renal disease among the first-degree relatives of ethnic minority populations with ESRD. A number of substantial collections of DNA from probands with renal disease in ethnic minority populations are being established around the world with much potential for the definition of the genes responsible, particularly given newer technical approaches to genome-wide scanning. Even though epidemiological data suggest a broad increase in susceptibility to ESRD in South Asians in the UK, the enormous cultural, religious, and social variety in this population must be recognized. DNA collections must be of sufficient size and mix to allow the opportunity to distinguish any effects restricted to particular racial and ethnic groups. A study in Pakistan indicates that ethnic sub-group influences prevalence of proteinuria, but no such studies has yet been undertaken in the UK (36).

Many racial groups have increased susceptibility to renal disease, and this has particularly been discussed in the context of type II diabetes, as populations undergo rapid urbanization. One favored hypothesis is that these populations exhibit a "thrifty genotype" (37), which has become dominant through natural selection since it confers the capacity efficiently to lay down fat and carbohydrate stores in response to occasional plenty among prolonged periods of famine, and was therefore an ideal genotype for survival among hunter gatherers. When confronted with sustained plenty, such a genotype, unless environmentally rigorously controlled, creates susceptibility to the metabolic syndrome (obesity, insulin resistance, type II diabetes, and dyslipidemia), vascular disease, and with it an increased risk of kidney disease. Another view is a "thrifty phenotype," in which intra-uterine and early life environment creates an acquired metabolic state adapted for relative starvation but with increased susceptibility to the metabolic syndrome and its consequences when social and environmental circumstances allow increased access to food creating "catch up" in childhood and adult life (12). At present, there is insufficient information to provide insight into the contribution of these two notions to the susceptibility to renal disease in ethnic populations in the UK.

Other populations around the world may provide comparative information relevant to the migrant populations in the UK. The Pima Indians, for example, share with South Asians susceptibility to ESRD due to diabetic nephropathy, but there is the important difference that virtually all ESRD in the Pima population is due to diabetic nephropathy (38), whereas the susceptibility in South Asians is broader. The Zuni Indians, although less well studied, may provide a more appropriate comparison since they have a risk of ESRD equivalent to the Pima Indians yet diabetic nephropathy, glomerulonephritis, and other intrinsic renal diseases all contribute to this risk (39). South Asians, like Zuni Indians, therefore appear to have a "double jeopardy," in which susceptibility to type 2 diabetes is combined with an increased susceptibility to progressive renal disease of all etiologies, provoking a marked excess of ESRD. Comprehensive and accurate phenotyping will be crucial to the successful analysis of genetic information arising from future DNA collections, if they are to yield information relevant to both-susceptibility to kidney disease, and also susceptibility to progression of kidney disease once it is established.

Fetal Environment

The impact of the fetal environment on subsequent adult disease patterns is closely associated with the hypothesis of Barker and his colleagues. They propose that in utero "programming" contributes to adult disease (40). The basis of their hypothesis is epidemiological evidence in the UK and elsewhere that low birth weight, due to intra-uterine growth retardation rather than pre-maturity, is associated with increased adult risk of type II diabetes, insulin resistance, coronary heart disease, and hypertension; although the association with hypertension has recently been challenged (41). It is suggested that deprivation of specific nutrients may create this intra-uterine programming although it is of course difficult to distinguish between in utero effects and those of subsequent adverse environmental factors, which in early life may be closely associated with the same circumstances that provoke maternal under-nutrition. It was additionally proposed that low birth weight might reduce nephron number and increase susceptibilities to systemic hypertension (42), and there is evidence in Caucasians of a relationship between primary hypertension and nephron number (43). There is considerable indirect evidence that in utero programming may contribute to adult kidney disease. It is known that the kidney is particularly susceptible to fetal malnutrition because 60% of nephrons are formed in the third trimester. There is also some evidence from ultrasound studies that kidney size is disproportionately reduced in babies who are small for gestational age (44) although there are no data in this study on ethnicity. Recent autopsy studies also confirm an association between low birth weight and reduced nephron number (45). Furthermore, there is an association between low birth weight and increased glomerular size, a factor known in a variety of experimental studies to increase the risk of glomerulosclerosis (45). These autopsy studies however did not confirm any additional impact of ethnicity modifying the relationship between glomerular characteristics and birth weight, suggesting that it is low birth weight per se which carries that increased susceptibility (45). In the very high-risk Australian Aboriginal population studied by Hoy (46) and her colleagues, there is additional evidence that low birth weight is associated with increased risk of adult proteinuria. In the UK, it is known that birth weights are lower in South Asians compared to White urban populations, although social and environmental influences on this difference have not been excluded. Information on the birth weights of South Asians who now are developing ESRD in the UK would be informative, but the majority of these individuals were born outside the UK and no data are available.

OUTCOME OF RENAL REPLACEMENT THERAPY

While the long-term goal in these high-risk people is the prevention or delay of ESRD, the immediate public health issue is that those who develop

ESRD, regardless of ethnicity or other factors, should receive RRT of equivalent efficacy with equity of access. A number of studies in the UK have reviewed clinical outcomes with these concerns in mind. There are few data in African Caribbeans, but more information is available from studies of South Asians in a number of UK centers including Leicester, Coventry, Bradford, and London; and these are now discussed.

Acceptance rate for RRT does not necessarily equate to the meeting of demand if there is inequity of access. Access will be highly variable and dependent upon social and economic circumstances of the migrant population. A study of referral patterns of South Asians with CKD in Bradford, UK, in the late 1990s showed no difference in severity of renal impairment at referral or risk of presentation as a uremic emergency when a South Asian population was compared to the White population treated in the same unit (R. Jeffrey, unpublished observations). These data provide some assurance, at least in that unit, that there was equity of access, and experience in a well-established South Asian community in Leicester is similar (J. Feehally, unpublished observations). However, this is not confirmed in a study from Manchester in which 31% of South Asians with ESRD had presented late to specialist renal services compared to only 19% of Whites in the same area (47). In the Manchester study, the South Asian population had significantly more socioeconomic disadvantage than the White population, and it is likely that in a number of other poorer and rapidly increasing migrant populations in the UK (for example in East London), there may also be disadvantage due to late referral.

Dialysis

We have evaluated the outcome of RRT in South Asians compared to Whites in a cohort starting RRT in Leicester between 1982 and 1998 (J. Feehally, unpublished observations). The catchment area of the Leicester renal unit includes a large city center as well as extensive suburban and rural areas. The majority of South Asians live within the city, and therefore "postcode matching" was used to define the study populations. Five-year survival was superior in the South Asian population, which was significantly younger because of the age distribution of the population, but there was no difference in age-adjusted all-cause mortality between South Asian and White populations. In both populations age, diabetes, and pre-existing vascular disease were the dominant factors predictive of mortality. Recent data from West London (patients starting RRT between 1996 and 2001) also indicate that lower mortality in a significantly younger South Asian cohort on HD (82% 5-year survival) compared to Whites (60% 5-year survival) although age-adjusted survival data were not reported (48)

Early in the Leicester study (those who started RRT 1982–1991), it was striking that 84% of South Asians started peritoneal dialysis (PD) as their first treatment modality, compared to only 60% of Whites. Home hemodialysis was a very infrequent option in South Asians compared to Whites. These retrospective observations do not reflect defined clinical policies, but indicate the views of lead clinicians on the difficulties of training for home hemodialysis in those for whom English is a second language, the relative difficulty of establishing vascular access (particularly challenging in South Asian women in whom small diameter peripheral arteries and veins are typical) and the relative ease of training for PD. Later in the study period (those who started RRT between 1992 and 1998), changes in clinical approach resulted in a significant shift—70% of South Asians starting PD compared to 62% of Whites. By contrast, in the recent West London experience 86% of South Asians started HD as initial RRT compared to 91% of Whites (48), and in the north west of England initial choice of dialysis modality was not influenced by ethnicity (47).

In the Leicester study, ethnicity had no impact on complication-free technique survival on hemodialysis, nor on vascular access dysfunction or failure, nor on hospital admission rates. Although complication-free technique survival on CAPD did not differ overall between South Asians and Whites, it was significantly worse in South Asians who spoke no English in the earlier study period, with PD failure ascribed mainly to peritonitis. There were incremental improvements in dialysis-related care when increasing resources were made available to provide information about RRT for South Asians in their preferred language with multilingual written information, increasing numbers of staff with relevant language skills, and individualized training programs. Later in the period(1992–1998), the impact of these progressive service improvements meant that ethnicity no longer had any significant effect on complication-free technique survival, peritonitis or exit site infection, regardless of language skills. Nor were any significant differences in CAPD outcomes between South Asians and Whites reported in a study in Coventry (49).

Data on outcome of RRT in African Caribbeans in the UK are even more limited. However, the West London study does report 58% 5-year survival in African Caribbeans; no different to Whites (60%) and inferior to South Asians (82%) (48). Since the African Caribbeans, like the South Asians, were significantly younger than the White population, this implied inferior outcome although age-adjusted survival was not reported.

Transplantation

We have reviewed our experience of 500 consecutive cadaveric renal transplants performed between 1983 and 1996 under cyclosporine immunosuppression, of whom 80 recipients were South Asian (P. Butterworth, unpublished observations). One-, 5- and 10-year patient and graft survival did not differ between South Asians and Whites. Similar equivalence in transplant outcome has recently been reported in West London (50). However, to achieve equivalent HLA-DR matching in the Leicester experience, there was a three-fold increase in median waiting time for cadaveric transplantation in South Asians compared to Whites. A similar reduced chance of receiving a cadaveric transplant has been reported in Yorkshire, UK (51). The South Asian population who are never offered a kidney should not be forgotten in considering the implications of these data. Difficulties with HLA matching are compounded by ethnic variations in ABO groups, blood group B being especially common in South Asians. There will always be inequality of access to cadaveric kidneys for any minority population, which has different HLA patterns compared to the majority population, but in the UK the contribution of South Asians and Blacks to the cadaveric donor pool remains disproportionately small, despite extensive educational programs directed at the community to increase awareness of organ donation and its implications. These substantial inequities of access to cadaveric kidney transplantation require a special emphasis on the promotion of live donor transplant in this and other minority communities if equity is to be approached.

Quality of Care and Quality of Life

It is relatively straightforward to obtain numerical data on the outcome of RRT from clinical records and databases. It is much less straightforward to make a meaningful evaluation of the quality of care and quality of life (QoL) for patients with RRT. Disease-specific QoL evaluation tools are now available for renal disease and have been extensively evaluated. However, these are almost exclusively written in English, and developed and tested in White Caucasian populations. Data from Coventry, UK, indicate that, using such evaluation tools, South Asians report reduced QoL compared to Whites with all modalities of RRT (52). Such studies are limited by the use of evaluation tools which have not been developed in light of the cultural, religious and social differences in ethnic minority communities, nor have they been able to take account of the important differences which may emerge when questionnaire-based QoL assessment relies on the use of health professionals, interpreters, and family members for patients in whom languages skills preclude the use of the primary tool. Such approaches continue to be necessary since a substantial proportion of minority ethnic populations in the UK do not speak, read, or write English. Ethnicity-specific QoL evaluation tools for renal disease are not yet validated.

Treating ESRD is expensive if it is to be delivered to the standards expected by contemporary society. Treating renal failure properly in a multiethnic, multicultural setting will be even more expensive because of the support programs and additional staff training required to deliver it with excellence. While language issues will slowly become less important as a stable migrant population increasingly speaks English, this will be a gradual process. These factors must be taken into account now when planning health services.

PUBLIC HEALTH IMPLICATIONS

The high rate of ESRD among ethnic communities in the UK will have a disproportionate impact on the need for RRT provision for a number of reasons, including the age distribution of ethnic minority populations, the exaggerated increase in the incidence of ESRD with age in ethnic populations, and the low rate of transplantation in ethnic minorities.

The age structure of all ethnic populations in the UK is younger than that of Whites. ESRD from all causes rises with age and this appears to be disproportionately so among ethnic communities (5,53). Therefore, unless preventative strategies are implemented effectively, there will be an epidemic of ESRD as the South Asian and African-Caribbean communities age. The impact of RRT for the ageing ethnic population will be particularly felt in urban areas with large ethnic populations. In 1997, Raleigh predicted that the number of older people in ethnic minorities in the UK would triple between 1991 and 2011 and that these changes in age structure would lead to a 45% increase in the incidence of ESRD in South Asian and African-Caribbean patients, so that they would account for 40–50% of all new recipients of RRT in London by 2001 (54). These predictions are probably an underestimate—for instance, at Hammersmith Hospital in 2001, 56% of prevalent patients were either South Asian or African Caribbean (Lightstone, personal communication).

In 1996, Roderick reported that although South Asians and African Caribbeans accounted for only 3% and 1.9%, respectively, of the total population in the 1991 English census, they accounted for 7.7% and 4.7% of the English dialysis population (8). From 1991 to 2001, the proportion of minority ethnic groups in England rose by 50% with particular increases in South Asians, African-Caribbean, and Black African people (53,55). These may appear small numbers in relation to the overall UK ESRD program. However, in the context of urban areas with large ethnic communities, the local impacts are much greater in certain boroughs and cities; for instance, Indians comprise only 2% of the population of England and Wales but account for 26% of the population of Leicester. Bangladeshis, one of the most deprived communities in England and Wales, account for 0.5% of the total population but 33% of one London borough. Blacks of African or Caribbean origin account for more than 10% of the population of eight London boroughs. As already mentioned, the double whammy of high take on rates and low transplantation rates mean that the prevalence of ethnic patients on local ESRD programs will continue to be disproportionate unless both of these issues are tackled (56). Recent data from London suggest that the excess of ESRD in ethnic communities continues unabated with incidence for Whites, Asians, and Blacks being 58, 221, and 163 pmp/yr, respectively (6). Perhaps the most striking influence on the proportion of patients on RRT is seen in the Northern city of Bradford, which has the largest Pakistani (predominantly Muslim) population in the country and where 72% of the patients on RRT in 2003 were of Asian origin (57). It is also clear that there is an additive effect of ethnicity and social deprivation, increasing the rate of ESRD still further.

What are the predictions for the next 10 years? Available evidence indicates no plateau in the prevalence of RRT in the U.K. As Roderick et al. (7,8,53) have highlighted for a number of years, the growing ethnic communities will continue to have a major impact on take on rates for RRT. Roderick's most recent model predicts a substantial growth in the RRT population to 2010 to a prevalence approaching 1000 pmp, with a steady state not being reached for at least 25 years (58). For all the reasons discussed, the rates among ethnic communities will rise even more unless effective prevention strategies are implemented; or unless the competing influence of premature death from cardiovascular disease in the South Asian community prevents patients surviving to ESRD. It needs to be recognized, however, that advances in the prevention of cardiovascular disease morbidity and mortality may compound the future burden of ESRD in this population.

THE CHALLENGE OF EARLY DETECTION AND PREVENTION OF RENAL DISEASE

The impact of ESRD in ethnic communities can only be minimized if there is a new focus on the prevention and early detection of CKD, with interventions to delay progression (59). This will include primary prevention of diseases which cause ESRD, for example diabetes; secondary prevention, for example of the renal complications of hypertension or diabetes; and effective management of established CKD.

Primary Prevention

There is increasing evidence that effective interventions are now available. A global health priority is to reduce the incidence and prevalence of type 2 diabetes and its complications (60). The combination of modest lifestyle changes (weight loss and exercise) and metformin has been shown to reduce the incidence of new onset type 2 diabetes in 58% of patients with impaired glucose tolerance, an effect independent of ethnicity (61). Since the prevalence of type 2 diabetes among South Asians is 5 to 10 times higher than in Whites, it is reasonable to predict that targeting such populations should have a rapid and high impact in reducing new onset type 2 diabetes (61). These studies are limited by their relatively short-term follow-up and the intensive nature of the care required to deliver the interventions successfully. Future emphasis will have to be on developing interventions which can be effectively applied in primary care and the community. The government has an important role in supporting public health initiatives which, for example, are aimed at reducing obesity and smoking, and increasing exercise. A recent study has shown that treating patients with type 2 diabetes, hypertension, and no microalbuminuria with an ACE inhibitor significantly delayed the onset of microalbuminuria in comparison to groups treated with either a placebo or verapamil (62). The long-term data are awaited but the suggestion will be that this simple intervention may significantly reduce cardiovascular and renal risk in these patients. Ethnicity of the patients was not given but since the study was from Italian centers, it is reasonable to assume the majority, if not all, were White. However, there is no a priori reason to assume that these interventions would not be equally effective in similar patients from the Indian-Asian and African-Caribbean communities, but such a strategy needs to be specifically evaluated in these groups.

Secondary Prevention

There are now UK guidelines on the effective management of type 2 diabetes and of hypertension (63–66). These guidelines and standards draw on the substantial evidence that rigorous control of blood pressure, particularly using renin–angiotensin system blockade, can reduce diabetic renal disease (67). Are such interventions as effective in ethnic communities? It is certainly the case in African Americans, who are more susceptible to the renal adverse effects of hypertension (68), and in whom ACE inhibitors were shown to be safe and effective (69) despite the concern that hypertension in African Americans is salt sensitive, associated with low renin levels, and therefore may not be suitable for treatment by renin–angiotensin blockade. Although there is scant direct evidence among South Asians, there is no a priori reason to suspect that the interventions would not also be effective.

In most cases, these interventions will only start once renal damage is established (identified by microalbuminuria or overt proteinuria with or without impaired GFR). Here there is also substantial evidence that control of blood pressure combined with reduction in proteinuria delays progression of nephropathy, regardless of the underlying cause (70). The cornerstones of management are low blood pressure targets achieved primarily by the use of ACE inhibitors and/or angiotensin-receptor blockers (ARB). The AASK trial has shown that such interventions are effective in African Americans (71). In the absence of specific evidence in ethnic communities in the UK, it seems appropriate to assume that the same interventions will be at least of similar benefit. Whilst the implementation of these strategies should be evaluated prospectively, ideally within the setting of a randomized control trial, it would now seem unethical to not treat ethnic patients deemed to be of similar risk with inhibition of the renal-angiotensin system. The research questions should focus on whether standard regimens are adequate or require finessing according to ethnic differences in disease progression. As mentioned earlier, extrapolation from similar prevalence rates of CKD suggests that ethnic patients progress to ESRD more rapidly. Hence, the influence of interventions might be expected to be seen more rapidly.

Finally, although prevention of onset and progression of renal disease must be the prime target in all at risk communities, increasing the number of transplant donors from ethnic communities, both cadaveric and living donors, must also have high priority if those suitable are to be transplanted rather than remain on dialysis. Therefore, the interventions required at all stages of the pathway to renal failure are clear. Much less clear is how effectively to implement the interventions—how to identify those at risk, how to increase awareness among those at risk, and how to ensure that healthcare providers, especially in the community, are aware of the high-risk patients in their midst and can optimize delivery of preventative interventions, as well as make timely referral to renal services where required.

There is insufficient evidence that general population screening for renal disease is cost effective though recent studies such as those from the PREVEND cohort suggest that screening for albuminuria may provide an important target not only for identifying those at risk of CKD and CVD but also for treatment (72–74). It has been argued that in the developing world, the focus has to be on screening for albumunuria as at that stage of CKD interventions are affordable and cost effective—dialysis is simply not an option for most individuals in such communities (75). What is much less contentious is screening among those with conditions predisposing towards CKD and CVD, i.e., those with hypertension and/or diabetes. Recent health economic analysis of key trials using ARB in either established diabetic nephropathy or in diabetic patients with microalbumuria demonstrated the benefits seen in reduction of CKD progression predicted substantial cost savings using Markov-based Monte Carlo simulation (76,77). Therefore, screening patients with type 2 diabetes for albuminuria should be mandatory for all ethnic groups and indeed is enshrined in the relevant guidelines. Screening for CKD in patients from ethnic communities with these conditions is likely to be cost beneficial as they have high rates of diabetes and hypertension, high risk of CKD and CVD, and there is evidence of sub-optimal care in these high-risk groups (78). Preliminary data from the population survey in West London suggest that screening all those with known diabetes, or hypertension, or cardiovascular disease will identify the great majority of South Asians and Whites with CKD (L. Lightstone, unpublished).

However, raising awareness of the risk of renal disease among ethnic communities is not straightforward. How can such communities be effectively accessed? What are the religious, cultural, and social beliefs and norms that might hinder the application of effective interventions? Several studies have shown quite different use of healthcare services by different ethnic communities in the UK. For example, among South Asians, gender, religion, and literacy profoundly influence awareness and self-management of diabetes (79–81). The UK National Kidney Research Fund (NKRF) has developed a campaign to raise awareness of the risk and presentation of renal disease among UK ethnic communities, and to promote research within these communities aimed at improving knowledge on epidemiology of renal disease and delivery of the treatment of CKD. The NKRF "ABLE" Campaign (A Better Life through Education and Empowerment) launched in December 2001 set out a blueprint for tackling the key issues (82) (www.nkrf.org.uk), and is funding projects in South Asian and Black communities to evaluate understanding of CKD and barriers to optimal care, and to develop appropriate educational tools to increase awareness. The UK experience will undoubtedly benefit from the work done by the NKDEP and NKF KEEP programs in the United States, where high-risk members of ethnic communities (those with diabetes, hypertension and/or a family history of renal disease) are being targeted both directly and via education of their primary care physicians (for details see http://www.nkdep.nih.gov and http://www.kidney.org/keep/index.cfm).

As well as identifying CKD in order to delay and prevent ESRD, this will also give the opportunity to address risk reduction for cardiovascular disease (72,83). This is particularly important in UK South Asians who have very high rates of cardiovascular disease (73,84) as well as CKD. A practical advantage of emphasizing the links between CKD and cardiovascular disease is to promote an integrated approach to the management of cardiovascular risk by primary care physicians that includes CKD, rather than to emphasize CKD as a distinct problem requiring a separate organizational approach, which may not receive sufficient priority when primary care in the UK has limited resources. A pessimistic view would be that increasing survival by reducing cardiovascular events would increase future costs, as patients would survive to ESRD. However, a recent flurry of publications have highlighted that CVD and CKD go hand in hand—it is more likely that preventing CVD will simultaneously reduce the onset or progression of CKD and vice versa (e.g., Refs. 83, 85–87).

CONCLUSION

The increasingly multicultural population of the UK is now manifesting the major increase in the incidence of ESRD seen in all other developed countries with substantial ethnic minorities. The challenges this presents to the UK healthcare system are formidable if the immediate needs of those with ESRD are to be met, and also strategies to minimize the future rates of ESRD are to be effective. At the same time, the opportunities must be grasped to learn more from this population of the etiology and pathogenesis of the increased risk of ESRD.

REFERENCES

1. Feehally J, et al. Disease variations in Asians in Leicester. Q J Med 1993; 86:263–269.
2. Lightstone L, et al. High incidence of end-stage renal disease in Indo-Asians in the UK. Q J Med 1995; 88:191–195.
3. Sakhuja V, Sud K. End-stage renal disease in India and Pakistan: burden of disease and management issues. Kidney Int Suppl 2003; 83:S115–S118.
4. Clark TJ, Richards NT, Adu D, Michael J. Increased prevalence of dialysis-dependent renal failure in ethnic minorities in the west Midlands. Nephrol Dial Transplant 1993; 8:146–148.
5. Higgins RM, Edmunds ME, Dukes DC. End-stage renal failure in Indo-Asians. Q J Med 1995; 88:523–524.
6. Ball S, et al. Why is there so much end-stage renal failure of undetermined cause in UK Indo-Asians? Q J Med 2001; 94: 187–193.
7. Roderick PJ, et al. Population need for renal replacement therapy in Thames regions: ethnic dimension. BMJ 1994; 309:1111–1114.
8. Roderick PJ, Raleigh VS, Hallam L, Mallick NP. The need and demand for renal replacement therapy in ethnic minorities in England. J Epidemiol Community Health 1996; 50:334–339.
9. Cass A, Cunningham J, Wang Z, Hoy W. Regional variation in the incidence of end-stage renal disease in Indigenous Australians. Med J Aust 2001; 175:24–27.
10. Dyck RF, Tan L. Non-diabetic end-stage renal disease among Saskatchewan aboriginal people. Clin Invest Med 1998; 21:33–38.
11. Dyck RF, Tan L. Rates and outcomes of diabetic end-stage renal disease among registered native people in Saskatchewan. Can Med Assoc J 1994; 150: 203–208.
12. Buck K, Feehally J. Diabetes and renal failure in Indo-Asians in the UK—a paradigm for the study of disease susceptibility. Nephrol Dial Transplant 1997; 12:1555–1557.
13. Cruickshank JK, et al. Hypertension in four African-origin populations: current 'Rule of Halves', quality of blood pressure control and attributable risk of cardiovascular disease. J Hypertens 2001; 19:41–46.
14. Burden AC, McNally PG, Feehally J, Walls J. Increased incidence of end-stage renal failure secondary to diabetes mellitus in Asian ethnic groups in the United Kingdom. Diabet Med 1992; 9:641–645.
15. Riste L, Khan F, Cruickshank K. High prevalence of type 2 diabetes in all ethnic groups, including Europeans, in a British inner city: relative poverty, history, inactivity, or 21st century Europe? Diabetes Care 2001; 24:1377–1383.
16. Pazianas M, Eastwood JB, MacRae KD, Phillips ME. Racial origin and primary renal diagnosis in 771 patients with end-stage renal disease. Nephrol Dial Transplant 1991; 6:931–935.
17. Frassinetti Fernandes P, et al. Causes of end-stage renal failure in black patients starting renal replacement therapy. Am J Kidney Dis 2000; 36:301–309.
18. Morgan SH, Eastwood JB, Baker LR. Tuberculous interstitial nephritis—the tip of an iceberg? Tubercle 1990; 71:5–6.
19. Benn JJ, Scoble JE, Thomas AC, Eastwood JB. Cryptogenic tuberculosis as a preventable cause of end-stage renal failure. Am J Nephrol 1988; 8:306–308.

20. Ball S, et al. The diagnosis and racial origin of 394 patients undergoing renal biopsy: an association between Indian race and interstitial nephritis. Nephrol Dial Transplant 1997; 12:71–77.

21. Moghal NE, Milford DV, Hulton SA, Taylor CM. The prevalence and treatment of end-stage renal disease in an Asian child population. Nephrol Dial Transplant 1997; 12:2517–2520.

22. Samanta A, et al. High prevalence of systemic disease and mortality in Asian subjects with systemic lupus erythematosus. Ann Rheum Dis 1991; 50:490–492.

23. Samanta A, Roy S, Feehally J, Symmons DP. The prevalence of diagnosed systemic lupus erythematosus in whites and Indian Asian immigrants in Leicester city, UK. Br J Rheumatol 1992; 31:679–682.

24. McKinney PA, Feltbower RG, Brocklebank JT, Fitzpatrick MM. Time trends and ethnic patterns of childhood nephrotic syndrome in Yorkshire, UK. Pediatr Nephrol. 2001; 16(12):1040–1044.

25. Feehally J, Kendell NP, Swift PG, Walls J. High incidence of minimal change nephrotic syndrome in Asians. Arch Dis Child 1985; 60:1018–1020.

26. Chaturvedi N, et al. Differences in mortality and morbidity in African Caribbean and European people with non-insulin dependent diabetes mellitus: results of 20 year follow up of a London cohort of a multinational study. BMJ 1996; 313:848–852.

27. Mather HM, Chaturvedi N, Fuller JH. Mortality and morbidity from diabetes in South Asians and Europeans: 11-year follow-up of the Southall Diabetes Survey, London, UK. Diabet Med 1998; 15:53–59.

28. Mather HM, Chaturvedi N, Kehely AM. Comparison of prevalence and risk factors for microalbuminuria in South Asians and Europeans with type 2 diabetes mellitus. Diabet Med 1998; 15:672–627.

29. Earle KK, Porter KA, Ostberg J, Yudkin JS. Variation in the progression of diabetic nephropathy according to racial origin. Nephrol Dial Transplant 2001; 16:286–290.

30. Koppiker N, et al. Rate of decline in renal function in Indo-Asians and Whites with diabetic nephropathy. Diabet Med 1998; 15:60–65.

31. Feest TG, Mistry CD, Grimes DS, Mallick NP. Incidence of advanced chronic renal failure and the need for end stage renal replacement treatment. BMJ 1990; 301:897–900.

32. John R, Webb M, Young A, Stevens PE. Unreferred chronic kidney disease: a longitudinal study. Am J Kidney Dis 2004; 43:825–835.

33. Jones CA, et al. Serum creatinine levels in the US population: third National Health and Nutrition Examination Survey. Am J Kidney Dis 1998; 32:992–999.

34. Lightstone L, et al. Systematic screening of patients in primary care to compare the prevalence of chronic kidney disease (CKD) in UK Indian Asians (IA) and Northern Europeans (NE). The Renal Association, 2004. http://www.triangle3. org.uk/cgi-bin/absdb/absdb_view.cgi?AbstractID=RA4603.

35. Coresh J, et al. Prevalence of chronic kidney disease and decreased kidney function in the adult US population: Third National Health and Nutrition Examination Survey. Am J Kidney Dis 2003; 41:1–12.

36. Jafar TH, et al. Ethnic differences and determinants of proteinuria among South Asian subgroups in Pakistan. Kidney Int 2003; 64:1437–1444.

37. Neel JV, Weder AB, Julius S. Type II diabetes, essential hypertension, and obesity as "syndromes of impaired genetic homeostasis": the "thrifty genotype" hypothesis enters the 21st century. Perspect Biol Med 1998; 42:44–74.

38. Nelson RG, et al. Incidence of end-stage renal disease in type 2 (non-insulin-dependent) diabetes mellitus in Pima Indians. Diabetologia 1988; 31:730–736.

39. Shah VO, et al. Epidemic of diabetic and nondiabetic renal disease among the Zuni Indians: the Zuni Kidney Project. J Am Soc Nephrol 2003; 14:1320–1329.

40. Barker DJ, et al. Type 2 (non-insulin-dependent) diabetes mellitus, hypertension and hyperlipidaemia (syndrome X): relation to reduced fetal growth. Diabetologia 1993; 36:62–67.

41. Huxley R, Neil A, Collins R. Unravelling the fetal origins hypothesis: is there really an inverse association between birthweight and subsequent blood pressure? Lancet 2002; 360:659–665.

42. Mackenzie HS, Brenner BM. Fewer nephrons at birth: a missing link in the etiology of essential hypertension? Am J Kidney Dis 1995; 26:91–98.

43. Keller G, et al. Nephron number in patients with primary hypertension. N Engl J Med 2003; 348:101–108.

44. Konje JC, et al. Human fetal kidney morphometry during gestation and the relationship between weight, kidney morphometry and plasma active renin concentration at birth. Clin Sci (Lond) 1996; 91:169–175.

45. Hughson M, et al. Glomerular number and size in autopsy kidneys: the relationship to birth weight. Kidney Int 2003; 63:2113–2122.

46. Hoy W. Renal disease in Australian Aborigines. Nephrol Dial Transplant 2000; 15:1293–1297.

47. Trehan A, et al. End-stage renal disease in Indo-Asians in the North-West of England. Q J Med 2003; 96:499–504.

48. Prasad S, et al. Ethnicity and survival on dialysis in west London. Kidney Int 2004; 66:2416–2421.

49. Bakewell A, Higgins R, Edmunds M. Nutrition, adequacy of dialysis, and clinical outcome in Indo-Asian and White European patients on peritoneal dialysis. Q J Med 2002; 95:811–820.

50. Loucaidou M, et al. Outcome of renal transplantation in South Asian recipients is similar to that in non-Asians. Transplantation 2004; 78:1021–1024.

51. Jeffrey RF, et al. Indo-Asian experience of renal transplantation in Yorkshire: results of a 10-year survey. Transplantation 2002; 73:1652–1657.

52. Bakewell AB, Higgins RM, Edmunds ME. Does ethnicity influence perceived quality of life of patients on dialysis and following renal transplant? Nephrol Dial Transplant 2001; 16:1395–1401.

53. Roderick P, et al. Estimating demand for renal replacement therapy in Greater London: the impact of demographic trends in ethnic minority populations. Health Trends 1998; 30:46–50.

54. Raleigh VS. Diabetes and hypertension in Britain's ethnic minorities: implications for the future of renal services. BMJ 1997; 314:209–213.

55. ONS, Ethnicity data from 2001 census, in http://www.statistics.gov.uk/census2001/profiles/commentaries/ethnicity.asp, 2001.

56. Lightsone L. End-stage renal failure in Indo-Asian in the UK: a double whammy. Transplantation 2002; 73:1533–1534.

57. Ansell D, Feest T, Byrne C, Ahma A. UK Renal Registry, The Sixth Annual Report December 2003. U.R. Registry, ed. UK Renal Registry Reports. Bristol: UK Renal Registry, 2003; 43–62.
58. Roderick P, et al. Simulation model of renal replacement therapy: predicting future demand in England. Nephrol Dial Transplant 2004; 19:692–701.
59. Lightstone L. Preventing renal disease: the ethnic challenge in the United Kingdom. Kidney Int Suppl 2003; 83:S135–S138.
60. Ritz E, Rychlik I, Locatelli F, Halimi S. End-stage renal failure in type 2 diabetes: a medical catastrophe of worldwide dimensions. Am J Kidney Dis 1999; 34:795–808.
61. Molitch ME, Fujimoto W, Hamman RF, Knowler WC. The diabetes prevention program and its global implications. J Am Soc Nephrol 2003; 14:S103–S107.
62. Ruggenenti P, et al. Preventing microalbuminuria in type 2 diabetes. N Engl J Med 2004; 351:1941–1951; Epub 2004 Oct 31.
63. Williams B, et al. Guidelines for management of hypertension: report of the fourth working party of the British Hypertension Society, 2004-BHS IV. J Hum Hypertens 2004; 18:139–185.
64. Clinical Care of Adults with Diabetes—Standards, in National Service Framework for Diabetes. London: Department of Health, 2001.
65. Preventing nephropathy in patients with type 2 diabetes. Manag Care Interface 2002; 15:72–75.
66. (NICE), N.I.f.C.E. Management of type 2 diabetes—renal disease, prevention and early management. In: NHS, ed. Management of Type 2 Diabetes, National Institute for Clinical Excellence, ISBN: 1-84257-147-8 2002 (www.nice.org.uk) 2002.
67. Brenner BM, Zagrobelny J. Clinical renoprotection trials involving angiotensin II-receptor antagonists and angiotensin-converting-enzyme inhibitors. Kidney Int Suppl 2003; 83:S77–S85.
68. Hebert LA, et al. Effects of blood pressure control on progressive renal disease in blacks and whites. Modification of Diet in Renal Disease Study Group. Hypertension 1997; 30:428–435.
69. Cohn JN, et al. Clinical experience with perindopril in African-American hypertensive patients: a large United States community trial. Am J Hypertens 2004; 17:134–138.
70. Ruggenenti P, Schieppati A, Remuzzi G. Progression, remission, regression of chronic renal diseases. Lancet 2001; 357:1601–1608.
71. Wright JT Jr, et al. Effect of blood pressure lowering and antihypertensive drug class on progression of hypertensive kidney disease: results from the AASK trial. JAMA 2002; 288:2421–2431.
72. Verhave JC, et al. An elevated urinary albumin excretion predicts de novo development of renal function impairment in the general population. Kidney Int Suppl 2004; 92:S18–S21.
73. de Zeeuw D, et al. Albuminuria, a therapeutic target for cardiovascular protection in type 2 diabetic patients with nephropathy. Circulation 2004; 110:921–927; Epub 2004 Aug 09.

74. de Jong PE, Brenner BM. From secondary to primary prevention of progressive renal disease: the case for screening for albuminuria. Kidney Int 2004; 66: 2109–2118.

75. Correa-Rotter R, et al. Demographic and epidemiologic transition in the developing world: role of albuminuria in the early diagnosis and prevention of renal and cardiovascular disease. Kidney Int Suppl 2004; S32–S37.

76. Alexander CM, et al. Losartan and the United States costs of end-stage renal disease by baseline albuminuria in patients with type 2 diabetes and nephropathy. Kidney Int Suppl 2004; 92:S115–S117.

77. Palmer AJ, Rodby RA. Health economics studies assessing irbesartan use in patients with hypertension, type 2 diabetes, and microalbuminuria. Kidney Int Suppl 2004; 92:S118–S120.

78. Kissmeyer L, et al. Community nephrology: audit of screening for renal insufficiency in a high risk population. Nephrol Dial Transplant 1999; 14:2150–2155.

79. Hawthorne K. Asian diabetics attending a British hospital clinic: a pilot study to evaluate their care. Br J Gen Pract 1990; 40:243–247.

80. Hawthorne K, Mello M, Tomlinson S. Cultural and religious influences in diabetes care in Great Britain. Diabet Med 1993; 10:8–12.

81. Hawthorne K. Accessibility and use of health care services in the British Asian community. Fam Pract 1994; 11:453–459.

82. Lightstone L. Preventing Kidney Disease: the Ethnic Challenge. Peterborough, England: National Kidney Research Fund, 2001.

83. Hostetter TH. Chronic kidney disease predicts cardiovascular disease. N Engl J Med 2004; 351:1344–1346.

84. Kooner JS. Coronary heart disease in UK Indian Asians: the potential for reducing mortality. Heart 1997; 78:530–532.

85. Go AS, et al. Chronic kidney disease and the risks of death, cardiovascular events, and hospitalization. N Engl J Med 2004; 351:1296–1305.

86. Segura J, Campo C, Ruilope LM. Effect of proteinuria and glomerular filtration rate on cardiovascular risk in essential hypertension. Kidney Int Suppl 2004; 92:S45–S49.

87. Mann JF, Yi QL, Gerstein HC. Albuminuria as a predictor of cardiovascular and renal outcomes in people with known atherosclerotic cardiovascular disease. Kidney Int Suppl 2004; S59–S62.

14

Chronic Kidney Disease in Aboriginal Australians

Wendy E. Hoy and Srinivas Kondalsamy Chennakesavan
Discipline of Medicine, Centre for Chronic Disease, University of Queensland, Herston, Queensland, Australia

Stephen P. McDonald
Nephrology & Transplantation Unit, The Queen Elizabeth Hospital, Adelaide, South Australia, Australia

Alan Cass
Renal Program, The George Institute for International Health, Sydney, New South Wales, Australia

Gurmeet R. Singh
Menzies School of Health Research, Causuarina, Northern Territory, Australia

John F. Bertram
Department of Anatomy & Cell Biology, Monash University, Clayton, Victoria, Australia

Michael D. Hughson
Department of Pathology, University of Mississippi Medical Center, Jackson, Mississipi, U.S.A.

INTRODUCTION

Aborigines living in remote areas are in epidemiologic transition, marginalized and poor. They have sub-standard living conditions, poor education, poor nutrition, few employment opportunities, and inadequate services of all types.

Their health profile reflects lingering "third-world" conditions and the onset of the lifestyle diseases, considered part of "westernization." Life expectancy of adults in their prior traditional lifestyle is not known, but we know from written histories and photographs that adults were very lean. In a 1957 survey of 713 people in one remote community (the first community described in detail in this chapter), Dr. John Hargraves found people "in the best of health from the nutritional point of view": only one person was considered obese and one hypertensive (unpublished report). Sudden death of natural causes in young adults, now commonplace (1), was then almost unheard of. Since the mid-1980s, an epidemic of chronic diseases, including cardiovascular disease, type 2 diabetes, hypertension, and chronic kidney disease has appeared. Standardized adult mortality rates are 3–6 times those of non-Aboriginal Australians, with cardiovascular disease the leading cause (2,3). Premature death in young and middle-aged adults is contributing to family, community, and cultural breakdown. Our challenge is to understand the genesis of this epidemic, the coexistence and connections of the morbidities, and to promote and design strategies for its prevention and amelioration.

This chapter provides an overview of renal and related chronic diseases in the Aboriginal population. It breifly reviews end stage renal disease (ESRD), then moves to kidney morphology. Next, findings from epidemiologic studies in two high risk communities are developed in some depth; the significant associations defined to this point are described and the links of renal to other chronic disease are emphasized. The benefit of systematic screening and treatment applied in one of these communities is then addressed. Finally, the attempted application of more systematic chronic disease care in other communities is described, along with the derived health profiles, and the implications of the findings for health services resourcing and policy are discussed.

END-STAGE RENAL DISEASE (ESRD)

The burden of renal failure in the Australian population is still underestimated. The Australian New Zealand Dialysis and Transplant (ANZDATA) Registry documents people beginning treatment for ESRD but misses renal deaths of people who do not come to dialysis. Death certificates substantially underestimate people dying with ESRD, even among those in the ESRD treatment program! (4,5). About one person in six with ESRD the Aboriginal communities we have studied has declined or been assessed as unsuitable for such treatment, while many others die with chronic kidney disease as a comorbidity.

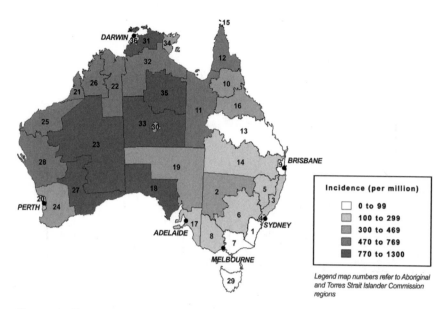

Figure 1 Treated ESRD among Indigenous Australians by ATSIC regions, 1993–1998.

There is regional variation of ESRD rates among Aboriginal people across Australia, as shown in Figure 1 (6). Nationwide, the incidence of ESRD in Aborigines is about 10 times that of non-Aboriginal Australians, and, up through the late 1990s, was increasing every year (7). Rates increased among Aboriginal people in every region in the Northern Territory (NT) over the last two decades, as shown in Figure 2. In 2002, incidence rates exceeded 1300 per million overall, with an age-adjusted rate of about 2070 pm, (vs. 90 pm for non-Aboriginal people nationwide) (8). Aboriginal people with ESRD are younger than their non-Aboriginal counterparts, and there is a female predominance (7,8).

The variation of ESRD rates by region largely reflects differences in socioeconomic status (SES). Cass et al. have shown that an index of SES disadvantage that includes measures of house-crowding, low birth weight, educational attainment, employment, and income is strongly correlated with ESRD in Aboriginal people, shown in Figure 3. SES disadvantage is also associated with ESRD among the much lower rates of non-Aboriginal Australians (9–11). Less comprehensive data suggest that mortality of Aboriginal people follows a similar regional pattern (3).

Currently, Aboriginal people from most remote communities must move to metropolitan centers to access ESRD treatment, although the recent establishment of some regional dialysis units means that some patients do not have to relocate quite so far from home. The disruption

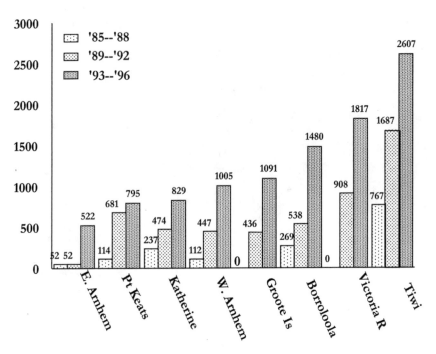

Figure 2 Average annual ESRD incidence in Aboriginal people in the Top End of the Northern Territory, per million.

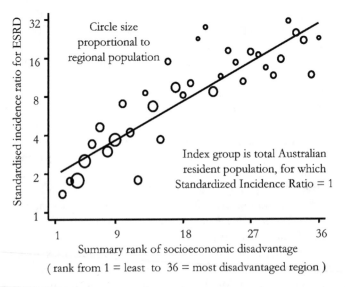

Figure 3 Socioeconomic disadvantage and indigenous ESRD incidence by ATSIC region.

to individual, family and community life, and the rigors and complexities of the sickness and treatment itself, are often devastating (12).

Aboriginal people on hemodialysis are less likely to move onto other forms of treatment, and are especially less likely to be referred for, or to receive, a kidney transplant (7,11,13). Between 1996 and 1998, it cost $112,648 per year to maintain a person an Aboriginal person on hemodialysis in the Top End of the NT: $71,000 for the treatments themselves and $41,648 for inter-current hospitalizations (14). Death rates of treated ESRD patients are 70% higher than that of non-Aboriginal people (7), in part due to are serious comorbidities. The median survival of Aboriginal people on ESRD treatment in the NT in the 1990s was only 3.3 years (8).

RENAL MORPHOLOGY

Aboriginal people with chronic kidney diseases usually have moderate to heavy proteinuria, sometimes with hematuria and/or hypertension. They often have a non-revealing work-up except for a frequent family history of renal disease and the variable presence of diabetes. Prior to recent heightened awareness, they were often picked up late in their course, and progressed rapidly to renal failure.

Features of kidney biopsies in indigenous people around Australia probably differ by region, just as their ESRD rates do. In biopsies already studied in the NT, where ESRD rates are among the highest, all the usual morphologic diagnoses are represented to some degree; some, such as infection-related amyloidosis, are in apparent excess, while many show non-specific mesangiopathic change (15,16). However, the striking findings are glomerulomegaly in two-thirds or more of the biopsies (Fig. 4) and various degrees of glomerular sclerosis, with which glomerular size is strongly correlated (17,18).

In a multiethnic study of kidneys of adults undergoing coronial autopsy without advance suspicion of kidney disease (19–21), we found that Aboriginal people from the NT, had, on average, smaller kidneys than non-Aboriginal people and fewer nephrons, and their mean glomerular volume was larger (Table 1). We postulated that reduced nephron endowment, which results in compensatory hypertrophy of existing nephrons, is a predisposing factor to susceptibility to renal disease and its progression in this population. We have also shown that one of the causes of reduced nephron number is intrauterine growth retardation (IUGR), reflected in lower birth weight (20).

EPIDEMIOLOGIC STUDIES

We have studied renal disease in some detail in two remote Aboriginal communities in the NT with high rates of ESRD and cardiovascular deaths (3,8). In one island community off the coast of Darwin, a cross-sectional study was performed on 90% of all people aged 5+ years, followed by long-

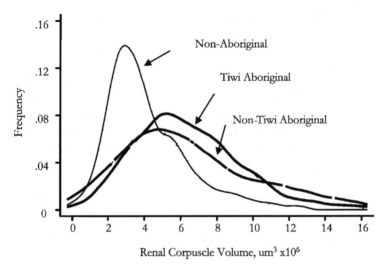

Figure 4   Distribution of mean glomerular corpuscle volume in diseased renal biopsies, Northern Territory Aboriginal versus non-Aboriginal.

itudinal follow-up, now in its 12th year. In another coastal community in East Arnhem, 700 km distant from the first, a cross-sectional study was performed on 60% of adults, using an updated menu of tests. The albumin/creatinine ratio (ACR, gm/mol) on a random urine specimen was used as the renal disease marker in these studies, and glomerular filtration rate (GFR), was estimated from creatinine-based formulae (22–26).

Population Distribution of Albumin Creatinine Ratio (ACR)

Pathologic albuminuria was very common in both communities. Subtle levels were evident in some of the youngest children (5+ years), and there was a relentless increase in rates and intensity with increasing age (Figs. 5 and 6). The median levels in adults are remarkable, given that levels <1.1 gm/mol are generally considered "normal". Overall, 28% of adults

Table 1   Autopsy Study, Right Kidney, Adults 18+ years, Aboriginal Adults vs. Non-Aboriginal, Adjusted for Age and Gender, Mean (SD)

	Aboriginal (n = 17)	Non-Aboriginal (n = 143)	
Kidney mass (g)	159 (15)	206 (13)	$p = 0.025$
Glomerular number	683,174 (66,440)	885,318 (58, 385)	$p = 0.036$
Mean glomerular corpuscle volume ($\mu m^3 \times 10^6$)	10.2 (0.7)	8.1 (0.5)	$p = 0.026$

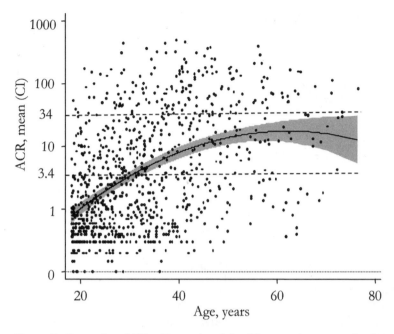

Figure 5 Increasing ACR with age in adults (18+ years), community 1.

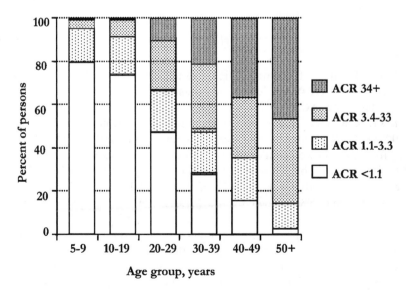

Figure 6 ACR category, gm/mol by age group, community 1.

Table 2 Correlations of Urine Dipstick Test for Protein with Simultaneous ACR in Adults, $n = 879$

	Sensitivity (%)	Specificity (%)	Correctly classified (%)
Dipstick protein trace+ for ACR 3.4+	72.5	79.7	76.2
Dipstick protein trace+ for ACR 34+	90.9	66.8	71.9
Dipstick protein 1+ for ACR 34+	85.6	81.4	82.3

had microalbuminuria and 21% had overt albuminuria in Community 1 (4), and the respective rates in Community 2 were 31% and 13%.

Technical Issues in Detecting Proteinuria

The urine ACR in individuals was very stable to glucose challenge and to protein and water loading (27). Urine protein by dipstick correlated well with the ACR on the same urine, although with less sensitivity, as shown in Table 2. Dipstick trace+detected more than 70% of people with ACR 3.4+ (microalbuminuria threshold), and correctly classified 76% of them. Dipstick protein 1+ detected 85% of people with overt albuminuria (ACR 34+) and correctly classified 82%. This good result might reflect, in part, concentrated urines and therefore higher absolute albumin concentrations in many participants, due to the tropical heat and humidity.

Excretory Renal Function

As shown in Figure 7, there was a significant increase in GFR, estimated from inverse serum creatinine levels and adjusted for age and sex, at subtle levels of increasing ACR ($p < 0.001$), as well as an inverse relationship between GFR and ACR starting in the early overt albuminuria range ($p < 0.0001$). GFR estimates by Cockroft Gault (CG) and the modified MDRD formulae showed similar relationships but with much lower explanations of variance. Table 3 shows estimated GFRs by gender and by ACR category for these methods. Estimated GFR was $<60 \, mL/min/1.73 \, m^2$ in 17% of women and 5% of men by the MDRD formula and in 10% of females and 4% of males by the CG formula, possibly reflecting the female predominance of renal disease in this population. The overall rates were not substantially worse than the aggregate rates in non-diabetics in the NHANES 111 study and Ausdiab study (28,29), but the Aboriginal population is substantially younger than these other populations and the data are not age-adjusted.

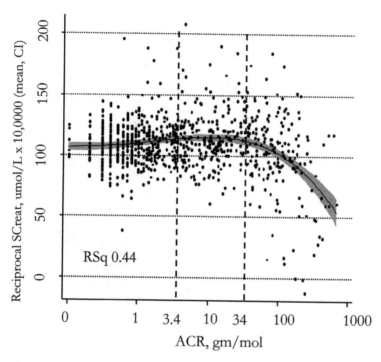

Figure 7 Relationship between reciprocal of serum creatinine and urine ACR in adults.

There are no validation studies of creatinine-based GFR estimates in Aboriginal people. They probably underestimate levels of renal insufficiency in many, who have conspicuously lower muscle mass, at least in the extremities. Nor do we know whether adjustments for gender and for "Black race" are appropriate.

Table 3 GFR Estimates by Modified MDRD and Cockcroft Gault Formulae, by Gender and Baseline ACR Category Without the Modification for "Black" in MDRD

	N	MDRD (mL/min/1.73 m²)	Cockcroft-Gault (mL/min/1.73 m²)
Females	398	87 (84–90)	103 (100–106)
Males	438	91 (89–92)	94 (92–96)
ACR <3.4	429	90 (87–92)	100 (98–101)
ACR 3.4–33	229	92 (82–96)	102 (98–106)
ACR 34–99	104	80 (74–87)	95 (89–101)
ACR 100+	74	72 (65–80)	81 (73–89)

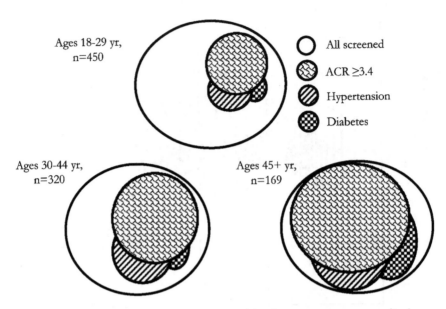

Figure 8 Overlapping and coexisting morbidities, by age group, community 1.

Integrated Morbidities

Hypertension and type 2 diabetes were also common, and they, too, increased with age. They were intimately linked to albuminuria, but albuminuria was more common than hypertension and diabetes in every age group (Fig. 8).

Factors Correlating with ACR

ACR was significantly correlated with many factors. Age was the single strongest determinant. We cannot dissect the contribution of age itself from that of risk factors that increase with ageing, but the effect appears to be mediated through loss of nephrons, which occurs throughout all of adult life (19). Females had higher ACRs than males in childhood and early adult life, which were reflected in higher urine albumin concentrations as well as ACR calculations, but ACR levels in males were equal to those of females by middle age.

After age, Syndrome X features had the strongest correlations with ACR in adults. Markers of body fat as well as blood pressure, cholesterol and triglycerides, and glucose or HbA1c levels and frank diabetes were all significant independent predictors of albuminuria. ACR was also inversely related to serum albumin levels and to hematocrit, and, in the overt albuminuria range, was directly correlated with homocysteine levels (24,30,31).

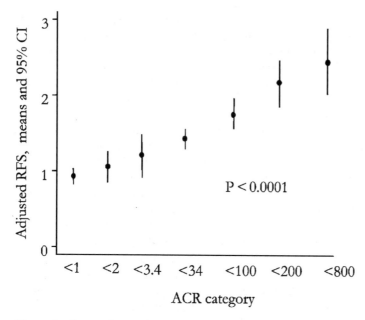

Figure 9 Composite cardiovascular risk factor score (RFS) and baseline ACR in adults in community 1.

Thus, a large component of chronic renal disease in adults is associated with the metabolic syndrome and thus with cardiovascular risk. Figure 9 shows this association through a cardiovascular risk factor score summed through the "traditional" risk factors of overweight, hypertension, high cholesterol, and high triglyceride levels. This was supported by an association of ACR with carotid intimal media thickness, a structural marker of cardiovascular risk (32).

Skin infections, related to crowding, poor hygiene and nutrition, high humidity, insect bites and minor injuries, are very common in this environment, and post-streptococcal glomerulonephritis (PSGN) is both endemic and epidemic. There are also high rates of persistent and recurrent infections of most other organ systems, with viral, bacterial, mycobacterial, fungal, and parasitic agents. ACR and microscopic hematuria were significantly correlated with the presence of skin sores and scabies at the time of examination, with persisting antibody to the M protein of Group A streptococcus (33), and with a remote history of PSGN, a mean of 14.6 years previously (34). ACR was also correlated with seropositivity to *H. pylori* (which also correlated with the metabolic syndrome), with increasing titres of combination *H. pylori* and *C. pneumoniae* antibodies, and with high titre CMV antibodies (35–38). Evidence of *H. pylori* infection was also associated with a doubling of risk of renal death! (38). ACR was also significantly correlated with total IgG levels and with levels of C reactive protein, which, on average, were very high, as well as with fibrinogen levels. While specific nephropathic mechanisms, as for PSGN, are possible, the broader slew of associations probably means that the overall burden of infection is contributing to renal disease. This mirrors the associations of cardiovascular disease with chronic infection rediscovered in the past decade or so.

The association of albuminuria with heavy drinking, marked by high GGT levels, appeared to be independent of blood pressure or lipid changes.

The family clustering of renal disease is marked, but still anecdotal. We are attempting to ascertain the relative contributions of environment and genotype to this phenomenon. The D allele of the angiotensin converting enzyme gene, differently represented in the two major study communities, is probably not the major determinant of renal disease expression (39). However, a polymorphism in the p53 gene associates strongly with albuminuria in smokers in both communities, as shown in Figure 10, as well as with HbA1c levels (40). We could not define associations of albuminuria with the MTHFR or eNOS gene alleles. Because consent in these studies was for candidate gene analyses rather than broad genome analysis, we will need to await additional hypotheses before doing more genetic probes.

Finally, albuminuria was inversely correlated with birth weight (41–43). Although not regularly recorded until the 1960s, birth weights in these communities have been low which largely reflects intrauterine growth retardation (IUGR). This is a complex problem, related to pregnancies in vulnerable teenagers maternal hunger, micronutrient deficiency, infection, smoking,

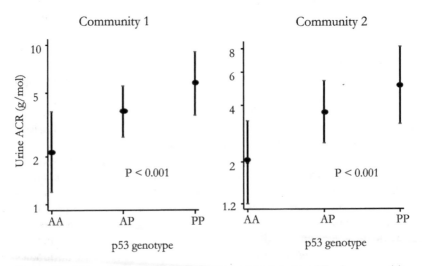

Figure 10 Urine ACR level and p53 genotype in two Aboriginal communities.

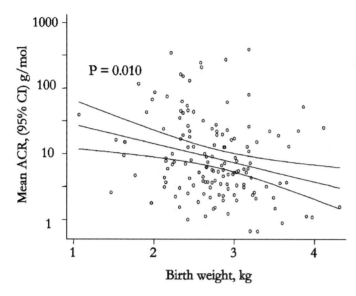

Figure 11 Birth weight and urine ACR in females, adjusted for age and weight. Predicts 41% (CI 19-64%) reduction in ACR per kg increase in birth weight.

drinking, family and social stress, and poor antenatal health care. In Community 1, birth weight was inversely correlated with ACR and overt renal disease in young female adults, of whom 20% had been low birth weight (<2.5 kg) (Fig. 11). Birth weight was also inversely correlated with fasting insulin levels in young female adults, as well as with blood pressure, as shown in Figure 12. Lower birth weight children also had smaller kidney volumes, estimated by ultrasound (44), and people with smaller kidneys, in turn, had higher blood pressures and urine ACR levels (45). A separate study in children suggests that maternal alcohol use during pregnancy also impairs kidney development in the offspring (46). These support and extend Barker's hypothesis that IUGR predisposes the chronic disease in later life (47) and provide another link between renal and cardiovascular disease in this environment.

The identification of several categories of risk factors led us to propose that renal disease in the Aboriginal community setting is multideterminant (23). In such a model, a variety of nephropathic factors operating simultaneously in a high-risk environment progressively amplify the increase in albuminuria and loss of renal function that accompany increasing age. Our models predict a fairly low prevalence of renal disease in people with no risk factors, and the almost inevitable presence of overt albuminuria by middle life in people with a full menu of risk factors. Nenov and associates have subsequently postulated a "multi-hit" model of chronic renal disease, which embodies the same concept (48).

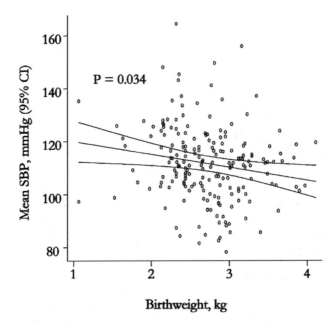

Figure 12 Birth weight and systolic blood pressure in young adult females, adjusted for age and weight. Predicts 4.3 (CI 0.3-8.3) mmHg reduction in SBP per kg increase in birth weight.

Although conveniently demonstrated through categories of ACR and categorical diagnoses such as "overweight," "low birth weight," "diabetes," "hypertension," and ACR correlated with each putative risk factor over a continuum (e.g., weight, birth weight, degree of glycemia, blood pressure), showing the limitations of categorical definitions in illuminating pathophysiology or defining risk.

Natural History

ACR increased and GFR fell in individuals with time, at rates that were strongly correlated with the severity of baseline disease (49). As shown in Figure 13, people without albuminuria had fairly stable renal function over the course of the observations, while those with the heaviest albuminuria (ACR 200+) were losing more than 12 mL/min of GFR per year.

Baseline ACR also predicted hospitalizations, including, but not restricted to, those related to cardiovascular diagnoses (35) (Fig. 14).

Overt albuminuria predicted all the cases of renal failure developing over the follow-up period. Pathologic ACR also predicted non-renal deaths,

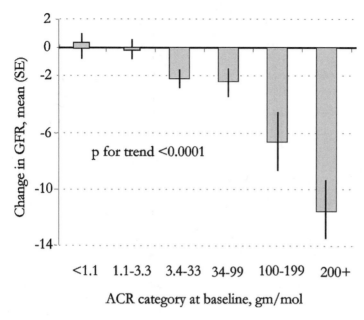

Figure 13 Annual loss of GFR, ml/min, by baseline ACR category.

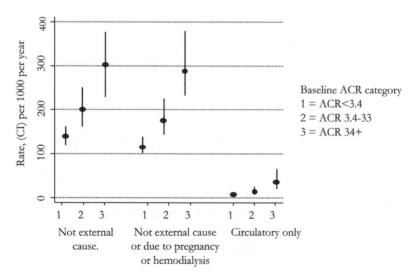

Figure 14 Hospitalizations in adults, by baseline ACR category, adjusted for age and sex.

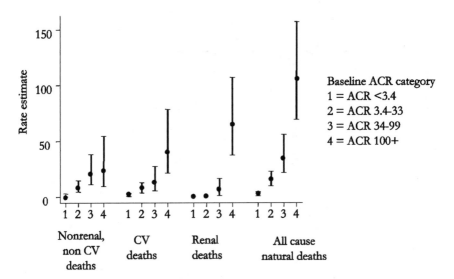

Figure 15 Rates (95% CI) of terminal events per 1000 person years, by baseline ACR category.

including, but not restricted to cardiovascular deaths, over a continuum, as shown in Figure 15 (35,50). Urine protein by dipstick also predicted natural deaths, shown in Figure 16, although with less discrimination among categories (27).

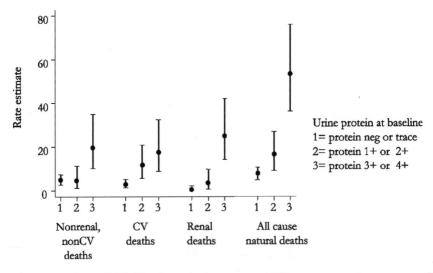

Figure 16 Rates (95% CI) of terminal events per 1000 person years by category of urine protein by dipstick at baseline.

TREATMENT PROGRAM

A systematic treatment program was introduced into Community 1 in late 1995 (51–53). Treatment, offered to people with pathologic albuminuria and/or hypertension, was centered around the use of a long-acting angiotensin converting enzyme inhibitor (Coversyl, Servier), blood pressure control and attempted control of glucose and lipids where needed. Despite an estimate that only two-thirds of people were taking their medicine with any regularity, there was dramatic and sustained fall in blood pressure and stabilization of renal function on a group basis. Over a mean treatment period of 3.4 years, renal deaths fell by two-thirds and non-renal deaths by 50% in people with ACR 34+ at baseline, with benefit at every levels of overt ACR (Fig. 17). The number of people with overt albuminuria needed to treat (NNT) over that interval to avoid one terminal event was only 9.5, despite the two-thirds "compliance." Reductions in community-based rates of ESRD and natural deaths supported the estimates of endpoint reductions. The cost of the program was calculated at about $1200 Aus per person for the first year of treatment, and much less thereafter, and savings of several million dollars were estimated in dialysis delayed or avoided alone (54).

In its fourth year, this program was handed over to the newly constituted local Health Board. The program's intensity diminished when

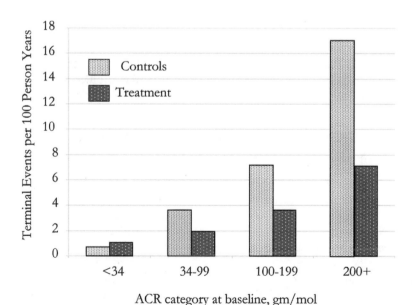

Figure 17 Rates of all-cause natural death, by baseline ACR category, controls vs. treatment cohort.

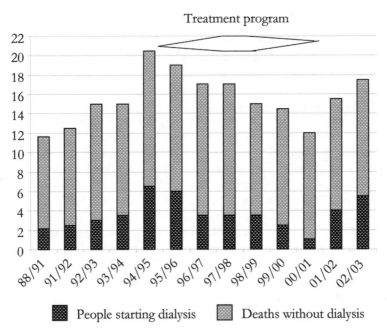

Figure 18 Terminal events of natural causes in adults age 18+ year in community 1, annual rolling average.

health services funding later fell short—blood pressures and ACR levels rose and estimated GFR fell, and followed by a rebound in terminal events in the community as a whole, as shown in Figure 18 (55). Thus continued systematic surveillance and treatment are essential for sustained good outcomes.

THE ABORIGINAL CHRONIC DISEASE OUTREACH PROGRAM

Principles and Obstacles

This program was started in 1999 to help improve awareness and management of renal and related chronic diseases in other Aboriginal communities (56–58). Its central tenets are that regular screening and appropriate treatment for chronic diseases and their risk factors should be core elements of primary health care, that those functions must be integrated, rather than "disease specific," and that these activities be run by local health workers. These are the only members of health care teams in remote areas with any geographic stability, and they have the community connections to advise on program structure and to encourage participation.

In this program health workers follow algorithms for testing and treatment, backed up by nurses or doctors, mostly from a distance. Testing protocols are simple, brief, and cheap. They emphasize point-of-care testing where possible: participant inudveneut in the exam, education, and immediate feedback. Minimal elements of testing include a brief history, weight (and height, once only), blood pressure, skin exam, random glucose on a capillary finger stick sample, and urine dipstick test for protein and blood and markers of infection. Other tests follow only where dictated by algorithms, e.g., urine ACR if urine dipstick is positive for protein or if the participant is diabetic or hypertensive, serum creatinine only if there is overt proteinuria or albuminuria or dangerously high blood pressure, HbA1c where diabetes is present or suspected, and lipids if other problems are under control and compliance with multiple drugs seem feasible, etc. Treatment protocols encourage prompt introduction and upward titration of a restricted menu of medicines. We have used a web-base chronic disease database for communities with no current information systems, which allows timely review of data by nurses and doctors from a distance and endorsement of assessments and treatment decisions taken by the health worker.

Obstacles are many. Lack of resources is the most critical. Space, plumbing, furniture, phone lines, refrigerators, centrifuges, computers, medical and diagnostic equipment and reagents are often absent or in short supply. Trained health workers are few, and work attendance is often very poor. This is a complex issue, to which family and community events and responsibilities, poor working conditions, unempowered roles, poor pay, and a different work ethic contribute. In addition, health workers are often recruited away from chronic disease tasks into other clinical activities perceived to be more urgent. Rapid turnover of nonAboriginal staff, related to hardships of remote placement, does not help. Travel to remote areas is very expensive and floods and cyclones often impede access. Finally, in one Outreach community, the treatment needs for the burden of chronic disease exposed by systematic testing overwhelmed the scantily resourced service. In the not so distant past, such a situation was used by government agencies as an argument against systematic testing!

Community Profiles

The Outreach Program has run for two to three years in three additional remote communities in the NT. Participation ranged from 67% to 100% of the adult populations, with a total of 1070 people age 18+ years tested.

Adults in those three NT communities had impressively different body habitus. Waist measurements in females, even those of modest BMIs, were significantly higher than those in non-Aboriginal Australians (59). Rates of suspected morbidities, were excessive in all, but differed two-fold or more, among communities as shown in Figure 19. Some of this variation are parallels differences in body weight, but some remains unexplained. There was a

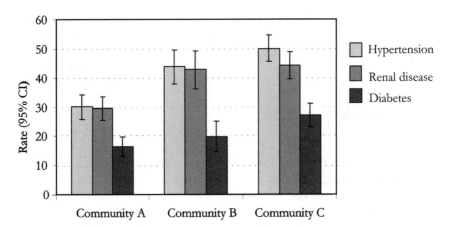

Figure 19 Rates of morbidities by outreach community, adjusted for age and sex.

powerful increase in prevalence of every condition with increasing age (Fig. 20). However, due to the youthful age structure of these groups, the majority of people with problems were young or middle-aged adults (Fig. 21). Finally, morbidities occured more commonly together than in isolation (Fig. 22). Proteinuria was an early and central element of the symptom complex, while diabetes was a late and variable development. These findings parallel those defined by the more sensitive use of the urine ACR in Community 1, described in an earlier section.

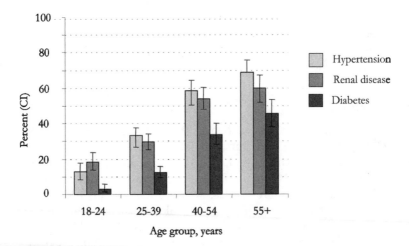

Figure 20 Rates of morbidities by age in outreach communities.

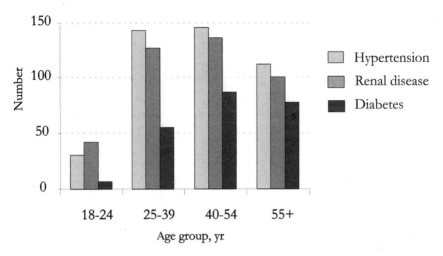

Figure 21 Number of persons with morbidities by age in outreach communities (of 1070 screened).

Outcomes

Despite the difficulties, health workers have become increasingly confident in chronic disease care and educating others in regional and national workshops. Adherence to testing and treatment protocols have improved markedly. The number of people diagnosed with renal disease increased by 110%, with hypertension by 19% and with diabetes by 24%. Antihypertensive or

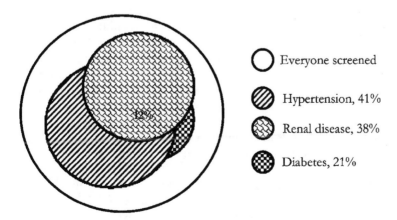

Figure 22 Overlapping morbidities in people age 18+ years, outreach communities.

renal-sparing agents, generally ACEi, were started or the dose was modified in 23% of the population, with a final coverage of 31% of everyone tested (and in 82% of diabetics), and coverage of diabetics with hypoglycemic agents increased from 56% to 72%. In people with BP ≥ 140/90 in whom ACEi treatment was introduced or increased, mean SBP dropped 14 mm Hg and mean DBP by 11 mmg Hg. However, responses among hypertensive females in Community C, where there was a female nurse coordinator and a female health worker, were much better, with a mean fall in SBP of 24 mmg Hg and DBP of 14 mm Hg. These responses, if sustained, should translate into reduced progression of renal disease and rates of renal failure, and, more importantly, to major reductions in cardiovascular complications and deaths (51–53,60).

DEVELOPING A STRATEGIC FRAMEWORK FOR CHRONIC DISEASE SERVICES

Most of these concepts about testing and treatment for chronic disease (61) are now incorporated into standard care guidelines for Aboriginal health (62–64). However, current resources, which are not standardized across states, regions, or communities, much less indexed to burdens of disease, do not cover their systematic application.

We are exploring use of community profiles for informed, needs-based health services planning. The increase in disease rates with age means that repeated testing needs to occur throughout life to detect treatable conditions as they develop. They can probably also suggest the optimum frequency of such testing, which would avoid excessive use of resources but pick up most newly appearing morbidities reasonably early. The age-related pattern also allows predictions of future burdens of disease as the population ages. The predominance of young and middle-aged people among those with morbidities anticipates many years of treatment and intensified follow-up, if they are to have a reasonable life expectancy. The different rates of morbidities among communities mean that pilot data are needed to plan resources to deal with chronic disease in individual sites. This process might be as simple as a review of existing clinic records. The coexistence of morbidities justifies integrated, rather than disease-specific, chronic disease screening, and suggests that most people will be on multiple drugs by middle age. It also implies that these conditions arise out of a common environment and will be susceptible to the same menu of primary and secondary prevention strategies.

Application of the HBG/HRG (Health Benefit Group/Health Resource Group) conceptual framework to these profiles, expanded to include categories of severity conditions, is an additional area to explore (65–67). This allows projections of clinical benefit and cost savings from each stage of intervention, which will advance the case for up-front planning and adequate resourcing. One challenge will be development of an approach that integrates all the common conditions which can be prevented or ameliorated, and is focused on individuals rather than specific diseases.

Arguments based on improved clinical outcomes, and cost savings from hospitalizations and dialysis avoided can be used to advocate with government for better resources. Allocation of a monetary value to a year of death postponed for people in the prime of life is an additional argument, although the more human perspective is better preservation of community and family stability.

CONCLUSIONS

Chronic kidney disease is but one manifestation of the chronic disease epidemic in Aboriginal people. Albuminuria is a sensitive marker, and creatinine-based estimates of GFR, while perhaps not ideal, are sensitive enough to serious renal insufficiency.

Renal disease is multideterminant, educed by a number of factors operating in a high-risk environment. Some people are probably predisposed through a relatively lower nephron endowment: this might have been adaptive in the first instance, in water and salt-depleted environments and with subsistence diets. IUGR is an additional important determinant.

Albuminuria provides a link between renal disease and other related chronic conditions and marks the risk for premature mortality in this population. The identification of relatively novel risk factors for renal disease, such as non-cutaneous infection, inflammation and low birthweight is compatible with the expanded risk factor base now recognized for cardiovascular disease in the general population. These relationships support a unified approach to prevention and treatment.

The emergence of the chronic disease epidemic in this population seems to be due, in part, to the dramatically improved survival of low-birth-weight babies in the last four decades, due to better hospital care of sick infants who are now surviving to adult life at high risk for chronic disease. Following a classic "life course" trajectory, the high risk postnatal environment, characterised by sedentary ways, poor diet, high rates of smoking and hazardous drinking, dirty, crowded, poorly maintained housing, and poor community infrastructure, educes or accentuates disease manifestations. The continued gradual improvement in Aboriginal birth weights provides one element of hope that disease rates might ultimately stabilize or fall in this complex situation.

Many of these findings might be generalized to other high-risk populations (68). An explosion of chronic disease will present a great burden of renal failure in developing countries and will exacerbate the premature adult mortality associated with poor nutrition and infections, most especially AIDS. The weightings of risk factors for renal disease might differ in different populations, but multideterminant causation and the integration of chronic disease probably still apply.

Prevention and disease modification in this environment are real possibilities. For persons already afflicted, chronic disease is easily diagnosed and progression is dramatically altered by standard interventions within our reach. For those at risk, but currently disease-free, pharmacologic prevention is an intriguing possibility. True primary prevention depends on sustained improvements in socioeconomic circumstances and community infrastructure, as well as health services and birthweights, and health care providers should advocate for the fundamental multisectoral changes needed to bring these changes about.

ACKNOWLEDGMENTS

This review is derived from an ambitious project that was started in 1989 by Professor John Mathews, Dr. David Pugsley, and Dr. Paul Van Buynder. We thank the laboratory and Renal Unit staff at Menzies, the laboratory staff at the Royal Darwin Hospital and Western Diagnostic Pathology, and all our multidisciplinary collaborators for their efforts. We especially thank the people of the communities for their participation and their Land Councils and Health Board for their support and oversight. The program has been supported by funds from the National Health and Medical Research Council, the Stanley Tipiloura fund, the Australian Kidney Foundation, Rio Tinto, Servier, Australia, Janssen Cilag, Territory Health Services, the New Children's Hospital in Sydney, Australia, Flinders University NT Clinical School, NT Cardiac Services, APMA-AMA Aboriginal Health Initiative, the Office of Aboriginal and Torres Strait Islander Health Services, and the Colonial Foundation of Australia.

REFERENCES

1. Young MC, Fricker PA, Thomson NJ, Lee KA, Dempsey KE, Condon JR. Sudden death due to ischaemic heart disease in young Aboriginal sportsmen in the Northern Territory, 1982–1996. Med J Aust 1999; 170(9):425–428.
2. Dempsey KE, Condon JR. Mortality in the Northern Territory, 1979–1997. Darwin: Territory Health Services, 1999. Enquiries to epidemiology@nt.gov.au.
3. The Health and Welfare of Australia's Aboriginal and Torres Strait Islander People, 2001. Australian Bureau of Statistics. ABS Catalogue no 4704.0, August 2001. www.aihw.gov.au.

4. Li SQ, Cass A, Cunningham J. Cause of death in patients with end stage renal disease: assessing concordance of death certificates with registry reports. Aust N Z J Pub Health 2003; 27:419–424.

5. Li SQ, Cunningham J, Cass A. Renal-related deaths in Australia 1998–1999. Intern Med J 2004; 34:259–265.

6. Cass A, Cunningham J, Wang Z, Hoy WE. Regional variation in the incidence of end stage renal disease in indigenous Australians. Med J Aust 2001; 175: 24–27.

7. McDonald SP, Russ GR. The burden of end stage renal disease among indigenous peoples in Australia and New Zealand. Kidney Int 2003; 63S: S123–S127.

8. Spencer JS, Silva D, Hoy WE. An epidemic of renal failure among Australian Aborigines. Med J Aust 1998; 168:537–541.

9. Cass A, Cunningham J, Snelling P, Wang Z, Hoy WE. End-stage renal disease in indigenous Australians: a disease of disadvantage. Ethnicity Dis 2002; 12(3):373–378.

10. Cass A, Cunningham J, Snelling P, Wang Z, Hoy WE. Beyond the biomedical perspective: the social determinants of end stage renal disease. Annual Report for 2002, ANZDATA Registry, 2003.

11. Cass A, Cunningham J, Wang Z, Hoy WE. Social disadvantage and variation in the incidence of end stage renal disease in Australian capital cities. Aust N Z J Pub Health 2001; 25:322–326.

12. Cass A, Lowell A, Christie M, Snelling P, Flack M, Marrnganyin B, Brown I. Sharing the true stories: improving communication between Aboriginal patients and health carers. Med J Aust 2002; 176:466–470.

13. Cass A, Cunningham J, Snelling P, Wang Z, Hoy W. Renal transplantation for Indigenous Australians: Identifying the barriers to equitable access. Ethnicity Health 2003; 8(2):111–119.

14. You J, Hoy WE, Zhao Y, Beaver C, Eager K. End-stage renal disease in the Northern Territory: current and future treatment costs. Med J Aust 2002; 176(10):461–465.

15. Howard D, Davis J, Pugsley JD, Seymour A, Hoy WE. Morphologic correlates of renal disease in a high risk Australian Aboriginal community. Kidney Int 1997; 51:1318.

16. Lloyd ML, Moore L, Pugsley DJ, Seymour AM. Renal disease in an Australian Aboriginal population: a pathologic study. Nephrology 1996; 2:315–322.

17. Bertram JF, Young RJ, Kincaid Smith P, Seymour AE, Hoy WE. Glomerulo-megaly in Australian Aborigines. Nephrology 1998; 4(suppl iii–iv):S46–S53.

18. Hughson M, Johnson K, Young RJ, Hoy WE, Bertram JF. Glomerular size and glomerulosclerosis: relationships to disease categories, glomerular solidification, and ischemic obsolescence. Am J Kidney Dis 2002; 39(4):679–688.

19. Hoy WE, Douglas-Denton RN, Hughson M, Cass A, Johnson K, Bertram JF. A stereological study of glomerular number and volume: preliminary findings in a multiracial study of kidneys at autopsy. Kidney Int 2003; 63(S83): S31–S37.

20. Hughson MD, Farris AB, III, Denton-Douglas R, Hoy WE, Bertram JF. Glomerular number and size in autopsy kidneys: the relationship to birth weight. Kidney Int 2003; 63:2113–2122.

21. Douglas Denton R, Hoy WE, Bertram JF, Hughson MD. Kidney mass, glomerular number, mean glomerular corpuscle volume and total renal corpuscle volume in Aboriginal and nonAboriginal Australians at autopsy. Nephrology 2003; 8(S):P20, A59.

22. Hoy WE, Norman RJ, Hayhurst BG, Pugsley DJ. A health profile of adults in a Northern Territory Aboriginal community, with an emphasis on preventable morbidities. Aust N Z J Pub Health 1997; 21:121–126.

23. Hoy WE, Mathews JD, Pugsley DJ, McCredie DA, Hayhurst BG, Rees M, Walker KA, Kile E, Wang Z. The multidimensional nature of renal disease: rates and associations of albuminuria in an Australian Aboriginal community. Kidney Int 1998; 54:1296–1304.

24. McDonald SP, Maguire GP, Hoy WE. Renal function and cardiovascular risk markers in a remote East Arnhem Aboriginal community. Nephrol Dial Transplant 2003; 18:1555–1561.

25. Cockcroft D, Gault MK. Prediction of creatinine clearance from serum creatinine. Nephron 1976; 16:31–41.

26. Levey AS, Greene T, Kusek JW, Beck GJ. The MDRD Study Group. A simplified equation to predict glomerular filtration rate from serum creatinine. J Am Soc Nephrol 2000; 11:A0828.

27. Hoy WE, McDonald SP. Albuminuria, marker or target in indigenous populations. Kidney Int Suppl 2004; 92:S25–31.

28. Clase CM, Garg AX, Kiberd BA. Prevalence of low glomerular filtration rate in nondiabetic Americans. Third National Health and Nutrition Examination Survey (NHANES 111). J Am Soc Nephrol 2002; 13:1338–1349.

29. Chadban SJ, Briganti EM, Kerr PG, Dunstan DW, Welborn TA, Zimmet PZ, Atkins RC. Prevalence of kidney damage in Australian adults: the Ausdiab Kidney Study. J Am Soc Nephrol 2003; 13:S131–S138.

30. McDonald SM, Maguire G, Duarte N, Wang XL, Hoy WE. C reactive protein, cardiovascular risk, and renal disease in a remote Australian Aboriginal community. Clin Sci (Lond) 2004; 106:121–128.

31. McDonald SP, Hoy WE, et al. Homocysteine, renal disease and cardiovascular disease in a remote Australian Aboriginal community. Intern Med J 2005; 35(5):289–294.

32. McDonald S, et al. Carotid intimal media thickness and renal and cardiovascular risk factors in a remote Australian Aboriginal community. Atherosclerosis 2004; 177(2):423–431.

33. Goodfellow AM, Hoy WE, Sriprakash KS, Daly MJ, Reeve MP, Mathews JD. Proteinuria is associated with persistence of antibody to streptococcal M protein in Aboriginal Australians. Epidemiol Infect 1999; 122:67–75.

34. White A, Hoy WE, McCredie DA. Childhood post-streptococcal glomerulonephritis is a risk factor for chronic renal disease in later life. Med J Aust 2001; 174:492–496.

35. McDonald SP. Renal Disease, Cardiovascular Disease and Shared Risk Markers in Remote Aboriginal Communities. PhD thesis, NT Clinical School, Flinders University and the Menzies School of Health Research, Darwin NT, Australia, 2004.

36. Hoy WE, Coles K. *Helicobacter pylori* infection increases renal disease risk and the metabolic syndrome: findings in an Aboriginal Community. JASN 2001; 12:68A; A 0360.

37. Hoy WE, Coles K. Noncutaneous infections and renal disease. Association of infections with *Chlamydia pneumoniae* and *Helicobacter pylori* infections with chronic renal disease in Australian Aborigines. JASN 2001; 12:A 1084, 209A.

38. Hoy WE, Nichol J, Coles K. *Helicobacter pylori* seropositivity correlates with renal disease and renal deaths in Australian Aborigines. Submitted, Am J Kidney Dis, May 2005.

39. McDonald S, Panagiotopoulos S, Smith T, Hoy W, Mathews JD. Angiotensin converting enzyme (ACE) polymorphisms and renal disease in Aboriginal Australians. Nephrology 2000, 5: PA69.

40. McDonald SP, Hoy WE, Maguire GP, Duarte N, Wilcken DEL, Wang XI. The p53Pro72Arg polymorphism is associated with albuminuria among Aboriginal Australians. J Am Soc Nephrol 2002; 13:677–683.

41. Hoy WE, Kile E, Rees M, Mathews JD. Low birth weight and renal disease in Australian Aborigines. Lancet 1998; 352:1826–1827.

42. Hoy WE, Kile E, Rees M, Mathews JD. A new dimension to the Barker hypothesis: low birth weight and susceptibility to renal disease: findings in an Australian Aboriginal community. Kidney Int 1999; 56(3):1072–1076.

43. Singh GR, Hoy WE. The association between birthweight and current blood pressure: a cross-sectional study in an Australian Aboriginal community. Med J Aust 2003; 179:532–535.

44. Spencer JS, Wang Z, Hoy WE. Low birth weight and reduced renal volume in Aboriginal children. Am J Kidney Dis 2001; 37(5):915–920.

45. Singh GR, Hoy WE. Blood pressure and kidney volume: findings in an Australian Aboriginal community. Am J Kidney Dis 2004; 43:254–259.

46. Singh GR, Sayers SM, Hoy WE. Maternal alcohol ingestion during pregnancy predisposes to albuminuria and smaller kidney in Aboriginal children: findings in an Aboriginal birth cohort. Nephrology 2004; 9(Suppl 1):75.

47. Barker DJ. The developmental origins of adult disease. Eur J Epidemiol 2003; 18:733–736.

48. Nenov VD, Taal MW, Sakharova OV, Brenner BM. Multi-hit nature of chronic renal disease. Curr Opin Nephrol Hypertens 2000; (2):85–97.

49. Hoy WE, Wang Z, Baker PRA, McDonald S, van Buynder PB, Mathews JD. The natural history of renal disease in Australian Aborigines, Part 1. Progression of albuminuria and loss of glomerular filtration rate over time. Kidney Int 2001; 60:243–248.

50. Hoy WE, Wang Z, Baker PRA, McDonald S, van Buynder PB, Mathews JD. The natural history of renal disease in Australian Aborigines, part 2. The

predictive value of albuminuria for premature death and renal failure. Kidney Int 2001; 60:249–256.

51. Hoy WE, Baker P, Kelly A, Wang Z. Reducing premature death and renal failure in Australian Aborigines: results of a community-based treatment program. Med J Aust 2000; 172:473–478.

52. Hoy WE, Baker PRA, Kelly A, Wang Z. Sustained reduction at four years in natural deaths and renal failure from a systematic renal and cardiovascular treatment program in an Australian Aboriginal community. Kidney Int 2003; 63(S83):S66–S73.

53. Hoy WE, Wang Z, Baker PRA, Kelly AM. Secondary prevention of renal and cardiovascular disease: results of a renal and cardiovascular treatment program in an Australian aboriginal community. J Am Soc Nephrol 2003; 14(7 suppl 2): S178–S185.

54. Baker PR, Hoy WE, Thomas RE. Cost-effectiveness analysis of a kidney and cardiovascular disease treatment program in an Australian Aboriginal population. Adv Chronic Kidney Dis 2005; 12(1):39–48.

55. Hoy WE, Kondalsamy–Chennakesavan S. Resurgence of deaths and end stage renal disease in a high risk Australian Aboriginal community. Nephrology 2003; 8(suppl):A59; Abs P19.

56. Hoy WE, Kondalsamy–Chennakesavan S, Scheppingen J, Sharma S. Kidney and related chronic disease profiles and risk factors in three remote Australian communities. Adv Chronic Kidney Dis 2005; 12:64–70.

57. Davey R, Gokel G, Hoy WE. Obstacles to good management of chronic disease in remote Aboriginal Australia. 38th Annual Scientific Meeting of ANZSN, September 1–4, 2002. Nephrology 2002; 7(suppl):A79.

58. Hoy WE, Scheppingen J, McKendry K, Sharma S, Kondalsamy–Chennakesavan S. Planning services for noncommunicable chronic diseases in Australian Aboriginal communities. 39th Annual Scientific Meeting of the ANZSN, 2003. Nephrology 2003; 8(suppl):A59; Abs P18.

59. Cameron AJ, Welborn TA, Zimmet PZ, Dunstan DW, Owen N, Salmon J, Dalton M, Jolley D, Shaw JE. Overweight and obesity in Australia: the 1999–2000 Australian Diabetes, Obesity and Lifestyle Study (AusDiab). Med J Aust 2004; 180(8):418.

60. Lawes CM, Rodgers A, Bennett DA, Parag V, Suh I, Ueshima H, MacMahon S. Asia Pacific Cohort Studies Collaboration: blood pressure and cardiovascular disease in the Asia Pacific region. J Hypertens 2003; 21:473–475.

61. Hoy WE. Screening and treatment for renal disease: the community model. Nephrology 1998; 4(suppl iii–iv):S90–S95.

62. CARPA Standard Treatment Manual Standard Treatment Manual. 3rd ed. http://crh.flinders.edu.au/collaboration/remote.htm (from the Central Australia Rural Practitioners Association) Mail P.O. Box 4066, Alice Springs 0871, Northern Territory, Phone: 08 8951 47770, Email, crh@flinders.edu.au.

63. Couzos S, Murray R. Aboriginal Primary Health Care—An Evidence-Based Approach. 2nd ed. Oxford University Press, Nov 2003.

64. The National Aboriginal & Torres Strait Islander Health Clearinghouse, Edith Cowan University, WA. www.healthinfonet.ecu.edu.au

65. Beaver C, Zhao Y, Skov S, Morton H. Health Benefit and Healthcare Resource Group classifications: linking health care needs to resource requirements across the health care sector. CASEMIX 2000; 2(2):61.
66. Mountney L, et al. The Use of Population Need Groupings in the Measurement of Care Outcomes, National Casemix Office, 2001. http://www.sis.port.ac.uk/~norrist/hic97lm.html
67. Benton PL, Evans H, Light SM, Mountney LM, Sanderson HF, Anthony P. The development of Healthcare Resource Groups—version 3. J Pub Health Med 1998; 20:351–358.
68. Hoy WE. Reflections on the 15th International Congress of Nephrology: renal and cardiovascular protection in the developing world. Nephrol Dial Transplant 2001; 16:1509–1511.

15

ESRD in Russia

Natalia A. Tomilina and Boris T. Bikbov

Department of Nephrology Issues of Transplanted Kidney, Research Institute of Transplantology and Artificial Organs, Moscow, Russia

ABBREVIATIONS

ESRD	end-stage renal diseases
RRT	renal replacement therapy
HD	hemodialysis
PD	peritoneal dialysis
CAPD	continuous ambulatory peritoneal dialysis

INTRODUCTION

The history of the Russian nephrology community dates back to the early 1960s. Not long before, the first artificial kidney treatment was administered to a Moscow patient with acute renal failure in 1958. In 1965, the first kidney transplantation from a living related donor was performed in Moscow. In the same year, the Society of Nephrology of the Soviet Union was founded. Nevertheless, until the beginning of perestroika in the mid-1980s, Soviet authorities devoted little attention to the problem of end-stage renal disease (ESRD). In 1998, the Russian Dialysis Society was founded with the objective of creating the country's first national registry of ESRD patients. Thus, information about the prevalence and distribution of ESRD has only been available since 1998.

The development of RRT in Russia depends not only on the economic conditions but also on the geographic features as well. The territory of Russia covers more than 17 million square kilometers—about one-seventh of the world's land mass—and is home to about 145 million people. Population density is extremely non-uniform, being low in many parts of Siberia, in the North and in the Far East, and equivalent to Western European levels throughout European Russia and the Urals.

The Russian Federation is composed of 89 territorial entities, each administrated by its own regional government and budget. While the Soviet healthcare system was financially centralized, Russia's local healthcare budgets and policies are determined by regional authorities. This has proved favorable to solving the ESRD treatment problem.

However, even though Russia's standard of living has improved over the past decade, economic indicators are still troublingly low. With an average income per capita of only $2140 (1), the expenditures per capita per year equal just $115 on health care (2). Thus, Russia is a huge country with big population, but its difficult economic conditions have generally prevented the development of RRT.

RENAL REPLACEMENT THERAPY: GENERAL DATA

Today, Russia has more than 1300 active nephrologists (8.2 nephrologists pmp). As a rule, they are located in the larger cities, where they work out of nephrological departments or dialysis units. The number of nephrologists working in outpatient clinics in Russia is small. As a part of regular rotations, all medical students take courses in nephrology, going on to specialize further in post-graduate courses if they choose it as their specialization. It used to be that physicians had to first get experience working in nephrology departments, after which they would enroll in 16-week post-graduate courses. In 2002, the system changed. Now, post-graduate courses last 3 years total, including 1 year of internal medicine followed by 2 years of nephrology residency.

At last count in 2002, ESRD patients could receive treatment in 258 renal units around the country—not a significant change from the number of renal units in 1998 (3). But over the same period, the number of patients receiving renal replacement therapy (RRT) has increased by 40% (Table 1). With an average growth rate of 8.8% per year, RRT gain in Russia to some extent exceeds RRT gain in many other countries (4). This high rate might be due to more intensive work on the part of the dialysis units, as well as to an increase in the number of hemodialysis machines.

Most importantly, however, Russia would not have witnessed such a sharp gain in RRT were it not for the decentralization of the healthcare system. In the face of economic fallout from the post-Soviet economic reforms, local authorities took on the job of financing the treatment of most of the

Table 1 Prevalence Rate for Different RRT Modalities in Russia, 1998–2002

Year	1998	1999	2000	2001	2002
Number of patients					
All RRT	8,227	8,747	9,513	10,821	11,517
HD	5,786	6.089	6,601	7,690	8,233
PD	424	416	486	538	569
Tx	2,017	2,242	2,426	2,599	2,715
Rate pmp					
All RRT	55.3	59.0	65.8	74.7	79.3
HD	38.8	40.9	45.6	53.1	56.7
PD	2.8	2.8	3.4	3.7	3.9
Tx	13.7	15.3	16.8	17.9	18.7
Increment to previous year (%)					
All RRT	–	6.3	8.8	13.7	6.4
HD	–	5.2	8.4	16.5	7.1
PD	–	−1.9	16.8	10.7	5.8
Tx	–	11.2	8.2	7.1	4.5

country's ESRD patients. In some regions, private dialysis units have recently been founded. The local governments reimburse all their expenditures, while patients receive their treatment for free.

In 2002, the total number of patients receiving RRT reached 11,517, an increase from the 8227 patients counted in 1998. Of these, 2715 (23.6%, 18.7 pmp) were living with a functioning kidney graft, 8233 (71.5%, 56.7 pmp) were undergoing hemodialysis (HD), and only 569 (4.9%, 3.9 pmp) were being treated with peritoneal dialysis (PD, mainly CAPD) (Table 1). Thus, the average prevalence of ESRD treatment increased from 56.1 pmp in 1998 to 79.3 pmp in 2002.

Unfortunately, the fact that there is no state national program for developing RRT contributes to markedly lower rates of dialysis and transplantation in Russia's distant regions. Depending on the state of the local economy, the prevalence rate of RRT ranges from less than 10 to 273 pmp, with highest rates being found in Moscow. In St. Petersburg, as well as in cities in the Urals, Tatarstan and in Russia's Northwest and Volga regions, the prevalence of RRT patients is already more than 100 pmp, and steadily increasing. This is in sharp contrast to the half of the country's provinces where the prevalence of RRT patients has yet to reach 60 to 70 pmp. Nevertheless, the number of regions with such a low rate is steadily decreasing, while the number of regions whose prevalence is closer to the country's average rate is on the rise.

Every year, about 2000 patients begin RRT. With 1763, 2271, and 2134 patients starting dialysis therapy in the years 2000, 2001, and 2002, respectively, the incidence rate in the year 2002 was 13.7 pmp for HD, and only 1.0 pmp for PD.

For economic reasons, mainly, HD has emerged as Russia's predominant dialysis treatment modality. First and foremost is the fact that it is cheaper in many provinces than PD treatment. At the same time, PD solutions cannot be obtained in many local regions, and, where it is accessible, local nephrologists and patients often resist trying this modality. The low rate of PD treatment results in a very significant impediment for the treatment of the majority of Russia's population living in small towns and settlements, since such areas also lack HD equipment.

In 2002, the PD growth rate was much lower than the HD growth rate, and, by the end of the year, the percentage of PD patients among the dialysis population had yet to top 5% (Table 1). The two cities where PD modality is developing most successfully are Moscow and St. Petersburg, more than half of the whole PD population is being treated.

As a rule, in the cohort of PD patients CAPD is used as a first treatment modality. But the practice of beginning PD after a few weeks of HD treatment has also been used to success among a minority of patients, most particularly among late referrals for whom HD had been the only efficient first treatment modality. Even more rarely, in cases when HD stations had also been lacking, both modes of treatment have been applied at once. Besides PD has been successfully used as the second dialysis modality in 2.9% of HD-patients, who, for reasons such as unsolvable problems of vascular access, could no longer be treated with HD.

As has been mentioned above, kidney transplantation has been performed in Russia since 1965, initially with donations from living relatives. Later, cadaveric kidney transplantation became the norm, although donations from living relatives have resumed in recent years. It is illegal in Russia to transplant kidneys from living non-relatives.

Kidney transplantation is especially important in the North, East Siberian, and Far East regions of Russia, where population density is low, and hemodialysis units are lacking or too far away. PD treatment is most expensive in these remote areas, since the severity of the climate often makes it difficult to transport dialysis solutions. For this reason, the best way to provide RRT is kidney transplantation, and there are 42 kidney transplant centers in large cities such as Moscow, St. Petersburg, Ekaterinburg, Novisibirsk, and Omsk.

Unfortunately, however, due to contradictory legislature and a shortage of donor organs, kidney transplantation has decreased in recent years. Only 409 renal transplantations were performed in 2002, 20 of them coming from living related donors. Still, while the rate of kidney transplantation is slowing down, 2002 figures still show the raise of kidney graft recipients of 34.5% from the rate in 1998 (Table 1).

RENAL REPLACEMENT THERAPY: PATIENT STATE

Russian patients on RRT differ in many respects from RRT patients in Europe and the United States. Younger to begin with, they also show a different pattern of ESRD causes, due, for the most part, to the lack of HD stations.

In 2002, men accounted for 54% of Russians on RRT. As much as only 6.7% of patients on HD were above the age of 65 (3), and most patients receiving HD treatment were between the ages 20 and 64 (Fig. 1). These tendencies became even more prominent among patients with a functioning kidney graft and patients on PD.

Statistics also revealed the leading cause of ESRD among dialysis populations to be glomerulonephritis, though this was rarely proved by biopsy (Fig. 2). Diabetic nephropathy accounted for 9% of current incident patients and 5% of all patients, while hypertension accounted for 5.2% among incident patients and 2.3% of prevalent patients. Meanwhile, the prevalence of congenital uropathies among children was higher than among the rest of RRT patients, as did pyelonephritis, hypertensive and diabetic nephropathies among the older population. These trends were characteristic of statistics polled in 1998.

Another important feature of HD patients in Russia is that in most of them the treatment starts late, only to encounter a shortage of HD machines. The median creatinine clearance for patients who started HD in 2002 was 8.0 mL/min (calculated according to the Cockroft–Gault formula), and the prevalence of hypertension (blood pressure above 140/90 mmHg) among these patients was 80%.

Erythropoietin (EPO) therapy has been available in Russia since the year 2000, but there is still a significant shortage of erythropoetin in many of the regions. For economic reasons, the practice of pre-dialysis EPO treatment has not been implemented either. These circumstances have led to very low hemoglobin levels in the majority of patients starting HD. In 2002, these levels ranged widely—with a quarter of patients registering

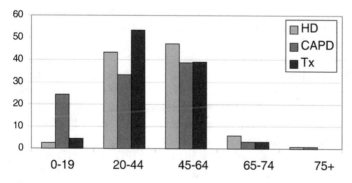

Figure 1 Age distribution of prevalent patients, by RRT modality.

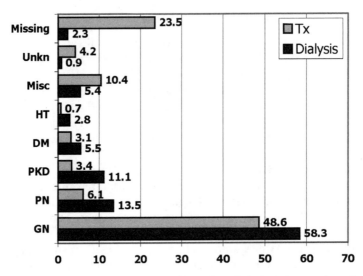

Figure 2 Primary renal disease in prevalent dialysis and transplanted patients (GN–glomerulonephritis, PN–pyloneophritis, PKD–Polycystic kidneys, DM–Diabetes mellitus, HT–Hypertension, Misc–Miscellaneous, Unkn–Unknown).

hemoglobin levels of less than 70 g/L, and 17.2% of patients at more than 100 g/L. However, as EPO therapy has become more accessible, hemoglobin levels have increased to 100 g/L and higher among 40% of the prevalent population.

HD is adequate among only half of prevalent patients, according to data figured by calculating the ratio of urea reduction, and among two-thirds of the HD population for whom Kt/V was calculated as an index of delivered dialysis dose.

In spite of the fact that dialysis is often started late, the 1-year survival rate of incident HD patients is rather high—90.2% in the year 2002, as compared to 87.6% in the year 2000—due, perhaps, to the recent abandonment of the cuprofan membrane in almost all of the dialysis units, as well as to modernization of HD equipment and the spread of bicarbonate dialysis throughout the country.

In 2002, Moscow accounted for as much as 18% of HD patients and 48% of PD patients in Russia overall. According to a more detailed analysis of patient survival on different dialysis modalities in Moscow, the 5-year survival rate of HD patients in cohort treated between the years 1995 and 2002 was 51.9%, and 46.7% among patients treated with PD (Fig. 3). Noteworthy, that in the whole cohort of patients during the first 4 years of treatment, statistics were significantly higher for PD than HD among both diabetic and non-diabetic patients, as well as among the patients of all ages (Table 2). And these data are similar to the results published by

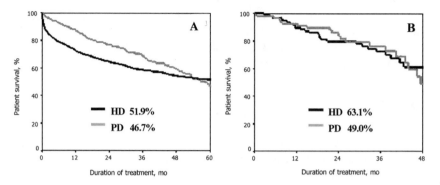

Figure 3 Survival probability of incident patients, by dialysis modality (Moscow RRT registry, 1995–2002). A–unadjusted ($n = 3241$, $p < 0.0005$), B–adjusted for age, sex, comorbidity status and laboratory measurements ($n = 230$, $p = 0.8$), by the Kaplan-Meier analysis.

others (5). But in a more detailed analysis of the survival rate in groups of patients adjusted for age, sex, comorbidity status, and laboratory measurements, no difference in survival between HD and PD was found: 1-year survival rates were 90.5% and 91.2% on HD and PD respectively, and the figures by the end of each following year equaled 79.7% and 83.8%, 72.4% and 76.4%, 63.1% and 49% on HD and PD, respectively (Fig. 3). Meanwhile, the 5-year technique survival among patients under peritoneal dialysis was 48%. The rate of peritonitis ranged from one episode every 24 patient-months to one every 28.

Table 2 Survival Probability of Incident Patients, by Dialysis Modality, Age and Presence of Diabetes Mellitus (Moscow RRT Registry, 1995–2002, $n = 3241$), Unadjusted

	Survival (%)							
	12 months		24 months		36 months		48 months	
	HD	PD	HD	PD	HD	PD	HD	PD
Total*	74.8	90.5	66.7	82.8	61.3	74.5	57.2	47.4
Age								
≤49 years**	80.8	95.5	73.6	86.9	69.8	75.5	67.2	56.9
50–64 years***	72.6	83.8	64.4	78.9	59.3	73.3	53.1	25.1
≥65 years***	58.9	94.4	50.8	67.3	39.9	67.3	39.4	67.3
DM*	60.5	92.6	47.0	79.4	40.2	66.1	32.7	33.1
No DM*	77.7	91.2	70.7	83.8	65.7	76.4	61.9	49.0

*The difference between survival rate on HD and PD statistically significant in all groups: **$p < 0.001$ by log-rank test; ***$p < 0.001$ by Breslow test; *$p < 0.01$ by log-rank test.

In most cases, death among dialysis patients was due to cardiovascular disease, regardless of the treatment modality. The mortality rate due to cardiovascular diseases was 43%, while infectious diseases accounted for 4.4% and discontinued dialysis for 5.5%.

DISCUSSION

Russia is a massive country with an extremely non-uniform population spread and relatively complicated economic conditions. In spite of these factors, renal replacement therapy has been developing rather quickly in recent years—quicker, in many cases, than in other countries (4). Nevertheless, the level of RRT is still insufficient, having yet to overtake levels in many parts of Central and Eastern Europe (6).

One possible way to improve RRT supply would be the institution of a new system by which local governments reimburse expenditures of local private dialysis units. This approach was successfully applied in Moscow, resulting in a two-time increase of HD patients over the last 4 years. Currently, about half of Moscow's HD patients are being treated in private dialysis units.

Given the gap between required and supplied RRT, another means of improvement would be to direct the attention of local health authorities to the problem and actively work with them to solve it. To this end, epidemiological studies and registries, both national and local, that count patients with CKD, chronic renal insufficiency, and ESRD, are indispensable. So far, such a registry only exists in Moscow, but similar data collection systems have recently been organized in other large cities such as Novosibirsk, Irkutsk, and St. Petersburg. To date, no data from these registries have been published.

However, much of Russia's nephrological situation can be discerned from the available Moscow data. In August 2004, 10,819 patients with CKD were registered in Moscow—a prevalence rate of 104.5 per 100,000, or 0.1% of the entire population. Among them, 3549 (32.8%) have chronic renal insufficiency and 2078 (19.2%) have ESRD. However, the official count of patients with CKD is undoubtedly underestimated, since there is currently no ongoing program specially geared toward detection of CKD, meaning that the available data are based only on active referral. Significantly, over the past few years, the number of registered CKD patients has jumped by an annual mean increment of 18%. This is a powerful indicator of growth in the number of patients and increased attention paid to problems of CKD.

The third and likely most effective way to address the problem would be further development of renoprotection, using angiotensin-converting enzyme inhibitors (ACEI), throughout the country. For several years already, the ACEI most widely available have been enalapril and monopril.

While these two drugs have been prescribed to patients with diabetes mellitus for quite some time, they have recently become regular treatment for patients with other forms of CKD as well.

Further development of RRT will be much more effective in the presence of a state-funded program, the resolution of the legislative contradictions in the field of transplantation, the establishment of local manufacturers of PD solutions, and, last but not least, a general improvement in Russia's economic situation.

REFERENCES

1. http://econ.worldbank.org/wdr/wdr2004/ (accessed May 2004).
2. http://www.who.int/country/rus/en/ (accessed May 2004).
3. Bikbov BT, Tomilina NA. Report on the state of renal replacement therapy in Russia on behalf of the registry of Russian dialysis society [in Russian]. Nephrologia i Dializ 2004; 6:4–42.
4. Moeller S, Gioberge S, Brown G. ESRD patients in 2001: global overview of patients, treatment modalities and developing trends. Nephrol Dial Transplant 2002; 17:2071–2076.
5. Fenton SSA, Schaubel DE, Desmeules M, Morrison HI, Mao Y, Copleston P, Jeffery JR, Kjellstrand CM. Hemodialysis versus peritoneal dialysis: a comparison of adjusted mortality rates. Am J Kidney Dis 1997; 30:334–342.
6. Rutkowski B. Changing pattern of end-stage renal disease in central and eastern Europe. Nephrol Dial Transplant 2000; 15:156–160.

16

Nephrology in China: A Specialty Preparing for the 21st Century Challenge

Shanyan Lin

Division of Nephrology, Hua Shan Hospital, Fudan University, Jiangwan, Shanghai, China

Bicheng Liu

Zhongda Hospital, Southeast University, Nanjing, China

Fanfan Hou

Nanfang Hospital, The First Military Medical University, Guangzhou, China

Jiaqi Qian

Renji Hospital, Shanghai Second Medical University, China

The origin of nephrology in China can be traced up to 200 B.C.; at that time some kidney diseases were recorded as "jiang" in "52 prescriptions." As documented in "Suwen," one of the Chinese earliest ancient medical works written about 100 B.C., our ancestors have realized the kidney's role in the body as an organ regulating water and tissue fluid. If the kidney is impaired, the patient will manifest increasing urine output or reduction of urine excretion, and even edema. Furthermore, traditional Chinese medicine had noted the relationship between bone metabolism disturbance and the kidney. They believed a doctor could judge a patient kidney's function from the appearance of the hair and face. If the kidney doesn't work well, bones will be fragile and easy to fracture, and the patient will suffer weakness and backache. During the Donghan dynasty (about A.D. 200), Zhang Zhong-jing suggested that the treatment of edema should be divided into two parts: when the edema was mainly in the lower limbs, diuretics could be prescribed, while when the edema was mainly in the face, sudatories would be more appropriate. However, we must note that the Chinese "kidney" is not equivalent to the meaning of kidney we are familiar with in the western book. Actually, what Chinese doctors thought was that "kidney" might include many functional parts of the human body. In the hundreds years fighting with renal disease, Chinese doctors diagnosed and treated the patients based on its unique theory, which mostly are empirical.

The practice of modern nephrology commenced in China in the late 1950s. Since 1980s, with the opening of China to the outside World, nephrology has greatly developed. Chinese nephrologists have gradually become active members of the international nephrology community. The first committee of the Chinese Society of Nephrology (CSN) was established in 1980 and the Society held its first academic congress in 1982. The Chinese Journal of Nephrology was first formally published in Guangzhou in 1985. Efforts to develop a comprehensive registry for dialysis and transplantation in China began in 1998.

Nephrologists are faced with a great mission and momentous challenges in China, a vast country with a huge population of 1.3 billion and a broad territory of 9.6 million square kilometers.

NEPHROLOGY SPECIALIST IN CHINA

Since the 1980s, nephrology has been gradually becoming an independent specialty in most large hospitals, including teaching hospitals affiliated to medical universities/colleges, province level hospitals, and the highest ranked hospitals in the metropolis (Beijing, Shanghai, Guangzhou, Nanjing, Wuhan, Shenyang, etc.). Although there is no specified nephrology division in many hospitals in medium-sized cities, there are always specialized groups taking care of renal patients. From June 1999 to June 2000, a registration organized by CSN found that the number of divisions of nephrology in province-level, city-level hospitals was 864, and the average number of doctors was 4.09 per million population (pmp), nurses 6.66 pmp, and technicians 0.53 pmp. There are 708 doctors specializing in nephrology within traditional medicine, accounting for 14.0% of overall nephrologists. Regarding the educational levels of doctors, 85.8% graduated from university, bearing Bachelor degree of medicine. Among them, 14.7% were awarded Masters or Doctorate degrees. For nurses and technicians, only 1.4% and 19.0% received standard university education, respectively, and 24.6% and 39.5% were actually educated in a specialized professional college (1).

The geographical distribution of medical services in the whole of China is quite imbalanced. The most deprived regions are in the Northwest and Southwest of China, and great effort should be taken in the future to improve medical services there.

CLINICAL NEPHROLOGY

Diagnosis of Renal Disease

Renal biopsy is commonly performed in major renal centers in China since 1980s. According to incomplete statistics (up to the end of 1998), 77,953 patients had a renal biopsy in China (1). The renal pathologists who interpret these biopsies have good clinical background. The renal tissue is routinely examined by light and fluorescence microscopy. Electron microscopic analysis is available in hospitals affiliated to medical schools. Thus, morphological diagnosis of renal diseases is essential, especially for cases of rapidly progressive glomerulonephritis or acute allograft rejection in most academic renal centers. However, due to the economic status and shortage of medical resources, renal biopsy cannot be performed in rural and relatively small city hospitals. So both clinical and pathological classifications of primary glomerulonephritis (GN) are applied in evaluating the renal patients.

Distribution of Renal Disease in China

Renal biopsy was performed routinely in China in the last 20 years. However, a nationwide renal registry has not yet been organized. The largest single-center analysis including 13,519 cases was reported by Li and Liu (2) recently. As many patients came from various regions all over the country, it might be taken as an illustration of the epidemiology of renal disease in China. In total, 13,519 cases were collected during the period of January 1979 to December 2002. Among them, 7752 cases (57.3%) were male and 5767 cases (42.6%) were female. Their age averaged 32.7 ± 12.2 (9–83) years. Primary GN accounted for 68.64%, secondary GN accounted for only 24.84%, tubular-interstitial diseases accounted for 3.43%, hereditary or congenital renal diseases took up 0.97%, and unclassified renal diseases took up 0.87% (Table 1). It was clearly shown that primary GN remained the most important and prevalent kidney disease in China. The ratio of primary to secondary GN as a whole was 2.75:1 (9278/3380). However, this ratio is progressively decreasing in the past two decades. It started from 3.61:1 (78.3–21.7%) in 1979 to 1985 and dropped steadily to 2.01:1 (66.8–33.2%) in 1998 and 1999. There was an increase in the incidence of secondary glomerular diseases such as diabetic nephropathy and nephrosclerosis. In addition, this change might be due to more cases of secondary GN diagnosed owing to improvement in the recognition of these diseases and more sophisticated diagnostic skills. In general, many cases of this category such as lipoprotein glomerulopathy, obesity-related glomerulopathy, and Fabry's disease were identified only in the past decade. Obviously, some of them might have been missed before. Most cases of the Alport syndrome were diagnosed in the past 5 years after the introduction of type IV collagen

Table 1 Pathological Classification of 13,519 Cases of Renal Diseases (1979–2002, Nanjing)

Pathological classification	Cases	Percentage (%)
Primary glomerulonephritis	9,278	68.64
Secondary glomerulonephritis related to:	3,359	24.84
Systemic disease	2,673	19.77
Lupus nephritis	1,824	13.49
Henoch-Schönlein purpura glomerulonephritis	685	5.07
Metabolic disease	345	2.55
Diabetic nephropathy	222	1.64
Amyloidosis	76	0.56
Vascular disease	244	1.80
Infections	97	0.72
Hereditary and congenital renal disease	131	0.97
Tubulo-interstitial disease	464	3.43
Rare renal diseases[a]	37	0.27
Sclerosing glomerulonephritis	132	0.98
Unclassified renal disease	118	0.87

[a]Obesity-related glomerulopathy, lipoprotein glomerulopathy, fibrillary glomerulopathy, Niemann Pick disease, Fabry's disease, POEMS syndrome.

chains staining. Therefore, the real frequency of these diseases should be higher than that shown in Table 1 and need to be further evaluated (2).

Among the primary causes of GN diagnosed by renal biopsy, IgA nephropathy is the leading cause (45.26%), followed by mesangial proliferative lesion (MsPL, 25.62%), membranous nephropathy (MN, 9.89%) and focal segmental glomerulosclerosis (FSGS, 6.00%) (2).

The pattern of secondary glomerular diseases seen in China is clearly quite different from that of the Western countries. Lupus nephritis is the most common and important renal disease in China, while diabetic nephropathy, the most common renal disease occurring in the United States, currently represents less than 7% of this group of patients. No doubt, this tendency might change in the next few decades, as the incidence of diabetes mellitus is progressively increasing in China.

Common Nephropathies in China

IgA Nephropathy (IgAN)

IgA nephropathy (IgAN) is the most prevalent pattern of primary glomerular disease in Asia-Pacific countries. The pattern of primary glomerular diseases occurring in China is unique in its high prevalence of IgA nephropathy (IgAN). It accounts for 30–40% of all primary glomerular diseases. Whether the high prevalence is related to genetic background, environmental factors, or frequent infections (either bacterial or viral) is uncertain.

Hao et al. (3) analyzed the clinical presentation and pathological feature of 524 cases with IgAN retrospectively. Among them, 289 cases (55.2%) were male and 235 cases (44.8%) were female. Their age averaged 28 (4–69) years, and youths and adults account for the most part of IgAN patients. In children group ($\leq$15 years, 20.6%), the incidence of recurrent gross hematuria was 47.2% and renal impairment 4.6%. Malignant hypertension as the first presentation associated with serious renal impairment occurred in 3.8% patients of youth and adult group (16–49 years, 74.6%). Higher incidence of nephrotic syndrome and acute renal failure was found in elder group (50–69 years, 4.8%), accounting for 35.0% and 8.0%, respectively. The incidence of hypertension in IgAN was 39.62%, which may be associated with many factors including familial history of hypertension, degree of proteinuria, level of serum creatinine, and degree of renal arteriolar lesion (4). In patients with IgAN, vascular lesion parallels the blood pressure, serum triglyceride, urine protein, serum creatinine, etc. Of 1005 IgAN patients, 54.6% were with vascular lesions. Multivariate logistic regression analysis showed that the influencing factors on vascular lesions included hypertension, high serum uric acid, global glomerular sclerosis ($\geq$50%), interstitial inflammation ($\geq$50%), and pathological grade III–V. It reflects the disease degree and can be used as an important histological prognostic indicator (5).

Interestingly, some doctors studied the relationship between the pathological form of IgAN and TCM manifestations (6). They classified the symptom in four TCM types. A multicenter, prospective study proved that the TCM syndrome type of patients with IgAN was significantly correlated with the grade and severity of their renal pathological changes. Patients of Pi–Fei Qi deficiency type (type 1) and both Qi–Yin deficiency type (type 2) showed rather milder pathological changes, by Lee classification, most of them belong to grade I–III (72.3%, 70.2%). Patients of Gan-Shen Yin deficiency type (type 3) had severe pathological change and majority of them belong to grade III–IV (84.6%). And the most severe pathological change was shown in patients of Pi–Shen Yang deficiency type (type 4), and the Lee's grade IV–V was dominant (88.0%) in these patients. Percentage of glomerular sclerosis in patients of type 4 was higher than that in patients of the other three types. The TCM syndrome type showed definite referential importance to conclude the severity of renal pathological changes in patients with IgAN (6).

Treatment options that slow the progression of IgAN are becoming available in China. For patients with only minor urinary abnormalities but without hypertension, the general consensus in China is not to offer specific treatment but to follow up the patients over many years. For those with proteinuria and/or hypertension, preventing this kind of renal disease from progressing to end-stage renal disease (ESRD) by using angiotensin-converting-enzyme inhibitors (ACEI), or angiotensin II type 1 receptor blocks (ARB) is recommended. Shi et al. (7) reported a randomized controlled trial in Chinese people by using ACEI. One hundred and thirty-one cases with IgAN diagnosed by renal biopsy, whose 24-hours proteinuria excretion over 0.5 g/d, serum creatinine (SCr) level below 3 mg/dL, were randomly divided into two groups: ACEI group (benazepril 10–20 mg/d) and non-ACEI group (calcium channel blockers, beta adrenergic receptor blockers, and/or alpha adrenergic receptor blockers) as control. After 18 months of treatment, the level of pro-teinuria decreased significantly and the endogenous creatinine clearance rate (Ccr) was stable in the ACEI group, while in the control group the proteinuria level increased and the Ccr decreased. In ACEI group, it was shown that nor-mal blood pressure, normal renal function, I–II degree of Lee's grade, and mild glomerular sclerosis predicted better response than those with hyperten-sion, renal insufficiency, V degree of Lee's grade. ACEI should be used as ear-lier as possible (7). Chen et al. (8) divided 71 cases of IgAN, Lee's grade ≥III and with fibrinogen deposits, into two groups to be treated for 12 months with either urokinase + benazepril (UK + BZ) or BZ alone. After 12 months of treatment, 25 of 35 patients (71.4%) in the UK + BZ group and 16 of 36 (44.4%) in the BZ-alone group had a ≥50% decrease in 24-hours urinary protein excretion compared with the baseline, and the therapeutic efficiency of UK+BZ was better than that of BZ alone. The Ccr was stable in the UK+BZ group, while Ccr declined significantly at 12 months in the BZ-alone group compared with baseline. Combined therapy with UK and BZ was more effective than with BZ alone in reducing proteinuria and protecting renal func-tion in patients with severe IgAN. Corticosteroids, and other immunosuppres-sive agents are only used in patients with nephrotic range proteinuria in China, while its use in non-nephrotic proteinuria is still controversial. A randomized controlled trial has proven that treatment with steroids could reduce protei-nuria and slow the decline of renal function (9). Recently, it has been reported that mycophenolate mofeil (MMF), a novel immunosuppressive agent, is more effective in reducing proteinuria and serum lipid than the currently wide-spread use of prednisone therapy in IgA nephropathy, and has less adverse effects with good tolerance (10). Chinese herbs, such as tripterygium, emodin, have also been prescribed by Chinese nephrologists for the treatment of IgAN with proteinuria for many years. In a retrospective study, 44 patients with advanced IgAN received a combined regime with tripterygium, emodin, and benazepril; the results showed that this combined regime could effectively reduce proteinuria and preserve renal function (11). Xu et al. (12) reported a combined regime of tripterygium wilfordii (TW) plus benazepril and emodin on IgAN, whose 24-hours proteinuria excretion over 1.0 g/d, serum creati-nine (SCr) level below 3 mg/dL, and pathological lesion was grade III or IV according to Lee's histological grading systems. Twelve patients (the herbs group) received the combined regime (TW, emodin, and ACEI) and the other 12 patients (control group) received treatment with prednisone and ACEI. After following up for 12 months, the amount of proteinuria was significantly decreased in the herbs group than in the control group, and no significant change of SCr was observed. Repeated renal biopsy study showed that glomerular index (GI) was significantly attenuated in the herbs group, while tubular-interstitial index (TI) and vascular index (VI) tends to decrease although it has not reach statistical significance. Combined regime of TW plus benazepril and emodin was effective in patients with IgAN by reducing proteinuria, improving renal function, and preventing the progression of renal fibrosis in patients with IgAN. However, it must be noted that there is no placebo-controlled randomized clinical trial on the long-term efficacy of herbs in IgAN so far.

Lupus Nephritis (LN)

Lupus nephritis is one of the most common forms of secondary GN in China. In south China, the occurrence of renal damage was more than 80%, which takes up the highest incidence among all clinical manifestations in SLE (13). The ratio of male LN to female LN was 1:5.2. Compared with female LN, arthritis and positive rate of ANA were more commonly occurred in male LN. Other clinical and pathological features of LN were similar in male and female patients (14). In a study with 48 patients with obvious clinical manifestation of renal damage, renal biopsy showed that most of them were Class IV (67%), followed by Class III (19%), Class II (13%) (15).

During the clinical course, it was seen that the renal pathological classification of LN was changing in certain patients. A retrospective study showed that 16 cases had pathologic class changed in 48 repeated biopsies. Seven cases changed to Class IV, five to class II, three to Class V from other classes, and one to Class III from Class II (16). Thus, the histologic classification of renal morphology at initial presentation did not fully predict the outcome.

As in other countries, induction treatment includes corticosteroids, cytoxic agents, and plasma exchange in the acute phase of the disease, and while corticosteroids, cytotoxic agents, and other newer forms of immunosuppressive agents have been used in the chronic phase of LN as maintenance therapy. In a study of 23 patients with biopsy-proven membranous lupus nephropathy, Hu et al. (17) reported the effect of cyclosporine A (CsA) in combination with prednisone on type V LV, after following up for 6–36 months (mean 16.8 ± 8.4 months), 12 patients (52.2%) achieved complete remission, 10 patients (43.3%) achieved partial remission after CsA treatment, and one patient showed no response. At the end of following up, all the patients had a normal SCr. Relapse occurred in 33.3% of the patients after withdrawing CsA for 4 to 24 months (17). Recently, an open-labeled prospective trial showed that MMF was more effective in Chinese patients in controlling the clinical activity of diffuse proliferative lupus nephritis and renal vascular lesions as compared with cyclophosphamide (CYC) pulse therapy (18). MMF therapy seems more effective in reducing proteinuria and hematuria. It was also suggested that MMF seems more effectively inhibiting the auto-antibody production (especially anti-dsDNA) and decreasing serum cryoglobulin levels. Following up for 3–6 months, repeated renal biopsy suggested that MMF significantly attenuate the renal pathological lesion (including reduction in glomerular immune deposits, less glomerular necrosis, microthrombi, crescent formation, and vascular changes) as compared to that in CYC group. The incidence of infection, especially viral infection in MMF group was remarkably lower than that in CYC group. Interestingly, some Chinese nephrologists have more likely used herbs to treat LN and generated some precious clinical experience. Guo et al. (19) demonstrated that using herbs appropriately in addition to immunosuppressants in active LN could significantly reduce the side effects of immunosuppressants and enhance the remission rate. Furthermore, herbs together with steroids might reduce the recurrence rate. As in treating other diseases, using herbs in LN is still empirical, and the effectiveness is fully based on doctor's own experience and the prescription may be different from patients to patients. It is compulsory to design randomized controlled clinical trials to explore the effective therapies.

Diabetic Nephropathy (DN)

Diabetic nephropathy (DN) is a leading cause of ESRD in Western societies. Diabetes is the single largest cause of ESRD in the United States and in some European countries, accounting for over one-third of all patients beginning renal replacement therapy. Patients with type 2 diabetes comprise the largest and faster growing single-disease group requiring renal replacement therapy. Fortunately, it is not the case currently in China. However, we must note that the rising incidence of diabetes and the increasing proportion of cases of ESRD induced by DN. DN only took up 1% in 1980s, 4.9% in 1985, but had strikingly increased to 10.6% in 1999 and even 17.6% in 2000 in China. Furthermore, the increasing obesity in Shanghai and other major cities (<30% in children aged 8–12 in 2000 in Shanghai) suggests the future preponderance of DN among cases of progressive renal failure in China. A survey of diabetes prevalence in the middle-aged and elderly Chinese from 12 areas of China showed that the prevalence of diabetes was 5.89% (95% CI: 5.62–6.16%), and that of IGT was 5.90% (95% CI: 5.63–6.17%). There were significant variations of standardized prevalence of diabetes among 12 areas in China. The prevalence of diabetes (urban: 6.8%, rural: 3.8%) varied significantly about one-fold in urban population than that in rural populations (20). Currently, diabetic nephropathy constitutes 10–20% of the cases of secondary glomerulopathy in China. So the prevention of diabetic nephropathy and the management of these patients have become a great challenge in China.

As it in other countries, treatment of this disease in China mainly focuses on the prevention of progression of the disease and reducing the complications during the later stage of this disease. Antihypertensive agents, specifically ACEIs and ARBs, have been widely recommended in treatment of diabetic nephropathy. Liu et al. (21) demonstrated that irbesartan exerted early renal protective role in diabetic nephrology, possibly through inhibition of renal hypertrophy and renal expression of connective tissue growth factor. In recent years, patient's education has been emphasized as one of the integrated therapies of DN in most diabetes center. More recently, some investigators found that rhein, an effective compounds from Chinese herb, could ameliorate hypertriglyceridemia and hypercholesterolemia, reduce the excretion of urinary protein, and markedly improve the structural lesions of glomeruli including mesangial expansion, diffuse glomerulosclerosis, and thickening of glomerular basement membrane in diabetic rats with type 2 diabetes mellitus (22). However, there are no convincing data on its efficacy in human diabetic nephropathy yet.

Nephrotic Syndrome (NS)

In China, the most frequently diagnosed pathological form of NS is mesangial proliferative lesion (MsPL, 29.3%), followed by MN (16.0%) and IgAN (15.1%) (23). Both ACEIs and ARBs are generally accepted as a basic treatment for NS, so long as there is no significant contraindica tion. Treatment of NS in China is basically based on the pathological classification in teaching hospital. However, it is still an empirical-based practice in most county hospitals to treat NS without pathological guidance. Most immunosuppressants are available and their choices generally adopted the international guideline or commensurate. More recently, new type of immunosupressants such as cyclosporine, MMF, and FK506 have been tried in Chinese patients. The combined treatment of MMF/prednisone decreased the urine protein and elevated the serum albumin significantly among 41 patients with primary nephrotic syndrome in Beijing. More interestingly, the side effects were tolerable and renal function remained stable during the treatment with this drug (24). Another prospective and multicenter clini cal study also demonstrated that MMF combined with oral prednisone was effective in treating primary nephrotic and well tolerated by the Chinese patients (25).

It is the generally accepted practice to add some herbs to NS patients aiming at reducing the side effects of immunosuppressant and increasing remission rate, although there is no convincing randomized controlled clinical trial to demonstrate that. Recently, a meta-analysis of Radix

Astragali, a Chinese herb, on primary nephrotic syndrome in adults in China has been done (26). There were 14 randomized controlled trials with 524 cases involved. It was shown that Radix Astragali could enhance the therapeutic effect of prednisone and immunosuppressant for primary nephritic syndrome and reduce its recurrence. Radix Astragali also had an effect in decreasing 24-hours proteinuria content and the plasma levels of total cholesterol and albumin. The definite effect of Radix Astragali for NS should be further confirmed by multiple-center, large-sample randomized controlled trial.

Acute Renal Failure (ARF)

ARF is an important and common clinical problem that is encountered frequently by most practicing clinicians both in China and the other parts of the world. ARF is not a single disease entity but rather a syndrome caused by a multiplicity of different diseases and pathophysiologic mechanisms. Chen et al. (27) reported a group of data suggesting that among the etiology of ARF, 16% were pre-renal, 5.6% post-renal, and 78.4% renal parenchymal ARF. For the parenchymal ARF, 80.6% were acute tubulointerstitial lesions. And infection and shock were the leading cause of ARF (24.8%), drug-induced ARF took up 22.4%. Wang et al. (28) has retrospectively analyzed the etiological changes of ARF in the past 18 years; it was suggested that ARF caused by renal parenchymal diseases and tumor was increased in 1991–2000, accounting for 26%, while it was only 8.3% in 1983–1990. Recently, the importance of renal biopsy in assisting to diagnose the ARF has been increasingly recognized by Chinese nephrologists. Statistics from Jinling Hospital showed zero case in 1984, two cases from 1985 to 1986, 49 cases from 1997 to 1998. ARF was observed chiefly in glomerular disease (35.9%), tubular-interstitial disease (48.0%), and secondary renal disease (16.2%). The most common glomerular diseases associated with ARF were crescentic glomerulonephritis and diffuse proliferative glomerulonephritis (accounted for 42.3% and 18.3% of glomerulonephritis, respectively). Acute interstitial nephritis (63.2%) and acute tubular necrosis (36.8%) were responsible for the ARF induced by tubular-interstitial lesions. The secondary renal diseases included vasculitis, microangiopathy, and cast nephropathy (29). The incidence and mortality of ARF remain high, early diagnosis may be beneficial in improving the prognosis of ARF.

Treatment of ARF in China is the same as other part of the world. Early dialysis for severe cases has been widely accepted to improve the survival rates. With the increasing of MODS, modalities of continuous renal replacement therapy (CRRT) have been introduced more aggressively, and it has been accepted as a regular therapy for MODS in most teaching hospitals, although the exact benefit of this therapy is still to be confirmed.

End-Stage Renal Disease (ESRD)

ESRD in China was most often associated with IgAN making up 26.70% of all such cases, followed by renal vasculitis (14.33%), LN (10.88%), and FSGS (9.60%) (2). Since the mid-1980s, there has been a marked increase in the incidence of ESRD across the world. From 1999.1.1 to 1999.12.31; the registration of dialysis was performed by CSN, using questionnaire. In total, 41,755 patients underwent maintenance dialysis and the point prevalence was 33.16 pmp, and the annual incidence rate was 15.3 pmp. Meanwhile, in Shanghai, the point prevalence was 180 pmp and the annual incidence rate is 102 pmp (1). It was clear that the annual incidence rate and the point prevalence in Shanghai were more than the average in whole China. However, the prevalence rate of ESRD seems lower than the developed World. Although the exact reason is unknown, it appears to us that in vast rural areas of China, ESRD has not been appropriately diagnosed and treated due to the shortage of resources and finance.

According to the Chinese registry data, the first cause of chronic renal failure was glomerulonephritis (49.9%), and then diabetic nephropathy (13.3%), hypertensive nephrosclerosis (9.6%), polycystic kidney disease (2.8%, Fig. 1) (1). In one group of maintained hemodialysis patients in Jinling Hospital, the leading cause of ESRD was primary GN (66.1%), in which IgAN was the most common type. Secondary GN accounted for 17.1%, and lupus nephritis, DN, and hypertensive nephrosclerosis were the top three common types (6.1%, 4.9%, 2.1%, respectively) (30).

As compared with the figures from developed countries, the prevalence of glomerulonephritis as the chief cause of ESRD in China is very striking, which is quite different from the fact that diabetic nephropathy is the leading cause of ESRD in developed countries. However, the situation has been

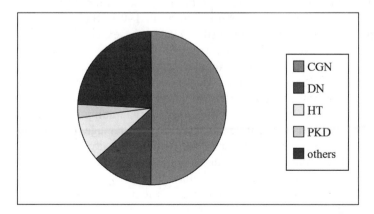

Figure 1 Cause of ESRD in China.

changing with the rising incidence of diabetes in China. Incidence of diabetes has risen from 1% in the 1980s to 3.25–5.95% in 2003, and this disease is estimated to more than 40 million people in the whole country. Diabetic nephropathy occupied 3% of all ESRD cases in the 1980s, while the figure has dramatically grown to 10–20% now (1).

Both dialysis and transplantation are the currently available therapy in China, although its development is quite unbalanced in different areas in this country. Due to the unaffordable financial support, a reluctant, conservative, non-dialytic treatment is widely used in most patients. Low-protein/low-phosphate diets, the use of ACEIs and ARBs, together with recombinant human erythropoietin (rhEPO) are widely used to mitigate the symptom of ESRD patients in China.

Traditional Chinese Medicine (TCM) in the form of herbal decoctions has been used extensively in the treatment of uremic patients for many years and remains the cornerstone of treatment in rural areas, although its exact effectiveness is still uncertain. In the past, herbal medicine has been prescribed for ESRD on an exclusively empiric basis. Strenuous efforts have been made in recent years to screen the effectiveness and therapeutic action of various individual herbs. An uncontrolled study suggested that rhubarb could reduce protein excretion in urine and slow the progression of human ESRD. Besides, it was shown that rhubarb attenuated mesangial cell proliferation and fibronectin production. It also delayed the progression of glomerular sclerosis by inhibiting hypertrophy of glomeruli and production of extracelluar matrix in diabetic rats. Although a number of experimental data suggested its benefit in the treatment of chronic renal diseases, it is still a challenge to recruit a large-scale clinical trial on the evidence-based medicine for this potential drug. It has been reported recently that Astragali and Angelica (A&A) also had inhibitory effect on lipid metabolites in rat nephrotic and glomerulosclerotic models (31). Also it decreased the accumulation of extracellular matrix in glomeruli, tubules, interstitium, and down-regulating the protein and mRNA expression of TGF-β in these rats (32). However, efforts must be taken to further clarify the exact mechanisms and testify their effectiveness by clinical trials.

In the long-term fighting to the renal diseases, Chinese nephrologists have taken great effort to find drugs from thousand of herbs, which has been suggested to benefit the renal patients. However, some Chinese herbs have been associated with severe toxicity. Inappropriate administration of Chinese herbs may cause negative effects. Kidney damage caused by inappropriate use of some Chinese herb drugs is not clinically uncommon.

The so-called Chinese herbs-related nephropathy is a new clarified type of sub-acute interstitial nephritis induced by herbs. Many studies revealed that Chinese herbs-related nephropathy is actually related to taking of Mu-tong, which contains aristolochic acid (AA), and have been inadvertently included in slimming pills (33–35). AA existed in many herbs, including Ma-dou-ling, Guan-mu-tong, Guang-fang-ji, Qing-mu-xiang, Tian-xian-teng, Xun-gu-feng, Zhu-sha-lian, etc. Since the toxic component has been clarified by Chinese doctors, it should be accurately named as aristolochic acid-related nephropathy (AAN), not Chinese herbs-related nephropathy. Clinically, AAN presented with three types: (1) acute AAN: the main presentation is tubular necrosis and acute renal failure; (2) sub-acute AAN: the main pathological and clinical manifestations were tubular degradation with atrophy, and renal tubular acidosis and/or Fanconi syndrome; (3) chronic AAN: the dominant pathological and clinical findings were renal interstitial fibrosis and chronically progressive renal failure. The main type of AAN is chronic AAN, which is taking up 80% of all AAN patients (33,34). Steroid therapy was tried to treat some patients with AAN, and it appears that steroids might have some beneficial effects in some acute and sub-acute AAN (33,34). Although kidney damage associated with Chinese herbs is not rare, no phenomenon is as extensive as that observed in Belgium and other countries (36). Stengel found that no association with Chinese herb using was found in any of ESRD patients, although the same drugs prescribed at the same doses had been widely distributed in France as in Belgium. The mechanism is still not clear. One hypothesis is a susceptibility to AAs, which is considered to be a causative agent, may be different among races. Another is that there could be some other toxic substances affecting the clinical findings although they are not identified at present. Further studies must be undertaken to clarify these differences.

DIALYSIS AND RENAL TRANSPLANTATION IN CHINA

Dialysis and kidney transplantation were introduced to China in the 1960s. In 1982, 196 hospitals were equipped with dialysis machines, and approximately 1500 patients were being treated by HD. The number of blood purification center has grown rapidly from 245 in 1984 to 305 in 1987. In 2000, the number had reached to 412. At the same time, the total number of dialysis machine in China had risen from 3874 sets in 1999 to 5040 sets in 2000. Most dialysis machines in major Chinese dialysis centers are in the brand of Fresenius, Gambro, and Baxter, while a few of them are of Nikiso Toray or B. Braun or locally made, etc. (1). Hemofiltration (HF), hemodiafiltration (HDF), and on-line HDF have been introduced to major hospitals and tended to expand further.

Continuous ambulatory peritoneal dialysis (CAPD), introduced in 1979, was rapidly adopted throughout China because of its simplicity and easy availability. However, the high frequency of peritoneal infection hindered the development of this technique. The total number of PD patient was 3763 in 1999 and 4445 in 2000 (1), which accounted for less than 10% of ESRD patients.

In 1999, 37,375 HD patients were registered, including 17,217 new cases within 1999. The annual incidence rate was 13.7 pmp and point prevalence (1999.12.31) was 29.68 pmp. In all, 4380 PD patients were registered in 1999 including 2051 new cases within 1999.

The annual incidence rate was 1.6 pmp and point prevalence (1999.12.31) was 3.48 pmp. In Shanghai, 97% patients underwent HD with autologous arteriovenous fistula. For those patients with PD, 82.8% received CAPD; 83.8% hospitals used Baxter peritoneal dialysate and 43.2% hospitals used peritoneal dialysate produced in Shanghai. Incidence of peritonitis was one time per 41.4 patient-month in cases with twin bag set (1).

It is noted that 5-year survival on HD accounted for less than 10%, and on PD less than 5% in whole China. While in Beijing, the 5-year survival rate was 19%, 17% in HD and PD, respectively (1). In Nanjing, however, the 5-year survival rate reached 64.2% in HD patients (30). Although it greatly varies from city to city, the lower survival rate is obviously related with the financial situation. The health insurance system has been establishing recently in most cities, but the capability of medical reimbursement is quite different from city to city based on the local economic situation. In most cities, patients have to pay quite large amount of money for the routine dialysis after the insurance covering, which may constitute their huge economic burden, and finally induce them to give up the therapy. So it is really a big gap that we have established a competitively technique for the patients in one hand, but on the other hand, many patients could not afford and enjoy the technical advancement. That's why we have quite good average Kt/V value, and many modern dialysis facilities, but the 5-year survival rate is very lower than the other parts in the world.

The most frequent causes of death in patients underwent maintenance dialysis were heart failure and cerebrovascular accident, accounted for 32% and 19%, respectively (Fig. 2). Besides, 16% of patients died by giving up dialysis due to financial problem.

Cardiovascular disease (CVD) is highly prevalent among ESRD patients in China and is the main reason for their high mortality and morbidity rates. It is the leading cause of death in dialysis patients, accounting for 32.20% in HD and 25.5% in PD, respectively (1). The prevalence of CVD is already very high at the beginning of renal replacement therapy (RRT). A study performed by Hou et al. (37) suggested that both clinical and echocardiographic manifestations of CVD were found to be highly prevalent in patients starting RRT in South China area. Among them, 9.1% had coronary artery disease, 39.4% had cardiac failure, and 69.3% had left-ventricular hypertrophy (LVH).

The average frequency of dialysis is 2.3 times per week. According to the data from Shanghai, the mean URR value was 0.63 (1285 cases) and the mean Kt/V was 1.34 (1227 cases) in HD patients and the average value of Kt/V was 1.7 for CAPD. The Kt/V was less than 1.2 and more than 1.6,

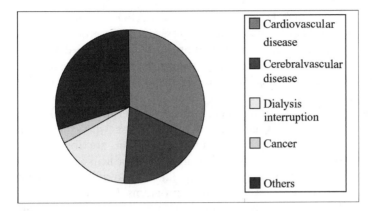

Figure 2   Cause of death in maintenance dialysis patients in China.

both accounted for 21.8% in 2626 HD patients. Inadequate hemodialysis was found in a certain part of cases (1).

According to a cross-sectional study performed in Shanghai on December 31 of 1999, the positive rate for HBV markers was 14.1% in HD patients and 14.4% in PD patients, while the positive rate for anti-HCV antibody was 28.6% in HD patients and 8.0% in PD patients. In Beijing, the situation seems to be better than in Shanghai. The positive rate for HBV markers was 3% in HD patients and 6% in PD patients. The positive rate for HCV markers was 7% in HD patients and 4% in PD patients. It was found that both HBV and HCV infection rates are closely related to the times and volume of blood transfusion and the treatment time for dialysis (1).

Anemia is a common complication of ESRD. Recombinant human erythropoietin (rhEPO) has been widely used as the alternative therapy in most patients since 1990s. However, due to the heavy economic burden, only one third of ESRD patients are treated with rhEPO. The average level of hematocrit in all patients was obviously less than normal. Although there are more than 20 bio-pharmaceutical companies producing rhEPO in China, and the pricing is much competitive (equivalent to one-third of the cost of imported products), the hematocrit levels of most cases are less than ideal (average 29.6% in HD patients and 26.7% in CAPD patients). One of the most important reasons for this may be the fact that intravenous iron preparations have not been widely used in mainland China. There were 36.83% of HD patients on oral iron treatment (1). About three-fourths of them received antihypertensive agents to control blood pressure.

Cost of RRT in Mainland China

Maintenance dialysis for patients with ESRD is one of the most expensive medical treatments in mainland China. The average annual cost for HD was US$6202–11,669, and US$9558–12,488 for CAPD, which is almost equivalent to 6–13-folds of the per capita gross domestic product. These rates are obviously much cheaper than those available in the developed nations. Nonetheless, this is still a heavy burden on the public health and social security systems of China. Inadequate hemodialysis was frequently found in a quite large part of cases in China. The financial support for dialysis comes mainly from government sources. Government employees, who work in government-owned enterprises and those who can obtain enrollment in the government health insurance program, are able to gain reimbursement for the costs of their treatment. The principle reason for non-acceptance onto dialysis programs is the inability to afford treatment for those who do not have access to insurance programs. It is now quite rare to find areas in China where dialysis is not available for lack of trained staff and facilities.

Renal Transplantation in China

The first renal transplant in China was performed in Beijing in 1960. Renal transplantation is performed by the qualified surgeons, and most of them have a background in urology. Most of the recipients of renal transplants are younger patients. Inability to pay for the procedure is still a barrier to kidney transplantation. For those with access to medical insurance, reimbursement of $100,000 Yuan (US$12,000) is available for the first year of transplantation. Cyclosporin, which is locally produced, together with MMF and prednisolone constitute the most widely used immunosuppressive regime, and tacrolimus and sirolimus also are available for application, and the cost of these agents can be reimbursed also. Monoclonal antibodies are available, but the cost of their use is not reimbursed.

By the mid-1980s, the total number of renal transplants performed exceeded 1300. The technique developed rapidly in 1990s. There had been totally 5040 transplant operations performed in 2000 and 4130 in 2001. Only less than 10% of these were from living donors. The principle source of organs is from brain-dead cadavers. There are laws enacted to govern this process and there is strict adherence to these in this country. The 12-month graft survival rate is over 80%, although there are regional differences. From 1972 to 2000, 2200 renal transplantations were performed in 1908 patients with end-stage renal failure in Beijing (38). Since the introduction of cyclosporin A (CsA) to China in 1985, the graft survival rates at 1, 3, 5 years were increased to 87.3%, 80.2%, and 60.7%, respectively. Pneumonitis was the dominant factor inducing death after renal transplantation, with an incidence of 4.49% and a mortality rate of 34.62%. The incidence of positive cytomegalovirus (CMV) infection after renal transplantation was up to 40.3%, while mortality is 8.0%. The incidence of tumor after renal transplantation was 1.5%. The most frequent site of tumor was urological system.

DISEASE REGISTRATION

The registration system in China has been established, although it is still in its infancy and the available date are incomplete. Data for the years 1999 and 2000 were published in the Chinese Journal of Nephrology in 2001. It is still a challenge to establish a nationwide network to register the patients of ESRD for the Chinese Society of Nephrology.

RESEARCH

The national nephrology research funding mainly comes from the National Science Foundation, and the Ministries of Health and Education. Besides, the National Chinese Medicine Administration Bureau also releases funds to researches on combined therapy of Chinese and Western medicine and on the application of Chinese traditional medications. Apart from the above funding, each province or city has its own research funding to support local medical researches. There is intense competition for these sources of funding. With the development of the nation's economy, the finance of the above funding is much strengthened.

EPILOGUE

Modern nephrology in China originated in late 1950s and spread quickly to nationwide in the 1980s and progressed rapidly in the 1990s. Now the basic frame of modern nephrology has been constructed. Except very few districts, almost all hospitals of province level or above have nephrology divisions, and the team of nephrology specialists is growing quite fast in most hospitals. Dialysis has become regular treatment to patients with renal failure. Our researches are catching up with international advances in some areas. However, the development of nephrology is not even in China. Due to economic status, many modern techniques for diagnosis and treatment cannot be widely used in some areas. Controlling the high incidence and studying the genetic and environmental mechanisms possibly related to the high incidence of renal disease, and establishing a nationwide network to apply guidelines for chronic kidney diseases, dialysis, and transplantation in a fashion relevant to real situations in China are major challenges to the Chinese nephrologists.

REFERENCES

1. Committee of Chinese Society of Nephrology. Chinese Dialysis and Transplantation Registration Report in 2000. Chin J Nephrol 2001; 17:72–104.
2. Li LS, Liu ZH. Epidemiologic data of renal diseases from a single unit in China: analysis based on 13,519 renal biopsies. Kidney Int 2004; 66:920–923.

3. Hao CL, Chen JJ, Zhang HX, et al. Clinical presentation and pathologic future of 524 patients with IgA nephropathy. Chin J Nephrol 2000; 16:324–327.
4. Zhuang YZ, Chen XM, Zhang YP, et al. Multivariate analysis of influencing factors for hypertension in patients with IgA nephropathy. Chin J Intern Med 2000; 39:371–375.
5. Wu J, Chen XM, Shi SZ. Significance of vascular lesions in IgA nephropathy and their influencing factors, a study of 1005 cases. Chin Med J (Zhonghua Yi Xue Za Zhi) 2003; 83:289–293.
6. Chen XM, Chen YP, Chen YP, et al. Multicenter prospective study on relationship of TCM syndrome type and renal pathology in 286 patients with IgA nephropathy. Chin J Integrated Med (Zhongguo Zhong Xi Yi Jie He Za Zhi) 2004; 24:101–105.
7. Shi XY, Chen XM, Liu SW, et al. The effect of angiotensin converting enzyme inhibitor on IgA nephropathy and the influencing factors. Chin J Intern Med 2002; 41:399–403.
8. Chen X, Qiu Q, Tang L, et al. Effects of co-administration of urokinase and benazepril on severe IgA nephropathy. Nephrol Dial Transplant 2004; 19:852–857.
9. Pozzi C, Andrulli S, Del Vecchio L, et al. Corticosteroid effectiveness in IgA nephropathy: long-term results of a randomized controlled trial. J Am Soc Nephrol 2004; 15:157–163.
10. Chen X, Chen P, Cai G, et al. A randomized control trial of mycophenolate mofeil treatment in severe IgA nephropathy. Chin Med J (Zhonghua Yi Xue Za Zhi) 2002; 25:796–801.
11. Xu MZ, Hu WX, Chen HP, et al. Evaluation of a combined regime with tripterygium, emodine and benazepril for patients with advanced IgA nephropathy. J Nephrol Dial Transplant 2002; 11:223–227.
12. Xu MZ, Hu WX, Liu ZH, et al. Prospective clinical study of a combined regime of tripterygium wilfordii plus benazepril and emodin in treatment of IgA nephropathy. J Nephrol Dial Transplant 2004; 13:19–24.
13. Chen XH, Ye RG, Yang NS, et al. Systemic lupus erythematosus: characteristics of clinical and immunologic manifestations in 720 patients. Chin J Nephrol 1999; 15:24–31.
14. Li H, Li XW, Chu GX, et al. A clinic analysis of 62 male patients with lupus nephritis. Acta Acad Med Sini (Zhongguo Yi Xue Ke Xue Yuan Xue Bao) 2000; 22:395–397.
15. Leng N, Zhu P, Wu ZP, et al. Relationship between clinical features and pathological changes of kidney in patients with systemic lupus erythematosus. Chin J Rheumatol 2004; 8:288–291.
16. Shen K, Yu Y, Tang Z, et al. The prognosis of biopsy-proven lupus nephritis in Chinese patients: long term follow-up of 86 cases. Chin Med J 1997; 110: 502–507.
17. Hu WX, Liu ZH, Shen S, et al. Cyclosporine A in treatment of membranous lupus nephropathy. Chin Med J 2003; 116:1827–1830.
18. Hu WX, Liu ZH, Chen HP, et al. Mycophenolate mofetil vs cyclophosphamide therapy for patients with diffuse proliferative lupus nephritis. Chin Med J 2002; 115:705–709.

19. Guo QY, Ye RG, Yang X, et al. Treatment of active lupus nephritis with integrated traditional Chinese herbs and modern medicine. Chin J Integrated Med (Zhongguo Zhong Xi Yi Ji He Za Zh) 2001; 2:36–38.

20. Research Cooperation Group of National 'the Ninth Five' Major Research Plan. A survey of diabetes prevalence in the middle aged and elderly Chinese from 12 areas of China. Chin J Endocrinol Metab 2002; 18:280–284.

21. Liu BC, Luo DD, Sun J, et al. Influence of irbesartan on renal hypertrophy and thickening glomerular basement membrane in streptozotocin induced diabetic rats. Chin J Intern Med 2003; 42:320–323.

22. Guo XH, Liu ZH, Ping A, et al. Rhein retards the progression of type 2 diabetic nephropathy in rats. Chin J Nephrol 2002; 18:280–284.

23. Zeng CH, Chen HP, Yu YS, et al. Clinical epidemiology of renal disease in China based on 10002 renal biopsy data. J Nephrol Dial Transplant 2001; 10:3–7.

24. Zhao MH, Chen XM, Chen YP, et al. Mycophenolate mofetil in the treatment of primary nephrotic syndrome. Chin Med J (Zhonghua Yi Xue Za Zhi) 2001; 81:528–531.

25. Lu FM, Ding XQ, Chen N, et al. Mycophenolate mofetile in treating primary nephritic syndrome: a prospective and multicenter clinical study. Chin J Nephrol 2004; 20:238–241.

26. Fan JM, Liu LS, Li Z, et al. A meta-analysis of Radix Astragali for prime nephritic syndrome in adult. Chin Med Clin Pharmacol (Zhong Yao Xin Yao yu Lin Chuang Yao Li) 2001; 3(14):62–66.

27. Chen N, Zhang W, Yu HJ, et al. Epidemiological survey of acute renal failure. Shanghai Med J 2001; 24:239–242.

28. Wang YL, Liu BC, Zhang XL, et al. An analysis of the clinical characteristic changes of ARF in past 18 years—the report of 145 cases. Clin Focus (Linchuang Huicui) 2002; 17:71–73.

29. Chen HP, Zeng CH, Li LS. Classification of acute renal failure according to histopathologic characteristics. Chin Crit Care Med 2000; 12:228–231.

30. Xie HL, Ji DX, Xu B, et al. Analysis of 25 years' maintenance hemodialysis practice in blood purification center of Jingling hospital for 25 years. J Nephrol Dial Transplant 2000; 9:405–410.

31. Wang HY, Li JZ, Pan JS, et al. The effect of Astragali and Angelica on nephritic syndrome and its mechanisms of action. J Peking Univ (Health Sci) 2002; 34:542–552.

32. Li XM, Wang HY. Opportunities and pot in renal diseases: from research to bedside. Chin Med J 1997; 110:499–501.

33. Li XM, Yang L, Yu Y, et al. An analysis of the clinical and pathological characteristics of Mu-Tong (a Chinese herb) induced tubulointerstitial nephropathy. Chin J Intern Med 2001; 40:681–687.

34. Chen W, Chen YP, Li A, et al. The clinical and pathological manifestations of aristolochic acid nephropathy—the report of 58 cases. Natl Med J China 2001; 81:1101–1105.

35. Chen W, Chen YP. Aristolochic acid nephropathy. Chin J Intern Med 2001; 40:426–427.

36. Stengel B, Jones E. End-stage renal insufficiency associated with Chinese herbal consumption in France. Nephrologie 1998; 19:15–20.

37. Hou FF, et al. Prevalence of CVD in chronic kidney diseases in South China. J Practical Hospital Clin 2005; 2(1):15–16.
38. Tang YW, Zhang YH, Jia BX, et al. Analysis of 2200 kidney transplantations. Chin Med J (Zhonghua Yi Xue Za Zhi) 2001; 18:82–85.

17

Renal Disease in Sub-Saharan Africa

Ebun L. Bamgboye

Dialysis and Transplant Unit, St. Nicholas Hospital, Lagos, Nigeria

Nomandla Madala

Department of Medicine, University of KwaZulu Natal, Durban, South Africa

Saraladevi Naicker

Division of Nephrology, University of the Witwatersrand, Johannesburg, South Africa

INTRODUCTION

Renal disease is more prevalent and tends to be more severe in Africa than in the developed world (1). Economic and manpower factors, however, impose severe restrictions on the detection and appropriate management of these patients (2). The paucity of trained personnel, absence of regional renal registries, poverty and lack of adequate governmental funding make it nearly impossible to determine precisely the epidemiology and prevalence of renal diseases in the region, a conservative estimate of 1000 new cases per million per year. Most documented studies are hospital-based and cannot truly represent the situation in the various communities (3).

ETIOLOGY OF RENAL DISEASE

Hypertensive Renal Disease

The South African Demographic Health Survey of over 13,000 adults is the largest and most geographically representative national cross-sectional study and was undertaken in 1998 to investigate the prevalence as well as treatment status of hypertension. This study showed a prevalence of hypertension in the South African adult population of 21.3% in both genders, using the WHO/International Society of Hypertension criteria (4). In addition, the study showed that hypertension in South Africans was characterized by low levels of awareness of the diagnosis and even lower levels of adequate blood pressure control, with less than 50% of hypertensives being treated and less than a third having achieved adequate control (4). Similarly in West Africa, low detection rates and inadequate treatment were noted even when detected (5).

Data from the South African Dialysis and Transplant Registry [with 3399 patients on treatment for end-stage renal disease (ESRD)] showed that hypertension was the most common cause of ESRD in Black South Africans and accounted for 34.6% of ESRD in this racial group. In contrast, hypertension was reported to be the cause of ESRD in 4.3% of Whites, 13.8% of Indians, and 20.9% in the mixed ancestry group (6). In a study to determine the pathological basis of ESRD in Black South Africans, Gold et al. (7) reported that essential malignant hypertension was the single commonest cause of ESRD, occurring in 49%.

Hypertension thus occurs more commonly in people of African descent when compared with people of other ethnic groups (8). This is often salt sensitive and not infrequently leads to an excess risk of hypertensive kidney disease in the Black population of sub-Saharan Africa (9). Hypertension, not unexpectedly, occurs as a major cause of kidney failure (6,10,11).

The Glomerulonephritides

These are more prevalent and more severe in Africa than in Western countries with nephrotic syndrome as the major mode of presentation (1). Aetiology is often undetermined, as is the histologic type, due to the infrequency of renal biopsies and absence of facilities for immunofluorescence and electron microscopy in many countries. However, the milieu of chronic parasitic, bacterial, and viral infections is considered to result in an increased prevalence of glomerular disease and hospital admissions. What is notable, however, is the paucity of minimal change lesions and the preponderance of focal segmental glomerulosclerosis and membranoproliferative lesions (12,13).

The pattern of renal disease in South Africa has recently been reviewed (14). In the study by Gold et al., chronic glomerulonephritis was the second most common cause of ESRD in Black patients and was present in 40% (7). In a study to investigate an association between hepatitis C virus (HCV) and idiopathic membranoproliferative glomerulonephritis (MPGN) in KwaZulu-Natal, a province on the east coast of South Africa, chronic renal failure was present at the time of diagnosis in 82.6% of those with idiopathic MPGN, with more than half of the patients requiring dialysis at the time of presentation or a few weeks thereafter; none of the patients were shown to have HCV infection (15). In an earlier report from the same province, idiopathic MPGN was the commonest type of glomerulonephritis in adult Black patients with nephrotic syndrome and was present in 35.7% (13). The HCV infection rate is variable in sub-Saharan Africa; 4.8% in dialysis patients and a blood donor prevalence rate of 0.2–0.7% in Durban, South Africa (16); 21% in hemodialysis patients (17) and 7.4% in renal transplant patients (18) in the Western Cape; and 6.3% in renal transplant patients in Kenya (19).

Hepatitis B virus (HBV) infection has been the major cause of chronic GN and nephrotic syndrome in children in endemic areas of Africa and South Africa in particular, presenting chiefly as membranous GN. Forty-three percent of 306 Black children with nephrotic syndrome had membranous GN; 86.2% were associated with HBV antigens (20). In a 14-year study of 70 Black children with nephrotic syndrome from Namibia, 29 (41.4%) were HBV carriers and 26 of them had membranous GN (21). The introduction of HBV vaccine into the Extended Programme of Immunisation in South Africa in 1995 has had a major impact in markedly reducing the prevalence of HBV-related renal disease in children in South Africa (22).

Chronic malarial infection plays an important role in nephrotic syndrome and chronic kidney disease in tropical Africa (23) and Sudan. Malarial parasitemia was present in 38.7% of 272 children with nephrotic syndrome in Nigeria (24).

HIV-associated nephropathy has been reported as the third major cause of ESRD in Black males aged 24 to 60 years in the USRDS (25). Considering the burden of HIV/AIDS in Africa (estimated at 28.5 million), there should be large numbers of patients with HIV-related renal disease. Renal disease was present in 51.8% of patients with AIDS in a study of 79 patients in Nigeria (26). A prospective study of 617 asymptomatic patients attending an HIV Clinic in Durban, South Africa, showed that proteinuria was present in 6% and HIVAN occurred in 86% of proteinuric subjects, including 85% of those with microalbuminuria (27).

Renal involvement is common in South African patients with systemic lupus erythematosus (SLE) and is a significant cause of mortality. Lupus nephritis has been reported in 65% of SLE patients (28). In a study of Black and Indian South Africans with SLE, renal involvement was associated with a mean serum creatinine of 202 μmol/L at entry and renal failure was the cause of death in almost 25% of patients (29). In a study to investigate a possible association between hypertension and renal function impairment in lupus nephritis, Naiker et al. (30) reported that impaired renal function was more frequent in those with hypertension at the onset of clinical lupus nephritis.

Progression of chronic glomerular disease to end-stage renal failure is not uncommon (31–33) as is relative unresponsiveness to steroids (34). It is thus not unexpected that chronic glomerulonephritis is responsible for the majority of patients presenting with ESRD in the region (2,33,35).

Acute Renal Failure

Major causes of acute renal failure in many parts of Africa are malaria, gastro-enteritis, HIV/AIDS, infections, and traditional medicines. Sepsis is largely the major cause of acute renal failure in the region (14,36). This is closely followed by obstetric and gynaecologic causes, a reflection of the poor standard of health care in the region as a whole. Toxic nephropathies, not infrequently, also occur as a sequel to the use of traditional herbal remedies (37,38). Other notable, though less frequently occurring causes, include complications of snake bites, cholera, and other severe diarrhoeal diseases and haemorrhagic fevers (39).

Schistosomiasis is an important cause of obstructive uropathy and acute renal failure in East Africa, together with genito-urinary tuberculosis (40).

The majority of the patients are young, aged less than 40 years, and mortality is quite high, particularly in those unable to take advantage of renal replacement therapy either because of non-availability or because they are unable to afford the cost of this treatment (39).

Chronic Renal Failure

This occurs even more commonly in the region with a conservative estimate of 1000 new cases per year (3). Hospital-based studies reveal that chronic renal failure (CRF) is responsible for up to 2–8% of medical admissions (3,11). The aetiology varies with the various studies but hypertensive nephrosclerosis and chronic glomerulonephritis both predominate in all the centres (3,6,7,10,11). Other causes peculiar to the region include sickle-cell nephropathy (in West Africa) and renal tuberculosis.

Diabetes occurs less frequently than observed in the developed world but a trend towards an increase with urbanization has been noted over the last decade (41,42) and is the third major cause of CRF in the region. The prevalence of diabetic nephropathy is estimated to be 14–16% in South Africa, 23.8% in Zambia, 12.4% in Egypt, 9% in Sudan, and 6.1% in Ethiopia (42), and it is anticipated to increase with the increasing burden of diabetes mellitus in these countries. In South Africa, it is currently estimated that there are 4 million diabetics; however, the burden of diabetic nephropathy is not known. Microvascular complications were studied in 219 patients who had long-standing diabetes mellitus. Persistent proteinuria was present in 25% of Blacks and 18.2% of Indians and almost 40% had a fall in glomerular filtration rate (GFR) (43).

Renal Replacement Therapies

The availability of these is limited in many countries of sub-Saharan Africa (1,44). Most of the countries have very few centres offering haemodialysis only and these are restricted to just the capitals of these countries (45). In the absence of state funding for RRT (which is mainly available in South Africa for specific categories of patients), very few individuals take advantage of the units even when they exist. Classically, the patients present late, are severely ill with comorbidities, and are often only able to afford few sessions of haemodialysis even though they require more.

CAPD is available mainly in Kenya, Nigeria, Sudan, Senegal, Namibia, Botswana, and South Africa with just a few centers offering acute and intermittent peritoneal dialysis in the rest of the region, with an unacceptably high incidence of peritonitis and cost, as the necessary fluids are imported with no local manufacturers available.

While renal transplantation (both living donor and cadaver) has been available in South Africa for several decades, it has recently become available in Nigeria (with three units now offering live-related kidney transplants), Sudan, and Kenya. This is however available mainly to just the wealthier members of society in most of the countries of Africa with the majority perishing for lack of funds.

CONCLUSION

There is a paucity of data regarding the true prevalence of chronic renal failure in sub-Saharan Africa. Epidemiological research is required to determine the prevalence of chronic kidney disease prior to the development of ESRD. Renal diseases are common in sub-Saharan Africa, are often undetected leading to late presentation of the patients. Resources for detecting and adequately managing ESRD are limited. There is a need for governments to seriously address the problems associated with the care of ESRD in their various countries. A focus on the establishment of renal registries, identification of the aetiology of ESRD and other renal disorders, and the development of preventive programs needs to be emphasized, as even the developed world with all the resources available to them have difficulty coping with the rising prevalence of ESRD.

REFERENCES

1. Naicker S. End stage renal disease in sub-Saharan and South Africa. Kid Int 2003; 63(suppl 83):S119–S122.
2. Akinkugbe OO. Nephrology in the tropical setting. Nephron 1978; 22(1–3): 249–252.
3. Akinsola A, Sanusi AA, Adelekun TA, Arogundade FA. Magnitude of the problem of chronic renal failure in Nigerians. Afr J Nephrol 2004; 8:24–26.

4. Steyn K, Gaziano TA, Bradshaw D, Laubscher R, Fourie J. Hypertension in South African adults: Results from the Demographic and Health Survey, 1998. J Hypertens 2001; 19(10):1717–1725.

5. Cappucio FP, Micah FB, Emmet L, Kerry SM, Antwi S, Martin-Peprah R, Phillips RO, Plange-Rhule J, Eastwood JB. Prevalence, detection, management and control of hypertension in Ashanti, West Africa. Hypertension 2004; 43(5): 1017–1022.

6. Veriawa Y, du Toit E, Lawley CG, Milne FJ, Reinach SG. Hypertension as a cause of end-stage renal disease in South Africa. J Hum Hypertens 1990; 4: 379–385.

7. Gold CH, Isaacson C, Levin J. The pathological basis of end stage renal disease in Blacks. S Afr Med J 1982; 20:263–265.

8. Cooper R, Rotimi C. Hypertension in blacks. Am J Hypertens 1997; 10(7 pt 1): 804–812.

9. Suying Li. Differences between blacks and whites in the incidence of end stage renal disease and associated risk factors. Adv Ren Replace Ther 2004; 1:5–13.

10. Plange-Rhule J, Philips R, Acheampong JW, Saggar-Malik AK, Cappuccio FP, Eastwood JB. Hypertension and renal failure in Kumasi, Ghana. J Hum Hypertens 1999; 13(1):37–40.

11. Mabayoje MO, Bamgboye EL, Odutola TA, Mabadeje AF. Chronic renal failure at the Lagos University Teaching Hospital: a 10 year review. Transplant Proc 1992; 24(5):1851–1852.

12. Abdurrahman MB, Babaoye FA, Aikhionbare HA. Childhood renal disorders in Nigeria. Pediatr Nephrol 1990; 4(1):88–93.

13. Seedat YK. Glomerulonephritis in South Africa. Nephron 1992; 60(3):257–259.

14. Naicker S. Patterns of renal disease in South Africa. Nephrology 1998; 4: S21–S24.

15. Madala ND, Naicker S, Singh B, Naidoo M, Smith AN, Rughubar K. The pathogenesis of membranoproliferative glomerulonephritis in KwaZulu-Natal, South Africa is unrelated to hepatitis C virus infection. Clin Nephrol 2003; 60(2):69–73.

16. Soni PN, Tait DR, Kenoyer DG, Fernandes-Costa F, Naicker S, Gopaul W, Simjee AE. Hepatitis C virus antibodies among risk groups in a South African area endemic for hepatitis B virus. J Med Virol 1993; 40(1):65–68.

17. Cassidy MJ, Jankelson D, Becker M, Dunne T, Walzl G, Moosa MR. The prevalence of antibodies to hepatitis C virus in 2 haemodialysis units in South Africa. S Afr Med J 1995; 85(10):996–998.

18. Moosa MR, Becker M, Cassidy MJD. Hepatitis C virus antibodies in renal allograft recipients. Saudi J Kidney Dis 1996; 7(suppl 1):S141–S144.

19. Ilako FM, McLigeyo SO, Riyat MS, Lile GN, Okoth FA, Kaptich D. The prevalence of hepatitis C virus in renal patients, blood donors and patients with chronic liver disease in Kenya. East Afr Med J 1995; 72(6):362–364.

20. Wiggelinkhuizen J, Sinclair-Smith C. Membranous glomerulopathy in childhood. S Afr Med J 1987; 72:184–187.

21. van Buuren AJ, Bates WD, Muller N. Nephrotic syndrome in Namibian children. S Afr Med J 1999; 89(10):1088–1091.

22. Bhimma R, Coovadia HM, Adhikari M, Connolly CA. Impact of HBV vaccine on HBV-associated membranous nephropathy. Arch Pediatr Adolesc Med 2003; 157:1025–1030.
23. Kibukamusoke JM. The nephrotic syndrome of quartan malaria. Med J Austr 1971; 23:187–191.
24. Okoro BA, Okafor HU, Nnoli LU. Childhood nephrotic syndrome in Enugu, Nigeria. West Afr J Med 2000; 19:137–141.
25. Szczech LA, Kalayjian R, Rodriguez R, Gupta S, Coladonato J, Winston J. Adult AIDS Clinical Trial Group Renal Complications Committee. The clinical complications and antiretroviral dosing patterns of HIV-infected patients receiving dialysis. Kidney Int 2003; 63:2295–2301.
26. Agaba EI, Agaba PA, Sirisena ND, Anteyi EA, Idoko JA. Renal disease in the acquired immunodeficiency syndrome in north central Nigeria. Niger J Med 2003; 12(3):120–125.
27. Han TM, Naicker S, Ramdial PK, Assounga AGH. Microalbuminuria is a manifestation of HIV-associated nephropathy in South African HIV seropositive patients. Abstracts of the EDTA/ERA Congress, May 2004.
28. Mody GM, Parag KB, Nathoo BC, Pudifin DJ, Duursma J, Seedat YK. High mortality with systemic lupus erythematosus in hospitalized African Blacks. Br J Rheumatol 1994; 33:1151–1153.
29. Seedat YK, Parag KB, Ramsaroop R. Systemic lupus erythematosus and renal involvement. A South African experience. Nephron 1994; 66(4):426–430.
30. Naiker IP, Chrystal V, Randeree IG, Seedat YK. The significance of arterial hypertension at the onset of clinical lupus nephritis. Postgrad Med J 1997; 73(858):230–233.
31. Akinsola W, Odesanmi WO, Ogunniyi JO, Ladipo GO. Diseases causing CRF in Nigerians—a prospective study of 100 cases. Afr J Med Med Sci 1989; 18(2):131–137.
32. Youmbissi TJ, Mbakop A, Eloundou. Extramembranous glomerulonephritis: clinicophathologic findings in a group of 45 Cameroonians. Arch Anat Cytol Pathol 1999; 47(1):48–52.
33. Ojogwu LI, Ukoli FA. A followup study of adult nephrotic syndrome in Nigerians: outcome and predictors of ESRF. Afr J Med Med Sci 1993; 22(2):43–50.
34. Seedat YK. Nephrotic syndrome in the Africans and Indians of South Africa. A ten year study. Trans R Soc Trop Med Hyg 1978; 72(5):506–512.
35. Anochie I, Eke F. Chronic renal failure in children: a report from Port Harcourt, Nigeria (1985–2000). Pediatr Nephrol 2003; 18(7):692–695.
36. Bamgboye EL, Mabayoje MO, Odutola TA, Mabadeje AF. Acute renal failure at the Lagos University Teaching Hospital: a ten year review. Ren Fail 1993; (1):77–80.
37. Kadiri S, Arije A, Salako BL. Traditional herbal preparations and acute renal failure in south west Nigeria. Trop Doct 1999; 29(4):244–246.
38. Swanepoel CR, Naicker S, Moosa R, Katz I, Suleiman SM, Twahir M. Nephrotoxins in Africa. In: De Broe, Porter, Bennett, Verpooten, eds. Clinical Nephrotoxins. 2nd ed. Dordrecht, Boston, London: Kluwer Acadeimic Publishers, 2003:603–610.

39. Kadiri S, Ogunlesi A, Osinfade K, Akinkugbe OO. The causes and course of acute tubular necrosis in Nigerians. Afr J Med Sci 1992; 21(1):91–96.
40. Otieno LS. Genito-urinary tuberculosis at Kenyatta National Hospital 1973–1980. East Afr Med J 1983; 60:232–237.
41. Alebiosu CO. Clinical diabetic nephropathy in a tropical African population. West Afr J Med 2003; 22(2):152–155.
42. Amos AF, McCarty DJ, Zimmet P. The rising global burden of diabetes and its complications. Estimates and projections to the year 2010. Diabet Med 1997; 14:S7–S85.
43. Motala AA, Pirie FJ, Gouws E, Amod A, Omar MA. Microvascular complications in South African patients with long-duration diabetes mellitus. S Afr Med J 2001; 91(11):987–992.
44. Bamgboye EL. Haemodialysis management problems in developing countries, with Nigeria as a surrogate. Kid Int 2003; 83:S93–S95.
45. Fogazzi GB, Attolou V, Kadiri S, Fenili D, Priuli F. A nephrological program in Benin and Togo (West Africa). Kidney Int 2003; 83:S56–S60.

18

A Global Renal Disaster Relief Task Force

Norbert Lameire, Wim Van Biesen, and Raymond Vanholder
Renal Division, Department of Medicine, University Hospital Ghent, Ghent, Belgium

Mehmet Sukru Sever
Department of Nephrology, Istanbul School of Medicine, Istanbul, Turkey

Jan Weuts
Artsen zonder Grenzen (Médéçins sans Frontières), Brussels, Belgium

INTRODUCTION

Crush injury-induced acute renal failure (ARF) following traumatic rhabdomyolysis is a major and frequent complication when earthquakes occur in urban regions with multistory stone or concrete buildings. Occurrence of ARF is best understood in the case of earthquakes, but also other disasters may be associated with crush-induced ARF. Concussive or explosive events (bombings, hurricanes, or tornadoes) may inflict major structural damage as well, causing crush and thermal injuries. Examples are napalm bombings (in Vietnam) and pipeline explosions like that occurring near Ufa, the former Soviet Union, in June 1989 (1,2).

The major source of ARF in disasters, however, is the massive damage caused by seismic events. The incidence of ARF caused by crush syndrome after major earthquakes is highly variable. Following the Kobe Earthquake in Japan, crush syndrome was observed in 372 out of 2702 (13.8%) injured and subsequently hospitalized patients (3). Acute renal failure developed in 202 (54.3%) of these 372 patients; thus, the incidence of renal problems was

7.5% (202/2702) when all injured victims were considered. Following the Marmara earthquake, the largest number of documented crush syndrome victims with renal problems ever reported was 639 among whom 477 were dialyzed (4). According to official reports, the number of injured victims was 43,953; thus, renal problems developed in 1.5% of all (mildly and heavily) traumatized victims, in a region which mostly contained concrete buildings. Overall, 9843 injured victims were admitted to the reference hospitals and 5302 of these were hospitalized in the Marmara earthquake. Therefore, renal problems on the basis of crush syndrome developed in 12% (639/5302) of all hospitalized victims, of whom 9% (477/5302) needed dialysis support. Major loss of lives occurs in areas where few of the sophisticated modern civil engineering and building techniques are available to create structures that can withstand seismic disturbances.

In addition, in many circumstances, the major services and local support systems are almost entirely destroyed, severely inhibiting the response time and causing delayed extrication of victims from under the rubble.

Also the moment at which the disaster occurs might have an impact. Overnight events where victims are recumbent increase the risk that non-vital organs are crushed with ARF as a consequence. In contrast, if the disaster occurs during the day, inhabitants can more easily escape into open areas but if they are hurt, a higher risk of cranial traumata in the upright position increases the mortality, relative to the occurrence of ARF.

The number of victims with ARF is thus not only determined by the magnitude of the earthquake (5).

The management of renal failure in a disaster setting requires an understanding of the events associated with a disaster that contribute to ARF and the impact of the disaster on patients with known chronic end-stage renal disease. ARF induced by traumatic rhabdomyolysis and crush syndrome is a well-known complication occurring in the wake of natural or man-made disasters (1,2,5–8). Early recognition of the crush syndrome and rapid initiation of fluid replacement can dramatically reduce the incidence of dialysis-requiring ARF (9–15). However, because of surrounding damage or overwhelmed local medical capabilities, extrication of the victims and initiation of prophylactic measures may be delayed, leading to the development of ARF. In addition, existing dialysis facilities may be destroyed, leaving many chronic dialysis patients without treatment (16). The medical community may thus be confronted with a request to institute renal replacement therapy in tens to hundreds of patients. A rapid, appropriate, and effective international response can be achieved only by rational planning and the establishment of an infrastructure composed of trained personnel, equipment, supplies, and transportation that can be mobilized at a few hours' notice.

Isolated reports have over the last decades described the epidemiology and several factors that determine the incidence of crush-injured ARF in relation with major earthquakes (3,17–22). The highly destructive earthquake in Armenia (December 7, 1988) and the equally devastating earthquake in Iran (June 21, 1990) (17) have caused a worldwide humanitarian relief response and stimulated various organizations to initiate plans to deal with future natural disasters. Especially after the devastating Armenian earthquake, the international renal community responded with an unprecedented relief action, including extensive dialysis support (23–27). However, the experience in the Armenian earthquake also showed that poorly organized relief efforts result in a chaotic influx of people and material that overloads available distribution systems and interferes with the transport of necessary supplies. This often causes what the laypress calls a "second disaster." On the other hand, also valuable lessons were learned from the Armenian experience about disaster relief, in general, and management of ARF, in particular. This experience led in 1989 to the formation within the International Society of Nephrology (ISN) Commission of Acute Renal Failure of the Renal Disaster Relief Task Force (RDRTF) to provide a coordinated international response to the problem of renal failure after major disasters (28). The creation of this task force and its main "philosophy" have been described in a 1993 editorial (29). Its main purpose is to prevent and treat crush injury-induced ARF that occurs after traumatic rhabdomyolysis. The concept proposed was one of a dialysis advance team, which would assess the needs and possibilities for dialysis, to be followed by supportive manpower and material. At that time, and for organizational reasons, the geographical responsibilities of the task force were divided into three major areas: North and South America, the Far East and Australia, and Europe. Each of these task forces was primarily responsible for disaster relief in these three areas of the globe. The European Task Force was primarily responsible for Europe, the Middle East, and Africa. Under the auspices of the Latin American Society of Nephrology, a South American Task Force under the leadership of Dr. Younes-Ibrahim (Rio de Janeiro, Brazil) has been created.

This article describes the organizational aspects and the major interventions of the ISN Renal Disaster Relief Task Force over the last years. It will also briefly discuss the potential role of pre-hospital liaison organizations and summarize the current views on rapid fluid and resuscitation measures that could be taken in the impact zone prior to referring the victims to a hospital.

The ARF commission of the ISN, in conjunction with the National Kidney Foundation, organized a conference on Disaster Relief in Ohrid, Macedonia, in May 1996. At this conference, criteria were developed for the intervention of the task force based on the level of support required in different countries. Level I countries are those that have already well established dialysis programs and do not require any external assistance. Level II countries are those that would potentially benefit from support of the task force and education from the ISN. In level III countries, no established dialysis programs are present. Currently, an as yet incomplete database of the dialysis services available in the different countries, with details on the number and location of the dialysis units, the personnel and equipment available at the facilities, and their resources and support has been constructed. One of the aims of this effort is to update a list of key persons from all countries represented in the ISN, to interact with the task force leaders, and to establish contacts with the responsible health and government authorities of their respective countries. They have the responsibility of drawing up lists of physicians, nurses, and technicians who can volunteer to participate in a disaster relief mission and who are available to leave their commitments at short notice.

Financial support has been negotiated from governmental and non-governmental relief organizations and corporate sources. In the beginning years, the European branch of the RDRTF had agreements with the European Community Humanitarian Office (ECHO), a department of the European Commission that has the task of managing and allocating funds from the European Union for humanitarian purposes. ECHO collaborates with international governmental and non-governmental organizations or other bodies involved in humanitarian aid. To obtain the financial support of ECHO, the RDRTF participated in a joint venture with Médecins Sans Frontières (MSF, Doctors without Borders) (28). MSF is an internationally very well known, independent, politically strictly neutral, non-governmental organization with very large experience in supplying medical relief in numerous disaster circumstances. For their humanitarian actions, MSF was awarded with the Nobel Prize for Peace in 1999.

It was agreed that MSF would add the additional costs incurred by the RDRTF for the renal relief action to their overall budget. At present, the financial means of MSF are sufficient to support the interventions of the Task Force so that no other financial support from international or national organizations is needed. This of course does not exclude that in the future the financial capacities of MSF could be overwhelmed so that further support from international governmental organizations could be necessary. A further benefit of the collaboration with MSF is the facilitated access to and communications with foreign governments for the purpose of quickly obtaining visas, landing rights, and various other authorizations. Many dialysis corporations, including Baxter Healthcare Corporation, Fresenius Medical Care, Gambro, Nipro, and others have agreed to support the effort financially and/or logistically by providing the necessary equipment for initial relief. Lists of individuals to be contacted in emergency (Table 1) and lists with requirements for drugs, fluids, and dialysis machines have been drawn. Equipment that is primarily intended for prevention of ARF, such as rehydration fluids, plasma expanders, mannitol, and bicarbonate, is stockpiled at the MSF warehouse, whereas dialysis equipment is stockpiled at the Baxter and Fresenius warehouses in Belgium. However, in view

Table 1 List of the Most Important Nondialysis and Dialysis Industries Actually Cooperating with the RDRTF

Industry	Contact person	Telephone	Fax	Mobile	E-mail address
BARD Benelux n.v., Hagelberg 2, 2250 Olen	(a) Danny Heungens, Sales Specialist Surgery	(a) (014) 28.69.50 Private: (09) 349.03.71	(a) (014) 28.69.55	(a) (0475) 92.04.39	(a) danny.heungens@crbard.com
BAXTER World Trade S.A., Pleinlaan 5, 1050 Brussel	(a) Raymond Francot, RDRTF-Member, Marketing Director Europe Renal Products	(a) (02) 650.16.30	(a) (02) 650.17.76	(a) (0477) 44.84.01	(a) francor@baxter.com
	(b) Greet Van Overberghe, Product Specialist	(b) (02) 650.17.35	(b) (02) 650.17.96	(b) (0479) 29.86.46	(b) vanoveg@baxter.com
BELLCO SORIN BIOMEDICA sa/nv, Waterranonkelstraat 2F, rue de la Grenouillette 2F, 1130 Brussel/Bruxelles	(a) Dirk Nauwelaerts, Product Specialist BELLCO	(a) (02) 245.39.38	(a) (02) 245.40.67	(a) (075) 38.53.31	(a) dirk.nauwelaerts@advalvas.be
	(b) Jean Moulart, SNIA Group	(b) (02) 245.39.38	(b) (02) 245.40.67	(b) (475) 70.23.17	(b) MoulartJ@sorin.be

(Continued)

Table 1 List of the Most Important Nondialysis and Dialysis Industries Actually Cooperating with the RDRTF (*Continued*)

Industry	Contact person	Telephone	Fax	Mobile	E-mail address
B.BRAUN MEDICAL n.v./s.a., Woluwelaan 140 b, 1831 Diegem	(a) Hubert Moldermans, Marketing Manager, Medical	(a) (02) 725.50.60	(a) (02) 725.96.05		
	(b) Johan Bostoen, District Manager, Pharma	(b) (02) 725.98.58 Private: (051) 22.27.85	(b) (02) 725.96.05		
	(c) Administration and Answering Center				
DIRINCO BVBA, Moeremanslaan 29, 1700 Dilbeek (sells also Mecomp)	(a) Tjeerd Keizer, Commercieel Manager Benelux	(a) (02) 466.82.81	(a) (02) 466.93.88		(a) dirinco@ping.be
FRESENIUS nv, Pharma Division, Boomststeenweg 939, 2610 Wilrijk	(a) Luc and Kim Teerlinck	(a) (03) 825.11.88	(a) (03) 825.11.06	(b) (0475) 83.60.82	
Attention: no service on weekends and during night!!!	(b) Koen Bossart	(b) (03) 820.70.80			
GAMBRO, Groeneveldstraat 15, 3001 Leuven	(a) Luc Deswaef, Directeur Général	(a + b) (016) 29.87.50	(a + b) (061) 22.65.21	On duty—start with no. 1:	LucDeswaef@ gambro.com

(b) José Lepla, Sales Representative (c) Patrick V.D. Seuuwen, code-numbers, material On duty (start with number 1): See "mobile"	(b) (016) 29.87.60	(c) (016) 22.65.11	(1) Julien De Smet: (0475) 27.43.04 (2) José Lepla: (0475) 27.43.02 (3) Mr. P. Minder: (0475) 27.43.03 (4) Kathia Wellis: (0475) 27.43.00
HOSPAL Renal Intensive Care, Groeneveldstraat 13, 3001 Heverlee (catheters) (a) Hilde Dekerf	(a) (016) 31.10.34	(a) (016) 31.10.38	(a) (0475) 35.75.36
HOSPAL Renal Care Groeneveldstraat 13, 3001 Heverlee (membranes, bloodlines) (a) Jean-Jaques Nicolay	(a) (016) 31.10.24	(b) (016) 31.10.39	(a) (075) 65.60.93
MEDCOMP (see Dirinco, Nissho-Nipro) (b) Walther Mathijs	(b) (061) 31.10.20		(b) (075) 65.89.58

(Continued)

Table 1 List of the Most Important Nondialysis and Dialysis Industries Actually Cooperating with the RDRTF (*Continued*)

Industry	Contact person	Telephone	Fax	Mobile	E-mail address
NISSHO-NIPRO EUROPE nv Weihoek 3H, 1930 Zaventem (sells also Medcomp)	(a) General Number	(a) (02) 725.55.33	(a) (02) 725.70.41	(d) (0486) 42.55.49	(d) raymond.vanmulders@skynet.be
	(b) Nicole De Coster, Customer Service	(b) (02) 714.01.61			
	(c) Ingrid Delvaux, Costumer Service	(c) (02) 714.01.62			
	d) Raymond Van Mulders, Sales Manager	(d) (02) 714.01.65 Private: (02) 569.69.29			
SANOFI-SYNTHELABO, Metrologielaan 5, 1130 Brussel	(a) General number	(a) (02) 735.95.13	(a) (02) 715.95.30	(b) (0497) 51.46.93	
	(b) Mister Soetemans, contact person				
SORIN: see BELLCO					

of the rapid communication that currently is possible between the headquarters of the task force (the Renal Division at the Ghent University Hospital) and the major suppliers of dialysis equipment in Belgium, the role of the stockpiling has become less important. To realize rapid provision of equipment, the task force is very efficiently assisted by the pharmacy and the secretariat of the Renal Division of the University Hospital in Ghent.

As noted previously, dialysis teams should be self-sufficient. Therefore, the need for other equipment, such as communication devices, portable generators, water purification systems, portable blood analyzers, and portable ECG machines, has also been foreseen. The collaboration of the RDRTF with MSF is crucial in this area.

On the American continent, no stockpiling of supplies or equipment on a large scale currently exists.

The threat of a great earthquake has compelled California to develop a disaster plan for catastrophic medical events that calls for local response with state-coordinated mutual aid and casualty evacuation, if necessary. During the 1989 Loma Prieta earthquake that killed 63 people and injured 3700, local emergency medical services systems were busy but not stressed excessively. The medical mutual aid system delivered medical personnel, supplies, and blood. One hospital suffered severe non-structural damage, but it was able to treat large numbers of casualties. It appeared that the local disaster relief system performed very well in this limited response, but was hampered by difficulties with disaster intelligence, communications, emergency medical services dispatch, patient care records, hospital damage, and inadequate disaster training (30).

In a recent report by Drs. Blake and Parker, who were asked by the ISN to establish a North American organization, it was proposed that given the relative rarity of renal disasters in the Americas, it does not seem logical that North American and Latin American RDRTFs should operate independently in this region (31). They correctly proposed a single RDRTF for all the Americas. The combination of the relatively greater economic resources of the North American Nephrology Community with the medical skills and cultural and linguistic attributes of the Latin American Nephrology Community would surely make the best basis for an effective region-wide response to renal disasters. Although these authors are convinced of the value and benefits of an acute rapid international response under leadership experienced in nephrologic disasters, the problem in the Americas is that there is no coalition of groupings analogous to that put in place by the European RDRTF (31).

It appeared logical to have a single RDRTF coordination center for the whole world where existing expertise can be concentrated and developed. The center would ideally be the present one in Ghent and would use the same organizational coalition in the Americas that it has already developed for an immediate response in Europe and Asia. The North and

Latin American RDRTF should be merged and should prepare a cadre of volunteers and an inventory of required resources to respond to renal disasters, all under the ultimate leadership of the European-based RDRTF coordination center. After several years of efforts to create an American task force, it became clear that the difficulties associated with such organization were virtually unsurmountable and that the European Task Force should assume global responsibility.

After discussing this report at one of the routine meetings of the Task Force in Ghent, the European branch decided to follow this suggestion on April 21, 2004.

ASSESSMENT OF NEED

In the event of an actual disaster, the RDRTF leaders communicate with the designated key person of the affected country. The key person makes a rough estimation of the number of possible crush injuries and collaborates with the RDRTF leaders to compose relief teams and to coordinate transportation and communication. Attempts are made to communicate with the local key contacts in the region of the disaster and with disaster relief teams already in place. If required, an advance nephrologic team consisting of at least one to two nephrologists and two dialysis nurses is sent to the disaster region to evaluate and treat crush injuries and to assess the need for RRT. They would need to explore whether transportation, communications, and electric and power supplies have been destroyed or incapacitated by the catastrophe and to assess the capabilities of the local hospitals and dialysis facilities, if present. The planning of the interventions is schematically summarized in Figures 1 to 3.

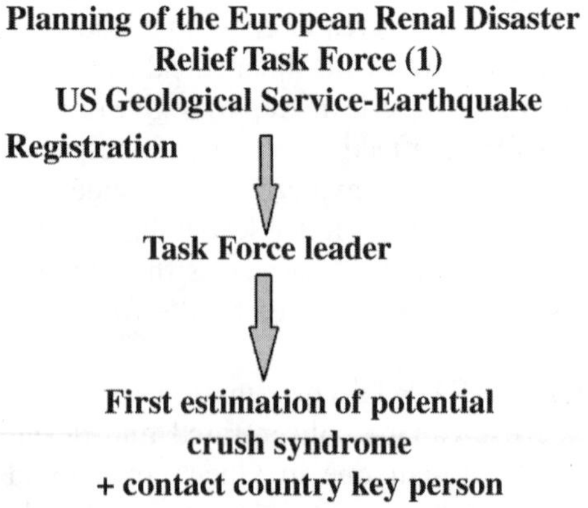

**Planning of the European Renal Disaster
Relief Task Force (1)
US Geological Service-Earthquake
Registration**

⇓

Task Force leader

⇓

**First estimation of potential
crush syndrome
+ contact country key person**

Figure 1   Planning of the European Renal Disaster Relief Task Force (1).

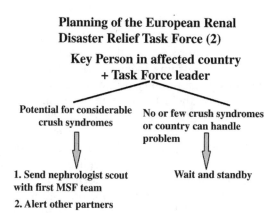

Figure 2 Planning of the European Renal Disaster Relief Task Force (2).

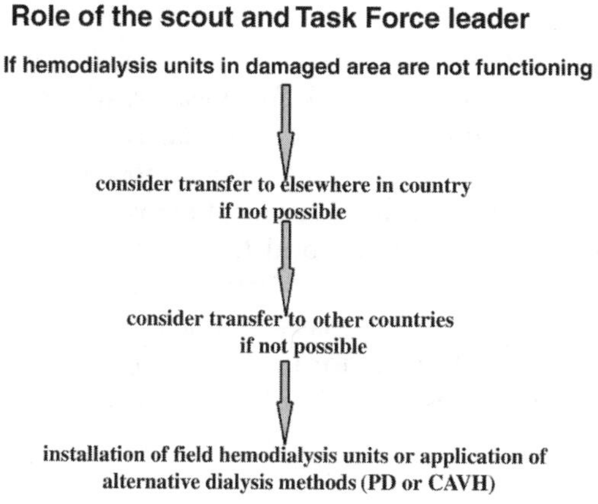

Role of the scout and Task Force leader

If hemodialysis units in damaged area are not functioning

consider transfer to elsewhere in country
if not possible

consider transfer to other countries
if not possible

installation of field hemodialysis units or application of
alternative dialysis methods (PD or CAVH)

Figure 3 Role of the scout and Task Force leader.

The RDRTF has an agreement with MSF that the advance dialysis team will be transported to the disaster area by any available carrier together with the pilot MSF team within the first 12 to 24 hours. When assessment teams arrive on the spot, they are coupled to local aid providers, to avoid misunderstandings based on linguistic or cultural differences.

The United Nations Office for the Coordination of Humanitarian Affairs (OCHA) realizes the difficulties in centrally controlling local disaster relief efforts and how to coordinate the Disaster Assessment and Coordination (UNDAC) teams. Efforts have been undertaken to install such "on-site operations coordination centers" (OSOCC) in an attempt to reduce the sometimes overwhelming influx of relief teams and equipment, further destabilizing the already "chaotic" situation in the disaster area (Dr. Jason van der Velde—chief medical officerBritish Civil Defence USAR Team, personal communication). The ISN Task Force recognizes the need for training search and rescue personnel as well as providing them with the necessary medical support but believes that this is the primary task of other international and national relief organizations. In fact, where in some circumstances the cooperation with for example, OCHA will be useful, the close liaison between the Renal Distaster Relief Task Force and MSF makes at present, the creation of a "third" party unnecessary. However, the Task Force has the duty to improve the contacts with the local nephrology communities in earthquake-prone countries and help them in disseminating the latest information on and in training local rescue teams in the prevention of crush-related ARF. To date, no international initiatives have succeeded in efficiently imposing standards of medical training on rescue personnel, focusing primarily on extrication of victims and team safety.

Mobilization of Resources

The primary information is relayed back to the task force leader, who can rapidly mobilize additional teams and supplies as needed. If dialysis support is required, it has to be deployed in a matter of no more than 3 to 4 days to be effective. It is important that the staff and the equipment arrive together in the disaster area, without the need to rely on local transport facilities, which may be completely overwhelmed. A permanent communication with the national key person and the task force leader is established, mostly via the Task Force own satellite telephone. A leader for the nephrology team is identified, and this person assumes the responsibility for coordinating the disaster relief effort locally.

RELIEF EFFORTS DURING THE DISASTER

The team leader at the site takes responsibility to triage the victims and to coordinate the distribution of resources. It is imperative that the team leader coordinates the care with other disaster relief teams already in the area.

Early administration of appropriate fluids has proven to reduce the number of patients with ARF (9–15,32). Pamphlets have been prepared in several languages to be distributed to the local rescue teams summarizing the quantities and composition of the fluid therapy that can be administered to a crush victim in the disaster area (Table 2). As soon as a venous access can be found even if the rest of the body is still buried under the rubble, fluid administration should be started before further attempts to extricate the victim should be made. Figure 4 illustrates how this was realized in the Maramara earthquake zone by one of the Israeli rescue teams.

Table 2 Fluid Administration Strategy in Patients with Impending or Ongoing Traumatic Rhabdomyolysis

- Find a vein in arm or leg even if the patient is still trapped
- Administer fluid as early as possible: start with 1 L before extrication
- Preferable fluid combination (for each 2 L)
  1 L of isotonic saline
  1 L of glucose 5% with 100 mmol bicarbonate
- Administer at least 3–6 L/d (in emergencies when supervision is not guaranteed) or up to 10 L/d or more if continuous supervision is available
- Add 10 mL of mannitol per hour if urine output is greater than 20 mL/hr

CS Therapy--on scene

- Therapy should begin while victim is still entrapped
- Address immediate life threats first
- Early IV fluid administration helps to prevent renal failure

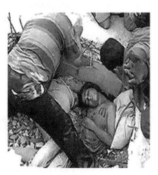

Figure 4 CS therapy—on scene.

If the demand for dialysis is overwhelming, patients with life-threatening hyperkalemia, acidosis, or fluid overload receive priority. Appropriate triage is one of the most important and difficult medical acts in a disaster setting. The medical team must alter its philosophy of care: it is no longer centered on the individual patient but must be readjusted to deliver the greatest good to the greatest number of people (33). Local authorities have ultimate control of the patient, and in every stage of the process, the local medical community should be involved as much as possible. Flexibility and sensitivity to the local customs, conditions, and political situation are essential to the success of the relief operation.

INTERVENTIONS IN TURKEY, INDIA, ALGERIA, AND IRAN

The major intervention of the ISN Disaster Relief Task Force has been in Turkey after the Marmara earthquake in 1999. The experience obtained

during this action has been extensively described (4,34–39) and this article
will only focus on the main results.

On Tuesday, August 17, 1999, at 3:01 A.M. local time, a major earthquake (7.4 on the Richter scale) struck Northwestern Turkey. The affected
zone covered a broad area surrounding the Marmara Sea. Mortality was
estimated at >17,000, with 35,000 wounded and 600,000 homeless. According to the official reports, the disaster caused 17,480 deaths and 43,953
wounded. Approximately 600,000 people became homeless, since 133,683
homes were partially or completely destroyed (Reports Turkish Prime
Ministry) (Crisis Center of the Turkish Prime Ministry. Earthquakes
1999, Press of Prime Ministry, Ankara, 2000, pp: 3–15). An unprecedented
number of 477 crush syndrome patients needing dialysis was observed.

A team from MSF landed at Istanbul Airport less than 22 hours after
the earthquake. One of the aims was to offer nephrologic support to patients
suffering from post-traumatic ARF, as a collaborative action between MSF
and the RDRTF of the ISN. The help consisted both of material and organizational support and the sending of personnel to decrease the workload
for the local medical professionals. In the Marmara earthquake, the proportion of dialyzed patients with nephrologic problems was unprecedentedly
high (37). At least one form of renal replacement therapy was administered
to 477 ARF patients. Of these, 437, 11, and four were treated solely by intermittent hemodialysis, continuous renal replacement therapy, and peritoneal
dialysis, respectively; 25 victims needed more than one dialysis modality. In
total, 5137 hemodialysis sessions were performed. Ninety-seven patients
(15.2%) died. The mortality rate of dialyzed victims was higher compared
with non-dialyzed patients with renal problems (17.2% vs. 9.3%). There
was a high need for blood transfusions that was dictated by the high incidence of muscle compartmental syndrome that led to a probably too-high
frequency of fasciotomies. The open wounds created by these fasciotomies
became frequently infected and were the main reason for sepsis in these
patients. The major cause of mortality was because of generalized septice-
mia. As recently pointed out in a lucid review (40), frequent fasciotomies
should be avoided and this advice will certainly be taken into account in case
of a next intervention.

As early as 12 hours after the arrival of the first team, it became clear
that some of the ARF patients were severely dehydrated. This was not surprising for the following reasons: (1) the chaotic conditions of extrication
and transport; (2) the outside temperatures, up to 38°C in the shade, with
most of the local hospitals destroyed so that patients were treated in open
air and in the sun; and (3) the severity of muscular damage, illustrated by
the fact that at least in 50% of the patients fasciotomy was performed. It
is known that many liters of extracellular volume can be sequestered in
severely damaged muscles (9,41).

Strategies were developed to pursue early rehydration. First, the general practitioners working with MSF in the dispensaries on the field were briefed about the characteristics of the crush syndrome as well as the appropriate fluid administration and referral procedure. They were asked to transmit this information to the local primary care doctors responsible for triage and first aid. Second, 400 pamphlets were made in Turkish language in which the same advice was given and distributed at locations where primary care and triage were taking place (see above).

Dialysis facilities in the most severely affected areas were not used for the treatment of ARF. The medical professionals in that zone concentrated on patient selection, referral, and immediate transfer rather than on complex secondary support measures. Intensive care units and surgical theaters were not operative. Also, in previous earthquakes, it appeared that crush patients who were treated in affected hospitals carried a mortality that was approximately three times higher than evacuated patients and that it was rewarding to transport them out of the affected area (19).

Medical and logistical problems related with chronic dialysis patients is another concern following mass disasters. This issue was analyzed in detail after the Marmara earthquake (16). Questionnaires asking about hemodialysis infrastructure, medical/social problems of chronic dialysis patients, and the fate of dialysis personnel after the disaster were sent to dialysis units located in the affected region (16). Data gathered from eight centers that responded to questionnaires were then analyzed. The number of centers and machines were 12 and 124, respectively, before the earthquake. The number of weekly HD sessions in the analyzed eight centers declined from 1093 before the disaster to 520, 616, and 729 1 week, 1 month, and 3 months after the earthquake, respectively. In the seven centers that remained active, the number of personnel was 112 before the earthquake, which dropped to 86 and 94, 1 and 3 months after the disaster, respectively. Overall, there were 439 patients in the analyzed eight centers before the disaster, whereas data were provided on 356 of them. Six patients died, and seven were seriously and 28 mildly injured by the direct effects of trauma. The percentage of patients who received once-weekly dialysis increased from 2.3% to 7.2% within the first week, with a return to lower figures (4.1% and 2.8%) 1 and 3 months afterward. Despite a decrease in the number of dialysis sessions, interdialytic weight gain decreased 1 week after the disaster and BP measurements did not change significantly before and after the earthquake. A total of 301 and 31 patients left their dialysis centers, temporarily and permanently. After catastrophic earthquakes, despite a decrease in the number of HD sessions, patients comply with disaster conditions, likely by strictly following dietary and fluid restrictions. Conceivably, only the least fortunate patients and those without family remained in the disaster area. The buildings in which dialysis took place were of dubious quality, with a risk for collapse when a new earthquake would occur.

It was therefore considered appropriate to construct new dialysis facilities, preferably low prefab buildings in safe areas. Quite quickly, the Turkish Society of Nephrology took initiatives in this matter. A total of 36 nephrologists, dialysis nurses, and technicians from outside Turkey were active in the Marmara area as members of the ISN Disaster Task Force over a 3-week period.

Several lessons were learned from this experience for the establishment of future strategies if disasters occur in areas where no dialysis facilities are available. The following options should be taken into consideration: (1) evacuation of ARF patients to more remote cities, if necessary abroad; (2) alternative transportation means (boat, plane, helicopter) because evacuation by road might impose problems; and (3) the construction of emergency dialysis units in tents or prefab buildings. We believe that in every earthquake-prone area, there is a need to organize a consensus with the several medical authorities of different neighboring countries to anticipate problems. Maps of the countries at risk and a complete list of all dialysis facilities in those countries have partly been prepared. Pamphlets with instructions on fluid administration are now available in advance in the different languages of the areas at risk so that they can be distributed from the moment the first assessment teams reach the damaged area. Periodic meetings regarding the first and second-line treatment strategies should be organized in potential distress areas, not only for the nephrologists but also for other specialists, general practitioners, and nurses.

In Turkey, mostly due to the efforts of the Turkish Society of Nephrology and the particular experience of one of us (M. S.), careful planing of an early "renal" intervention scheme in case of earthquake has been made. Quite successful application of such an intervention scheme and particularly of an "early hydration policy" to the victims of crush syndrome was realized after the Bingol earthquake in Turkey, that occurred on the first day of May 2003, at 03:27 A.M. Following this disaster, 16 victims (11 of whom were students trapped in the dormitory of their school) suffered from considerable crush injury (15). Fourteen victims were receiving isotonic saline at admission, which was followed by mannitol-alkaline fluid resuscitation. Except two cases, all were polyuric. The mean volume of administered fluids was 21.8 ± 2.7, 20.6 ± 7.6, and 9.2 ± 5.8 L/day within the first, second, and third days of hospital admission, respectively. One of the patients received even 26 L of fluids/day. Interestingly, corresponding mean volumes of urinary output were 8.8 ± 2.3, 10.2 ± 2.9, and 8.1 ± 3.2 L/day. Only four of the 16 (25%) victims needed hemodialysis support. Duration between rescue and initiation of fluids was significantly longer in the dialyzed victims as compared with the non-dialyzed ones. All patients survived and were discharged from the hospital with excellent renal function. The authors concluded that "early and vigorous fluid resuscitation followed by mannitol alkaline solution have played a key role in this encouraging outcome, by preventing ARF and related complications" (15).

In India, an earthquake occurred in the area of Gujarat on January 26, 2001, around 9 o'clock in the morning when most people were outside, explaining the high death toll (official number 19,727), but a total number of only approximately 60 to 70 ARF patients due to crush syndrome. A scouting team consisting of one nephrologist and one dialysis nurse were sent together with members of MSF to Gujarat. A recent report on the renal complications observed after this earthquake has been presented at the ISN/EDTA/ERA meeting of nephrology in Berlin 2003 (42). Out of 35 patients with ARF, admitted to IKDRC in Ahmedabad, 34 (97.1%) had crush syndrome and one patient had pre-renal ARF. Male:female ratio was 24:11.

Clinically ill patients presented with oligoanuria, 28 (80%) with smoky urine, and two (5.71%) with hypotension. Nineteen patients (54.29%) had a compartmental syndrome, and 11 of them (31.43%) required fasciotomy. Thirty-three (94.28%) patients required dialysis. Six patients died (17.14%). After a few days, it became clear that further help of the Task Force was no longer needed.

A major earthquake occurred on May 21, 2003 in Northern Algeria (Boumerdes-Thenia). A scouting team, consisting of one nephrologist and two experienced dialysis nurses arrived in Algeria on May 24. After several visits to the disaster area, together with the local nephrologists and the responsible MSF members, the team came to the conclusion that the local Algerian nephrologists were able to control the situation and that no further international help was needed. Although no precise number of ARF patients could be provided, it could be estimated that a total of maximum 20 patients needed renal replacement therapy for post-crush ARF. It should be noted that the earthquake occurred while a number of chronic patients were dialyzing in the hospital of Thenia, the epicenter of the earthquake. The patients fled the unit in panic but could later be dialyzed in other centers in Algeria. Some equipment, mostly dialysis catheters, were donated to the Algerian units. The team returned to Belgium on May 26, 2003.

The most recent intervention of the Task Force occurred in Iran at the occasion of the Bam earthquake on December 26, 2003. This earthquake caused several thousands of death and wounded patients. As soon as the earthquake was announced in the press, contacts were made between the Task Force headquarters in Ghent, MSF, and the president of the Iranian Society of Nephrology (Prof. Broumand). It was decided to send a scouting team, consisting of one nephrologist and two experienced dialysis nurses to Iran; they made contact with the renal staff at the Kerman hospital, approximately 150 km from Bam (epicenter of the earthquake). Most of the crush-induced ARF patients (approximately 60 patients) were transferred to this city since the hospital in Bam was completely destroyed. Approximately another 40 patients were dialyzed in several other Iranian cities as far as Isphahan and Tehran. Several pieces of equipment, including dialysis machines, dialysate, catheters, and antibiotics were transported by MSF to the Kerman hospital. After several days of hard work in collaboration with the local nephrologists in Kerman, the situation seemed to become stable and the scouting team decided that no further help from the task force was needed. They returned on January 5, 2004.

Upon request of the Iranian Nephrology Society, a post-earthquake meeting was organized in Tehran on April 16–17, 2004, where the different scientific and organizational aspects of the intervention were analyzed. This highly successful meeting will lead to a number of measures within Iran to a better preparedness for eventual later disasters.

CONCLUSIONS

We believe that nephrologists have the moral obligation to intervene in case an epidemic of ARF occurs in disaster circumstances. The quite successful intervention of the ISN Renal Disaster Relief Task Force in the Marmara earthquake and on a lesser scale in India, Algeria, and Iran proves that many lives can be saved and that the moral as well as the financial and logistic support from the international community has helped the local nephrologists and nurses to cope with the immense problems with which they had been confronted (43). We have called this new field of acute disaster nephrology "seismo-nephrology." (44). Although we all hope that devastating disasters will never occur in the future, we also know that this hope is unrealistic and that the nephrologic community should be prepared to help whenever it is needed.

We are very grateful that besides our medical, nursing, and technical volunteers, mostly coming from the European Dialysis Transplantation Nurses Association (EDTNA) and ORPADT, the Flemish and French-speaking dialysis nurses organizations in Belgium, also the ISN, the dialysis industry and, above all, our partner MSF are willing to provide this continuing support. The acceptance of the European branch of the RDRTF to take the responsibility for the renal interventions in disasters on a global scale is most certainly a major challenge, but we are sure that the international nephrology community will support us in case we need their help.

REFERENCES

1. Better OS. History of the crush syndrome: from the earthquakes of Messina, Sicily 1909 to Spitak, Armenia 1988. Am J Nephrol 1997; 17(3–4):392–394.
2. Better OS, Rubinstein I. Post-traumatic acute renal failure with emphasis on the muscle crush syndrome. Molitoris BA, Finn WF, eds. Acute Renal Failure—a Companion of Brenner&Rector's the Kidney. Philadelphia: W.B. Saunders, 2001:227–235.

3. Oda J, Tanaka H, Yoshioka T, Iwai A, Yamamura H, Ishikawa K, Matsuoka T, Kuwagata Y, Hiraide A, Shimazu T, Sugimoto H. Analysis of 372 patients with Crush syndrome caused by the Hanshin-Awaji earthquake. J Trauma 1997; 42(3):470–475; discussion 475–476.

4. Sever MS, Erek E, Vanholder R, Akoglu E, Yavuz M, Ergin H, Tekce M, Korular D, Tulbek MY, Keven K, Van Vlem B, Lameire N, Marmara Earthquake Study Group. The Marmara earthquake: epidemiological analysis of the victims with nephrological problems. Kidney Int 2001; 60(3):1114–1123.

5. De Vriese AS, Mehta R, Vanholder R, Lameire N. Renal failure in disasters. Molitoris BA, Finn WF, eds. Acute Renal Failure—a Companion of Brenner&-Rector's the Kidney. Philadelphia: W.B. Saunders, 2001:236–245.

6. Better OS. The crush syndrome revisited (1940–1990). Nephron 1990; 55(2):97–103.

7. Bywaters EG, Beall D. Crush injuries with impairment of renal function. Br Med J 1941; 1:427–432.

8. Noji EK. Disaster epidemiology. Emerg Med Clin North Am 1996; 14(2):289–300.

9. Better OS, Stein JH. Early management of shock and prophylaxis of acute renal failure in traumatic rhabdomyolysis. N Engl J Med 1990; 322(12):825–829.

10. Better OS, Rubinstein I, Winaver J. Recent insights into the pathogenesis and early management of the crush syndrome. Semin Nephrol 1992; 12(2):217–222.

11. Better OS. Post-traumatic acute renal failure: pathogenesis and prophylaxis. Nephrol Dial Transplant 1992; 7(3):260–264.

12. Better OS, Rubinstein I. Management of shock and acute renal failure in casualties suffering from the crush syndrome. Ren Fail 1997; 19(5):647–653.

13. Ron D, Taitelman U, Michaelson M, Bar-Joseph G, Bursztein S, Better OS. Prevention of acute renal failure in traumatic rhabdomyolysis. Arch Intern Med 1984; 144(2):277–280.

14. Shimazu T, Yoshioka T, Nakata Y, Ishikawa K, Mizushima Y, Morimoto F, Kishi M, Takaoka M, Tanaka H, Iwai A, Hiraide A. Fluid resuscitation and systemic complications in crush syndrome: 14 Hanshin-Awaji earthquake patients. J Trauma 1997; 42(4):641–646.

15. Gunal AI, Celiker H, Dogukan A, Ozalp G, Kirciman E, Simsekli H, Gunay I, Demircin M, Belhan O, Yildirim MA, Sever MS. Early and vigorous fluid resuscitation prevents acute renal failure in the crush victims of catastrophic earthquakes. J Am Soc Nephrol 2004; 15(7)1862–1867.

16. Sever MS, Erek E, Vanholder R, Kalkan A, Guney N, Usta N, Yilmaz C, Kutanis C, Turgut R, Lameire N. Features of chronic hemodialysis practice after the Marmara earthquake. J Am Soc Nephrol 2004; 15(4):1071–1076.

17. Atef MR, Nadjafi I, Broumand B, Rastegar A. Acute renal failure in earthquake victims in Iran: epidemiology and management. Q J Med 1994; 87(1): 35–40.

18. De Bruycker M, Greco D, Lechat MF, Annino I, De Ruggiero N, Triassi M. The 1980 earthquake in Southern Italy—morbidity and mortality. Int J Epidemiol 1985; 14(1):113–117.

19. Kuwagata Y, Oda J, Tanaka H, Iwai A, Matsuoka T, Takaoka M, Kishi M, Morimoto F, Ishikawa K, Mizushima Y, Nakata Y, Yamamura H, Hiraide A, Shimazu T, Yoshioka T. Analysis of 2,702 traumatized patients in the 1995 Hanshin-Awaji earthquake. J Trauma 1997; 43(3):427–432.

20. NadJafi I, Atef MR, Broumand B, Rastegar A. Suggested guidelines for treatment of acute renal failure in earthquake victims. Ren Fail 1997; 19(5):655–664.
21. Noji EK, Kelen GD, Armenian HK, Oganessian A, Jones NP, Sivertson KT. The 1988 earthquake in Soviet Armenia: a case study. Ann Emerg Med 1990; 19(8):891–897.
22. Whittaker R, Fareed D, Green P, Barry P, Borge A, Fletes-Barrios R. Earthquake disaster in Nicaragua: reflections on the initial management of massive casualties. J Trauma 1974; 14(1):37–43.
23. Collins AJ. Kidney dialysis treatment for victims of the Armenian earthquake. N Engl J Med 1989; 320(19):1291–1292.
24. Eknoyan G. Acute renal failure in the Armenian earthquake. Ren Fail 1992; 14(3):241–244.
25. Richards NT, Tattersall J, McCann M, Samson A, Mathias T, Johnson A. Dialysis for acute renal failure due to crush injuries after the Armenian earthquake. BMJ 1989; 298(6671):443–445.
26. Tattersall JE, Richards NT, McCann M, Mathias T, Samson A, Johnson A. Acute haemodialysis during the Armenian earthquake disaster. Injury 1990; 21(1):25–28.
27. Van der Reijden HJ, Van der Neut F. Guidelines for dialysis aid in Yerevan. MSF Med News Int 1989; 6:1–2.
28. Lameire N, Vanholder R, Clement J, Hoste E, Van Waeleghem JP, Larno L, Lambert MC. The organization of the European Renal Disaster Relief Task Force. Ren Fail 1997; 19(5):665–671.
29. Solez K, Bihari D, Collins AJ, Eknoyan G, Eliahou H, Fedorov VD, Kjellstrand C, Lameire N, Letteri J, Nissenson AR, et al. International dialysis aid in earthquakes and other disasters. Kidney Int 1993; 44(3):479–483.
30. Haynes BE, Freeman C, Rubin JL, Koehler GA, Enriquez SM, Smiley DR. Medical response to catastrophic events: California's planning and the Loma Prieta earthquake. Ann Emerg Med 1992; 21(4):368–374.
31. Blake PG, Parker TF III. Report of the International Society of Nephrology: North American Renal Disaster Response Task Force. Adv Ren Replace Ther 2003; 10(2):100–103.
32. Atef-Zafarmand A, Fadem S. Disaster nephrology: medical perspective. Adv Ren Replace Ther 2003; 10(2):104–116.
33. Waeckerle JF. Disaster planning and response. N Engl J Med 1991; 324(12): 815–821.
34. Erek E, Sever MS, Serdengecti K, Vanholder R, Akoglu E, Yavuz M, Ergin H, Takce M, Duman N, Lameire N, Turkish Study Group of Disaster. An overview of morbidity and mortality in patients with acute renal failure due to crush syndrome: the Marmara earthquake experience. Nephrol Dial Transplant 2002; 17(1):33–40.
35. Sever MS, Erek E, Vanholder R, Ozener C, Yavuz M, Kayacan SM, Ergin H, Apaydin S, Cobanoglu M, Donmez O, Erdem Y, Lameire N. Lessons learned from the Marmara disaster: time period under the rubble. Crit Care Med 2002; 30(11):2443–2449.
36. Sever MS, Erek E, Vanholder R, Akoglu E, Yavuz M, Ergin H, Turkmen F, Korular D, Yenicesu M, Erbligin D, Hoeben H, Lameire N. Clinical findings

in the renal victims of a catastrophic disaster: the Marmara earthquake. Nephrol Dial Transplant 2002; 17(11):1942–1949.

37. Sever MS, Erek E, Vanholder R, Koc M, Yavuz M, Ergin H, Kazanciogu R, Serdengecti K, Okumus G, Ozdemir N, Schindler R, Lameire N, Marmara Earthquake Study Group. Treatment modalities and outcome of the renal victims of the Marmara earthquake. Nephron 2002; 92(1):64–71.

38. Sever MS, Erek E, Vanholder R, Ozener C, Yavuz M, Ergin H, Kiper H, Korular D, Canbakan B, Arinsoy T, VanBiesen W, Lameire N, Marmara Earthquake Study Group. The Marmara earthquake: admission laboratory features of patients with nephrological problems. Nephrol Dial Transplant 2002; 17(6):1025–1031.

39. Vanholder R, Sever MS, De Smet M, Erek E, Lameire N. Intervention of the Renal Disaster Relief Task Force in the 1999 Marmara, Turkey earthquake. Kidney Int 2001; 59(2):783–791.

40. Better OS, Rubinstein I, Reis DN. Muscle crush compartment syndrome: fulminant local edema with threatening systemic effects. Kidney Int 2003; 63:1155–1157.

41. Vanholder R, Sever MS, Erek E, Lameire N. Rhabdomyolysis. J Am Soc Nephrol 2000; 11(8):1553–1561.

42. Viroja D, Shah P, Trivedi HL, Shah V, Vaniker A. Management of crush syndrome following Gujarat earthquake. Proceedings World Congress Nephrology, Berlin, 2003:W357.

43. Sever MS, Erek E. Sincere thanks of Turkish nephrologists to their European friends. Nephrol Dial Transplant 2000; 15:1478–1480.

44. Vanholder R, Sever MS, Erek E, Lameire N. Acute renal failure related to the crush syndrome: towards an era of seismo-nephrology? Nephrol Dial Transplant 2000; 15(10):1517–1521.

19

Community-Based Approach to Prevention of Chronic Kidney Disease: The Chennai Experience

Manjula Datta

Department of Epidemiology, Tamil Nadu Dr. MGR Medical University, Chennai, India

M. K. Mani

Apollo Hospital, Chennai, India

India is a country in transition. Infant mortality has come down to about 75 per thousand, and the life expectancy of men has gone up to above 65 years and that of women to above 60. It is estimated that about 10–15% of India's population are today above the age of 60. This demographic transition inevitably leads to an epidemiological transition. As the population ages, the diseases of life style such as diabetes and hypertension also increase. This is happening while the healthcare system is still struggling to control infectious diseases such as tuberculosis and malaria, malnutrition and maternal deaths. This "double burden" of infectious and life style diseases imposes a severe strain on the health budget.

Consider this against the economic situation. India has shown significant economic growth in the last decade and a half, but most of the economic gains have been overshadowed by the burgeoning population. Although it has been shown that health expenditure can be viewed as an investment opportunity (1), spending on health in India has remained among the lowest in the world (2). Several estimates, including that of the

World Health Report have shown that diabetes, hypertension, and coronary artery disease are likely to increase and will be among the top five causes of death in India by the year 2020. Yet, there is no allocation for the control of these diseases in the 10th plan. Estimates for the number of patients with renal damage or chronic kidney failure (CKF) in India are not available. Therefore, it is difficult to even suggest what kind of allocation should be made in the health budget.

Chronic kidney disease (CKD) and failure are among the most common of complications of diseases such as diabetes and hypertension (3,4). It has also been reported that these two diseases account for 40% of cases of CKF seen in a tertiary care clinic (5). Pyelonephritis accounts for another 10%, and thus preventable causes appear to account for a large proportion of CKF. Identifying patients with these risk factors and keeping these conditions under control is a good way to prevent CKD in the community.

Seventy percent of India's population lives in rural areas. Hence, any program aimed at the rural people can have the maximum impact in reducing the burden of illness in the population. Presented below are the details of a project, which has been carried out by the Kidney Help Trust in a rural area of a South Indian District for the past 8 years. Although carried out in a very small area, the project has yielded information on the burden of illness, and also provides a very simple and cost-effective methodology for the prevention of CKF in the community.

THE ECONOMICS OF TREATING CHRONIC KIDNEY FAILURE (CKF)

India is a poor country with a per capita income of US $460/year. Only 3.2% of the population earn more than $1100 a year, and 29% are below the poverty line and earn less than $110. Government provides medical care free of cost, both in cities and in villages, but the expenses on health of the State and Central Governments together average $8 per capita per year. This sum covers public health, sanitation, and immunization besides the treatment of disease. Government pays for just 18% of healthcare costs. It has been estimated that 82% of health expenses is met by patients from private sources. The least expensive form of renal replacement therapy (RRT) is renal transplantation, and this would cost $6500 to perform, and around $220/year for immunosuppressive treatment, even if only prednisolone and azathioprine are used. If, as is done with the majority of transplants these days, cyclosporine is also used, the cost rises to $2000 a year. Maintenance hemodialysis in a hospital, or CAPD at home, costs around $5000 a year. With a per capita income of $460, it is clear that neither the average Indian nor the government can afford the treatment of end-stage renal disease (ESRD) (5).

Despite the bleak economic picture, India has efficient programs for dialysis and transplantation. A few Indians are wealthy enough to pay for treatment out of their own family funds. Some industries and the government itself meet the expenses of transplantation for their employees. Government-run medical colleges run transplant programs to enable the teaching of nephrologists and transplant surgeons, and treatment is provided free of costs, but the budget will provide funds only for very small numbers, which have no impact on the common man. We have no reliable estimates, but perhaps 100,000 Indians reach ESRD each year, and just 3000 of them are treated.

The only treatment available for end-stage kidney failure is dialysis or transplantation. Several private and corporate centers offering this form of treatment have come up, particularly in the urban areas of India. This is testimony to the fact that chronic renal failure is a significant problem in the community. However, as described above, such treatment is expensive and can be afforded by only a small section of the patients requiring them. The economic burden due to ESRD has been discussed in detail in a previous paper (6). Suffice it to say here that the government spends US $8 per capita on health, and the initial cost of one transplantation is US $6500. Thus, each transplant carried out by our government deprives several thousand people of basic healthcare amenities. It is clear that the government cannot afford to provide renal replacement therapy for all those who need it. The per capita income of the average Indian is less than US $1000 a year and renal replacement is unaffordable. The few who can afford it face a substantial depletion of resources as a consequence. Hence, prevention is not only the best approach; it appears to be the only one.

THE KIDNEY HELP TRUST

The Trust was originally formed by a group of five doctors and two lay persons who had renal patients in their family. The Trust is registered with the Government of India, and donations to the Trust are exempt from income tax. The Trust is also cleared by the Government of India to receive money from abroad. The intention was to help poor patients defray the expenses of renal transplantation. Donations were received from members of the public, mostly wealthy patients of one of the founders. However, it soon became clear that the cost of transplantation was so high that the corpus accumulated after 2 years would only cover the costs of 15 patients. With thousands of poor patients needing financial support, it was clear that a fortunate handful would benefit and the vast majority would languish and die for lack of the wherewithal to pay for treatment.

The Trust then took a decision to find more effective ways to use its limited funds to benefit a larger number of people with kidney disease. Diabetes, hypertension, and pyelonephritis together account for more than

Table 1 Causes of Chronic Kidney Failure at Apollo Hospital
(7686 patients in 20 years)

Disease	Percentage
Diabetic nephropathy	31.29
Chronic interstitial nephritis	19.69
Chronic glomerulonephritis	17.77
Arteriolar nephrosclerosis	11.76
Chronic pyelonephritis	10.49
Focal and segmental glomerulosclerosis	3.89
Autosomal dominant polycystic disease	2.41
Sum of these seven causes	97.29

50% of patients with CKF in this part of the country (Table 1). Urinary infections do not lead to renal failure unless there are underlying anatomical abnormalities. The availability of effective antibiotics means that the acute episodes are often easily controlled and no attempt is made to find underlying lesions, which ultimately lead to the decline in renal function. It was felt that these three conditions offered a reasonable prospect of preventing CKF. Early detection of other renal diseases would also help to reduce the burden of ESRD, and good control of hypertension, whatever the cause, should slow the decline to the end stage and at least procure a few more years of useful life to the patient (7). Control of diabetes has also been shown to prevent the onset of complications (8). The Trust therefore changed its focus to the prevention of CKD using an approach of early detection and treatment of renal disease, and of hypertension and diabetes.

THE COMMUNITY PROJECT OF THE KIDNEY HELP TRUST

The Trust selected a rural community because 70% of the country's population resides in its villages, which are relatively less well served by the medical profession. While government runs primary health centers (PHCs) that have the aim of preventing diseases as well as curing them, the accent has been on therapy. Patients have to go to the center and wait in line for a week's supply of medicine. Rural areas are poorly connected by roads, and the poor cannot afford to pay for transport even for the average distance of 10 km to the PHC. The trip to the PHC for a week's supply of medicine means the loss of a day's wage, which the rural family cannot afford. Patients will therefore seek treatment only for an illness that prevents them from working anyway, a high fever or an unbearable pain, and chronic diseases, which do not incapacitate them from working, are neglected. Testing and treatment have to be provided to the villager close to his or her home, and often in the home itself, and our accent has been on domiciliary care.

Being aware that India is one of the poorest countries in the world, the Trust has concentrated on keeping costs low without sacrificing efficiency. Therefore, social health workers rather than doctors have been employed for the main work, and the cheapest drugs available have been selected for the major goals, the control of diabetes and hypertension. No support has been sought from any other agency, and even the donations received have been made of the donor's own volition and have never been sought. The funds received have been adequate for the limited area for which coverage has been undertaken so far.

THE PROJECT DESCRIPTION

This project is being carried out by the Kidney Help Trust from June 1996 (for the past 8 years), located in a part of Sriperumbudur Taluk, which is predominantly a rural area and is done in conjunction with the Tulsi Trust, which is another voluntary agency providing basic health care to the people. The project covers a population of about 22,000 people spread over 26 villages. There are 13 female healthcare workers and eight mini health centers with an equal number of peripheral health centers. These female healthcare workers are from the local area, have completed their schooling, and have received a further 6 months training in basic health care. They provide antenatal care, maternal, and child health, and also provide medicines for simple ailments under the supervision of a doctor, who visits each health center once a week.

TRAINING OF THE HEALTH CARE WORKERS

The primary healthcare workers employed by the Tulsi Trust have completed 12 years of schooling and have subsequently undergone 6 months of training in basic health care at a multipurpose healthcare worker training school. The major portion of this training involves maternal and child care. Thus, they had already developed competency in the recognition of the sick, in taking blood pressure and in carrying out urine examinations, in the process of antenatal care. They were also aware of the concept of "high-risk approach" in the management of disease.

A 1-day training program was held for these female healthcare workers at their place of work. They were initially given a talk on CKD and how a large part of it can be prevented. They were then told about the diseases like hypertension and diabetes and how these diseases can be largely controlled with regular low-cost medication. They were given refresher training in taking blood pressure, and in urine examination using Benedict's solution for reducing substances and sulfosalicylic acid for albumin. Simple user-friendly definitions using non-medical terms for the common symptoms suggestive of kidney disease had been developed by the Trust (Fig. 1).

1.Frequency of micturition: The need to pass urine more than
        twice in an hour; It is often but not always
        accompanied by pain.
2. Dysuria: Pain while passing urine either in the urethral region
        or the lower abdomen.
3. Haematuria: Passing blood along with urine.
4. Pyuria: Passing pus along with urine
5. Oedema: Swelling of the body, mostly involving the lower
        limbs; but can involve the face or lower limbs.
        Seen over the back in bedridden persons. Firm
        pressure with the thumb over a bony point leaves
        a depression
6. Nocturia: The necessity to wake up at night from sleep in order
        to pass urine
7. Renal Pain: Pain in the back at a point just below the place
        where the last rib meets the backbone. This pain
        can be dull and continuous or occur in sharp
        stabs.
8. Difficulty in breathing: Getting short of breath while attending
        to normal daily activities

Figure 1 Symptoms referable to renal disease.

A laminated card with these symptoms and their definitions was given to each healthcare worker. These symptoms were explained to the female healthcare workers and they were thus equipped to screen the population for early kidney involvement and its risk factors.

In the new area, there were no female healthcare workers, and this was a major hurdle. In this area, female volunteers who had finished 12 years of schooling and were waiting to enter university were selected, based on their willingness to carry out the field work. They were then given a 3-day training. On the first day, they were given an orientation about the old area by one of the senior health workers in the old area. Then they were given talks about the importance of CKD and the role of diabetes and hypertension in contributing to CKD.

On the second and third day, they were given intensive hands on training in taking blood pressure and in examining urine. Each volunteer performed at least 10 tests on other volunteers. They were then taken to the field and their performance assessed. Retraining was provided where necessary. Female healthcare workers from the old area assisted in training the volunteers; this also trained them to be trainers.

This was supplemented by in service training by one of the Trust staff in the form of periodic supervisory visits and regular review meetings. Ten percent of the tests done in the field was repeated by a doctor or a senior health worker. None of the persons reported as normal turned out to have raised blood pressure or sugar in the urine; however, about 2% of those reported to have raised blood pressure turned out to be normal. There were no false positives in the urine examination.

Tools

In a pilot project before the start of the main program, urine dipsticks had been found to be unreliable. A number of subjects reported to have albuminuria when tested in the field were found to be quite normal when the test was repeated in the hospital. It is possible that transport and storage of the strips under the hot conditions and open sunlight in the field rendered them less reliable. Therefore, the standard and time-tested methods of sulfosalicylic acid for protein and Benedict's reagent for glucose were used and the results have been found to be reproducible when the patients are brought to the hospital for detailed investigation.

Blood tests for the subjects selected on screening are done free for the project at Apollo Hospital, Chennai. Blood samples are collected in the field and transported back to Chennai, using the hospital's collection tubes.

THE SURVEY METHOD

A house-to-house survey was undertaken using these healthcare workers, and all individuals were screened for symptoms and urine sugar and albumin. Blood pressure (BP) was taken for all individuals above the age of 5 years using a mercury sphygmomanometer. Those found to have a BP of 140/90 mmHg were checked again an hour later. All persons, with a blood pressure of 140/90 mmHg or higher, albumin or sugar in the urine, or answered yes to any one of the symptoms, were examined by a doctor of the Kidney Help Trust.

The doctor uses the mini health center of the Tulsi Trust in villages where it is available. In the other villages, a temporary center is set up at a convenient location such as a school, the panchayat union office, the veranda of a house or even under an old tree. For those who are unable to come even to these centers, the doctor visits them at home. Thus maximum compliance is ensured.

A thorough clinical examination is done and the screening tests are repeated for all those who had either a raised blood pressure or sugar or albumin in the urine in the house-to-house survey. Blood is collected for investigations like random blood sugar, urea, creatinine, protein, and lipid profile, and glycated hemoglobin for those who are found to be abnormal in this second screen. Subjects having a blood pressure of 140 mmHg systolic and/or 90 mmHg diastolic are asked to wait and their blood pressure is checked after 1 hr. If their blood pressure remains above 140 systolic or 90 diastolic, they are labeled as hypertensive and treatment is initiated immediately. For those with reducing substances in the urine, blood is collected in heparinized tubes for investigations. This blood is centrifuged in the mini-health center and the plasma is transported to the Apollo Hospital. Treatment is started if the blood results show a random glucose of above 200 mg/dL or a glycated hemoglobin of above 7%. Patients showing a serum creatinine above 1.5 mg/dL are taken to the hospital for further tests like ultrasound and renal biopsy. They are managed as per the instructions of the nephrologist. Six such surveys have been completed over an 8-year period.

MANAGEMENT

Treatment is initiated only by the doctor who visits each mini health center once a fortnight. Hypertension (as defined above) is treated with a combination of hydralazine and reserpine, with hydrochlorothiazide where necessary. Diabetes (as defined above) is treated with glibenclamide and metformin. These medications are started at a low dose and gradually increased until the optimum dosage is obtained. They are then maintained on this dosage. The healthcare worker checks the blood pressure once a week, or more often in case of symptoms, and is allowed to adjust the dose.

In case the patient has a family physician and is desirous of continuing his treatment with him, he is not dissuaded. However, if the patient is indifferent to his health, he is visited by the health worker and doctor, and is persuaded to take the treatment. Blood tests for glycated hemoglobin are carried out every 3 months and the dosage adjusted accordingly. This is done only by the doctor. The target is to maintain the blood pressure below 140 systolic and 90 diastolic, and to achieve reductions in blood sugar, ultimately getting the glycated hemoglobin below 7%.

The healthcare workers are trained to recognize adverse events such as hypoglycemia and sudden fall or rise in blood pressure. Medicines are stopped and the doctor informed immediately in case of hypoglycemia. The patients are seen at least once a month by the doctor, and more often when needed. Patients developing albuminuria, edema or a high serum creatinine are taken to the nephrologist for further management. In case of any emergency, the patients are taken to the nearest tertiary care center, where they are managed. They are also visited by the Kidney Help Trust doctor and the details of the treatment given are noted. Patients who develop a non-renal event such as a coronary or cerebro-vascular event are also assisted in getting tertiary care.

No separate awareness campaigns are conducted, but education is given to the patients and their family members in the clinics. One-to-one counseling and advice is provided for all those who seek it.

After the program had been in existence for 8 years, an adjacent area was surveyed using a similar methodology. This new area had a similar population size and was very similar in demography and other characteristics to the population in the project area. This was done in order to compare the situation in the project area with that of an area without the intervention.

In the new area, specialized healthcare workers were not available. Therefore, community volunteers were selected and given training for 3 days, in eliciting symptoms, taking blood pressure and in examining urine. Periodic in-service training was continued, and their findings were randomly checked by the doctor or an experienced health worker to ensure that errors were minimal. This procedure of using community health volunteers was much less expensive than using trained health workers.

A flow chart of this project is given in Figure 2.

RESULTS

There were about 21,000 individuals in each of the areas (Table 2). The survey is ongoing, and therefore all data are incomplete. It will take several weeks to achieve complete coverage. It can be seen that the number of individuals who became eligible for the blood collection after the second screen was not much different from the first screen. This is a measure of the competence of the healthcare workers.

The coverage has been high with 89.61% of the population cooperating for the survey. Those who did not participate were mostly young boys, and very old people who had become indifferent to their health. Of those diagnosed to have diabetes or hypertension, only 30.34% had known of it earlier. Seventy-five percent of patients accepted the treatment offered and over 90% continued treatment. 24.6% of those with disease preferred to be treated by their own practitioners initially, but in later years, as the community gained confidence, most of the patients preferred to take treatment with the project. Of the 78.91% who cooperated for treatment, hypertension was controlled to less than 140/90 in 95.77%. Glycated hemoglobin was brought down to 7% or less, which would qualify as tight control, in only 52.13% of the population, which is not as good. However, there was a reduction of 10% in glycated hemoglobin in 76.79% of the patients, so the vascular complications of diabetes, including renal failure, could be reduced at least to some extent.

The effectiveness of the program was assessed by comparing the proportion of the population with reduced glomerular filtration rate in the intervened area and the new area. This is shown in Table 3. Unpublished observations of over 2000 live donors in the Apollo Hospitals, Chennai,

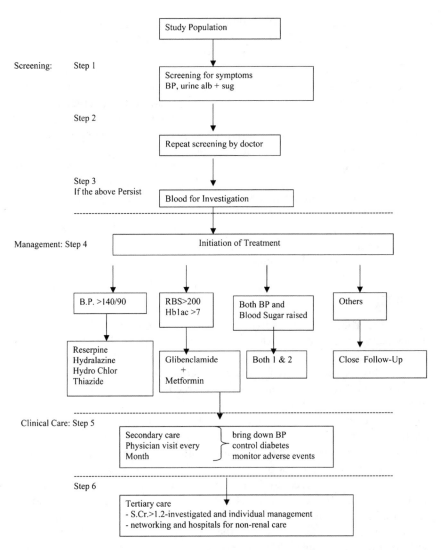

Figure 2   Flow-chart of activities referable to renal disease.

have shown that the normal GFR in Indians is between 80 and 95 mL/min. It can be seen that the number of persons with GFR below 60% of normal (severe reduction in GFR) was reduced by half in the intervened area ($p < 0.00002$, relative risk 0.51, CI 0.38–0.70) and that of persons with GFR below 80% of normal (moderate reduction) was reduced by almost five times ($p = 0.0000001$, relative risk 0.24, 95% confidence interval 0.2–0.28). This suggests that the program may have prevented or delayed the onset of renal failure in 25 subjects per 1000 population.

Table 2 Population and Coverage

	Intervened area	New area
Total population	21,062	20,701
Total screened (coverage)	19,888 (94%)	17,521 (85%)
Number with screening abnormalities	590	1,385
Eligible for blood collection (screening abnormalities confirmed at second examination)	534	1,033
Blood collected	458	673

The cost of achieving such a reduction is given in Table 4. It is seen that entire program could be carried out at a cost of 31 cents per capita. The government expense on health care is US $8 per capita.

DISCUSSION

Prevention is not yet a concept that is thought of in association with CKD. Yet the cost of managing CKF is so high that the only approach that would work is prevention. Presented here is a model of prevention of CKF well worth emulating in other parts of the country and of the world. The program was started in an area where healthcare facilities were meagre; hence, the community welcomed it and readily participated. Coverages have been very high for all the investigations and treatment and this has been main-

Table 3 Glomerular Filtration Rates by MDRD Short Formula

	Original area	New area
Population screened	19,888	17,521
Number selected by screening	534	1,034
Blood results available for	398	500
Number with GFR <60 mL/min	47	52
Projected for total selected	63 for 534	108 for 1,034
Prevalence/1000 population	3.17	6.16*
Number with GFR <80 mL/min	115	279
Projected for total selected	154 for 534	577 for 1034
Prevalence/1000 population	7.74	33**

*$p < 0.00002$, RR 0.51 CI 0.38–0.70.
**$p < 0.0000001$, RR 0.24, CI 0.20–0.28.
MDRD short formula (9): GFR in mL/min for males $= (170 \times (S.\ \text{creat}(mg/dL))^{-0.999}) \times (age^{-0.176}) \times ((S.\ \text{urea nitrogen}(mg/dL))^{-0.170}) \times ((albumin(g/dL))^{+0.318})$. GFR in mL/min for females = above result $\times 0.762$.

Table 4 The Costs of the Rural Program of the Kidney Help
Trust (US $ per Annum)

Medicines and supplies	4,210
Salaries	775
Transport	1,320
Cost of survey	215
Cost of project per capita	0.31
Government expenses per capita	8
Each renal transplant costs	6,500
Cost of maintaining a transplant per year	220

tained over 8 years. There has been an increasing demand for such a program from neighboring areas. Indeed, in the old area, about 20% of the
patients treated were from outside the study area, with people traveling
5 to 10 km to seek treatment. It is possible that the reasons for this success
have been the modest and relatively simple goals, and especially the domiciliary program, which goes to the villagers in their homes without waiting
for them to seek attention.

Relatively simple tools have been used, especially for screening for
diabetes. It is likely that several diabetics and certainly all the impaired glucose tolerance cases would have been missed. However, it is neither feasible
nor economical to use a glucometer for screening. Similarly, fasting glucose
is definitely a better indicator of the diabetic state, but in a rural area most
people work in the fields and eat very early. In resource poor settings, the
technology that works best is the one that is the simplest.

The drugs used here are also deliberately chosen for their low cost.
Reserpine and hydralazine have been given up in most parts of the world.
The reasons for this are unclear. They have very few side effects, and are
effective. In this area, there were very few patients who were given other
drugs; and in most instances, this was because they had a coronary or
cerebral event and the consultants in the city had prescribed these more
advanced drugs.

The 1999 WHO-International Society of Hypertension Guidelines (7)
say that a prolonged 5 mmHg fall of the usual diastolic BP reduces the risk
of stroke by 35–40%, of major coronary heart disease events by a lesser
amount, and of chronic renal failure by one-quarter. The DCCT (8) showed
that for every 10% reduction in glycated hemoglobin there is a 40% reduction in vascular complications, which includes nephropathy. Even if tight
control cannot be achieved in all the patients, some degree of control is
possible.

Is reserpine adequate as a hypertensive agent? This is an Indian
drug, and older physicians have extensive experience with it, though it has

fallen into disuse. This has been shown to be an effective agent. Kronig et al. (10) found it more effective than some of the modern favorites. Besides preventing hypertensive nephropathy, control of hypertension should slow down decline in renal function in all other diseases. Much of this work has been done with ACE inhibitors, which are expensive. It is hoped that reserpine and the combinations we use will also prove useful in this regard.

The PSHW monitors blood pressure once a week and is allowed to modify the dose of the drugs within limits. The doctor sees them once a month, and is responsible for major changes and for diet advice. Diabetics are treated only by the doctors, who modify doses with the aid of glycated hemoglobin readings once in 3 months. The PSHW is taught to recognize hypoglycemia and correct it, and will then stop the drug and call on the doctor to modify treatment on his next visit. Severe hypoglycemia has not been encountered in the project area as yet, with the oral agents and our method of gradually increasing the dose.

The cost of 31 cents per capita is well within the average of US $8 per capita spent by the central and state governments on health, and could easily be incorporated into the activities of the PHC. There may be other benefits, which have not been specifically looked for, in prevention of cerebral, coronary, and peripheral arterial disease, since control of hypertension has been excellent and of diabetes fairly good. It has been relatively easy to implement the program using unskilled workers from the area, and provides them some supplemental income with no need for relocation from their own homes.

When is a preventive program worth implementing? Some questions have to be answered:

1. *Is the disease prevalent in the community?* There is no doubt that large numbers of Indians suffer from diabetes and hypertension and their consequences.
2. *Are the effects serious enough to warrant the effort?* Renal failure, strokes, coronary artery disease, peripheral vascular disease are all deadly.
3. *Is it easy to detect?* A simple urine test and a recording of blood pressure are easily done. There has been very good cooperation from the population for such a program. The presence of such a program also makes it possible for the community to approach the project staff in between surveys, and get diagnosed and treated.
4. *Can it be easily prevented?* Primary prevention of diabetes and hypertension is just being considered. The recommendations for this are still not clear. But this program has shown that good control of hypertension and reasonable control of diabetes can be established in the community, and the incidence of CKF can be reduced.

5. *Is the cost of screening and prevention affordable, and cheaper than treating the established disease?* It has been demonstrated that this project can be implemented with a small fraction of government's health budget, and, it is quite possible that the cost saved from the cases of CKD prevented by this program will be more than adequate to pay for it.

The resources for health care in India are minuscule, and the problems are colossal. The greatest good for the greatest number at the least cost should be the aim of research into primary healthcare delivery.

This project has, as far as we are aware, demonstrated for the first time in the world that with very little effort and expense it is possible to achieve reasonable results at community level. Although this has been done in a very small area, it has been possible to do this without much difficulty, and the model that has emerged is easily replicable. Lateral thinking and a sense of commitment have been the key elements of success. It is remarkable that there was total cooperation from the community, and practically no hurdles in implementing this project. This project now needs to be scaled up and incorporated into government policy. While this could be a long and uphill process, it could easily be replicated, at least by NGOs working in health.

Guidelines for Others Planning Such Programs

The important point is to make a clear and simple goal, and not get distracted by nebulous possibilities. There has been some temptation as well as pressure by many to expand the scope of the program to cover other conditions, or to add more expensive medicines, but this will inevitably call for more manpower and money and make it difficult to implement. It is essential that the expenses be kept to a reasonable level, in keeping with the economy of the society in which the program is implemented. The success of any program depends on the commitment of the members, and this will inevitably get diluted as the work gets spread out and more people are involved. This program can be efficiently duplicated by small groups in different areas, rather than by a massive monolith on a national scale.

It is essential that the supply of medicines is maintained and the needs of the population are served, thus presenting a healthcare program that yields research results that can be applicable generally. The people should not get a feeling that we are only interested in a study and not in them. The Indian villager is shrewd enough to know when a medical team has a publication as its main goal, and we are sure this will apply to any developing nation.

Domiciliary care is very important, especially for diseases that do not cause major symptoms and do not force a patient to seek relief. With a little persuasion and a minimum of inconvenience, it has been shown that we can obtain compliance from most people.

ACKNOWLEDGMENTS

The field work described in this paper has largely been coordinated by Dr. Manjula Datta and Dr. Vijay K. Gupta of the Kidney Help Trust, and by Mr. C. S. Dorai of the Tulsi Rural Development Trust. Dr. Nirmala Chandrasekar, Dr. Lalitha Balakrishnan and Dr. R. Govindaraju have done most of the actual work, and Dr. S. Bhaskaran has provided nephrological guidance. We are grateful to the numerous donors who gave us the wherewithal to undertake this work, and to the Apollo Hospital of Chennai for investigating all our patients free of cost.

REFERENCES

1. Murray C. The World Development Report, Investing in Health, 1993.
2. Living standards. Economist 1996; 340(7975):94.
3. Ramachandran A, Snehalatha C, Satyavani K, Latha E, Sasikala R, Vijay V. Prevalence of vascular complications and their risk factors in type 2 diabetes. J Assoc Phys India 1999; 47(12):1152–1156.
4. Mohan V, Meera R, Premalatha G, Deepa R, Miranda P, Rema M. Frequency of proteinuria in type 2 diabetes mellitus seen at a diabetes centre in southern India. Postgrad Med J 2000; 76(899):569–573.
5. Mani MK. Prevention of chronic renal failure at the community level. Gupta SB, ed. Medicine Update 12. Mumbai: API, 2002:768–713.
6. Mani MK. Experience with a program for prevention of chronic renal failure in India. Kidney Int 2005; 67(Suppl 94):S75–S78.
7. Chalmers J, MacMahon S, Mancia G, Whitworth J, Beilin L, Hansson L, Neal B, Rodgers A, Ni Mhurchu C, Clark T. 1999 World Health Organization-International Society of Hypertension Guidelines for the management of hypertension. Guidelines sub-committee of the World Health Organization. Clin Exp Hypertens 1999; 21:1009–1060.
8. The Diabetes Control and Complications Trial Research Group. The effect of intensive treatment of diabetes on the development and progression of long-term complications in insulin-dependent diabetes mellitus. N Engl J Med 1993; 329:977–986.
9. Levey AS, Bosch JP, Lewis JB, Greene T, Rogers N, Roth D. A more accurate method to estimate glomerular filtration rate from serum creatinine: a new prediction equation. Modification of Diet in Renal Disease Study Group. Ann Intern Med 1999; 130:461–470.
10. Kronig B, Pittrow DB, Kirch W, Welzel D, Weidinger G. Different concepts in first-line treatment of essential hypertension. Comparison of a low-dose reserpine–thiazide combination with nitrendipine monotherapy. German Reserpine in Hypertension Study Group. Hypertension 1997; 29:651–658.

20

Academic and Clinical Collaboration Between Individuals, Departments and Institutions: The Ghana Experience

J. B. Eastwood and J. Plange-Rhule

Departments of Renal Medicine and Transplantation, and Community Health Sciences, St. George's, University of London, London, U.K. and Department of Medicine, Komfo Anokye Teaching Hospital, Kumasi, Ghana

INTRODUCTION

In the field of health and medicine, there is a tradition of collaboration between developing countries and Western nations. These collaborative efforts have embraced teaching, research, and provision of training and personnel, as well as donations of resources and technological help (1).

There are now serious issues in the context of collaborative ventures. Are inputs and outputs equal? How much of any assistance that has resulted has been based on the needs of, and at the request of, the recipient health worker or institution? How has the "information gap" been reduced? How can the problem of "without funds you cannot carry out good research but without good research you cannot attract funds" be solved?

We believe that links formed as a result of an "invitation" by individuals or institutions in developing countries have the most chance of success. Such links can broaden the hopes and aspirations of doctors and other health workers practicing in developing countries whether working in village settings, district hospitals, or medical schools.

In all developing (as in many developed) countries, medical schools have considerable difficulty recruiting teaching staff. This means that career development opportunities are likely to be limited. Similarly, research opportunities, if available, may only be short-term. There are also likely to be considerable difficulties providing clinical care.

GETTING THINGS STARTED

International collaborative links usually start with two individuals (Fig. 1). They are unlikely to be sustained unless there are identifiable achievable gains for both parties involved. What are these gains? What is needed at each end of the link (Fig. 1)?

Less-Developed Country

A link with a sister institution in a developed country has the potential to contribute in three areas—teaching and education, research, and the clinical care of patients. Once the link is established, there may be spin-offs for undergraduates and postgraduates, both medical and nursing. There should be enhancement of the learning environment, and other benefits may accrue, e.g., library enhancement, computing facilities, etc. Small advances in these areas can create an environment where students and young doctors—hopefully including the most academic—can take pride in their work and aspire to a long-term medical career in their own country. Such individuals will become role models for their successors.

More-Developed Country

Any health professional contemplating a link with a colleague in a less-developed country will need to commit himself to the collaboration

---

- Regular personal contact between the individuals at the two ends
- Mutually agreed, locally relevant aims which might include clinical priorities, research objectives or staff development, or a mixture of all three
- Clear written guidelines, preferably at institutional level, as to how the link will be fostered and supported
- Acceptance that the scope of the collaboration will not be limited by the priorities of Western funding agencies
- Bilateral annual visits
- The vision of a long time scale (10 + years) with a view to a lasting collaboration, not a transient one
- Training of individuals from developing countries taking place in their own country as much as possible
- Ability to respond to a changing environment at either end
- Involvement of nurses and other health workers in the collaboration
- Consider Honorary contracts for individuals taking part in established links; these can strengthen the link
- Early planning as to the means of securing future funding
- Independence from commercial sources of funding, avoiding possible future conflicts of interest and ability to publish the results of research
- Foster the development of other links and contribute to an international philosophy of links in general

Figure 1   Components of a successful link.

for a number of years. Much of the medicine practiced in the West, because of increasing specialization is limited in variety, both medical and geographical. Indeed, it is quite common now to spend one's whole career, from year 1 medical student to House Officer to permanent post, within a radius of no more than 20 miles. For many doctors, a link with a clinician working in a country with different culture, climate, range of diseases, and health system is an opportunity to expand their horizons.

The opportunities for collaboration in high-quality research and involvement in teaching of overseas undergraduates and postgraduates will undoubtedly enhance performance in the clinician's own specialty at home. For the institution, there is the opportunity to share some of its resources with another less well off, and to benefit from broadening the experience of its staff.

Financial Aspects

Many medical societies and institutions in developed countries make special provision for fostering links with developing countries. The ISN through the Commission for the Global Advancement of Nephrology (COMGAN) is a good example. In the U.K., the Royal Colleges as well as both the Association of Physicians of Great Britain and Ireland and its surgical counterpart allocate funds to generate overseas links. Indeed, our own collaboration started in 1994 with a grant from the Association of Physicians' *"Links with developing countries"* initiative.

OUR LINK IN DETAIL

Institutional Aspects

From the mid-1980s, there has been collaboration at institutional level between the School of Medical Sciences, Kwame Nkrumah University of Science and Technology, Kumasi, Ghana, and St. George's Hospital Medical School, London, U.K. The first link was in hematology (1986) and others followed (infectious diseases, pediatrics, and microbiology). Arising out of these the two medical schools drew up a Code of Practice for the partnership.

In 1994, the wish of one of us (J. P. R.) to initiate a link was facilitated through an individual with an existing link in hematology. The two individuals (J. P. R. and J. B. E.) forming the developing link drew up a list of areas of common interest and possible collaboration, and applied for funding, as above. The funds were used to set up a blood pressure clinic, to fund future visits, and to make suitable arrangements for reliable communication. This meant the purchase of a laptop computer with Internet access.

Where possible, visits have been annual in each direction, those to London lasting on average 6 weeks and those to Kumasi around 2 weeks. Objectives and a program (always flexible) are agreed before each visit and a report written at the end.

Communication

Communication issues are probably the most testing element of any link. It should be remembered that in many developing countries some of the standard means of communication taken for granted in Western countries are severely restricted. In Kumasi, for example, the hospital telephones are limited in number, and more or less restricted to clinical areas, and the junior doctors have neither bleeps nor pagers. Fax machines, photocopiers, and clinical secretaries are normally the privilege of Heads of Department. It is easy to see how isolated individuals can become. A budding clinician or research worker may have access to few facilities, and will find that it is necessary to go to the main Post Office or city center to pay for the use of a telephone, fax machine, or photocopier.

There remain four further forms of communication—e-mail, mobile telephone, the postal service, and international couriers. E-mail, though very effective, is not uncommonly difficult to access from developing countries, particularly from sub-Saharan Africa. In our experience, mobile telephone conversations, while useful for rapid clarification and discussion, end for over 50% of conversations by being cut off. Ordinary post remains very useful for paper transfer. For research projects, international couriers such as TNT, DHL, etc. are invaluable.

Components of the Link

Teaching

It is useful for students and teachers to meet colleagues from other cultures and other health systems, and where there is a different spectrum of disease. It is valuable too for visitors to see for themselves the difficulties doctors and nurses face in treating patients, as well as the differences between different curricula and teaching establishments.

Research

Our research plans evolved in ways not envisaged at the start. Indeed, of the four projects proposed at the very beginning of our collaboration, only one has materialized. On the other hand, our close association, coupled with intermittent visits, has enabled other research ideas to take root. Perhaps, the most important element in this formative process has been the opportunity for equality of "inputs" (ideas) from both ends of the link as regards projects and their time scales. Similarly, we have striven to maintain equality of "outputs" in terms of authorship and publications as far as possible.

The Association of Physicians grant was followed by a substantial grant from The Wellcome Trust (U.K.) for a community project on stroke in a number of villages in the vicinity of Kumasi. Other charities have provided small amounts of funding from time to time. Twelve peer-reviewed papers and two chapters have been published to date and others are in preparation.

Clinical

Although the original basis for forming the link was to enhance teaching, training, and research, there have been clinical spin-offs. In Kumasi, the most obvious nephrological problem was the lack of diagnostic ultrasound. This was corrected by the Teaching hospital in the late 1990s, so attention can now be focused on other needs. The hospital is now actively developing dialysis facilities, especially for patients with acute renal failure.

Training

Because of our own collaborative link, ISN-COMGAN saw an opportunity to come to the West Africa sub-region for the first time. There was a COMGAN-sponsored postgraduate meeting in Accra in December 2003, and a delegation of speakers to the 16th Nigerian Association of Nephrology in Jos in February 2004. There have been bilateral links in nephrology for some years, but there is no doubt that new links have been fostered by the interest of the International Society of Nephrology. Individual nephrologists are now members of the ISN and European Renal Association, and receive regular supplies of journals. Units with existing links have through ISN, the opportunity of achieving "ISN Renal Sister Center" status—one unit being in a developing country, the other in a developed country. Benefits focus especially on educational initiatives—including help with Fellowship training, student exchange, visiting Professorships, and clinical investigation.

CAREER ENHANCEMENT

Links such as the one described here can enhance the careers of both partners in the link. Perhaps, unexpectedly career enhancement was similar at both ends of the collaboration, not just in the developing country, i.e., there is mutual benefit.

- The need to focus primarily on needs identified in Africa; the health workers usually already know what is required
- Committed and influential champions at both ends of the link are essential
- Ensure equality of inputs and outputs as much as possible
- Remember communication difficulties: the system is more likely to be at fault than the individual
- Before establishing a link, determine what other links there are in the institution; it is useful to know about these

Figure 2 Lessons learned from the Kumasi-St. George's link.

A WAY FORWARD FOR LINKS BETWEEN HEALTH PROFESSIONALS

Links exist at least five levels—individual links between two collaborators, departmental links, institutional (hospital/health facility) links, College links, and Ministry of Health links.

Links between two individuals once established do seem to continue for many years. The development of trust over a long time is not easily eroded. In such a link, loss of one of the partners of the link would bring the link to an end (Fig. 2). On the other hand, if there are several collaborative links in the same institution, they will provide strength when a link is threatened or becomes less active. Both departmental links and institutional links lend support that can foster the exchanges, and provide material benefits. There are examples of the Chief Executives of two institutions—one in the developing world and one in the developed—agreeing on aims and objectives as well as on the conduct of the collaboration. Such collaboration brings benefit to both sides.

It is easy to see how Colleges of Physicians and Surgeons can facilitate collaboration between countries. Ministries of Health too can be of invaluable assistance.

Long-term links between institutions in countries that differ so significantly in their geographical, climatic, political, cultural, and religious characteristics provide enormous opportunities for mutual benefit and understanding, and for the development of enduring professional and personal friendships. In the current international atmosphere, the need for such links is more pressing than ever.

ACKNOWLEDGMENTS

Support from the Deans of the School of Medical Sciences, Kwame Nkrumah University of Science and Technology, Kumasi and St. George's, University of London, as well as from the Chief Executive of Komfo Anokye Teaching Hospital, Kumasi, has been invaluable. The constant support of Dr. John Dirks, Chairman of ISN-COMGAN, has been unwavering for many years.

REFERENCE

1. Eastwood JB, Plange-Rhule J, Parry V, Tomlinson S. Medical collaborations between developed and developing countries. Q J Med 2001; 94:637–641.

21

Nephrology in the Republic of Benin (West Africa)

Giovanni Battista Fogazzi
U.O. di Nefrologia e Dialisi, Ospedale Maggiore, IRCCS, Milano, Italy

Attolou Vénérand
Centre d'Hemodialyse, Centre National Hospitalier Universitaire, Cotonou, Benin Republic

Aouanou Guy
Division de Pédiatrie, Hôpital Saint Jean de Dieu, Benin Republic

BENIN: AN INTRODUCTION

The Republic of Benin is a country of West Africa, which lies between 12° and 7° latitude North, and 1° and −4° longitude East. It borders on Nigeria in the East, Togo in the West, Burkina Faso and Niger in the North, and the Gulf of Guinea in the South (Fig. 1). While the South is a plain with a tropical climate and environment, the North is a dry and hilly savannah.

Benin is a small country, with a surface of 112,622 km² and about 6.5 million inhabitants. They belong to several ethnic groups such as Fon (39%), who prevail in the South, Yoruba (12%), Adja (11%), Houeda (8.5%), Bariba (8%), Fulbe (5.5%), and several others (16%) (1). Animism and traditional beliefs are the prevailing religions (62%), followed by Catholicism (21%), Islam (12%), and others (5%) (1).

Until 31st of July 1960, Benin was a country belonging to Western French Africa with the name of Dahomey. Today, it is a francophone independent

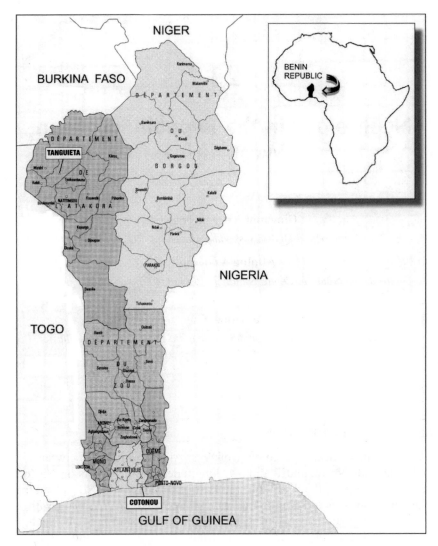

Figure 1   The map of the Republic of Benin.

republic with two main political parties (RB, *Renaissance du Benin*—Rebirth of Benin, and PRD, *Parti du Renouveau Démocratique*—Party for Democratic Renewal), and other minor parties. Administratively, the country is divided into 12 departments, each of which includes several sub-regions (Fig. 1). The capital of the country is Porto-Novo, but the most important town is Cotonou, on the Gulf of Guinea, with approximately 650,000 inhabitants.

The economy of the country is based mainly on agriculture (Benin is the 16th most important producer of cotton in the world), with a small industrial production of beer, palm and copra oil, sugar, and cement. The currency is the CFA (*Communauté Financière Africaine*, African Financial Community) franc, which Benin shares with several other countries of the region, and which has a fixed rate of exchange with the Euro (€) (1).

The main demographic and social indicators, shown in Table 1, clearly indicate that Benin belongs to the many poor developing countries of the world. From the medical standpoint, it is important to note the data concerning the very high child and maternal mortality, the short life expectancy, the chronic shortage of doctors and hospital beds, the low calorie intake, and the scarce access to drinkable water.

Due to this poor socioeconomical situation, nephrology is very undeveloped and exists only at an embryonic level, with the consequence that the vast majority of renal patients have very few possibilities of being treated adequately.

In this chapter, we describe the nephrological situation of Benin as seen from the point of view of two health institutions, one being the University Teaching Hospital (*Centre Nationale Hospitalier Universitaire* or *CNHU*) at Cotonou, the other the *Hôpital St Jean de Dieu* at Tanguiéta, which is located in a small town of the far North of the country, in the middle of a savannah area. We also describe a voluntary-based nephrological program,

Table 1 The Main Demographic and Social Indicators of Benin Republic as Compared to Those of France (1)

Indicator	Benin Republic	France
Birthrate (‰)	44.3	13
Fecondity[a]	6.3	1.9
Overall mortality (‰)	13.6	9
Child mortality (‰)	98	4.3
Maternal mortality[b]	500	10
Life expectancy in years (M/F)	52/56	76/83
Gross national product per head (in US $)	368	23,197
Index of human development[c]	0.411 (161)	0.925 (17)
Illiteracy (%)	61.4	—[d]
Number of doctors/1000 inhabitants	0.1	3
Number of hospital beds/1000 inhabitants	0.2	8.5
kcal available/day/inhabitant	2,558	3,591
Access to drinkable water (%)	63	—[d]

[a]Average number of children/woman of child-bearing age.
[b]Number of women who die from delivery every 10^5 children born alive.
[c]Derived from: longevity, knowledge (education and information), and purchasing power (the figure in parentheses indicates the rank among the countries of the world; Norway has the highest score, 1, whilst Sierra Leone has the lowest, 159).
[d]Information not available.

which was recently set up at Tanguiéta hospital and beyond, and finally analyze the main factors, which hamper the development of nephrology in Benin and in the region.

NEPHROLOGY AT CENTRE NATIONAL HOSPITALIER UNIVERSITAIRE (CNHU) OF COTONOU

The CNHU is the only teaching hospital of Benin, of which it is the main institution for the treatment of the sick and for biomedical research. Founded in 1963, it has today 609 beds for 24 specialties or subspecialties. Twelve of these, including nephrology, cover the main areas of internal medicine, seven are surgical, and five are diagnostic (three for radiology, one for laboratory medicine, and one for pathology). CNHU has a partnership with the Creteil Hospital in Paris for the permanent education of its personnel.

With a staff of 106 doctors and 650 nurses, CNHU in 2003 had 17,000 hospitalizations (for a total of 165,000 days of hospitalization), and 60,000 outpatient visits (data forwarded to the authors by the Management of CNHU).

As in all other hospitals of Benin, the cost of hospitalization is almost totally borne by the patients themselves. For instance, 1 day of hospitalization costs 1800–10,000 F^{CFA} (2.7–15.2 €), according to the level of accommodation chosen, to which the costs of *each* diagnostic test and drug have to be added. In fact, with the exception of only a few drugs such as diuretics, β-lactam, or aminoglycosidic antibiotics, which are supplied by the hospital, all other drugs must be bought by the patients themselves.

Since December 1997, CNHU has had a Dialysis Unit (*Unité de Dialyse*). This is run by one of us (A. V.), who at present is one of the two nephrologists active in Benin, with the help of a junior doctor and a staff of 15 well-trained nurses. The unit has 12 modern dialysis machines (Fresenius 4008B), 10 of which are in actual use, whilst two are kept as a spare capacity. Hemodialysis (HD) is available for both acute (ARF) and end-stage renal disease (ESRD).

About 10 patients with ARF are treated by HD/year, with a 90% survival rate. The main causes of ARF are dehydration, followed by sepsis and nephrotoxic drugs, which include indigenous remedies. Dialysis is given only to patients who can afford it (cost per dialysis session: approximately 107 €). Unfortunately, at present there are no remedies to this highly discriminatory and unjust situation. The patients and their families are left alone to face this dramatic problem. The costs of dialysis are too high for both government and private citizens to be available to all who need it. Even religious organizations, which in countries such as Morocco support maintenance HD programs (2), cannot be of any help in Benin.

As to maintenance HD, this is possible only for selected patients, the selection being based on both clinical and economical criteria. Clinically, the excluded patients are those with severe comorbidity, such as HIV infection, severe cardiovascular complications, or life-threatening neoplasia. Economically, only the patients who can sustain the financial burden of dialysis for 3 to 4 months are admitted, this period of time being necessary for the Ministry of Health to evaluate whether the patient is fit for dialysis and whether he/she qualifies for financial coverage. Once the patient is admitted to maintenance dialysis, all the related expenses, including the costs for recombinant epoetin beta, are covered by the government (estimated cost/patient/year: 18,300–21,960 €). Clearly, these rules discriminate against patients with ESRD who cannot afford the first months of renal replacement treatment.

When ESRD is diagnosed, the family of the patient is informed about the need for HD and its cost for the time necessary to know whether the government will give coverage. Since this cost is far beyond the possibilities of the vast majority of patients, in most instances they are discharged without dialysis and with conservative treatment only.

This dramatic situation is common to the whole region including Nigeria, in which for the impossibility to sustain the cost of dialysis most ESRD patients are left to die after being treated with HD for only few weeks (3).

With such a policy, at CNHU there are today 70 patients on chronic HD, whose main clinical features are shown in Table 2. All patients receive standard bicarbonate dialysis, biofiltration techniques not being available. Various types of filters with polysulphone membrane are used, but due to the lack of appropriate facilities their reuse is not possible. For the evaluation of renal bone disease, the measurement of serum alkaline phosphatase levels can be performed, but not that of parathyroid hormone. All patients have a good rehabilitation, as demonstrated by the fact that 61 of them (87%) are able to continue with their jobs or activities (44 patients working as officials, 12 as traders, four as students, and one as a craftsman). Interestingly, 5 years ago even an *association* of the patients on chronic dialysis was set up, which is still active today. This association has been instrumental in creating a feeling of mutual aid among dialysis patients and in representing them before the management of CNHU and the Ministry of Health. It also offers some aid to the families of patients in case of necessity. However, by no means it has the financial possibility to promote prevention programs or to cover the dialysis cost for the poor.

At the time of writing, these 70 patients with six others, who are on maintenance HD in a private center of Cotonou, represent the whole dialysis population of the country. Another public dialysis unit, with 10 new machines, is due to open in 2004 in Parakou, a town with about 128,000 inhabitants located in the center of the country. This new unit, which will be run by a doctor who has just returned from Cuba where he received

Table 2   The Main Clinical Features of the Patients on Maintenance
Dialysis at the Dialysis Unit of CNHU at Cotonou

No. of patients	70
M/F	47/23
Age	
Mean ± SD (range)	40 ± 4.2 (17–78)
Median	48
Cause of ESRD	
Hypertension	34 (48.5%)
Malignant hypertension	14 (20%)
Chronic glomerulonephritis	13 (18.5%)
Diabetic nephropathy	6 (8.5%)
Chronic interstitial nephritis	2 (3.0%)
Polycystic kidney disease	1 (1.5%)
With arteriovenous fistula	70 (100%)
With a history of tuberculosis	0
Positive for hepatitis B (HBsAg)	6/67 (8.9%)
Positive for hepatitis C (anti-HCV antibodies)	19/68 (27.9%)
On recombinant epoetin beta	67 (96%)
Dialysis schedule	
2 dialyses/week (5 hr/session)	54 (77%)
3 dialyses/week (4–4.5 hr/session)	16 (23%)
Duration of dialysis (months)	
Mean ± SD (range)	34.7 ± 21.4 (3–73)
Median	31.5

a training in nephrology for 4 years, will give access to dialysis to patients living in an area which is far from, and poorer than, Cotonou.

Due to the lack of financial resources and appropriate facilities, peritoneal dialysis and renal transplantation are not available in Benin. A few patients have recently been transplanted in France, and are now looked after locally.

Considering that Benin has approximately 6.5 million inhabitants with 76 patients on renal replacement therapy, and that in European countries there are 110 (the Netherlands) to 192 (Germany) ESRD patients on renal replacement therapy per million population (4), it is easy to estimate how many hundreds of patients are excluded from dialysis in Benin. However, it should be noted that compared to 2001, when the patients on chronic dialysis at CNHU were 50 (5), efforts have been made to increase the availability of dialysis in the country.

A larger development of dialysis programs in Benin has been hampered by several factors, all of which are equally important. There is shortage of qualified personnel, both at medical and paramedical level, and of adequate technology, without which the regular supply of electric power and water and the regular service of the equipment is impossible. Dialysis needs a strong laboratory support, but well-equipped laboratories are extremely rare in Benin (see also "Comment").

In addition, it must be considered that Benin is a country in which infectious diseases (mainly due to parasites and HIV) are still the main cause of morbidity and mortality. For this reason, health programs are addressed to this field rather than to dialysis, which supports relatively small numbers of patients at a very high cost.

Therefore, we believe that an expansion of dialysis programs could be achieved only with the solution of the problems mentioned above.

An integral part of the renal service is a nephrological ward with 18 beds and a clinic.

In 2003, in the ward there were 216 hospitalizations with a 15% mortality rate, and 501 patients were seen in the renal clinic. The renal diagnoses for 371 of such patients are shown in Table 3. These were obtained by using the facilities available at CNHU, which include the basic diagnostic tests, such as serum creatinine, BUN, serum and urine electrolytes, urinalysis, urine culture, serum and urine protein electrophoresis, i.v. pyelography, ultrasonography, CT scan, and Doppler of renal arteries. However, other tests, such as C3 and C4 serum levels, serum immunoglobulins, anti-DNA antibodies, ANCA, acid–base balance, and renal angiography, which in the developed world are taken for granted, are not yet available. This holds true also for *renal biopsy*, a fact that greatly limits the adequate handling of renal patients, especially those with ARF or glomerular diseases, conditions by no means rare at CNHU (Tables 2 and 3).

Table 3 The Renal Diagnoses Made in the Renal Ward and Clinic at CNHU of Cotonou in 2003

Renal disease	Number (%)
Chronic renal failure	175 (47.2)[a]
Acute renal failure	98 (26.4)
Nephrotic syndrome	17 (4.6)
Glomerulonephritis	13 (3.5)
Diabetic nephropathy	12 (3.2)
Interstitial nephritis	9 (2.4)
Urolithiasis	9 (2.4)
Nephroangiosclerosis	5 (1.3)
Perirenal abscess	4 (1.1)
Polycystic kidney	3 (0.8)
Others	26 (7.1)
Total	371 (100)

[a] 23/175 (13.1%) with uremic encephalopathy at presentation.

As to drugs, the main categories of antihypertensive agents including diuretics, beta-blockers, calcium channel antagonists, and ACE-inhibitors can all be found on the market. β-Lactams, and aminoglycosides are the most used antibiotics, whilst oral prednisone, prednisolone, and azathioprine are the only immunosuppressive agents used.

In spite of all these limitations, a number of good-quality scientific publications have been obtained from the patients under the care of the CNHU renal services. They have often been published in local and national journals highlighting issues of importance to the community. Among these, it is worth mentioning the studies on the prevalence of ARF in patients with sickle cell disease (6), the electrolyte disorders in patients with ARF (7), the renal syndromes in patients with HIV infection (8), the prevalence of urinary tract infections (9), hypertension (10), and vascular renal syndromes (11) in pregnant women, the risk factors for eclampsia (12), the prevalence and causes of both ARF and CRF (13), the clinical aspects of the nephrotic syndrome and of post-infectious glomerulonephritis in Benin children (14,15).

NEPHROLOGY AT HÔPITAL ST JEAN DE DIEU (HSJD) AT TANGUIÉTA

The HSJD at Tanguiéta serves the population of a large rural territory in the northern part of the country (the so-called *"le pays profond"* "the deep country"), close to the border with Burkina Faso (Fig. 1).

Built in 1970 by the friars of the religious order of Saint Jean de Dieu, it is recognized today by the National Health System as a referral hospital of the Atakora Subregion, an area of 20,459 km^2 and more than 400,000 inhabitants. It has 237 beds distributed in five pavilions, which include Medicine, Surgery, Intensive Care, Gynecology, and Pediatrics, and other services such as the Emergency unit, the Laboratory, the Radiology unit, the Rehabilitation center, the Clinic for the outpatients, and the Pharmacy.

Ten doctors, nine of whom are Africans, and 106 paramedicals work in the hospital, where in 2002 more than 7700 patients were hospitalized (2842 of whom were children), 1842 interventions of major surgery were performed, and 11,560 patients were seen in the clinics (16,17).

For its peripheral and rural location, the HSJD is frequented by patients who differ from the average patients of CNHU. In fact, they are mostly peasants, shepherds, and small traders of low, or very low, social condition, who are often illiterate, belong to different ethnic groups, and often speak languages poorly known even to the local personnel of HSJD. For all these reasons, very frequently it is impossible to outline the clinical history of patients, with obvious limitations on the handling of the clinical problems. Finally, quite often patients turn to the hospital only after failing to obtain relief of symptoms by traditional healers, with delays in presentation, which can be very harmful for the patients themselves.

Similarly to what happens at CNHU and in all the other public hospitals of the country, also in this case the patients have to pay for their medical needs. However, due to the religious nature of HSJD, the fees are much lower than in the government institutions, and patients are treated even when they cannot sustain, partially or even entirely, the financial burden. This is made possible through the financial support of the religious order of Saint Jean de Dieu and of a number of voluntary organizations mainly from France, Italy, and Switzerland.

Malaria due to *Plasmodium falciparum* is endemic in the area of HSJD, with 10% mortality among the hospitalized patients, as are tuberculosis and HIV infection, which affects 12% of the local population (17). Periodic epidemics such a meningitis, which in 2002 caused 24 deaths out of 72 hospitalized children, and typhoid fever, which in 2003 caused bowel perforation in a high proportion of patients (17), are not uncommon. However, the most frequent life-threatening disorders remain pulmonary infections and diarrhea, the latter being associated with a very high parasitic load, including schistosomiasis (187 positive cases in the year 2000) (5).

Thus, at HSJD renal diseases do not represent a priority, even though they do exist. In an unpublished report of 1992 by one of us (A. G.), it was found that the children affected by glomerulonephritis, nephrotic syndrome, or renal failure represented 0.9% (53/5863) of the medical pediatric patients hospitalized in a 4-year period (1989–1992) (18). More recently, by analyzing the laboratory files for the year 2000 we found, among adults, 176 patients with serum creatinine ≥ 2.0 mg/dL and 52 patients with $\geq +++$ albuminuria, who represented 4.9% and 1.4% of the total adult admissions. Among children, those with serum creatinine ≥ 2.0 mg/dL were 17, and those with $\geq +++$ albuminuria were seven, who represented 0.8% and 0.3% of the total child admissions (5). Unfortunately, with our analysis it was not possible to obtain information about the nature of the renal disease. However, in 2003 we were able to review the case histories of 36 adult hospitalized patients with renal insufficiency and found that the most frequent causes of renal insufficiency were arterial hypertension (50%) and diabetes mellitus (33.3%). For children, the most frequent nephropathies were nephrotic syndrome and acute glomerulonephritis (Table 4).

What are the facilities for the management of renal patients at HSJD? From the diagnostic standpoint, serum creatinine, BUN, urinalysis, plain x-rays of the abdomen, i.v. pyelography, kidney and bladder ultrasonography are all available. However, other crucial tests such as the measurement of Na^+ and K^{+*}, urine culture, acid–base balance, the immunologic tests, and the renal biopsy cannot be done.

$^*Na+$ and $K+$ measurements have successfully been introduced in October 2005 (method: flame photometry).

Table 4 The Main Clinical Features and Diagnoses of the Renal Patients Hospitalized in the Pediatriac Ward of HSD of Tanguiéta in 2003

Sex	Age	Screat (mg/dL)	Urine albumine	Blood pressure	Kidney ultrasounds	Diagnosis
M	18	·1.4	++++	130/80	Normal	Cortico-resistant NS, responsive to cyclophosphamide
F	14	0.6	++++	120/60	Normal	Cortico-dependant NS
F	7	0.9	+++	100/80	Normal	Cortico-sensitive NS
F	3	1.7	+++	100/50	Normal	Acute GN from unknown cause
M	2	1.4	++	90/60	NA	Acute GN after tonsillitis
M	6	2.0	++	110/30	NA	Acute GN from unknown cause
F	2	3.6	+	NA	NA	ARF due to hemoglobinuria caused by malaria
M	15	1.9	++++	110/60	NA	CRF + NS unresponsive to corticoids and cyclophosphamide

Abbreviations: NS, nephrotic syndrome; GN, glomerulonephritis; ARF, acute renal failure; CRF, chronic renal failure; NA, not available.

Also therapeutically there are many limitations, which are due to the difficulty to supply drugs, which are too expensive for the local situation. These include ACE-inhibitors, fluoroquinolones and, especially, dialysis. The latter is not available at all at HSJD nor in the rest of the country with the exception of CNHU.

Based on our knowledge of the country, we believe that the situation described for HSJD is similar to that of other peripheral public hospitals of Benin.

A NEPHROLOGICAL PROGRAM AT HSJD AND BEYOND

In 1997 a voluntary-based nephrological program was set up with the aim of improving the Nephrology at HSJD (5) and of creating in-country capacity (19). This program, which included periodical visits to HSJD by one of us (F. G. B.), was based on several points (Table 5),

Improvement of Urinalysis

The detection of urine proteins with the sulfosalicylic method was replaced with a 10-pad dipstick, which besides albumin allowed the detection of other

Table 5 The Main Features of Our Program of Cooperation with HSJD

A personal commitment over the years
Regular visits to the institution where the program was set up
Regular contacts
Identification of the local clinical priorities and needs
Identification of the persons who carry out the program locally and their permanent education
Supply of instrumentation (which has to be solid, easy to use and maintain with low operating costs, and possibly new)
Regular supply of reagents
Written documents and guidelines based on clear and essential information

important analytes such as urine pH, specific gravity, glucose, hemoglobin, leukocyte esterase, and nitrites. In addition, traditional urine microscopy was replaced with a more sophisticated technique based on the use of phase-contrast microscopy coupled with polarizing light when needed and a continuous through-the-year education of two laboratory technicians. Today, they are able to identify with confidence all the particles of the urine sediments as well as the different urine profiles, and to alert the physicians when findings suggesting serious renal diseases are seen. This has improved the capability to diagnose renal diseases, especially glomerulonephritis and nephrotic syndrome.

This program was made possible, thanks to funds collected in Italy among friends, colleagues, and relatives. These allowed the *regular supply* of dipsticks (number of urinalyses/year: approximately 5000) and slides for microscopy. In addition the Italian NGO *Gruppo Solidarietà Africa* allowed us to purchase a microscope for urine sediment examination.

Dipsticks, however "cheap" they may appear to our eyes (about 0.20 €/strip), are still seen as a "luxury" in sub-Saharan Africa, where their use is extremely limited. To reduce their cost, we use to cut with scissors the strips in two parts longitudinally, so that with one strip two samples can be analyzed.

As to the microscope, we purchased a phase-contrast instrument because it allows the best identification of the urine particles whilst maintaining the possibility to examine blood and stool samples with conventional light simply by switching the condenser to the appropriate position. We equipped the microscope also with a double co-observation device, because we consider this of the highest importance for teaching and discussing with others the findings.

Another clue for the success of this program was a *continuous contact* with our "pupils," who were educated not only during "on-site" visits but also through exercises of identification and interpretation of urine findings, which were sent them by mail several times a year, and for which they received both comments and scores.

Introduction of Electrolyte Measurement

In 1998, two flame photometers for the measurement of Na^+ and K^+ were purchased thanks to the financial support of the Italian NGO mentioned above. However, due to some drawbacks in the method itself and the poor quality of the gas, this part of the program resulted in complete failure. Thus, to date, the measurement of Na^+ and K^+ continues to be missing at HSJD. Today, very simple and reliable methods based on dry chemistry are available on the market. However, the high operating costs (approximately 1 €/single measurement) make them too expensive to use at HSJD (see footnote at page 425).

Improvement of the Treatment of Renal Patients

This was developed through written documents and guidelines on the approach to the renal patient, integrated with demonstration at bedside. In addition, we introduced drugs which were almost unknown locally, such as ACE-inhibitors to protect kidney function, the K^+ sparing compound hydrochlorothiazide + amiloride, the 500 mg tablets of furosemide, and the sublingual nifedipine for hypertensive crises. Furthermore, modern therapeutic schemes for the treatment of nephrotic syndrome, especially in children, were supplied. Today, one of us (A. G.) is in charge of all nephrotic patients seen in the hospital, and looks after them also after discharge (seven children and three adults at present). This has improved the short-term outcome and has reduced the rate of patients lost to follow-up, which in the past exceeded 50% (18).

Written documents and guidelines have always been prepared by keeping in mind the local facilities and patient population.

Over the years, the following documents have been produced:

Urinalysis. This included instructions for a correct urine collection, advantage and pitfalls of urinalysis by dipsticks, the particles of the urine sediment, the integration of dipstick results with microscopy findings, the main urine profiles (proliferative and non-proliferative glomerulonephritis, nephrotic syndrome, diabetic nephropathy, acute tubular necrosis, urinary tract infection including schistosomiasis, contamination of urine from genital secretions), the adjustment, maintenance, and repair of the microscope.

Na^+ and K^+ disorders. Unfortunately, this document after being discussed with the doctors could not be used for the failure in introducing the electrolyte measurement.

Approach to the renal patient. This described the importance of integrating the figures of plasma creatinine with the findings obtained by urinalysis and ultrasonography of the urinary tract. In a situation in which it is very often difficult to obtain the clinical history from patients (see paragraph 3), ultrasonography is of particular importance, especially in distinguishing acute from chronic renal diseases.

The main antihypertensive drugs. This described the action and the side effects of the antihypertensive agents regularly available at HSJD (diuretics: hydrochlorothiazide, hydrochlorothiazide + amiloride, furosemide; calcium channel antagonists: nifedipine; ACE-inhibitor: enalapril; antiadrenergic agents: methyldopa, clonidine).

The documents were always simple and practical, and based on essential information, since at present there is no room for academic or sophisticated nephrology at HSJD as well as in many other health institutions of the region.

Improved Documentation

A registry for the record of all renal patients hospitalized in the pediatric and internal medicine ward was set up in 2004 with the aim of obtaining sound epidemiological data, which are lacking at present.

An epidemiological community-based program for the detection and prevention of chronic kidney disease is also envisaged. However, such a project needs funds and facilities to support a permanent local task force, which are not available at the moment.

Educational Aspects

In February 2003, a 2-day course on basic nephrology was organized with the financial and logistic support of the Ministry of Health of Benin and of the Commission for the General Advancement of Nephrology (COM-GAN) of the International Society of Nephrology (ISN).

This was the first national postgraduate course ever organized in the country (Fig. 2), and was held first at HSJD and was then repeated in the town of Ouidah in the South. Faculty included two of us (A. V. and F. G. B.),

---

REPUBLIQUE DU BENIN

MSP/MESRS

PREMIER COURS NATIONAL POST-UNIVERSITAIRE DE NEPHROLOGIE

A TANGUIETA DU 06 AU 08 FEVRIER 2003

ORGANISE PAR LA SOCIETE INTERNATIONALE DE NEPHROLOGIE.

Figure 2 The badge of the First National Postgraduate Course of Nephrology ever held in the Republic of Benin.

a diabetologist from CNHU (Djorolo François) and a nephrologist from Ibadan University Teaching Hospital, Nigeria (Kadiri Solomon). The program covered several aspects of basic nephrology, such as epidemiology of the renal diseases in the region, glomerular diseases with focus on the forms associated with infections, blood hypertension, diabetes mellitus, acute renal failure with particular attention to the forms caused by indigenous remedies, and chronic renal failure. The aim of the course was to bring to the attention of the 22 attendees, mostly general practitioners working on the territory or in hospitals, the importance of preventing renal failure and of slowing down its progression. Due to the extremely limited resources available for the treatment of ESRD, we consider this part of the program to be of the highest importance and worth repeating in the future with a larger audience.

Contacts with Other Nephrologists of the Region

These were developed to know the nephrological situation around Benin and to establish contacts with the view of a possible common program for the future. To date, contacts have been established with nephrologists of Nigeria and Burkina Faso.

In Nigeria, where there are several centers of nephrology and an active national society of nephrology, the situation is much more advanced than in Benin. However, due to poverty, the access to drugs and dialysis is still a major problem for the vast majority of the renal patients (20). In spite of some recent positive contacts between the renal unit of CNHU and the renal unit of Ibadan run by Solomon Kadiri (5), intercourse between Nigeria and Benin and the rest of francophone Africa seems to be difficult especially due to language barriers, Nigeria being an anglophone country.

As to Burkina Faso, the nephrological situation is very similar to that of Benin. In fact, there is only one nephrologist and one hemodialysis unit for the whole country, located in the *Centre Hospitalier Universitaire "Yalgado Ouédraogo"* at Ouagadougou, which is the capital of the country. As in Benin, diagnostic and therapeutic facilities are very scarce and insufficient for an adequate handling of renal patients. In addition, at the time of writing only 24 patients are on maintenance dialysis in a country with more than 10 million inhabitants (A. Lengani, personal communication, 2004).

Due to the similar situation, common language and recent history—Burkina Faso also belonged to Western French Africa—a program encompassing the francophone countries of the region (Benin, Burkina Faso, Niger, Mali, and Togo) seems to be possible and advisable. Therefore, in the last few months we have started working on this new project.

COMMENT

In this chapter, we have described the nephrological reality of Benin, a small developing country of West Africa, and given two examples.

On the one hand, there is the CNHU, a University hospital located in the most important town, with a dialysis unit in which 70 ESRD patients are successfully treated at the expense of the government. On the other hand, there is the HSJD, a peripheral hospital that serves a large and poor territory, in which nephrological facilities are almost completely missing, as happens in all other hospitals of Benin with the only exception of CNHU.

This intra-country variation in hospital facilities is common in developing countries (21). However, in spite of the many differences between CNHU and HSJD, the two realities have several important features in common. We consider these features as an example of some of the problems, which nephrology faces in most countries of sub-Saharan Africa.

In our view, there are three main problems, which hamper the development of nephrology in the region, which are all due to poverty and underdevelopment:

The shortage of diagnostic facilities. The most striking of these is the lack, in the whole country, of a center in which renal biopsy can be performed. This situation is common to Burkina Faso and Togo, and involves even richer Nigeria, where renal biopsy is available, but usually without the possibility to perform immunofluorescence investigation (22).

Another major problem, at HSJD as well as in the majority of public hospitals of Benin, is the impossibility to obtain very basic tests such as the measurement of electrolytes or urine culture (see footnote at page 425). This confirms that functioning biochemistry and microbiology are rare in tropical developing countries and that the microscope remains the single most useful diagnostic tool (23).

These deficiencies undermine the practice of nephrology at a basic level. If a solution for the measurement of electrolytes might be possible in the short- or mid-term, and the lack of urine culture is often replaced by surrogates such as the use of Gram staining on the urine (24), the introduction of renal biopsy seems to be far ahead in the future. In fact, it requires expensive and sophisticated equipment, an inter-disciplinary approach, technical skills, and specific knowledge, which are difficult to have now.

The lack of access to treatment. With the only exception being the patients on maintenance hemodialysis at CNHU, all the expenses for the treatment of renal diseases must be paid by the patients themselves.

Together with a profound attachment to traditional medicine (25), the high costs of drugs and of health services explain why most renal patients only come to hospital as a last resort, when the disease is very advanced and the symptoms overwhelming (13,14), a fact which has been noticed in several other countries such as Burkina Faso (26,27), Morocco (2), and Nigeria (20,28). Interestingly, this behavior is maintained even when patients from developing countries emigrate to rich ones, where national health systems cover the costs (29), which we see as a residue of a habit acquired in the native countries.

Another consequence of the cost of treatment, which goes together with poor education, is the low compliance to the prescribed medications and the high rate of patients who do not come for medical controls (18).

Recently in Benin, several generic drugs including some antihypertensive agents such as methyl-dopa and clonidine have been introduced. This will certainly improve access to medications, even though the vast majority of the population, especially in the rural areas, will still continue to find the costs of treatment prohibitive, especially for chronic diseases such as arterial hypertension, diabetes mellitus, or renal failure. Therefore, national programs do not seem to be sufficient and should be supported by global programs and funds, aimed at improving the availability of drugs with protective effects on kidney function, such as ACE inhibitors (30).

Shortage of nephrologists. At present, there are only two nephrologists in Benin, only one in Burkina Faso, Togo, Niger, and Mali The presence of one nephrologist every several million inhabitants implies a heavy work load, shortage of time for studying and research, as well as professional and cultural isolation.

This problem, together with a dramatic shortage of doctors in all developing countries, is very difficult to solve. Some help can come from programs for the training of junior nephrologists, whilst isolation can be overcome by regional meetings and "on-site" visits of experts working on middle- or long-term programs such as those organized by COMGAN of the ISN.

At the moment, a "basic level of training" in nephrology of local medical students and general practitioners might represent a partial solution for the shortage of nephrologists. In our opinion, this training should be focused on the subject of the day, which is the early diagnosis and treatment of renal diseases and the prevention of renal failure, which to a certain extent might already be carried out with the tools available locally. However, for a full nephrological practice, there are no short cuts, a full nephrological education being mandatory, which at the moment can be obtained only by sending junior doctors abroad.

The improvement of health information is also very important, and this is now possible also in sub-Saharan Africa through an increased connectivity to the Internet and e-mail (31,32). In this respect, it is certainly encouraging that these facilities are now reaching also HSJD.

For now, this is one of the most important achievements, not only for the spreading of health information but also for the improvement of the links between "our World," in which the best and newest treatments are within almost everyone's reach, and the "other World," in which even the basic health services are a luxury for the vast majority of renal patients.

REFERENCES

1. Calendario Atlante De Agostini 2004. Novara: Istituto Geografico de Agostini, 2003:299–300.
2. Bourquia A. Etat actuel du traitement de l'insuffisance rénale chronique au Maroc. Néphrologie 1999; 20:75–80.
3. Arije A. Short-term dialysis. 16th Nigerian Association of Nephrology Annual Scientific and General Meeting, Jos, Nigeria, February 18–20, 2004.
4. Locatelli F, Valderrabano F, Hoenich N, Bommer J, Leunissen K, Cambi V. Progress in dialysis technology: membrane selection and patient outcome. Nephrol Dial Transplant 2000; 15:1133–1139.
5. Fogazzi GB, Attolou V, Kadiri S, Fenili D, Priuli F. A nephrological program in Benin and Togo (West Africa). Kidney Int 2003; 63:S56–S60.
6. Attolou V, Avode DG, Bigot A, Latoundji S, Houngbe F, Gninafon M, Zohoun I. Prevalence de l'insuffisance rénale chez les patients drépanocytaires hospitalisés dans le Service des Maladies du Sang du CNHU de Cotonou. Bénin Méd 1997; 6(bis):12–16.
7. Attolou V, Avode DG, Avimadje M, Houngbe F, Djrolo F, Addra B, Gninafon M, Monteiro B, Hountondji A. Perturbations hydroélectrolytiques au cours des insuffisances rénales aiguës en milieu hospitalier de Cotonou. Bénin Méd 1997; 6(bis):87–90.
8. Attololu V, Bigot A, Ayivi B, Gninafon M. Complications rénales associées à l'infection par le virus de l'immunodéficience acquise humaine dans une population hospitalisée au CNHU de Cotonou. Cahiers Santé 1998; 8:283–286.
9. Attolou V, Takpara I, de Souza J, Guedou F, Djimegne F, Alihonou E. L'infection urinaire chez la femme gestante Béninoise (Aspects bactériologiques et cytologiques). Bénin Méd 1998; 8:15–19.
10. Attolou V, Takpara I, Akpovi J, Avode G, Nida M, de Souza J, Agboton H, Alihonou E. Les différents types d'hypertension artérielle chez les femmes enceintes Béninoises admises au centre national hospitalier et universitaire (CNHU) de Cotonou. Cahiers Santé 1998; 8:353–356.
11. Akpovi J, Attolou V, Noukounwoui ER, de Souza J, Perrin RX, Alihonou E. Contribution à l'étude des syndromes vasculo-rénaux sévères à Cotonou. Bénin Méd 1998; 8:84–86.
12. Attolou V, Avode DG, Aguemon R, Takpara I, Akpovi J, Atchade D, de Souza J, Chobli M, Perrin R, Alihonou E. Facteurs de risque de l'éclampsie (A propos de 21 cas observés dans le Service Polyvalent d'Anesthésie et de Réanimation du CNHU de Cotonou). Bénin Méd 1998; 7:39–40.
13. Aguemon A, Attolou V, Kohossi L, Atchade D, Monteiro B. Contribution à l'étude de l'insuffisance rénale au CNHU de Cotonou. Bénin Méd 1998; 9:106–108.
14. Attolou V, Koumakpaï S, Toukourou R, Djrolo F, Sovigui G, Avode GD. Syndrome néphrotique pur chez l'enfant. Expériences Béninoises de dix ans. Bénin Méd 2000; 14:84–89.

15. Attolou V, Koumakpaï S, Avimadje M, Toukourou R, Djrolo F, Sovigui G, Avode GD. Les glomérolonéphrites post-infectieuses de l'enfant Béninois: aspect cliniques, thérapeutiques, et économiques (à propos de 41 cas). Bénin Méd 2000; 14:102–107.

16. Hôpital Saint Jean de Dieu de Tanguiéta. Rapport d'activité 2002–2003.

17. Zaongo D. Infezioni ed epidemie: le possibilità di diagnosi e terapia in un centro ospedaliero di una regione rurale in Africa sub-sahariana. In: Infettivologia a confronto: strategie di prevenzione e scelte di terapia nei paesi in via di sviluppo. Legnano, 18 ottobre 2003:76–79; Abstracts book.

18. Aouanou G, Gougbenou J. Prise en charge des néphropathies dans le Service de Pédiatrie à l'Hôpital St Jean de Dieu de Tanguiéta. Tanguiéta 1992; Thesis.

19. Editorial. Tropical medicine: a brittle tool of the new imperialism. Lancet 2004; 263:1087.

20. Bamgboye EL. Hemodialysis: management problem in developing countries with Nigeria as a surrogate. Kidney Int 2003; 63:S93–S95.

21. Smith MK. Hospitals in developing countries: a weak link in a weak chain. Lancet 1999; 354(suppl Lancet 2000):26.

22. Kadiri S, Osopbamiro O, Ogunniyi J. The rarity of minimal change disease in Nigerian patients with the nephrotic syndrome. Afr J Med Med Sci 1993; 22: 29–34.

23. White NJ. Practice of clinical medicine in the tropics. Lancet 1997; 349(suppl III):6–8.

24. Manual of Basic Techniques for a Health Laboratory. 2nd ed. Geneva: World Health Organization, 2003:251–252.

25. Kubukeli PS. Traditional healing practice using medicinal herbs. Lancet 1999; 354(suppl Lancet 2000):24.

26. Lengani A, Kabore J, Traore R, Ouedraogo C, Zoungrana R, Drabo J, Savadogo A. Epidémiologie de l'insuffisance rénale aiguë de l'adulte au Centre Hospitalier National Yalgado Ouedraogo de Ouagadougou. Burkina Méd 1998; 2(suppl 1):48–53.

27. Lengani A, Guissou P. Toxicologie des remèdes traditionnels au Burkina Faso: insuffisance rénale aiguë et plantes médicinales. Ann Université Ougadougou 1997; 5(serie B):111–120.

28. Mabayoje MO, Bamgboye EL, Odutola TA, Mabadeje AF. Chronic renal failure at the Lagos University Teaching Hospital: a 10-year review. Transplant Proc 1992; 24:1851–1852.

29. Fogazzi GB, Castelnovo C. Maintenance dialysis in patients from developing countries: the experience of an Italian Centre. J Nephrol 2004; 17:552–558.

30. Schieppati A, Perico N, Remuzzi G. Preventing end-stage renal disease: the potential impact of screening and intervention in developing countries. Kidney Int 2003; 63:1948–1950.

31. Godlee F, Pakenham-Walsh N, Ncayiyana D, Cohen B, Packer A. Can we achieve health information for all by 2015? Lancet; 364:295–300.

32. Editorial. A window of opportunity for Africa's health information. Lancet 2004; 1364:222.

22

International Aid and the Formation of Successful Chronic Kidney Disease Prevention Programs (CKDPP)

Ivor Katz

Dumisani Mzamane African Institute of Kidney Disease, Chris Hani Baragwanath Hospital, University of the Witwatersrand, Johannesburg, South Africa

INTRODUCTION

This chapter will investigate the general issues, practices, and problems for nephrologists and public health professionals in the developing world, when accessing international aid for the establishment of chronic kidney disease prevention programs (CKDPP). This will require an analysis of some existing international medical aid organizations and their activities after which the focus will shift to renal international aid organizations and their initiatives. It is here that the author will draw on personal experiences and focus on prevention initiatives in South Africa. The chapter will conclude with a helpful practical approach to access international aid and focus on practical tasks necessary when accessing international aid and for establishing prevention programs.

BACKGROUND

There is a realization in the nephrology community that we must have a more realistic approach to the existing and increasing burden of chronic kidney disease. In 2020, the contribution of chronic non-communicable

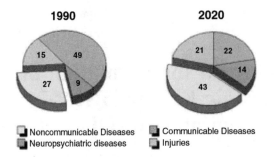

Global burden of disease 1990–2020 by disease group
in developing & newly industrialized countries

Figure 1 Changes in Noncommunicable disease distribution in developing countries. *Source*: The challenge of chronic conditions: WHO responds. Epping-Jordan J. BMJ 2001; 323:947–948.

diseases is set to rise from 27% in the 1990s to 43% (1) (Fig. 1). These conditions include non-communicable diseases such as diabetes, chest, and heart disease, mental health disorders such as depression, and certain communicable diseases such as HIV infection and AIDS. By 2020, the burden of diabetes and cardiovascular disease will have increased by 130% in Africa alone, affecting nearly 21 million and 1.3 million people, respectively, with concomitant similar increases in prevalence of end-stage renal disease (2). More patients will die of strokes, heart failure, and kidney failure all over the world but especially in Africa and the developing world (3,4). We also know that we are unable to afford the type of care required to manage our patients who develop ESRD in the developing. No nation will escape this burden unless its government and healthcare leaders decide to act: the prevalence's of all chronic conditions are growing inexorably and are seriously challenging the capacity and will of governments to provide coordinated systems of care (Table 1) (1). The burden of these conditions falls most heavily on the poor, and one-dimensional solutions will not solve this complex problem. People's health status and quality of life will not be improved solely by medication and technical advances; and thus healthcare systems will have to move away from a model of "find it and fix it" (Fig. 2). Lastly, these solutions cannot be delayed and the sooner governments invest in care for chronic conditions, the better. This realization has resulted in a number of initiatives by individuals, NGOs, and renal societies to establish CKDPP. However, it should be realized that establishing a CKDPP relies on the ability to acquire skills and access resources. So, we have to balance this enthusiasm with the practical reality, which recognizes that most of the countries needing prevention programs are also those in which they are most difficult to set up.

Table 1 Strategies to Improve Clinical Care and Outcomes for Chronic Conditions

Strategies to improve clinical care and outcomes for chronic conditions
Develop health policies and legislation to support comprehensive care
Reorganize healthcare finance to facilitate and support evidence-based care
Coordinate care across conditions, healthcare providers, and settings
Enhance flow of knowledge and information between patients and providers and
  across providers
Develop evidence-based treatment plans and support their provision in various
  settings
Educate and support patients to manage their own conditions as much as
  possible
Help patients to adhere to treatment through effective and widely available
  interventions
Link health care to other resources in the community
Monitor and evaluate the quality of services and outcomes
These strategies are based on WHO's review of innovative best practice and
  affordable healthcare models

Source: The challenge of chronic conditions: WHO responds. Epping-Jordan J. BMJ 2001; 323: 947–948.

INTERNATIONAL AID AND MEDICAL PRACTICE IN THE DEVELOPING WORLD

Existing International Aid Organizations—Aims and Projects

It would be important to evaluate and critically appraise some relevant international aid organizations in order to help us with the task of establishing chronic kidney programs.

The most well-known NGO worldwide is the *World Health Organization*, established in 1948. Its objective is the attainment by all people the highest possible level of health. It aims to achieve this by communicating

TYPICAL APPROCAH TO HEALTH CARE

'The Radar Syndrome'

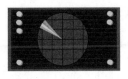

- Patient appears
- Patient is treated "find it and fix it"
- Patient is discharged

... then disappears from radar screen

Figure 2 'The Radar syndrome' approach to chronic diesase management. *Source*: Epping-Jordan J. The challenge of chronic conditions: WHO responds. BMJ 2001; 323:947–948.

evidence-based policy; managing information and stimulating research and development; catalyzing change through technical and policy support, to build sustainable national and inter-country capacity; negotiating and sustaining national and global partnerships; setting, validating, monitoring, and pursuing the proper implementation of norms and standards; stimulating the development and testing of new technologies, tools and guidelines for disease control; risk reduction; healthcare management; and service delivery (5).

These ideals are those of most organizations wishing to prevent kidney disease and establish projects for kidney and cardiovascular protection.

Another Foundation worth reviewing is the *Global Forum for Health Research* (GHRF) in Geneva. This organization has a strong focus on the developing world situation. Their central objectives include "correcting the 10/90 gap" by focusing on research and collaboration between partners in both the public and private sectors. Their motto includes promoting research to improve the health of poor people. They aim to achieve this by organizing annual meetings, helping to develop priority-setting methodologies, and by supporting networks in priority health research areas. Thus, this organization is focused on using research to develop health care and delivery by establishing support networks around these developments (6).

The Initiative for Cardiovascular Health Research in Developing Countries (IC Health) is another NGO, which shares similar interests with the renal care specialists. They work closer to the coal face than the previous two NGOs. IC Health receives funding from the World Bank and other partners whose aims are to prioritize resource-sensitive research and to address the growing burden of cardiovascular diseases in the developing countries. They also prioritize research on sustainable models of disease prevention through primary health care in resource-poor settings. These model programs deliver established safe and effective methods to reliably and affordably prevent cardiovascular disease. They acknowledge that even though these methods of prevention are known, e.g., ACE inhibitors, management of risk factors; they still need to be delivered in the developed world setting. They are therefore trying to develop large-scale cost-effective programs in low- and middle-income countries. The programs have surveillance and intervention components.

IC Health also recognizes the importance of capacity and skills development through "A Capacity Building and Institutional Strengthening project," which aims to develop capacity in institutions so that they can develop and manage prevention programs. This will ultimately lead to institutional strengthening and sustainability. They also offer short courses in epidemiology, biostatistics, and data management and as well as other fellowships to develop capacity. Recognizing the economics of health care and healthcare costs makes them focus on the macroeconomic consequences of cardiovascular diseases and diabetes in low- and middle-income countries. They have established a project known as Macroeconomic Consequences of Cardiovascular Diseases and Diabetes, which has been developed with Earth Institute at Columbia University, New York (7). These latter aspects of capacity building and economics are critical in winning support from developing country governments and for acquiring funding from international funding organizations and pharmaceutical companies.

It would be difficult to leave out an invaluable organization like *Médecins Sans Frontières* (MSF), which was established in 1970 and has been providing medical care to vulnerable populations for decades. They are a grass roots organization working on approximately 400 projects in 80 countries around the globe (8). Their focused activities include mainly emergency interventions providing assistance after natural disasters, epidemics, and armed conflicts. However, more recently, they have established epidemiological programs looking at Ebola virus and more recently have been involved in establishing relevant protocols for managing complex diseases like HIV/AIDS to resource-poor populations that have neither the means nor the technical knowledge to deal with these health calamities. The latter programs and their practical nature are therefore of particular interests to nephrologists trying to establish kidney disease programs.

Having reviewed some well-known international aid organizations and their activities, we must examine exactly what relevance they have for us, and what lessons we can learn.

Analyses of International Aid Organizations (IAO) and Their Initiatives

These IAO express these wonderful ideals, but they are not always possible. It is therefore important to recognize a few important facts. These include the reality that there is no substitute for formal health structures. An IAO may aim to provoke change and be a catalyst for change by passing on knowledge and skills, but this is difficult to achieve.

Although MSF, WHO, IC Health, and the Global Forum for Health Research aim to complement formal health sectors, there remains an ongoing moral dilemma in providing health care to vulnerable populations. Problems exist such as the development of dependence on external assistance, which can minimize a government's responsibility to deliver health care. These initiatives can be manipulated by existing governments or mask the real problems (9).

Problems Facing IAOs

Real problems therefore exist for an IAO. These include making their "intellectual resources" available to the people who most need them. The WHO summarizes this well by describing "making good management ideas travel" and ensuring medication and technical advances results in real quality of life improvement. In the Global report from the WHO, they emphasize the shifting from an acute, reactive, and episodic model of care, i.e., the "find it and fix it" model to one of organizing and simplifying the use of guidelines into a complex delivery model, which takes into account all the facets of a health system and the community which it serves (Figs. 2 and 3) (10).

There exist key problems for people and organizations trying to establish prevention programs, which include:

- accessing existing resources and available aid projects;
- establishing contact with international aid projects;
- accessing the funds for the development of the project and once it is established the management of these funds;
- planning and then sustaining the of projects;
- evaluating the role of research in international aid and medical practice both as a means of accessing resources and of managing the project.

Innovative Care for Chronic Conditions Framework

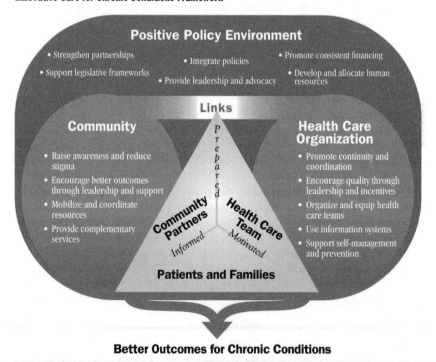

Figure 3 WHO innovative care for chronic conditions framework.

Ellen Einterz summarizes the above with a few simple questions. How do we convert "action plans" and intentions to real success? And how do we reduce the "plausible reasons" explaining failure, e.g., inflation, no stability, lack of political will, time and logistics, mismanagement, corruption, and theft by managers (9).

Lessons to Learn from International Aid Organization

In this section, the focus will be on the activities and focus of grass root organizations. Similar analysis could be applicable when evaluating the WHO.

The Global Forum for Health Research and IC Health has an active history of being involved in research-based projects. This strong emphasis on science does have a negative element, as it requires certain baseline research skills or support before starting such a project. IC Health has developed from the establishment of partnerships with international aid organizations like the World Bank and WHO. They have a strong focus in the primary care setting and emphasize qualitative as well as quantitative research. GFHR is focused on the core health issues and has a long-term outlook and commitment to disadvantaged communities.

These organizations face common problems of funding and donor shortages, which impacts on sustainability. Although their focus is on the developing world, these communities don't have easy access to these funds. Access depends on having the contacts with potential funders and the skills to write funding proposals. Grant funding requires significant skills and resources, especially time, and in the developing world clinicians are overburdened with clinical responsibilities.

Médecins Sans Frontières (MSF) is one of those grass root organizations with an excellent record in the developing world. They have a very strong culture of volunteerism. Their volunteers spend extended times in poor communities and they can transfer skills at the same time as conducting well-planned programs. Programs are also developed with the local community and local NGO input. MSF emphasizes the evaluation of local problems in the country together with local NGOs or government structures. An organization like MSF requires significant funding to support its programs, the fact that they can is very positive, emphasizing the importance of generating funding. This ability indicates that the organizational skills required to run such an organization. MSF have only recently entered the chronic disease management "market" and sustainability in this area is critical.

Key Components for the Management of Chronic Disease Illnesses

Having outlined what international aid organizations do, and how they can assist with the establishment of chronic disease programs, we now examine what mechanisms are needed to establish chronic kidney disease programs.

Table 2 Key Components to Establishing a Chronic Kidney Disease Program

- The support from government, local community organizations (NGOs), health workers and patients
- Securing some form of bridging assistance from an IAO, whether financial or other, such as equipment, human resources, or technical skills
- The establishment of a productive interaction between patients and the health practice team
- The establishment of an organized integrated program as compared with the "usual" standard "find it and fix it model" of care existing in most countries. Organized care has shown better outcome compared with standard care programs
- A strong primary healthcare focus with the PHC Nurse being critical especially in the developing and poorly developed countries (Yawn, 2000)

Among these include a strong primary healthcare focus with the PHC nurse being critical especially in the developing and poorly developed countries (Table 2) (11).

The WHO recognizes the difficulty to achieve ideal circumstances and therefore advises those in the developing world to follow a more practical approach. Therefore, one's approach should be modified according to one's capacity. Dr. Ruth Bonita, Director, NCD Surveillance Non-Communicable Diseases and Mental Health of the WHO, outlines the methods for achieving this (12). She highlights the need to develop a hierarchical framework to unify surveillance and prevention program activities, explaining that these should be flexible across a range of risks, conditions, ages, and areas. The program or research organizer is encouraged to develop standard methods and tools, which are adaptable to local settings. One needs to start with common core methods, tools, and treatments and then develop expanded and optional extras if possible or if resources arise. So if the only method available is lifestyle modification, then this is where one should start and not be discouraged to start from there. So the aim is to develop basic sentinel surveillance and treatment sites and then to add on to existing systems. One should remember the basic guiding principles on keeping it simple (Fig. 4).

INTERNATIONAL AID AND THE NEPHROLOGIST

Having provided the general principles and having given some background to aid organizations and establishing a sentinel surveillance site or chronic kidney program, we will now focus on the more specific task faced by nephrologists. At this point, it is important to recognize the two options facing a nephrologist in the developing world. Firstly a CKDPP could be established on its own with the primary focus being the kidney as the organ to treat. The second option could be for the kidney to fall under the gambit

Step1: Behaviors

- Tobacco and alcohol use
- Intake fruit and vegetables
- Physical inactivity

Step 2: Physical measures

- Height, weight, waist
- Blood pressure
- Pulse rate

Step 3: Blood samples

- Cholesterol
- Blood glucose

Next Steps: ... Expanded ... Optional etc.

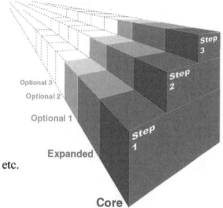

Figure 4 The WHO STEPS framework—integrating NCD surveillance into research on high blood pressure. Global Forum for Health Research 5, Arusha, WHO Non-Communicable Diseases and Mental Health, Geneva.

of all chronic illnesses recognizing that managing the key chronic illnesses risk factors such as hypertension and diabetes will have the greatest impact on reducing the progression of kidney disease. However, it can be said that even if one starts more specifically maintaining your own "organ identity," it will be unlikely and short sighted should you want to progress further to ignore all other cardiovascular and infectious disease known to cause chronic kidney disease and chronic disease. Ultimately stroke, heart failure, ischemic heart disease, and CKD will all be influenced by prevention strategies.

International Renal Organizations

There really is only one international renal organization, which has a focus on the developing world and the capacity to work in poorer countries, i.e., The International Society of Nephrology (ISN) and its flagship committee; The Commission for the Global Advancement of Nephrology (COMGAN). The COMGAN was founded in 1995. Its purpose is to bring advancements in nephrology to countries and regions of the world where the need for better renal care is foremost. It is through this commission that a great deal of networking has been established, a critical factor required to develop local skills and establish projects. It is through this networking that projects are developed, grant funding is sourced, and that global networks have developed to establish prevention strategies worldwide. The ISN flies the banner calling for "the prevention of renal diseases in the emerging world: toward global health equity." There are a few other local kidney foundations, the International Federation of Kidney Foundations (IFKF), and pharmaceutical companies that have similar goals but the ISN COMGAN would really be the only international renal organization, which could be classified as a global medical IAO. This is not to say that other foundations or organization do not exist. However, the ISN uses its international position to lobby foundations and the pharmaceutical companies to sponsor development and education worldwide. So whilst the organization exists, it probably does not have the same grass roots involvement like MSF, but it does have extensive networks. The ISN is involved in the arena of grass root chronic kidney disease development and aid, so the questions of sustainability and continuity are becoming important. There are many CKDP programs around the world and the ISN has managed through its own network to arrange a fairly loose network of these groups and has also published more recently the findings of these kidney disease prevention programs (13).

Establishing Kidney Disease Renoprotection Programs

With the background to medical and renal aid organizations, the chapter will now focus more specifically on the practical development and establishment of a CKDPP. The focus will be on the current existing programs. The author will attempt to critically appraise existing programs and then try and analyze their reasons for their successes and failures. This will hopefully help the reader to establish their own program or integrate these principles into their daily clinical practice. The chapter will also focus on the specific practical tasks and the suggested processes, which one should consider and which are needed when accessing international aid for such a medical project (Table 3).

Wendy Hoy in Australia is probably the person with the most experience of establishing kidney and cardiovascular protection programs. Her

Table 3 Practical Aspects to Establishing a Chronic Kidney Disease Prevention Program

Generally these specific skills include the following:
- Project planning
- Collaboration with international aid
- Funding of projects and developing sustainability
- Development of a data base to evaluate the aid project
- Data collection
- Establishments of systems to run the program
- Development of clinical algorithms
- Development of local teams and structures

team has developed a number of programs in the Australian Aboriginal community and collaborated with teams in the rest of the world including India, Nigeria, and South Africa. She has outlined the need to work together with communities to engage community interest in chronic illness management and prevention strategies to help assess needs in the community to then develop an agreement with the local community or health authority (14). Once these basic requirements have been met, then one can go on to help local staff implement the program, to try and ensure sustainability, and then to provide a mechanism or skills to evaluate processes and outcomes, which have been established. These are the fundamentals needed in the approach to develop chronic illness programs and a CKDPP.

THE MODEL FOR PREVENTION PROGRAMS

Focus on Current Programs in Nephrology Programs

The Kidney Disease Outcomes Quality Initiative Clinical Practice Guidelines for Chronic Kidney Disease draw on the results of NHANES III and the 1998 USRDS studies to establish the CKD stages. This staging protocol has significantly improved our focus for detecting, following, and managing CKD (15). However, what this protocol exposed was the hierarchical or pyramid shape to kidney disease. It indicated that most CKD patients fall into CKD stage 1or 2 and not stage 5 (ESRD). These are also the stages in which people are least likely to present with kidney disease. So the options when establishing a CKD program include either screening an entire population as in the Dutch PREVEND and the Australian Aboriginal studies or detect a cohort of people at the highest risk of kidney disease (16,17) (Fig. 5). It is clear that the former approach is more costly and less likely to be achieved in the developing world. However, one has to make this judgment according to local conditions and resources. A couple of CKD programs are critically evaluated below.

A Nephrological Program in West Africa

Giovanni et al. (18) published results from a hospital-based screening and treatment "program" in Benin and Togo. The program was more a detection program, with possible successes of the study being the raising of awareness of renal disease in the hospital. It was also obviously carried out according to existing resources. However, the criticisms would be that this is a small hospital-based program focusing on a limited number of people. It was not focused on prevention or early detection, it was treating those already with disease, i.e., "find it and fix it" model (Fig. 2).

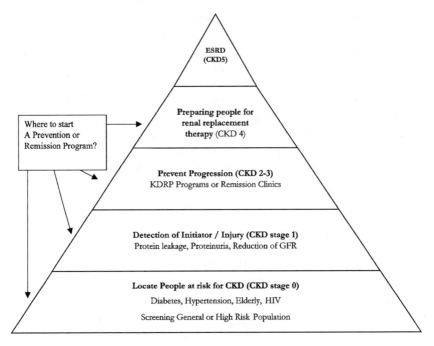

Figure 5   Kidney disease renoprotection programmes, where to start?

Kidney Help Trust Rural Project—India

Here Muthu K. Mani (19) established primary care chronic disease program, which focused on proteinuria, hypertension and diabetes, and other renal diseases. It was run by local community participants (health workers) and included a screening and treatment component. The *successes* of this very exciting project were its simplicity as stated by Dr. Mani himself, "We keep it simple." It was also a cheap mass screening campaign including 25,000 people and this was an early detection program. It also was primary health-care nurse driven as primary healthcare workers were used to detect disease and give basic treatment under supervision. The problems include the fact that there was no long-term quantitative data available and therefore he was unable to evaluate impact of his intervention. He also noted that only 8% took ongoing treatment and that they were only able to visit homes every 18 months.

The Bolivian Renal Disease Project

Here Plata and Remuzzi collaborative project with support of Bergamo Institute and ISN-COMGAN ran an educational campaign and mass screening for urinary disease in apparently healthy subjects (20). About

14,000 patients were screened and urinary abnormalities were detected in over 4000. These people were referred to local health centers and were to be followed up over the next 3 years. The successes of this project outlined the basis to starting all such programs, i.e., gaining a good understanding of local problems using a simple and cheap test. This study helped define the incidence of asymptomatic renal diseases in an unselected population. It showed that it is possible to screen a large population at relatively low cost (similar to Mani's Indian project), providing the framework for further action that may help in the prevention and timely diagnosis of renal diseases. It was also run in both urban and rural setting. The current question here will be the ability to sustain such a program, which requires mass screening of healthy people with good follow-up. There is also uncertainty in this program of primary nurse involvement, especially with follow-up. However, the program does have a follow-up component. Follow-up has proven to be a difficult task in most developing country projects.

Australian Chronic Disease Outreach Program

Wendy Hoy Australian Outreach program remains an ideal template on which to develop ones own program (17). It has both screening and ongoing integrated care program, which started in Tiwi Islands and extended to other Aboriginal areas in Australia and involves screening of entire community for high-risk groups and then the initiation of treatment and follow-up of these patients. The programs have from 5 to 15 years of experience in these communities. Wendy Hoy has also helped to establish programs in South Africa (see below) and India. The Kidney Disease Research Program (KDRP) has also made contact with potential program coordinators in Nigeria and Kenya. The successes include showing definite improvement from baseline and reduction in kidney and cardiovascular disease as well as all cause mortality (strokes, heart failure, etc.). It has influenced protocols and become a government lobby group and galvanized NGOs working in these communities. These include the replication of a first world economy-based program into the developing world. The Aboriginal communities remain an ongoing developing community in a developed country. The program relies on community support and has not been sustained by all communities as a result of poor support from local governing authorities in some areas. This appears to be changing due to the high success, which is becoming recognized by these communities and the authorities running them. However, despite successes, it is still slow to change and influence day-to-day practice throughout Australia and the Aboriginal people remain a marginalized minority relying on "paternalism" from the majority White Australians.

The Chronic Disease Outreach Primary Prevention Program in South Africa

The development of the South African CKDPP is an ideal example of utilizing international aid organizations. The author met Wendy Hoy in 1998 in Abidjan and quickly realized that the Australian Aboriginal project could be adapted for Soweto. This network was established with the assistance of the ISN. Soweto is a melting pot of people in transition, from a healthy traditional lifestyle to a Westernized one, now at high risk for chronic diseases including HIV-associated nephropathy (21). Against a known background of poor blood pressure and glucose control, the program was implemented in 16 primary care clinics in Soweto and nearby regional clinics. A tertiary hospital served as the focal point for data collection (surveillance) and management of the program (Fig. 6). The SA CKDPP is an integrated chronic illness program based on an understanding that adequate blood pressure control, diabetic control, and risk factor control will confer a specific effect (advantage) in preventing, reversing, or retarding diabetic, hypertensive, and proteinuria as well as those with established CKD (Fig. 7) (22). The program is developed around the Wagner Chronic Illness Care model, which focuses on creating a prepared and proactive health team and an informed patient (Fig. 8) (23). It does this by focusing on critical components of treating people with chronic diseases. These components contain simplifying the targets for blood pressure, glucose and proteinuria control, providing ongoing

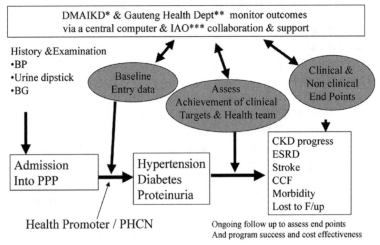

Figure 6 Outline of South African CKDPP. *Abbreviations*: BG, blood glucose; BP, blood pressure; PHCN, primary health care nurse; PPP, primary prevention program; CCF, congestive cardiac failure.

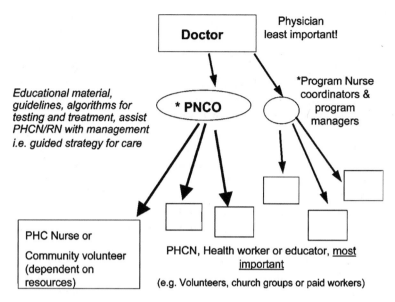

Figure 7 Chronic disease outreach program integrated care model. *Abbreviations*: PHCN, primary health care nurse; RN, registered nurse.

education and support with patient management, as well as regularly evaluating whether clinical targets are being achieved. The results of this analysis together with ongoing qualitative evaluation are hoped to ensure that chronic illness care are dynamic and meeting the needs of the population it serves. The focus is on a high-risk group recognizing the resource capabilities of the service. Phase 1 lasting 2 years served as the baseline surveillance assessment

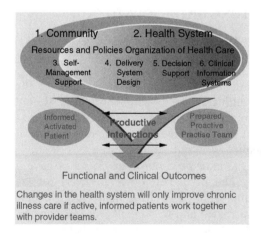

Figure 8 Wagner chronic illness care model.

of the community. The program focused on the kidney and on achieving quantitative clinical targets only. It achieved treatment success but was unable to assess endpoint improvements, e.g., reduction in ESRD, strokes, and heart failure. This will be the target in phase 2, which continues to get strong support from the Australian program, which includes assistance with data evaluation, direct skills training of local primary health care nurse program coordinators and nurses. The criticisms include poor planning in phase 1 against known existing resource shortages and inability to show cost effectiveness. Other common problems to the developing world communities included funding shortages, especially drugs and infrastructure; data capture quality and efficiency; inadequate long-term follow-up and evaluation of endpoints in phase 1 as well as only focusing on quantitative data and not qualitative data evaluating service quality, efficiency, and staff motivation.

The positive aspects include a better understanding of renal disease and cardiovascular risk, positive short-term treatment outcomes and a model of international aid assistance. It was noted that although problems existed, the program still showed benefit. It also showed that a program could be transportable, i.e., from Australia to South Africa. This assistance was set up through the ISN COMGAN network. There remains ongoing support from the Australian KDRP in the form of skills transference, data management, and analysis. The program is developing sustainability, as we are using existing staff and infrastructure and government is directly involved in sponsoring and providing staff and support for the program. There is an essential link between primary and tertiary care. There is skills transference to health workers. After 5 years, it demonstrates stamina "staying power," probably the most critical component for establishing a CKDPP.

PITFALLS ENCOUNTERED IN SETTING UP THE SOWETO CKDPP

There are important problems encountered when establishing a CKDPP and specifically in an urban developing world community like Soweto. However, these problems are relevant for any such program.

Consultation: There was inadequate consultation at the start of the project from experts in Public Health Care field. As nephrologists, we are entering a new realm and we do not have the necessary skills. After embarking on this project, we realized that we did not have a good understanding of the burden of disease, i.e., epidemiological data were poor.

Epidemiological skills: The specialty of nephrology does not have a strong tradition of epidemiology like in diabetology. However, we are now realizing that this is very important. Therefore, many more people qualified for the program than anticipated and we were ill prepared for this. We also had not planned for the cost of the screening investigations, e.g., blood and urine tests. A better knowledge of the conditions in which we were working would help with better planning. A good surveillance or pilot project is important.

Developing a model for your CKDPP: It is important to have a model around which to work and develop one's local program. Even if one has the resources and the appropriate numbers, it is important to make sure that the correct systems are established. This is where expertise was sought from both local experts and IAOs. The program was adapted for the local situation. Instead of screening and following all people of the population, we are focusing on cohorts of high-risk patients in each clinic. However, we are encouraging the use of the skills and knowledge acquired for other patients in the clinic population. We are using the data to influence the service delivery and priorities.

Support from local community people and structures: Follow-up of patients with problems is important, and contacting patients who fail to turn up is also vital. For this good systems needed to be established, this included a good database of patients and the support of the clinic health promoters (community-based health workers). The patient promoters could follow up on patients who did not return for check ups and outcomes could be determined, i.e., the patient had a stroke or had died.

Research and auditing skills: Research skills remain a problem amongst most primary healthcare nurses in developing countries. Training needed to be implemented in this regard and support for analysis of data was sought. PHC nurses did not realize the importance of entering data accurately and fastidiously. Clinical audit is not taken seriously and the importance this administrative skill is not emphasized. Health workers are also too focused on clinical care and do not consider this to be important. The Program Nurse Coordinators (PNCO) were sent for training in "Good Clinical Practice" and research skills.

Developing simplified guidelines: Although we have a good understanding of the methods to prevent or slow the deterioration of CKD, the approaches are not well documented from a practical perspective and especially for a primary care setting. Guidelines are also often completely inappropriate and too academic. One does not realize how many different protocols exist and how difficult it is for health workers to synthesize this vast amount of knowledge. Local protocols needed to be appropriately updated and one had to include local protocol groups so as not to alienate the PHCN and their teachers. Thus, the PHCN training school was incorporated into the CKDPP management. All educational materials are jointly reviewed and taught.

An alliance of community organizations: This latter point highlights the key aspect in a CKDPP of involving various appropriate health and community organizations in an alliance. The more groups involved the more likely the success.

Skills and resource development: The central surveillance site (Dumisani Mzamane African Institute of Kidney Disease) also did not have all the skills and expertise and resources to analyze data quickly and appropriately. Support needed to be sought from Australia from their epidemiology and statistical support team. It was hoped in fact that data could be entered on a web-based program. This would have made it easier and more efficient to analyze and communicate. However, we failed to realize the skills that were necessary. Despite the PHCNs being very skilled in delivering health care, they were not computer literate. Most developing communities have not had access to this technology. The development of skills serves as a great motivator for nurses. This lack of motivation and fatigue is a critical area, which needs attention. Many clinics also did not have the correct equipment that we take for granted, e.g., computers, modems, etc. Training has had to be started for this component and we are auditing all sites in order to upgrade them to develop the capacity in the future. Currently, the program is running on a paper-based system, whilst these necessary skills and resources are being developed.

Funding and financial skills: Funding is needed even if one has good support from local health authorities. Funding had to be found for transport for the PCNO to access clinics and to provide training and medical education for the local clinics. One also needs funding for development training and for the teaching materials. The government health authorities did not have a budget for these components and even if it was available accessing these funds or resources was often completely impractical. Therefore, assistance with fund raising was sought from professional fund raisers. This included developing skills to draw up a "funding proposal," which is essential when asking for funds. In this regard, both skills and support is needed for managing a CKDPP budget.

Communication: Many of these components were only realized after consulting both local and international experts from aid organizations. Thus, solutions to many of the pitfalls were available but just needed to be found. Communication on many levels remains a critical component to developing a CKDPP.

Patience and perseverance: This is probably the most necessary skill. Even when things are going wrong there is always time to correct them. One just has to start the process from the beginning again and go slowly, keeping it simple.

FUNDAMENTALS TO INTERNATIONAL AID AND ESTABLISHING A CKD PROGRAM

The above examples demonstrate clearly that it is possible to establish a CKDPP in the developing world. They also demonstrate the strong links needed with international aid organizations. They also demonstrate some of the fundamentals when managing chronic diseases in less developed

Table 4 Common Practical Principles for Doing it Right: A Beginners Guide!

1. *Consultation*: Good and careful project planning with experts, government, and the community
2. *Epidemiological Data*: Assess disease burden and community knowledge with a pilot project or research study
3. *CKDPP Model*: Development of local teams and structures and coordinators. Development of a database to evaluate the project quantitatively, qualitatively, and the cost effectiveness of the program. Developing a model and the establishments of systems to run the program, i.e., ensure efficiency and sustainability
4. *Primary Health and Community Focus*: Ensuring a well functioning, "happy" team, which includes the primary healthcare nurse, health workers, and the community
5. *Research and Audit Skills*: Data collection (using established 1st World scientific principles), this includes the development of the necessary research and audit skills
6. *Guidelines*: Development of clinical algorithms (*SIMPLIFIED!*), *e.g., WHO principles of Core, Expanded Core and Optional, summarize and simplify existing local or international guidelines*
7. *Skills and Resource Development*: Ensuring ongoing training and development as well as audition resources. Improving these for health workers helps with motivation and sustainability of the program
8. *Funding and Financial Skills*: Try and establish funding of projects or other means to develop sustainability as well as the resources, skills and support to source and manage the funding and funds of the project
9. *Communication*: Collaboration with appropriate international aid organizations, i.e., expert support and assistance
10. *Patience and Perseverance*: Persistent hard work—stamina! The most important component. Possible regional, national, or international adaptation

countries, the establishment of an informed and proactive health team and strong patient and community partnerships. These components remain as important as adequate funding. One has to focus not only on the technical aspects but also on supporting or caring for staff. The paradox being that continuing care delivered by a well-functioning team is the basis on which control of chronic disease must rest (1). Ultimately, one has to have the long-term commitment and stamina to build a chronic disease program. Some of the practical fundamentals including a list of dos and don'ts, which is advice and for people starting up a CKDPP, are summarized in Table 4.

REFERENCES

1. Epping-Jordan J. The challenge of chronic conditions: WHO responds. BMJ 2001; 323:947–948.

2. Schena FP. Epidemiology of end-stage renal disease: international comparisons of renal replacement therapy. Kidney Int 2000; 57:39.

3. Aubert RE KH, Herman WH. Global burden of diabetes, 1995–2025: prevalence, numerical estimates, and projections. Diabetes Care 1998; 21:1414–1431.

4. Reddy S YS, Ounpuu S, Anand S. Global burden of cardiovascular diseases: part I: general considerations, the epidemiologic transition, risk factors, and impact of urbanization. Circulation 2001; 104:2753–2756.

5. WHO. About the World Health Organisation. Vol. 2004. Geneva, World Health Organisation, www.who.int, 2004.

6. GlobalForumHR. Global Forum for Health Research http://www.globalforumhealth.org/pages/index.asp. Vol. 2004. Geneva: Global Forum for Health Research, 2004.

7. ICHealth. Initiative for Cardiovascular Health Research in the Developing Countries, Delhi, http://www.ichealth.org/, 2004.

8. Médecins Sans Frontières MSF. The MSF role in emergency medical aid. Electronic Source URL http://www.msf.org/ Access year 2004; Access date 6/23/2004.

9. Einterz EM. International aid and medical practice in the less-developed world: doing it right. Lancet 2001; 357:1524–1525.

10. WHO. In: (CCH) WHOHCfCC, eds. World Health Organisaion: Observatory on Health Care for Chronic Conditions. Vol. 2004. Geneva: World Health Organization: Health Care for Chronic Conditions (CCH), 2004:chronic disease website of WHO.

11. Yawn BP. West J Med 2000; 172:77–78.

12. Bonita R. Integrating NCD surveillance into research on high blood pressure. In: Arusha, ed. Global Forum for Health Research [Abstr]. Vol. 5. Geneva: WHO Non-Communicable Diseases and Mental Health, 2003.

13. Pugsley David J AL, Nelson Robert G. Renal disease in racial and ethnic Minority Groups. Kidney Int 2003; 63, s83:S1–S2.

14. Hoy WE SJ, McKendry K, Sharma S, Kondalsamy Chennakesavan S. Planning services for noncommunicable chronic disease (NCDs) in Aboriginal communities. In: Abstract. Berlin: ISN EDTA-ERA WCN, 2003.

15. NKF-K/DOQI. NKF-K/DOQI clinical practice guidelines for chronic kidney diseases: evaluation, classification and stratification. Am J Kidney Dis 2002; 39:S1–S266.

16. de Jong PE HH, Pinto-Sietsma SJ, de Zeeuw D. Screening for microalbuminuria in the general population: a tool to detect subjects at risk for progressive renal failure in an early phase? Nephrol Dial Transplant 2003; 18:10–13.

17. Hoy WE WZ, Baker PR, Kelley AM. Reduction in natural death and renal failure from a systematic screening and treatment program in an Australian Aboriginal community. Kidney Int 2003; 63:s66–s73.

18. Giovanni B. Fogazzi VnRA, Solomon K, Domenico F, Fiorenzo P. A nephrological program in Benin and Togo (West Africa). Kidney Int 2003; 63: S56–S60.

19. Mani M. Prevention of chronic renal failure at the community level. Kidney Int Suppl 2003; 83:S86–S89.

20. Plata RSC, Yahuita J, Perez L, Schieppati A, Remuzzi G. The first clinical and epidemiological programme on renal disease in Bolivia: a model for prevention and early diagnosis of renal diseases in the developing countries. Nephrol Dial Transplant 1998; 13:3034–3036.
21. Mohammed ES. In: Gauteng Health Department Report on Hypertension and Diabetes control at Soweto Clinics. Johannesburg: Gauteng Health Department, 2000.
22. Katz IJ LV, Butler O, Hopley M. An Early Evaluation of the Primary Prevention Program (PPP), a Kidney Disease Renoprotection Programme (KDRP) in Soweto, South Africa. In: South African Renal Society Bi-annual Congress, Bloemfontein, Department of Renal Medicine, Chris Hani Baragwanath Hospital, University of the Witwatersrand, Soweto, South Africa, 2002.
23. EH Wagner CD. In: Improving Chronic Illness Care (ICIC). Vol. 2004. Seattle: The Robert Wood Johnson Foundation, 2004.

23

Links Between Bolivia, Moldova, and Italy for Prevention of Chronic Nephropathies

Igor Codreanu
Department of Hemodialysis and Kidney Transplantation, Republican Clinical Hospital, Chisinau, Moldova

Norberto Perico, Agustina Anabaya, and Giuseppe Remuzzi
Department of Medicine and Transplantation, Asienda Ospedaliera Ospedali Riuniti di Bergamo—'Mario Negri' Institute for Pharmacological Research, Bergamo, Italy

INTRODUCTION

The growing global burden of non-communicable diseases worldwide has been neglected by policy makers, major aid donors, and academics. In 2003, there have been 56 million deaths globally, of which 60% were due to non-communicable diseases (1). These chronic diseases are the largest cause of the death in the world, led by cardiovascular disease (17 million deaths in 2002, mainly from ischemic heart disease and stroke), followed by cancer (7 million deaths), chronic lung disease (4 million), and diabetes mellitus (almost 1 million) (2). These leading diseases share key risk factors: tobacco use, unhealthful diets, lack of physical activity, and alcohol abuse (1). The global prevalence of these chronic diseases is increasing, with the majority occurring in developing countries and projected to increase substantially over the next two decades (3). It is increasingly recognized that the burden of chronic kidney disease (CKD) is not limited to its implication on demands for renal replacement therapy (RRT) but has major impact on overall population health (4). Indeed, patients with reduced kidney function represent a population not only at risk for progression of kidney disease and development of end-stage renal disease (ESRD), but also at even greater risk for cardiovascular disease (CVD) (5–7). This suggests that CKD patients who are advancing toward ESRD carry the heaviest burden of CVD and that this frequently leads to death before ESRD is reached. Cardiovascular and renal disease share common risk factors and markers, are linked clinically, and are susceptible to similar menu of interventions. Thus, a single coherent policy of containment would reduce morbidities of both conditions. Early renal disease and high cardiovascular risk factors are both easily diagnosed and can be modified by standard interventions, with dramatic reduction in renal failure, heart attack, stroke, and premature death over the short and intermediate term. Screening programs can be implemented with simple, cheap, and reliable tests, such as measurement of body weight, blood pressure, and dipstick urinalysis for protein and glucose. Examples already exist. On this line, we have established in the past linked prevention programs of renal disease with Bolivia and now we are working to extend this experience to the Republic of Moldova. Here we will briefly analyze these experiences.

THE PROJECT FOR RENAL DISEASES IN BOLIVIA

In 1992, the "Mario Negri Institute for Pharmacological Research" in Bergamo, Italy, on the behalf of the general project of "Mario Negri for Latin-America" through the support of the "Associazione il Conventino," Bergamo, Italy, and the cooperation of young doctors of the Ospedale Giovanni XXIII in La Paz (Bolivia) activated a specific project entitled "El Proyecto de Enfermedades Renales en Bolivia." The project established an initiative for Bolivia mainly directed to education and prevention in the field of renal diseases, bearing in mind that Bolivia is a developing country and the possibility to obtain renal replacement therapies, like dialysis or transplantation, is only for patients who earn over 1500 US $ monthly, whereas the majority of the people has a monthly salary lower than 70 US $. Therefore, the project was aimed to demonstrate that in emerging countries the strategies to be fulfilled for renal disease is prevention and early detection. The general objective was to give tools for advancement in nephrology in Bolivia that would help identify subjects at risk of developing renal diseases later in life, with the hope to provide the basis for building a regional and nationwide prevention strategy. After a proper training of local personnel at the Clinical Research Center "Aldo e Cele Dacco" of the Mario Negri Institute in Bergamo, Italy, an educational campaign entitled "First Clinical and Epidemiological Program of Renal Diseases"—under the auspices of the Renal Sister Center Program of the International Society of

Nephrology—was conducted in three selected areas of Bolivia, including tropical, valley, and plain areas (8). The goal was to define the frequency of asymptomatic renal disease in these areas by screening a large population of subjects at relatively low costs. The campaign was conducted by doctors, nurses, and social workers with the aid of brochures prepared for largely illiterate population. To this purpose, an information leaflet was distributed to 25,000 people. It explained the basic principles of kidney function and malfunction and the aims of the screening program in a very simple language and with the aid of cartoons. The screening was formally performed at the first-level health centers (Unidad de Salud). The study was conducted by 21 clinical centers distributed in three areas of the country, which represent three different geographical and socioeconomic environments. Apparently healthy people (14,082) were enrolled over a period of 7 months (Fig. 1). There were 6759 (48%) males and 7323 (52%) females. Urinary abnormalities were found at first screening in 4261 patients (Table 1). Patients were then invited to come back for a confirmatory urinalysis investigation, if needed. Only 1019 patients—23.9% of the group with positive dipstick test—were available for the follow-up. On the second urinalysis, 35% of subjects had no abnormalities. In the remaining positive group of subjects further investigations included biochemistry, microbiology,

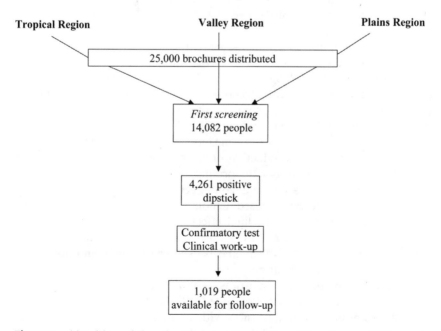

Figure 1 Algorithm of the educational and screening phases for renal diseases in Bolivia.

Table 1 Urinary Findings at First Screening

Urinary findings	Number of subjects	% of screened population
Hematuria	2010	14.3
Leukocyturia	1765	12.5
Proteinuria	298	2.1
Proteinuria and glycosuria	37	0.3
Proteinuria and hematuria	15	0.1

ultrasound, and intravenous pyelography, where indicated. The final diagnoses were as follow: urinary tract infection (48.4%); isolated hematuria (43.9%); chronic renal failure (1.6%); renal tuberculosis (1.6%); and other diagnoses 4.3% (kidney stones, 1.3%; diabetic nephropathy, 1%; polycystic kidney diseases, 1.9%).

This study shows that through an extended information campaign, mass screening of the population for renal ailments is feasible in a developing country, and can provide useful information on the frequency of renal diseases, as reflected by the abnormal dipstick findings.

The experience achieved with this initial screening program has represented the basis to plan pilot studies to prevent renal disease progression in selected target population in Bolivia (9). Bolivia is a country in which a large percent of the population live at high altitude. This prompted us to begin our research program in this country with a pilot experiment targeting these subjects. The aim was to demonstrate that polycythemia can be a risk factor for the development of proteinuria, and that pharmacologic intervention may help controlling high-packed cell volume and reduce urinary protein excretion, which eventually could translate in the prevention of renal disease progression. Indeed, people acclimatized to high altitudes have a raised concentration of hemoglobin that helps maintain oxygen delivery to tissues. This increase is mainly mediated by expansion in erythrocyte mass sustained by raised production of erythropoietin (10). In early phase of acclimatization, erythropoietin production is stimulated by decreased blood oxygen concentration and consequent decreased oxygen delivery to the kidney (11). However, raised hemoglobin concentration inhibits production of erythropoietin. The final effect of this negative feedback is a new equilibrium characterized by a normal blood oxygen concentration, increased volume of erythrocytes, and packed cell volume, and normal or slightly raised erythropoietin concentrations (12). In about 15% of cases, however, this compensated status is achieved at very high-packed cell volume levels (>55%) that are associated with high frequency (about 40%) of persistent proteinuria and possibly with an increased risk of cardiovascular complications. Inhibition of the renin–angiotensin system by angiotensin-converting-enzyme (ACE) inhibitors or angiotensin II receptor antagonists has proved effective for the treatment of another form of secondary polycythemia that follows renal transplant and is sustained by increased erythropoietin activity (13).

Here we aimed to investigate whether an ACE inhibitor could be beneficial in altitude polycythemia, another form of secondary erythropoietin-dependent polycythemia. Our primary endpoint was the effect of enalapril on packed cell volume, hemoglobin concentration, and urinary protein excretion rate. Secondary endpoints were the relations between packed cell volume and hemoglobin concentration and urinary protein excretion rate at study entry, and between reduction in packed cell volume or hemoglobin concentration and reduction in urinary protein excretion rate during treatment.

This was a prospective randomized study in 26 people of mixed Indian and European, mostly Spanish, ethnic origin, born at altitudes of 3200–4000 m, and who had lived in La Paz (3600 m) for at least 1 year. Diagnosis of polycythemia and persistent proteinuria was made, respectively, on the basis of packed cell volume greater than or equal to 55%, and urinary protein excretion rate greater or equal to 150 mg/24 hr, measured on two or more occasions, 2 months apart, in otherwise healthy people. Among exclusion criteria, diastolic blood pressure greater than 90 mmHg, diabetes, chronic pulmonary, or cardiac disease, polycythemia vera, renal insufficiency (serum creatinine >1.4 mg/dL), or an ultrasound suggestive of renal, renovascular, or urinary tract disease were considered. Patients with clinical or laboratory evidence of urinary tract infection were assessed after completion of a course of antibiotic treatment and a negative result from urine culture. All participants gave oral informed consent. Thirteen participants were assigned to the ACE inhibitor enalapril (5 mg/day) for 2 years (study group) and 13 subjects to no treatment (controls). Treatment allocation was open to patients and doctors. All patients were interviewed in person for treatment compliance and side effects every 3 to 6 months for 2 years. Because of economic constrains, laboratory assessments were repeated at 12 and 24 months' follow-up. Other antihypertensive drugs, but not ACE inhibitors, were allowed for patients who developed diastolic blood pressure of more than 90 mmHg.

In all participants, baseline packed cell volume was significantly and positively correlated with body weight ($r = 0.46$, $p = 0.02$) and systolic ($r = 0.49$, $p < 0.01$) and diastolic ($r = 0.40$, $p < 0.04$) blood pressure, and highly correlated with serum creatinine ($r = 0.61$, $p < 0.0009$) and urinary protein excretion rate ($r = 0.56$, $p < 0.003$). Correlation with age was of borderline significance. Systolic and diastolic blood pressure decreased slightly in the study patients and increased (not significantly) in controls. Packed cell volume, hemoglobin concentration, and urinary protein excretion significantly decreased in the ACE inhibitor-treated patients, but in controls packed cell volume and protein excretion rate increased. At

12- and 24-month follow-up, differences between the two groups in these three parameters were highly significant ($p < 0.01$). In study patients, but not controls, 12- and 24-month changes in packed cell volume were positively correlated with changes in systolic blood pressure and urinary protein excretion rate. Linear regression analysis done per patient found a positive and highly significant correlation between changes in packed cell volume and proteinuria ($r = 0.88$, $p < 0.0001$) at 6, 12, 18, and 24 months as compared to baseline.

In summary, our results showed that in patients with altitude polycythemia, long-term treatment with low doses of enalapril safely prevented increase in arterial blood pressure and progressively reduced packed cell volume and proteinuria. Reductions in packed cell volume were independent of changes in arterial blood pressure and renal function, and were positively correlated with reduction in proteinuria. The possibility exists that the decline of both packed cell volume and proteinuria should have an additive effect in decreasing the renal and cardiovascular complications of altitude polycythemia, and in the long term, should substantially reduce morbidity and mortality. Beside its scientific value, this study can be taken as an example of how by rationalizing resources and investing into research programs, the renal disease progression and cardiovascular risk may eventually improve, which ultimately would translate into better quality of life for patients. By reducing the need of dialysis and thus providing alternatives to the prohibitive costs of the renal replacement therapy, a general benefit would result to the national health system.

THE HURDLES IN IMPLEMENTING RESEARCH PROGRAMS IN THE DEVELOPING COUNTRIES

These studies shows that through an extended information campaign, mass screening of the population for renal ailments, as well as the pilot research studies, are feasible in a developing country, and can provide useful information on the frequency and treatment of renal diseases. However, the difficulties of such studies emerged when we tried to test for a second time those patients who had a positive dipstick at the first check. Among the rural population, traditional medicine is still much diffused and followed. The sorcerer quack doctor needs to visit the patient only once for diagnosis and treatment prescription. It is not in the custom to go back again for the same problem. Moreover, we were looking for asymptomatic renal abnormalities, and the people's concern was small. Therefore, only 24% of positive subjects returned for a second check. Nevertheless, our results show that among apparently healthy subjects in rural and metropolitan areas of Bolivia there is a considerable incidence of renal abnormalities, as reflected by the abnormal dipstick findings. These findings underline the need for educational campaigns and prevention programs for renal diseases in emerging countries such as Bolivia. Indeed, the major hurdle to the smooth development of the program relates to trained personnel involved in the project. Some Bolivian physicians and nurses have been trained in these years in our center in Bergamo, Italy, other locally. One problem sometime we found, and probably it may occur in the future—if no adequate initiative will be taken—is that at the end of training some people returned to Bolivia but did not belong anymore to the Project, looking for a more remunerative job in private practice and private clinics. Other left Bolivia for United States or Europe after training. This underlines the difficulty of having adequate number of trained people directly involved in the project in Bolivia, which is vital for its future survival and development.

The data from Bolivia recall a rather obvious truth: for an impressively large proportion of the world's population a basic knowledge of their needs is not available. The transformation of the pilot model from Bolivia into a systematic program has led us to attempt to cover the need of other invisible low/middle income countries, such as the Republic of Moldova.

THE EARLY DETECTION AND INTERVENTION PROGRAM FOR CHRONIC RENAL DISEASES IN THE REPUBLIC OF MOLDOVA

Moldova is a land-locked country of Southeastern Europe (14). Since its independence, the Republic of Moldova has faced serious economic challenges that have impacted on incomes and funding available for health and other social development activities. According to the Human Development Index, in 1998 the Republic of Moldova ranks as 113th in the list of 174 countries (15). In 2000, more than 90% of the population lived on less than US $1.00 per day, and real income has not even reached 80% of the 1997 level (16). At independence, Moldova was faced with a health system with numerous facilities and staff, but few resources to sustain them. In 2001, there were about 14,000 doctors and 32,406 nurses employed in the Republic of Moldova by the Ministry of Health, giving a rate of 3.3 doctors and 7.6 nurses per 1000 population (17). In 2000 life expectancy was 67.75. Infant mortality in 1999 were 18.54, a figure still three times that of the EU average of 6.07 (17). The main causes of death in the Republic of Moldova are diseases of the circulatory system followed by cancer, diseases of the digestive system, and injury and poisoning (18). Smoking, a contributory cause for circulatory diseases and cancer, is widespread with approximately 46% of the male and 18% of the female population estimated to smoke (19). Alcohol abuse is also widespread. An official survey found that more than 8% of the population had undefined health problems caused by excessive alcohol consumption (15).

Moldova lacks a kidney disease registry. The last epidemiological study concerning chronic renal failure prevalence in R. Moldova was performed in 1988, when the prevalence of ESRD in adult patients was of 212 patients per million of population (pmp) per year (20). Today, however, the exact incidence and prevalence of chronic renal failure in the population, its burden on the healthcare system, and the outcome of these patients remain ill defined. Currently, only 170 patients with ESRD benefit from renal replacement therapy, which represents approximately 18–19% of the needs. The mean age of dialysis patients is 45.2 years, with only a minority of patients older than 60 years. Among patients on dialysis therapy the most frequent causes of ESRD are glomerulonephritis (52.8%), pyelonephritis (20.8%), and autosomal dominant polycystic kidney disease (10.4%). Diabetic nephropathy represents only 4.8% of dialyzed population, due to a very low acceptance rate of those with diabetic nephropathy. Together, these observations indicate that very little information is available about the prevalence of pre-dialysis chronic diseases in the Republic of Moldova and that the programs for regular renal replacement therapy for all chronic kidney patients cannot be fully established because of its prohibitive costs.

Identification of subjects with or at risk of developing chronic renal diseases and activation of a prevention program of renal disease progression to ESRD at relatively low costs could be of great help for the patients and for the health system of this country. We believe that, with some efforts, screening program for chronic kidney diseases and intervention programs to prevent the progression of renal diseases with the combination of pharmacologic and non-pharmacologic approaches—shown effective in the developed countries—can be applied to the Republic of Moldova. To this purpose, an early detection and intervention program is currently developing for R. Moldova under the support and coordination of the Mario Negri Institute for Pharmacological Research in Bergamo, Italy, and will be locally coordinated through the Department of Hemodialysis and Kidney Transplantation, Republican Clinical Hospital, Chisinau (21). The project is designed to identify the rates of renal disease in subjects, aged 18 to 65 years, attending for a visit to medical units of primary, secondary, and tertiary healthcare facilities. It is foreseen to screen a group of 20,000 subjects over 12 months, living in the main towns, including Chisinau. Sample data are weighted appropriately to account for the complex design and unequal probability of selection of sample persons, to compute prevalence estimates of abnormal albumin excretion levels. Similar procedures are used to compute estimates for other sub-populations of special interest: all persons with hypertension, all persons with cardiovascular disease, all persons with physician-diagnosed diabetes, all obese persons.

An intervention program centered on the use of ACE inhibitors to prevent renal disease progression and alter renal and cardiovascular disease outcomes in subjects with a positive screening for albuminuria, hypertension, and diabetes is also planned. As premise to any pharmacological intervention, efforts will be done to properly educate patients toward healthy lifestyles, which include moderation of alcohol consumption, stop smoking, increase in physical activity, reduction of dietary sodium/salt, cut down protein intake, and weight reduction in those individuals who are over weight or obese.

Nevertheless, the implementation of such an ambitious program of prevention of renal diseases in these emerging countries can be realized only through a coordinated approach between local health authorities, National Societies of Nephrology, and ISN-COMGAN.

CONCLUSION

Medicine is developing evidence for non-communicable chronic disease, including cardiovascular and kidney diseases, but has no equity plan. A more concerted, strategic, and multisectorial approach, underpinned by solid research, is essential to help reverse the negative trends in incidence of these chronic diseases, not just for few beneficiaries but on a global health equity program. The Bolivian experience, however, also underlines that education and training of health professional is the first priority. A comprehensive training program for physicians and nurses should be established and carried out in selected institutions in developed countries. The opportunity to train in different societies is a rich experience for them. What is needed is an acknowledgment that institutions in developed countries have an ethical obligation to facilitate the return of health professionals to their own emerging countries. The plan is to impress on this health personnel, who will be mostly providing first-line medical care in their countries, the need for early diagnosis of kidney disease, and the use of preventive measures readily available in the country at present. Moreover, the aim of these developments must be the establishment of sustainable research and development partnership between emerging and developed word. This ultimately would require building research infrastructures in emerging countries as reference centers of the prevention program. Academia in the developed world must evolve lasting ties with its partners in the developing countries, which cannot survive another 10 years of neglect. However, the implementation of such an ambitious program of prevention of renal diseases can be realized only through a coordinated approach between local health authorities, national societies of nephrology and ISN-COMGAN, and the involvement of international agencies such as the World Health Organization (WHO) and World Bank (WB).

ACKNOWLEDGMENTS

Dr. Igor Codreanu is a recipient of the ISN-COMGAN Fellowship.

REFERENCES

1. WHO. The World Health Report 2002, World Health Organization, 2002.
2. WHO. The World Health Report 2003—Shaping the Future, World Health Organization, 2003.
3. Murray CJL, Lopez AD. The Global Burden of Disease. Boston, MA: Harvard School of Public Health, 1996.
4. Collins AJ. The hemoglobin link to adverse outcomes. Adv Stud Med 2003; 3:S14–S17.
5. Ritz E, McClellan WM. Overview: increased cardiovascular risk in patients with minor renal dysfunction: an emerging issue with far-reaching consequences. J Am Soc Nephrol 2004; 15:513–516.
6. Go AS, Chertow GM, Fan D, McCulloch CE, et al. Chronic kidney disease and the risks of death, cardiovascular events, and hospitalization. N Engl J Med 2004; 351:1296–1305.
7. Anavekar NS, McMurray JJV, Velazquez EJ, Solomon SD, et al. Relation between renal dysfunction and cardiovascular outcomes after myocardial infarction. N Engl J Med 2004; 351:1285–1295.
8. Plata R, Silva C, Yahuita J, Perez L, et al. The first clinical epidemiological programme on renal disease in Bolivia: a model for prevention and early diagnosis of renal diseases in developing countries. Nephrol Dial Transplant 1998; 13: 3034–3036.
9. Plata R, Cornejo A, Arratia C, Anabaya A, et al. Angiotensin-converting-enzyme inhibition therapy in altitude polycythaemia: a prospective randomised trial. Lancet 2002; 359:663–666.
10. Grover R, Weil J, Reeves J. Cardiovascular adaptation to exercise at high altitude. Exerc Sport Sci Rev 1986; 14:269–302.
11. Ou L, Salceda S, Schuster S, Dunnack L, et al. Polycythemic responses to hypoxia: molecular and genetic mechanisms of chronic mountain sickness. J Appl Physiol 1998; 84:1242–1251.
12. Cahan C, Hoekje P, Goldwasser E, Decker M, et al. Assessing the characteristic between length of hypoxic exposure and serum erythropoietin levels. Am J Physiol 1990; 258:1016–1021.
13. Gaston R, Julian B, Curtis J. Post transplant erythrocytosis: an enigma revisited. Am J Kidney Dis 1994; 24:1–11.
14. United Nations Cartographic Section. http://www.un.org/.Depts/Cartographic/map /profile/moldova pdf, 2004.
15. United Nations Development Programme. National Human Development Report, Chisinau, 2000.
16. European Commission. Moldovan Economic Trends. Chisinau: DGIA MS/Tacis Services, 2001.
17. World Health Organization. Health for All Database. WHO Regional Office for Europe, Geneva, 2002.
18. Scientific and Practice Centre of Health and Health Management. Public Health in Moldova 1999. Chisinau: UNICEF, 2000.
19. World Health Organization. The European Report on Tobacco Control Policy. Warsaw: WHO European Ministerial Conference for a Tobacco-free Europe, 2002.

20. Tanase A. Epidemiologia Insuficientei Renale Cronice Terminale si organizarea asistentei medicale specializate in R. Moldova. Ph.D. dissertation, Chisinau, Moldova, 1988.

21. Codreanu I, Tanase A, Perico N, Schieppati A, et al. A screening and prevention program for chronic renal disease (CRD) in Republic of Moldova. Conference on Prevention of Progression of Renal Disease [abstr], Hong Kong, June 29–July 1, 2004.

24

The Renal Sister Center: "Antwerp (Belgium)—Yerevan (Armenia)"

Marc E. De Broe

Department of Nephrology, University of Antwerp, Belgium

HOW IT STARTED

At 11.40 A.M. on the 5th of December 1988, an unpredicted severe earthquake destroyed three Armenian cities. Approximately 25,000 people died and more than 250,000 were injured. This dramatic event was the onset of an acute nephrology rescue intervention originating from many parts of the world, among them was the team of two nephrologists and three nurses from the department of nephrology of the University of Antwerp, the A. Z. Werken Glorieux Ronse, St. Jozef Hospital Turnhout, and St. Jans Hospital Brugge. As soon as the Armenian earthquake disappeared from the headline news and television screens, the international medical help faded away in parallel. The department of nephrology of the University of Antwerp was approached by "Medecins sans Frontieres" to take over their position in Armenia, since the activities of this particular organization is limited to acute help and their skills and experience in nephrology were almost nonexisting. This opened the possibility that renal replacement therapy introduced through the acute disaster of an earthquake should become available for patients with chronic kidney diseases (CKD). At that stage, it was impossible to even think about the initiative and support of such a chronic treatment program in a country, belonging to the poorest in the world and just stepping out of 50 years of Russian communist domination. We decided to limit our efforts to education and training in clinical nephrology of Armenian doctors, nurses, and technicians.

THE PROJECT

In the initial phase (1990–1998), we focused our efforts on the quality of different types of dialysis treatments by introducing better dialysis equipment via the Armenian Diaspora and some Flemish dialysis centers and confronting as well as informing our Armenian colleagues with a successful organ retrieval program in the province of Antwerp and kidney/kidney–pancreas transplantation program.

During the initial phase, we were fortunate to have the opportunity to train Armenian colleagues, nurses, and technicians who, in the majority of instances, had a good knowledge of basic medicine.

Our specific aim was to establish a polyvalent nephrology program consisting not only of dialysis treatment but also of renal transplantation. In the long term, we aim at prevention (early detection of CKD and intervention program) and the development of simple, feasible clinical research programs in the field of renal diseases.

In order to realize these objectives, NAF (Nephrology-Armenia-Flanders) was launched in 1995 by which the nephrology departments of the Antwerp University Hospital, General Hospital "Werken Glorieux" Ronse and the General Hospital "Maria Middelares" St. Niklaas joined their efforts. Later on, the Nephrology Department of the General Hospital "St. Jozef" Turnhout (Dr. Paul Arnouts) became also an important participant in NAF.

The stay of Dr. Ara Babloyan (urologist with interest in renal medicine) during 1 year in our department of nephrology/transplantation was a breakthrough for the project. It turned out that Ara Babloyan was not only a good clinician interested in improving his knowledge and attracted to new technologies but also that he had a rich personality. Once back in its country, he decided to use all his energy, skill, and intellect to improve the renal program in his country. His organizational talent and his motivating personality resulted in the attraction of several gifted young doctors (internist, surgeons) in his department. In 1995, he was asked to take over the position of Minister of Health of his country.

From 1988 to 2004, 35 Armenian doctors, nurses, technicians, and hospital administrators received training for several months in the above-mentioned hospitals.

MILESTONES

In 1999, the first kidney transplantations from a living donor were realized in Yerevan by a joint Antwerp–Yerevan team of surgeons, anesthesiologist, etc.

In 2001, a beautiful concert was organized by NAF in the Carolus-Borromeus church in the heart of Antwerp. Two renowned choirs gave their highly appreciated assistance.

In 2002, two more transplants were performed in September 2002 by the same team. During these 8 days, a multidisciplinary group of Flemish renal healthcare workers organized a clinical-teaching program: (1) living donor transplantation; (2) surgical and medical complications during and after transplantation; (3) metabolic complications during and after transplantation; (4) metabolic deficiencies of the dialysis patient; (5) anemia in renal failure; (6) diabetes and kidney failure; (7) technical and medical aspects of vascular access; (8) cyclosporine dosage and some other laboratory techniques; (9) bedside teaching. At the end of 2002, the Armenian transplant team in Yerevan performed autonomously their first living-related kidney transplantation.

In May 2003, a concert was organized in the Holy Mary Cathedral of Antwerp. Apart from three Armenian artists, Stanislas Deriemaeker played Bach on the Antwerp XXIIIth orgue. A visit to Yerevan was organized between 12 and 19 September consisting out of a delegation of Flemish doctors (G. Verpooten, M. De Broe, M. Van Laere, and T. Chapelle), a nurse (J. P. Van Waeleghem), a laboratory technician (W. Leyssen), and two U.S. colleagues M. Kashgarian (pathologist, Yale) and F. Finkelstein (nephrologist, New York).

A 5-day course/workshop was organized consisting in lectures, clinico-pathological confrontations and bedside teaching, covering topics selected by our Armenian colleagues.

Dr. T. Chapelle assisted Armenian surgeons in two living-related renal transplantations. A distal splenorenal shunt was constructed in a child with portal hypertension.

W. Leyssen implemented four new tests on the Cobas machine installed in 2002 and gave a course on quality control.

In 2004, a concert was organized in May at the St. Paulus church. Three renowned Armenian artists played music of Haendel, Shubert, and Rachmaninoff.

A visit to Armenia is scheduled (15–24 October 2004). The surgical program consists in the discussion of five patients with portal-hypertension, two of them candidates for surgery. Two living-related transplantations and clinico-pathological conferences dealing with renal transplantation are planned.

Wilfried Leyssen, our laboratory technician (Antwerp University Hospital), will install the recently sent photometer. He will introduce two new applications on the Cobas installed 2 years ago: ferritine and valproic acid determination. He will install the Coulter machine for hemoglobin and cytological analyses.

The teaching program consists in conferences dealing with vascular access, evaluation of the living-related donor, infectious complications in transplantation and new immunosuppressive drugs (J. P. Van Waeleghem, M. Helbert, D. Ysebaert) and bedside teaching.

Dr. Ashot Sarkissian (pediatric nephrologists, Yerevan) stayed during 4 months in the department in order to optimize his skills in renal transplantation. He was also involved in an experimental study dealing with the role of particular proteins (osteopontin, CD44), and hyaluron acid in the crystal adhesion to the epithelium in the distal nephron. He was taught the installment of the remnant kidney in the rat and involved in histomorphometric analysis. Finally, he was associated with the setup and writing of a protocol "early detection and intervention program for chronic renal diseases in the Republic of Armenia," an ISN-COMGAN (research committee—chair: G. Remuzzi) program for chronic renal diseases in the Republic of Armenia.

Dr. Ashot Sarkissian will be supported by NAF to attend a meeting in the Netherlands on prevention in nephrology organized by P. de Jong (ISN, 13–14 November 2004).

In 2005, a visit to Armenia is planned in January to discuss the implementation of the "early detection and intervention program for chronic renal disease in the Republic of Armenia" project, a new initiative of the ISN-COMGAN research committee.

During the spring time (April/May), several "sponsored biking tours" will be organized. The driving force behind this project is Dr. P. Arnouts (Turnhout).

A MODEL SISTER CENTER

The possible reasons why the Armenian-Flanders sister center became a "model" of the ISN Sister Center Program can be summarized as follows:

- Commitment of the Armenian doctors to their country. Well-educated colleagues, several of them spent some time abroad in top institutions, decided to stay and work in difficult conditions (logistic, financial) in their country instead of moving abroad towards a more "successful" career.
- The strong charismatic personality of the Head of the Department of Nephrology in Yerevan, Dr. Ara Babloyan, his organizational talent, his ability to motivate people from inside and outside to help him in improving the quality of medicine in his country.
- The sustained commitment (over many years) of several Flemish doctors (nephrologists, transplant surgeons, pathologists), nurses, lab technicians, secretaries towards the NAF (Nephrology-Armenia-Flanders) project.

- The growing personal relationship of several of us with many colleagues in Armenia, some of them became friends over the years. This allows to have discussions from time to time on delicate matters.
- The structural short- and long-term planning of the project whereby the limitations of both partners concerning time, manpower, technical facilities, and budget are carefully taken into account.
- The careful evaluation in spending the limit resources of the program towards the most relevant items after the discussion with our Armenian partner.
- The broad basis of interest and sympathy in the different collaborating hospitals where can be relied upon in order to collect the essential *yearly budget* of € 20,000–25,000. The realization of that yearly budget was until now possible through:

  - The organization of a concert in one of the beautiful churches (cathedral Holy Mother, Carolus Borromeus church, Sint-Paulus church) of Antwerp. This happening could only be realized, thanks to the help of many people and particularly three internationally renowned Armenian artists who performed on a voluntary basis;
  - The organization of sponsored sport activities (biking, walking parties, marathon running, etc.).

25

Introduction to Nephrology Training in the Developing World

Meguid El Nahas

Sheffield Kidney Institute, University of Sheffield, Sheffield, U.K.

Worldwide, the majority of patients with end-stage renal disease (ESRD) live in a few developed countries with economies able to meet the growing cost of renal replacement therapy (RRT) (Chapter Levin). Developing countries are often unable to meet the growing challenge of ESRD due to limited financial resources. Also, developing countries have limited manpower trained in the field of nephrology to meet the challenge of chronic kidney disease (CKD). These limitations and difficulties are highlighted by the contribution of Naicker and Barsoum that details the shortcomings in manpower and training in nephrology in sub-Saharan Africa. It also identifies new training objectives including more emphasis on preventive medicine and nephrology.

Provision of care for patients with CKD and ESRD in the developing countries will depend, over the next decade, on a new generation of nephrologists well trained and equipped to meet the demands of their community. As described by Naicker and Barsoum, these may involve changes in emphasis from curative to preventive nephrology. For that, training provisions will have to accommodate their clinical priorities and service requirements. These nephrologists will often depend on their training on regional or international resources. The training of these nephrologists will depend on the clinical environment they will practice in and the need of their community. For that, their training will have to be evolutionary in its planning, starting with limited resources and ambitions and evolving into a more comprehensive training package bearing similarities to those of their colleagues in the developed world.

In this section, El Nahas and Remuzzi define the requirements of the "emerging nephrologist" practicing in a deprived area/country where educational as well as clinical resources are limited. The training of physicians to meet the nephrological requirements of such community has to be realistic and gradual. On occasions, it may have to be minimalist. However, such training will have to evolve in time to provide an ever-growing nephrology service to meet the increasing demand of the community it serves. For that, the emerging nephrologist will have to gain more skills and fulfill new curricula along the lines of those highlighted by the International Society of Nephrology (ISN). Rastegar and Field in their chapter define the training requirements such a nephrologist will require. They are based on the recommendation of the ISN Commission for the Global Advancement of Nephrology (COMGAN)'s education committee. They aim to standardize nephrology training worldwide in order to guarantee minimal standards of good clinical care and governance. They acknowledge the difficulties that may face some emerging nephrologists to meet those training requirements and divide them into essential, desirable, and optional. Such a flexibility of training aims to provide a curriculum in nephrology adaptable to the environment the nephrologist will practice in within the developing countries.

Overall, the four contributions outlined below are complementary in their concept as they aim to meet the educational demands of those in developing countries and societies at different stages of medical and nephrological evolution.

26

Training and Education of Nephrologists Worldwide

Asghar Rastegar

Department of Medicine, Yale University School of Medicine, New Haven, Connecticut, U.S.A.

Michael Field

Northern Clinical School, University of Sydney, Sydney, Australia

BACKGROUND

The Emergence of Nephrology as a Medical Specialty

Nephrology became a recognized specialty only in the second half of 20th century. However, the foundations for the specialty were laid during the first half of the century, which saw great strides in elucidating the biochemistry, physiology, and pathophysiology of the kidney in health and disease. It was not until early 1950s that these developments encouraged several pioneers, especially Jean Hamburger and his colleagues at the Necker Hospital in Paris, to establish a unit devoted to the care of patients with renal disease (1). Although this pioneering event was the product of half a century of progress, several more recent developments were critical to its rapid recognition as a unique specialty worldwide. These included the development of dialysis and its first successful use by Wilhelm Kolff in 1945 (2), the description of acute renal failure as a potentially reversible disease by Bywaters and Beall in 1941 (3), the development of percutaneous renal biopsy by Muehrcke et al. in 1954 (4), the performance of the first transplant in man in Paris in 1954 (1), and the first successful transplant by David Hume et al. in Boston in 1955 (5). These developments created the need for training of physicians who were able to provide highly specialized care to patients with kidney disease, particularly end-stage renal failure (ESRF).

Over the next two decades, nephrology departments and divisions were organized in many academic centers worldwide, training an increasing number of specialists. In certain countries such as the United States, Canada, and certain European countries, this was quickly followed by the development of a process to certify these physicians as specialists in the recognized field of nephrology.

The Role of the International Society of Nephrology (ISN)

The further development of nephrology as a specialty is partly indebted to the creation of the International Society of Nephrology (ISN) as a professional organization that would bring together investigators and practitioners interested in kidney function in heath and disease, and would foster the development of this discipline worldwide. The first meeting of what was to become the ISN was held in Evian, France, under the leadership of Hamburger and his colleagues in Paris and Geneva. This set the stage for the creation of the charter and bylaws of the society. Although kidney disease was represented as part of other societies in different countries (e.g., as a section of the American Heart Association in the United States), there was a need for the establishment of such a society on the international stage, reinforcing the unique nature of this specialty. It is interesting that the establishment of the ISN preceded that of most national nephrology societies, and as a result ISN played a critical role in helping create many national and regional societies. During the same time, nephrology divisions within Departments of Internal Medicine or as independent units became commonplace in Europe, North America, and Australia, providing opportunity for the training of specialists in this field. The success of dialysis and transplantation as life-prolonging modalities had great impact on the desirability of the field to young physicians-in-training, and fueled its rapid expansion worldwide during the seventh and eighth decades of the 20th century.

ISN Commission for the Global Advancement of Nephrology (COMGAN)

In 1993, the ISN took a crucial step by establishing the Commission for the Global Advancement of Nephrology (COMGAN), under the leadership of Barry Brenner and John Dirks, and with strong support of the President and President-elect of the Society, to focus primarily on specific regions where renal care was felt to be deficient (6). ISN, primarily through COMGAN, developed many educational activities, such as regional conferences, a Fellowship program, visits by senior scholars to academic centers in developing countries, the Library Enhancement Program and Sister Center

Program, to enhance knowledge about, and skills to care for, patients with renal disease worldwide. Looking back, this effort has had a great impact on the development of nephrology, especially in regions of the world where this discipline was new and often underdeveloped.

The Education Advisory Committee (EAC) of COMGAN

Recognizing that physicians play a major role in the type and quality of care provided to patients with renal disease, ISN through COMGAN created an Education Advisory Committee in 1999 with the goal of enhancing the quality of nephrology training programs worldwide. The Committee, with membership from many regions of the world, initially set out to develop universally accepted guidelines for training of nephrologists, defined as physicians who are trained to provide comprehensive care to patients with a variety of renal diseases.

The Committee first collected data from representative countries in different regions of the world, regarding both the content and process of local nephrology training programs. These regions (and number of countries) are as follows: Africa (3), Western Europe (6), Eastern Europe (7), Middle East and CIS (4), South East Asia and Australia (8), North America (2), and Central and South America (4). Given that specialist training programs as a whole are quite variable in different regions, the Committee was surprised that, with few exceptions, there were considerable similarities among the countries surveyed (Table 1). All trainees were expected to have some training in internal medicine (12–72 months, with a median of 36 months) spending a defined period of time, from 12 to 48 months, focusing on nephrology.

Two clear exceptions were noted. In Russia and CIS countries, nephrology training, which follows a 24-month period of training in internal medicine, is class-based and of short duration (4–5 months). In sub-Saharan Africa (with the exception of South Africa) and in Central America (with the exception of Mexico), little or no formal training is available locally.

Table 1 shows the educational structure and content of nephrology training in the countries surveyed. The majority of the countries provide training in all areas of nephrology to ensure that their graduates are able to provide care to their patients with renal disease and associated specialized needs. Experience in continuous modes of dialysis therapy is only available in 28 (78%) of the programs. Most of the training programs also provide an opportunity for their trainees to engage in some type of relevant research, with 18 (50%) providing opportunity for both laboratory as well as patient-based research and 14 (39%) in patient-based research only.

Table 1 Educational Structure and Content of Training Programs Surveyed ($N = 36$)

I. Structure[a]	
A. Prerequisite training in internal medicine	12–72 months (median 36)
B. Length of training	12–48 months (median 36)
II. Content	
Consultative nephrology	36
Training in care of patients with ARF	35
Nephropathology	34
ICU nephrology	35
Fluid, electrolyte & acid-base	
Ambulatory consultation	31
Hemodialysis	36
CAPD	34
Transplantation	34
Continuous renal replacement therapy	28
Research training	
Patient-based only	14
Patient and laboratory-based	18
None	4

[a]Data from several regions are not included in this table. In Russia (and CIS countries), a 24-month training period in internal medicine is followed by two formal courses in nephrology lasting 12 and 6–8 weeks. In sub-Saharan Africa, formal training is only available in South Africa. In Central America, formal training is only available in Mexico.

Development of Universal Guidelines for Training in Nephrology

Training guidelines have been developed by several national organizations (7–9), some overseeing the training of nephrologists in those countries (7,8). These guidelines define both the resources needed for an academic center to train nephrologists as well as the content of training. In the United States, this function is divided between two separate organizations, with the Accreditation Council for Graduate Medical Education (ACGME), which represents major educational and professional organizations, overseeing the structure and resources of training programs (10), and the American Board of Internal Medicine (ABIM), defining the training a trainee must receive to be allowed to sit for the relevant specialty examination. In many other countries, such as Australia and the U.K., these two functions are handled by a single organization (8).

    After reviewing available guidelines from different regions of the world, the EAC decided to create a document that would set out both the specific expertise to be acquired by trainees, as well as the minimum resources needed to train nephrologists. The Committee felt that it was important initially to develop a universal definition for a specialist in this field before the development of specific training requirements. A nephrologist is defined by the EAC as a physician who is able to provide comprehensive care to patients with kidney disease. This individual is not only able to care for patients with different types of kidney disease, but also patients at different stages in the evolution of kidney disease. A nephrologist should therefore be able to manage a spectrum of patients, from those considered to be at risk for the development of kidney disease, to patients with ESRF being treated with a variety of life-extending modalities. In certain regions of the world, physicians are trained exclusively to care for a small population with ESRF often treated with hemodialysis. We do not believe that these individuals, who serve a very important and critical function in their health care systems, fit the definition of "nephrologist" as used in this document. We also recognize that in a few developed countries, some nephrologists trained to provide comprehensive care choose to sub-specialize and limit their practice to a specific domain such as transplantation or dialytic therapy. It is important to appreciate that this document only defines the guidelines for core training of nephrologists and does not deal with issues relevant to practice patterns in different regions of the world.

The guidelines, shown in Table 2, define the recommended duration of overall training as well as the fraction of time to be devoted to its major components, the clinical expertise and procedural skills required, as well as the resources needed to adequately train candidates. These recommendations are derived from the data collected through a survey undertaken by the EAC as well the consensus of the members of the EAC representing different regions of the world. The Committee also defined each element as *essential*, *desirable*, or *optional*, reflecting the importance of that specific element in achieving the overall mission of the training program. Essential elements *must* be available, while desirable elements *should* be provided. Optional elements, while enhancing the quality of training, are not considered to be universally critical to the training of clinical nephrologists. These judgments were based on input from EAC members and other contributors from many countries of the world.

Under these guidelines, the minimum total training time is defined as 4 years with at least 2 years devoted specifically to nephrology training. In view of the great variation in undergraduate as well as internal medicine training in different countries, the Committee felt that a 6-year training program with 3 years devoted to training in internal medicine and 3 years to nephrology is more desirable for most but not all regions of the world, especially given the broad knowledge base and skill demanded from nephrologists in providing comprehensive care. In addition, trainees should be able to maintain a high level of expertise as the field evolves during their professional life. Although research training is considered to be optional for training of clinical nephrologists, it was felt by the EAC that it was essential

Table 2   ISN Guidelines for Training in Nephrology

1. Objective: This document provides guidelines for the training of a nephrologist, defined as a physician who is able to provide comprehensive care to patients with kidney disease. These guidelines define the *minimum* requirements for training of nephrologists worldwide.

2. Duration of program
   a. Minimum 4 years; optimum 6 years (for internal medicine and nephrology training)
   b. Number of years devoted exclusively to nephrology training: minimum 2 years, optimum 3–4 years

3. Specific clinical expertise	Level of requirement
Trainees should gain expertise in diagnosis and management of:	
a. Acute kidney failure	Essential
b. Fluid/electrolytes/acid-base disorders	Essential
c. Renal parenchymal diseases	Essential
d. Hypertension and hypertensive kidney disease	Essential
e. Chronic kidney failure (CKD)	Essential
f. Acute PD	Desirable
g. Hemodialysis	Essential
h. CAPD	Essential/desirable[a]
i. Transplant workup	Essential/desirable[a]
j. Post-transplant patient	
Early management	Desirable
Long-term management	Essential/desirable[a]
k. Nutrition in patients with kidney disease and patients with ESRD	Essential
l. Urinary tract stone disease	Essential
m. Complicated urinary tract infection	Essential

4. Clinical training program	% Time allocation
Total training time devoted to:	
a. Management of patients with kidney disease (non-ESRD), in both inpatients (including ICU) and outpatients	~40%
b. Management of patients with ESRD, including chronic hemodialysis and/or CAPD	~40%
c. Transplant nephrology	~20%
d. Research	Optional

(Continued)

Table 2 ISN Guidelines for Training in Nephrology (*Continued*)

5. Procedures	Level of requirement
Trainee should gain expertise in the following procedures:	
a. Urinalysis and urine microscopy	Essential
b. Renal biopsy	Desirable
c. Placement of central lines/access	Essential
d. Connect patient for hemodialysis	Desirable
e. Placement of acute PD catheter	Optional
f. Placement of CAPD catheter	Optional
g. Urinary tract ultrasound	Desirable
h. Vascular access contrast study	Optional
i. Access/line declotting procedure	Optional
j. Vascular access angioplasty	Optional

6. Training program resources	Level of requirement
Training program should have the following resources:	
a. Renal pathology service	Essential (EM optional)
b. Acute hemodialysis	Essential
c. Acute continuous treatment (CVVH, CAVH)	Optional
d. Acute peritoneal dialysis	Optional
e. Chronic hemodialysis	Essential
f. CAPD	Essential
g. Ambulatory nephrology (outpatient clinic, consultation clinic)	Essential
h. Internet access	Desirable
i. Library with nephrology resources	Essential
j. Availability of imaging:	
Radiology, ultrasound	Essential
Nuclear medicine, CT scan	Desirable

7. Faculty support	Level of requirement
Level of support by faculty to the trainee:	
Continuous direct supervision	Desirable
Nephrologist contactable 24 hr/day	Essential

[a]Level of requirement depends on regional availability of CAPD and transplantation as treatment modalities.

for those who are involved in training of future nephrologists. However, it is critical that all trainees be well versed in research methodology and basic biostatistics to be able to evaluate clinical studies with a level of sophistication required to provide ongoing high-quality care in an evolving discipline. The EAC therefore believes that each program must develop a minimum curriculum to meet this objective (Table 2).

In putting forward these guidelines, the EAC acknowledges that many of the standards set here may not realistically be achieved in the near future in those areas of the world where economic and social factors impose severe limits on the resources available for delivering specialized clinical care to the population. While consideration was given to developing an alternative set of guidelines for such areas, with less ambitious targets for training conditions and resources, it was felt overall that only one set of standards should be created so that physicians in all regions could advocate to their governments and healthcare systems for moving towards an optimal system. This in no way diminishes the importance and impact of the work done under sub-optimal conditions in areas of Africa, Asia, and Central America, where care for patients with kidney disease is provided by doctors and other health professionals with less sophisticated training opportunities.

The ISN Core Curriculum

A further activity of the Education Advisory Committee of COMGAN has been the development of a core curriculum for postgraduate training in nephrology. This was intended to amplify the specific areas of content knowledge required in a training course satisfying the previously developed guidelines.

In developing this document, the Committee drew on, and referred to, several comprehensive curricula already published in the literature or on the Internet (9,11,12). However, these documents were designed for sophisticated medical centers in the developed world, and were not always appropriate for training programs in developing countries. Moreover, most published guidelines did not address many aspects of tropical and regional nephrology of relevance to many developing economies, and had relatively little emphasis on the epidemiological or population-based perspective of renal disease.

In order to develop a syllabus, which would be useful in guiding the selection of content to be included in training programs in all parts of the world, the EAC took the approach that it was most useful to define the *competencies*, which need to be developed by the nephrology trainee, and to relate these to relevant domains of required knowledge and specific skills. A feature of the curriculum is that it acknowledges the wider role of the specialist physician in the developing world by referring to both patient-based competencies and population-based competencies. The curriculum is also unique in providing scope for each competency to be refined in terms of the regional variations which might be relevant in a particular zone of the world, e.g., referring to AIDS nephropathy in Africa and parasitic nephropathy in the tropics. The population-based competencies draw attention to the need for the nephrologist to be able to design a research protocol to ascertain the burden of kidney disease in a national or regional population, and to implement a strategy for the prevention of renal disease in a defined patient population. To support these competencies, some instruction in basic research methodology, including biostatistics, is recommended for inclusion in the training syllabus (see K6). Finally, broader roles in advocacy for patients with kidney disease, including a role in the cost-effective management of health service resources, are also included.

Following definition of the required competencies for training, a checklist of required knowledge and skills is provided. Again, these sections allow for altered emphasis to be applied to enhance the relevance of the syllabus in different regions. Importantly, knowledge areas are also prescribed in relation to the competencies listed in the epidemiology and population health domains.

A final section of the core curriculum refers to appropriate methods of learning and assessment (evaluation) applicable to nephrology trainees. A wide range of teaching and learning approaches is recommended for maximum enrichment of the training experience. While conventional didactic lectures, use of library materials, and participation in journal clubs are all included, increasing emphasis should be placed on the use of current online resources, as these are more regularly updated than fixed print material. In this regard, the planned development by the ISN of its own educational website is very timely. Over the course of 2004, this ambitious project will be launched, aiming eventually to provide an accessible and powerful resource for access to outstanding educational materials in the field of nephrology for trainees in any part of the world.

The overall philosophy of the training defined by the core curriculum is that the program should empower the trainee to provide competent patient care under supervision, with growing responsibility for independent decision making. The specialized knowledge and skills to be obtained by trainees must also be matched by acquisition of the generic attributes of a consultant physician. These include the adoption of a patient-centered approach, the highest personal and professional ethical standards, a commitment to contribute to teaching of students and junior colleagues, and acceptance of the need to work with colleagues in a multidisciplinary team. Perhaps most important is the commitment to pursue lifelong continuing professional self-education, an activity that is supported by COM-GAN through its extensive program of educational visits to developing countries and through other means.

Again, it must be emphasized that the curriculum, like the guidelines, provides a template for an ideal program of education in nephrology, where sophisticated concepts in the basic sciences and recent developments in diagnosis and management are presented to trainees as part of their overall professional development. Clearly, such components of training must be seen in perspective in regions of the world where only basic medical services are available. In those settings, consultants should still be aware of areas where advances are currently being made, and should strive to gain access to sources of relevant contemporary information. However, realistically priorities will inevitably need to be set, both in training and in practice, such that the best possible care is provided to patients within the limitations posed by locally available resources.

Taken in conjunction with the wide range of other programs developed by COMGAN, it is hoped that the training guidelines and core curriculum developed by the Education Advisory Committee will provide sound leadership for nephrology training programs throughout the world.

ISN CORE CURRICULUM FOR POSTGRADUATE TRAINING IN NEPHROLOGY

Goals of Training

At the conclusion of a postgraduate training program in nephrology, the trainee should be competent to provide an independent consulting and management service for the care of patients with kidney disease, with disordered fluid and electrolyte balance (with or without kidney disease), or with hypertension.

In providing such service, the trainee should have acquired the specialized knowledge and skills detailed below, but also the *generic attributes* of a consultant physician. These include attitudes and behaviors consistent with

- high personal and professional ethical standards;
- an approach to practice, which is centered on patients' needs;
- a commitment to provide service and care to patients of all sociocultural and age groups;
- acceptance of the need to work with colleagues in a multidisciplinary team;
- a willingness to devote time to teaching students and junior colleagues;
- a commitment to continuing professional self-education.

Syllabus

I. REQUIRED COMPETENCIES

Competencies	Regional variations (examples only)
A. Patient-based competencies	
Make a clinical assessment and direct the management of a patient presenting with:	
1. Disturbed fluid and electrolytes balance, including hypervolemia,	Including the management of patients with cholera in Asia

Competencies	Regional variations (examples only)
hypovolemia, and abnormalities of plasma Na and K concentration	
2. Disturbed acid–base balance, with a particular emphasis on metabolic acidosis and alkalosis	Regional inherited forms of renal tubular acidosis in Asia
3. Disturbed bone and mineral metabolism, including abnormalities in plasma Ca, Mg and phosphate, renal osteodystrophy, and urinary tract stone disease	Regional variations in stone etiology
4. Urinary tract infection and/or obstruction	Renal tuberculosis Schistosomiasis in Africa
5. Tubulointerstitial diseases	Chinese herb nephropathy Leptospirosis
6. Glomerular disease: including primary glomerular disease presenting as nephritic syndrome, nephrotic syndrome, and asymptomatic hematuria/ proteinuria, as well as systemic diseases such as HCV, vasculitis, SLE, and amyloidosis	Parasitic nephropathy in the tropics Hemolytic-uremic syndrome in South America AIDS nephropathy in Africa
7. Diabetic nephropathy	Diabetic nephropathy in indigenous populations
8. Hypertension, particularly when associated with evidence for renal disease or dysfunction	
9. Renal functional impairment of uncertain etiology	Balkan nephropathy
10. Acute renal failure, including the critically ill patient in an intensive care setting	Tropical causes of ARF: toxins, venoms, infections (N.B. prevention)
11. Chronic kidney disease, including the management of pre-end stage disease as well as renal replacement therapy (modes of dialysis) for ESRF	
12. A request or indication for renal transplantation, or a functioning renal transplant (to include selection, preparation, post-op care, management of immuno suppression, common medical complications, etc.)	
13. Inherited renal disease	

Competencies	Regional variations (examples only)
B. Population-based Competencies	
1. Source and interpret the best available epidemiological evidence to guide the management of a patient presenting with kidney disease	
2. Design a research protocol to ascertain the burden of kidney disease in a national or regional population	
3. Implement a strategy for the prevention of kidney disease in a defined patient population	Diabetic nephropathy in indigenous populations Endemic stone disease
4. Promote the support by health systems of programs for treating patients with renal disease, and contribute to the cost-effective implementation of such programs	
5. Participate in the management of health services so as to achieve optimal allocation of resources for the care of patients with kidney disease	

N.B. Experience in relation to each of the above competencies should ideally be acquired in a range of patient groups, including

- children;
- pregnant women;
- the elderly.

II. REQUIRED KNOWLEDGE AND SKILLS

Knowledge

Trainees should be able to draw on a comprehensive knowledge base, sufficient to understand clinical problems and support optimum patient care decisions, in the following areas:

K1 Basic renal sciences

K1.1 Anatomy and histology of the normal kidney
K1.2 Embryology of the kidney and urinary tract
K1.3 Normal fluid and electrolyte homeostasis
K1.4 Physiology of glomerular filtration

K1.5 Physiology of tubular function

K1.6 Renal endocrinology, especially erythropoietin and Vitamin D

K1.7 Renal pharmacology, especially diuretic, immunosuppressive, and antibiotic agents

K1.8 Immunology of infection and transplant rejection

K1.9 Molecular biology and genetics

K2 Renal pathology, pathophysiology, immunology, and microbiology

K2.1 Patterns of abnormal microscopic structure in the kidney, including the basic histopathology of common renal diseases*

K2.2 Pathophysiology of disturbed metabolism of water, sodium, potassium, acid, calcium, magnesium and phosphate, due to renal and extra-renal diseases

K2.3 Immunopathology of glomerulonephritis and interstitial nephritis

K2.4 Pathogenesis of diabetic nephropathy and other systemic diseases affecting the kidney*

K2.5 Microbiology and pathogenesis of urinary tract infection

K2.6 Pathophysiology of urinary tract obstruction

K2.7 Pathogenesis of essential hypertension and hypertension in renal and endocrine disorders

K2.8 Pathophysiology of progressive kidney disease

K2.9 Etiological factors and pathogenesis relevant to environmental kidney disease

K2.10 Pathophysiology of renal transplant rejection

K3 Clinical manifestations and natural history of kidney disease and hypertension

K3.1 Patterns of clinical presentation of kidney disease, and the approach to differential diagnosis of common presenting syndromes

K3.2 Natural history of specific kidney diseases, both primary (especially glomerulonephritis) and secondary (especially diabetic nephropathy)

K3.3 Kidney disease and hypertension in pregnancy

K3.4 Pathogenesis of characteristic features of acute and chronic kidney failure

K3.5 End-organ disease and clinical consequences in hypertension

K3.6 The short- and long-term course of renal transplantation

---

*Note that in this and subsequent sections emphasis should be placed on conditions, which are common in the region where the trainee is working.

K4 Investigation and diagnosis of kidney disease and hypertension

    K4.1 Comprehensive renal function testing: assessing glomerular and tubular function

    K4.2 Immunological investigations in kidney disease

    K4.3 Rationale and interpretation of urinalysis, urine microscopy, urine culture, and sensitivity testing

    K4.4 Indications for and interpretation of renal biopsy

    K4.5 Hormone and cytokine assays in the investigation of kidney disease and hypertension

    K4.6 Radiological and other imaging modalities in the investigation of kidney disease and hypertension

    K4.7 Molecular biology in the diagnosis of kidney disease

K5 Treatment of kidney disease and hypertension

    K5.1 Nutrition and dietary management of kidney disease, before and after end-stage renal failure

    K5.2 Other non-pharmacological measures in the management of kidney failure

    K5.3 Drug therapies for kidney disease and its complications

    K5.4 Non-pharmacological measures and drug therapy of hypertension

    K5.5 Renal replacement therapy using dialysis: principles of prescribing and monitoring peritoneal dialysis (including CAPD) and hemodialysis

    K5.6 Renal transplantation: patient selection and preparation, immunosuppressive therapy, acute and long-term postoperative management

    K5.7 Published guidelines for management of common kidney disorders as well as complications of kidney failure

K6 Clinical epidemiology, prevention, and population health

    K6.1 The principles of evidence-based medicine: evaluation and application of findings from the clinical research literature

    K6.2 Epidemiology of disease in populations: outbreaks and trends

    K6.3 Research-based interventions in populations with kidney disease

    K6.4 Clinical trial design and implementation

    K6.5 Basic research methodology, including biostatistics

K7 Miscellaneous

> K7.1 Ethical issues in management of patients with ESRD (such as patient selection for dialysis and transplantation, donor selection, resource allocation, etc.)
> K7.2 Advocacy for cost effective care of patients with kidney disease
> K7.3 Public education focused on prevention of kidney disease

> *Skills*

Trainees should achieve competence and confidence in performing the following clinical skills (refer also to the *Postgraduate Training Guidelines*):

> S1 Perform a complete clinical history and physical examination of a patient presenting with kidney disease and/or hypertension (to include digital rectal examination and fundoscopy).
> S2 Integrate all clinical and investigative findings into a coherent diagnosis, with formulation of a differential diagnosis, management plan, and prognosis.
> S3 Perform a dipstick urinalysis, and fresh urine microscopy to detect cellular elements, crystals, and casts.
> S4 Perform a transcutaneous renal biopsy, under local anesthetic, on a native or transplanted kidney.
> S5 Place temporary intravascular lines for hemodialysis access.
> S6 Connect a patient to the hemodialysis circuit (desirable).
> S7 Place an acute peritoneal catheter (optional, as required by conditions).
> S8 Place a Tenchkoff catheter (or equivalent) for commencing CAPD (optional).
> S9 Perform a urinary tract ultrasound examination (desirable).
> S10 Assess and manage a poorly functioning vascular access device (shunt or fistula).

Methods of Learning and Assessment

Depending on local expertise and facilities, the following educational methods may be employed in the implementation and assessment of this curriculum. It is recommended that a range of teaching and learning methodologies be used for maximum enrichment of the training experience.

The overall philosophy of training is that it should empower the trainee to provide competent patient care under supervision, with growing responsibility for independent decision making.

> 1. Self-directed learning by use of Library materials (texts and journals) and on-line resources
> 2. Participation in Journal Clubs or equivalent formats for maintaining familiarity with current trial evidence and new advances

3. Formal teaching by lectures, tutorials, or demonstration sessions
4. Case presentations and discussions with supervisor and clinical department members
5. Maintaining a logbook of cases managed and procedures performed
6. Assessment of trainee competence should utilize more than one of the following tools:

- multiple choice questions;
- modified essay questions (case-based);
- review of clinical records kept;
- observation of consulting and procedural skills by senior colleague(s);
- survey of observations of trainee performance made by colleagues, non-medical staff and patients.

ACKNOWLEDGMENTS

We thank the members of the Education Advisory Committee for their contributions to the work presented in this chapter. They are (in addition to the authors): Drs. A. Al-Khader (Saudi Arabia), G. Capasso (Italy), R. Correa-Rotter (Mexico), S. Lin (China), P. Masssari (Argentina), Z. Morad (Malaysia), S. Naikar (South Africa), S. Pritchard (Canada), D. Rana (India), L. Rosivall (Hungary), N. Schor (Brazil), J. Seifter (United States), N.Tomalina (Russia) and R.Vanholder (Belgium). We would also like to thank other colleagues from around the world who contributed to the data in the initial survey reported in this paper.

REFERENCES

1. Robinson R. Crucible for birth of an idea, the first decade:1960–1969. Kidney Int 2001; 59(suppl 79):S-2–S-18.
2. Kolff WJ. New Ways of Treating Uraemia: the Artificial Kidney, Peritoneal Lavage, Intestinal Lavage. London: J&A Churchill, 1947.
3. Bywaters EGL, Beall D. Crush injuries with impairment of renal function. BMJ 1941; 1:427–432.
4. Muehrcke RC, Kank RM, Pirani CL, Schoenberger JA. Clinical value of percutaneous kidney biopsy. Clin Res Proc 1954; 2:96.
5. Hume DM, Merrill JP, Miller BF, Thorn GW. Experience with renal homotransplantations in human; report of nine cases. J Clin Invest 1955; 34:327.
6. Weening JJ, Brenner BM, Dirks JH, Schrier RW. Toward global advancement in medicine; the International Society of Nephrology experience. Kidney Int 1998; 54:1017–1021.
7. ACGME. Graduate Medical Education Directory 2002–2003. Chicago: American Medical Association, 2002:115–117.

8. Royal Australasian College of Physicians. Requirements for Physician Training in Australia: Adult Internal Medicine. Sydney, 2000.
9. Specialty Section in Nephrology, UEMS. Programme for harmonization of training in nephrology in the European Union. Nephrol Dial Transplant 1996; 11:1657–1660.
10. Accreditation Council on Graduate Medical Education. Program requirements for residency education in nephrology. www.acgme.org/Req_Print/148 print.asp, 2001.
11. Kumar R (for the Am Soc Nephrol Training Program Directors Committee). 1996 Nephrology Curriculum: American Society of Nephrology. J Am Soc Nephrol 1997; 8:1016–1027.
12. Joint Committee on Higher Medical Training (UK). Higher Medical Training Curriculum for Renal Medicine. www.jchmt.org.uk/renal/index.asp, 2003.

27

The Emerging Nephrologist: A Training Vision

Meguid El Nahas

Sheffield Kidney Institute, University of Sheffield, Sheffield, U.K.

Giuseppe Remuzzi

Department of Medicine and Transplantation, Asienda Ospedaliera Ospedali Riuniti di Bergamo—'Mario Negri' Institute for Pharmacological Research, Bergamo, Italy

THE GLOBAL SCALE OF CKD PROBLEM

Chronic kidney disease (CKD) is rapidly becoming a major and global public health problem. More than 1 million patients are currently requiring renal replacement therapy (RRT) worldwide (1). It has been predicted that the number of patients on RRT will continue to rise and double during the next decade (1,2). Of note, about 90% of patients treated by RRT come from developed nations able to assume the financial implications (3). By contrast, the developing world with a predictable equal, if not superior, burden of CKD is unable to meet the demands for RRT of the majority of its patients. In the United States, it has been estimated that the annual expenditure on end-stage renal disease (ESRD) will double in this decade to reach more than 27 billion U.S. dollars by 2010 (2). In Europe, dialysis consumes about 2% of the healthcare budget with only a small fraction (0.02–0.05%) of the population on RRT (3). There is a direct relationship between the gross national product (GNP) of a given country and the availability of RRT (3). Consequently, there is limited access to RRT in developing nations where the low GNP is unable to meet the increasing demands of healthcare and in particular the growing burden of ESRD. It is even doubtful that in the future the demands for RRT will be met by most nations.

With the above in mind, it is therefore highly imperative and timely to shift the emphasis of the global approach to CKD towards early detection and prevention rather than on the late management of ESRD and RRT. It is also timely to consider a shift in the emphasis of nephrology training from the current view of a highly specialized and technically demanding specialty to a more pragmatic and realistic approach based on local needs rather than universal guidelines designed and planned in the academies and societies of Western nations. The emerging nephrologists (EN) practicing in the emerging and developing world would have educational needs and objectives aimed to meet the clinical priorities that characterize their environment and available resources, which would often differ greatly from those of colleagues practicing in the West.

DETECTION AND PREVENTION (D&P) OF CKD PROGRAMS

One of the most urgent tasks of nephrology and emerging nephrologists over the next decades is to identify the actual burden of CKD in order to attempt to plan their health care and to prevent progression to end-stage renal failure (ESRF). Detection and Prevention (D&P) programs if well planned and thoroughly conducted can prove a very cost-effective investment for nephrologists worldwide aimed at preventing an imminent tragedy of untreated ESRD.

In order to identify patients at risk of progressive CKD, a number of screening strategies have been implemented. Some of the D&P programs have focused on the entire population, while others targeted a specific group within the population.

Whole Population CKD Evaluation Programs

The U.S.-based National Health and Nutrition Examination Survey (NHANES) III is a nationally based health survey carried out from 1988 to 1994 involving 15,626 adult participants (4). NHANES III estimated the prevalence of CKD among the population at 11% (representing about 19 millions U.S. adult) (4). The prevalence distribution pattern across the National Kidney Foundation (NKF)—kidney disease outcome quality initiative (KDOQI) stages of CKD (5) was: Stage 1 [defined by persistent albuminuria with a normal glomerular filtration rate (GFR)]: 3.3% of the U.S. population, Stage 2 (GFR: 89–60 mL/min/1.73 m^2): 3.0%, Stage 3 (GFR: 59–30 mL/min/1.73 m^2): 4.3%, Stage 4 (GFR 29–15 mL/min/1.73 m^2): 0.2%, and Stage 5/ESRF (GFR < 15 mL/min/1.73 m^2): 0.2% (4). This survey pointed to a large number of cases of asymptomatic CKD in the presumably normal general population.

The Australian Diabetes, Obesity and Lifestyle (AusDiab) study is a population-based cross-sectional survey aimed at determining the prevalence of diabetes mellitus, obesity, cardiovascular risk factors, and indicators of CKD in Australian adults (6). A representative sample of Australian adult population comprising 11,247 participants was studied from may 1999 to December 2000 and showed 11% to have significant renal impairment (GFR < 60 mL/min) whilst 3% had proteinuria (6).

In Japan, the Okinawa screening program carried out in 1983–1984 investigated more than 106,000 individuals and followed them up for 17 years to determine predictors of CKD (7). The study identified obesity, dyslipidemia, and smoking as significant risk factors for the development of albuminuria. It also identified proteinuria (8) and obesity (9) as major risk factors for the development of ESRF.

In Europe, the Prevention of End-Stage Renal and Vascular End-points (PREVEND) study was undertaken in the Dutch city of Groningen (10). It evaluated almost half the population (~40,000 individuals) in a cross-sectional cohort study to determine the prevalence of microalbuminuria. Around 7% of those screened had albuminuria. There was an association between the level of albuminuria and the incidence of cardiovascular death over 3 years (10). This observation highlighted the potential value of albuminuria as a predictor and marker of endothelial dysfunction, atherosclerosis, and cardiovascular morbidity and mortality.

In the Far East, the National Kidney Foundation of Singapore has set up a comprehensive national program for CKD prevention (11). It was initiated in 2000 and is currently ongoing with over 450,000 Singaporeans recruited from all ages and walks of life (11). The program detected significant urinary abnormalities (ranging from 5% to 8% proteinuria and/or heamaturia) in the general population and amongst high-risk individuals with family history of renal insufficiency (11).

In India, the Chennai community-screening program screened approximately 25,000 individuals and found around 6% with previously undiagnosed hypertension and 4% with diabetes mellitus (12). Intensive management of hypertensive and diabetic patients with readily available and cheap drugs when applied to this community achieved target values in the majority of patients (12). This program could well prove to be a template for similar action plans in the developing world. It was built on a nephrologist's initiative and leadership and relied for screening and delivery of care on well-trained and dedicated teams of rural health workers (12). (Discussed in details by Datta and Mani in Chapter 19).

Targeted CKD Screening Programs

Some screening programs targeted specific at-risk populations. In Australia, the inhabitants of the Tiwi islands are Aborigines whose quarter of all deaths is attributed to ESRD (13). Their annual incidence of ESRF is around 2760 per million of population (pmp) (15 times the incidence in the general Australian population). This may explain their very high incidence of cardiovascular mortality (five times that of the general population). In the Tiwi screening program, the overall prevalence of albuminuria was a staggering 55%, and when followed longitudinally it highlighted all future risks for renal deaths and cardiovascular morbidity and mortality. Of interest, intervention in this high-risk group with angiotensin converting enzyme inhibition reduced blood pressure, proteinuria, and overall mortality (13). This program may also prove to be a model for future intervention studies aimed at reducing renal and cardiovascular morbidity and mortality in high-risk populations (it is discussed in details by Wendy Hoy and colleagues in Chapter 14).

In the United States, Zuni Indians are affected by CKD due to glomerulonephritis and diabetic nephropathy and 2% have ESRD (a prevalence rate of 17,400 pmp) (14). The Zuni Kidney Project is a population-based, cross-sectional survey of the Zuni Indians that showed a prevalence of albuminuria ranging from 12% to 36% (14).

The Kidney Early Evaluation Program (KEEP) was piloted in 1997–1999 by the U.S. NKF to identify individuals at risk of CKD and the prevalence of early stages of CKD among at-risk population including relatives of patients with CKD (15). It is currently ongoing and by the end of the year 2003 had recruited over 22,000 participants. It revealed an overall prevalence of the different stages of CKD in about 50% of those studied (15). The KEEP program was well designed and may turn out to be a prototype of such exercises aimed at early detection of CKD in the developed world where logistics exist for such a targeting.

Detection and prevention programs will have to be tailored to the needs and infrastructure/resources available within the community. Different communities probably will have to adopt different methods that best suit their environment taking into consideration such factors as health's awareness and availability of human and material resources. Targeted population screening will suit well-developed health systems with accurate records and databases. Whole population surveys, on the other hand, may be better suited to less sophisticated health systems, where it would start by identifying those diseases underlying most nephropathies, namely, infections, diabetes, and hypertension. Interventions would follow to treat those diseases in the hope of minimizing their long-term complications including CKD.

Manpower Requirements for Implementation of D&P Programs

Detection and Prevention of CKD programs will require considerable resources both in term of manpower and funds. The implementation of far reaching D&P of CKD programs will require considerable infrastructure and staffing. It will depend primarily on the leadership of nephrologists worldwide. It will also depend on the training and availability of a new generation of dedicated nephrologists with an interest and training in epidemiology and public health. They will have to rely on well-trained and motivated community health workers. The formulation of such team has proved extremely effective and successful when applied in projects such as that of Chennai Community Screening project in India (12) or of the Tiwi islanders (13).

THE EMERGING NEPHROLOGIST (EN)

The implementation of D&P of CKD programs as well as the nature of renal services needed to be practiced in many of the developing world requires a serious and innovative look at the nature of nephrology training and even at the definition of a nephrologist in some part of the world.

Definition

The Western definition of a nephrologist is that of a physician who provides a competent and comprehensive range of renal services based on an in depth and lengthy training leading to a sound knowledge and expertise in the field. Many of these tenants are inapplicable in countries where nephrology is emerging along with the country itself. There, the "nephrologists" will not be providing a range of renal services as these are not available due to lack of funds and infrastructure. Instead, they will provide a limited service with little scope for expansion. For that their training requirements, knowledge, and skills may be very different from those of colleagues practicing in the more affluent West. For instance, many developing countries don't have renal replacement therapies (RRT). Dialysis, when available, may be limited to the management of patients with acute renal failure (ARF). In other countries, chronic hemodialysis may be available in a few centers catering for a small number of privileged patients, often for a limited and short period of time. CAPD is unheard of in the majority of developing nations where the social and economical conditions are not supportive of such a form of RRT. Renal transplantation is not an option in most developing nations.

Similarly, the in-depth training of potential nephrologists is unavailable either due to the fact that country itself has no nephrologists or that the resources including time and money to train such physicians are unavailable.

Even when training possibilities are available in slightly better off developing countries with some nephrological practice, the limited infrastructure hampers the quality of training and subsequent practice. For instance, histopathology is basic if at all available in many countries. Immuno-fluorescence and electron microscopy evaluation of renal biopsies is seldom an option. Therefore, the very nature of diagnosis of the most common nephrological problem, namely glomerulonephritis, is often wanting. Misdiagnosis, based on light microscopy alone, often leads to erroneous treatment.

Finally, management is hampered by the cost and unavailability of drugs. This applies to a range of medication from antihypertensive drugs such as angiotensin converting enzyme inhibitors (ACEI) and angiotensin2 receptor antagonists (ARB) to immunosuppressive drugs needed to treat glomerulone-phritides as well as antibiotics to treat the more chronic and pernicious of infections including HCV and HIV.

So can nephrology be practiced in these countries and what would the role of the nephrologists be? The answer is undoubtedly yes, nephrology can be practiced in these countries but the definition of the specialty and its practitioners has to be redefined in light of the local needs and infrastructure at variance with the Western template often based on unlimited resources. Nephrology has to start by being an area of expertise available to some internists. The emerging nephrologist would provide that expertise based on his/hers community geo-social healthcare requirements. There would be no universal template but a well-defined, albeit limited, mission namely, the detection, prevention, and management of the most common nephrological problems within that community. Additional knowledge would initially be superfluous.

THE BASIC TRAINING REQUIREMENTS OF THE EMERGING NEPHROLOGIST (EN)

The EN who will practice in countries with limited nephrological input and infrastructure will be a pioneer upon much depends. The EN will set up the required nephrological service. The EN will provide the training of the next generation of nephrologists who by then may be more than emerging, perhaps even emerged. The EN will be the link between the more conventional and experienced nephrologists in the area, country, continent, and West.

Setting up a Nephrology Service

This will vary and will have to be based on the community in which the EN practices rather than a broad definition made elsewhere of the emerging nephrologists job description. If the EN practices in a rural area where infection control is poor leading to a large number of infections-related nephritides, training will have to a large extent focus on infectious disease. The EN will have to be familiar with their nature, their prevention, detection, and management, and will also have to be familiar with the renal manifestations of these infections as well as their diagnosis and management. The EN will also have to be familiar with renal manifestations indirectly related to infectious disease including fluid and electrolytes disorders induced by fever and diarrheal diseases. Knowledge of the impact of the medication used to treat these infections on kidney function and structure will have to be acquired.

On the other hand, if the EN practices in an urban, albeit deprived, environment where systemic hypertension and diabetes are highly prevalent, the EN will be familiar with public health screening and detection methods. The EN should have knowledge of the epidemiology of these conditions and their impact on kidney structure and function. The EN should be able to implement early D&P programs for early detection of glucose intolerance/diabetes as well as pre- and well-established hypertensives states. They should be well acquainted with the manifestations and diagnostic means of detection of renal involvement in diabetes and hypertension. They should have a sound knowledge of their management to prevent their progression to chronicity worse still to ESRF. They should also be aware of the cardiovascular impact these conditions and kidney disease have in general on population health and outcome. Finally, these EN should have some knowledge of health economics as well as the cost effectiveness of drug therapies.

These two scenarios described above are likely to cover in some respect two-third of the practice of the emerging nephrologists; infectious diseases, diabetes, and hypertension. There remain the need to have a knowledge of drugs and the kidney and the potential nephroxicity of medication ranging from analgesics, non-steroidal anti-inflammatory drugs, as well as traditional herbal remedies. They should also be aware that antibiotics used to treat infections as well as antihypertensive drugs including ACEI/ARB are potentially nephrotoxic, thus warranting care in prescription and monitoring of side effects.

In geographical areas where other specific nephropathies prevail such as renal stone disease, training of EN will have to assimilate that knowledge.

It is also important to appreciate that the first, if not the sole, task of the EN will be to provide a "nephrology service" for the community. Nephrology service in that context means supporting the community healthcare by their expertise in nephrology and not in the Western sense of the provision of a centralized renal unit-based service. The EN may provide this service from a practice or on an ambulatory basis by visiting communities and advising their health carers. In that context, EN will not provide, in the first instance, a comprehensive renal service but an expertise targeted to address the nephrological needs of the community. Renal replacement therapy or investigative nephrological tests would not be an option or a priority.

The Training Requirements of the Emerging Nephrologist

As mentioned above, training's emphasis will vary from country/region to another. This will be taken into consideration by the trainers as described below. The emerging nephrologist would be expected to have had at least 3 years of internal medical training in his/her community after graduation from medical school. This would be followed by the nephrology training. For that, basic knowledge will be expected/acquired in:

1. anatomy and function/physiology of the kidney;
2. pathology of the kidney at macroscopic (radiological) and microscopic level;

3. geographically relevant infectious disease and their renal complications;
4. diabetes mellitus and hypertension and their renal complications;
5. glomerulonephritides (with emphasis on the relevant; if their knowledge of Alport's disease, Goodpastures'syndrome, ANCA associated vasculitis, or Finnish-type nephrotic syndrome is wanting this would/should have no serious consequences on the community they treat);
6. tubulointerstitial nephritides (with emphasis on the geographically common drugs, herbs-induced or related to renal stones and obstructive uropathies);
7. diagnosis and management of major fluid and electrolytes disorders;
8. drugs and the kidney; including dosage adjustments and nephrotoxicity;
9. epidemiology and public health methods of screening, data collection, and population research;
10. essential diagnostic tests relevant to the needs and available resources (serum urea and electrolytes as well as urinalysis absence of immunological tests may not be a disaster);
11. essential radiological investigations: renal ultrasonography;
12. principle of the kidney biopsy (experience may be less relevant as pathology analysis may seldom be available);
13. principles of renal replacement therapy (practical exposure initially unnecessary);
14. principles of renal transplantation;
15. health economics.

In addition, the emerging nephrologist will need to learn the skills of self-learning including literature and Internet searches. The EN will be taught problem-solving skills. This may include problem solving in the absence of comprehensive medical libraries or teaching resources and without access to the Internet. Problem solving may mean phoning a reference centre; linkage to a centre/colleague of more expertise.

Provision of Training for EN

The training of the EN may depend on many options. Where and when there is in the community the EN aspires to serve an experienced nephrologist, the training will become the responsibility of that nephrologist. If on the other hand, as often is the case, the EN would like to serve a community devoid on any previous nephrological input, a travel to a nearby center where such expertise is available is required. In the absence of such expertise in the country EN aspires to serve, a travel to the nearest facility where such training can be provided would be needed. This may be facilitated by the development of Regional Nephrology Schools (RNS). These could provide a training resource within an area/continent with limited training facilities.

The Regional Nephrology School (RNS)

Such training centre will pool the expertise of experts within the area/continent. The RNS would provide intensive crash training courses in nephrology ranging from 1 to 3 months. It will depend on the goodwill of experienced nephrologists and teachers on that continent. It could also depend on funding provided by a range of sources including governments, non-governmental organizations (NGOs) as well as the pharmaceutical industry. The International Society of Nephrology (ISN) and its Commission for the Global Advancement of Nephrology (COMGAN) can play a key role in developing these centers through its regional committees as well as those dedicated to training, education, and research within a given region/continent. The RSN should be centers networks of educational excellence with input from educationalists as well as well supported teaching facilities: library, Internet access, etc. The ISN training resources and courses would be made accessible electronically to these schools. The RNS may also have direct links with centers of training excellence in the developed world.

The school courses could be held once or twice a year depending on the availability of the regional faculty. It can involve overseas contributors and faculty. It could also stipulate some exchanges of trainees with Western centers of training excellence. Selected trainees completing the RNS training could be sent to Western centers to acquire additional and required skills. They would in turn return to their region as senior emerging nephrologists with a duty to contribute to the teaching and training programmes of their regional RSN.

The RSN Syllabus

The RSN syllabus will be based on the above-described training requirement. Emphasis will vary from region to region. Each topic will consist of one to three lectures with an additional self-learning exercise and essay/presentation by students encouraging mutual and horizontal teaching. Training will also consist of case studies and simulation clinical scenarios. The training will be interactive based on vertical transmission of knowledge from the teachers to the trainees but also horizontal amongst the trainees to harvest their respective skills and knowledge and amplify the training delivered within the limited resources of time and funds available.

At the completion of the RSN course, candidates would undergo some form of evaluative assessment. This should include an evaluation of their theoretical knowledge as well as simulated clinical training (case discussions). Successful candidates could be recognized as trained ENs with some national, regional, and international recognition. The ISN could give some of these an honorary fellowship and thus access to its Global Fellow Club (GFC) network. This would provide them with more opportunities for exchanges of knowledge with young colleagues/ISN fellows worldwide.

The EN Training Role

The EN would be expected to be the focus of the training of the next generation of EN and ultimately nephrologists (N) within the area, country, or region. For that the EN will need to acquire teaching and leadership skills.

These will include:

1. knowledge of teaching methods;
2. knowledge of communication skills;
3. knowledge of teaching resources and their accessibility;
4. knowledge of self-assessment methods;
5. knowledge of training evaluation;
6. quality assurance and audit issues.

The EN could acquire some of these skills during their training at the RNS. For that the RNS would have to recruit and call upon the skills and expertise of regional educationalists. Other ENs of proven potential can be selected at the end of the course for further training in centers of excellence in training and education in the West.

EVOLUTION FROM EMERGING NEPHROLOGIST TO NEPHROLOGIST

The evolution of emerging nephrologists to fully fledged nephrologists, in the larger and more conventional/Western sense of the definition, will depend on a range of circumstances and opportunities. These will be local, regional, and global.

At the local level, the evolution of the nephrology service from a practice-based or an ambulatory advisory and consultative service to a "nephrology center" may be evolutionary with time as the growing practice and reputation of the ENs will enhance the attendance and income of their practice. This may allow the setting up of basic investigation tools for urine testing and serum urea, creatinine, and glucose measurement. This may be complemented in due time by basic ultrasonography. Support from such developments may be sought from government, NGOs, and pharmaceutical sponsors. The ISN may choose to support a small number of thriving and successful centers by giving them an affiliation and providing them with access to the Internet and Kidney International. Visits and exchanges could also be envisaged through ISN COMGAN to the most promising and innovative of these centers, thus enhancing their profile and reputation within the community.

Some of these mini-nephrology centers will evolve in time into macro-nephrology centers, providing additional services including hemodialysis. For that, a small number of dialysis machines could be purchased and used judiciously by the coordinating nephrologist. The setting up of a macro-nephrology center will require additional training of the EN in the field of hemodialysis. This will see the completion of their evolution and that of their practice from EN status to N (Nephrologist).

ALTERNATIVE TO TRAINING NEPHROLOGISTS

It has been argued that it may be unrealistic to expect developing countries to train sufficient medical specialists including nephrologists to meet their requirements (16). It has also been suggested that trained medical and nursing specialists in developing countries seek employment in the developed countries where remunerations meet their expectations and those of their higher qualifications, thus further draining manpower resources away from developing countries that need them most; It has been estimated that 27,000 highly qualified Africans including doctors and nurses have emigrated between 1960 and 1975 (17). Since, the annual emigration rate has risen from 1800 skilled individuals per year in the 1970s to 20,000 in the 1990s (17). Bonding doctors to their native countries have failed due to limited punitive actions and the fact that health workers find ways to evade the system. Combining bonding of doctors and incentive strategies has been tried in some countries with some success.

Conversely, non-medically/nursing qualified health workers/auxiliaries find it much more difficult to leave their countries. Mostly, their qualifications are not internationally recognized and their skills are limited. However, healthcare workers can provide the backbone of an emerging rural nephrological service. They can be trained in a very short period of time, days (see Chapter Datta and Mani), to perform key medical tasks aimed at detection and prevention as well as treatment of common medical conditions predisposing to progressive CKD. For instance, these workers could be trained in hours to be competent in measuring blood pressure and test urine or blood for glucose. Hypertension and diabetes contribute to a large percentage of patients with CKD in the developing countries. The Chennai experience related in chapter 19 is a testimony to the valuable role of health workers in the detection of hypertension and diabetes. Health workers could also be trained in hours to test urine for protein/albumin, blood, and glucose. They could be effectively deployed to ensure the distribution of medication and compliance. They could monitor response to treatment. They could disseminate health advice and distribute relevant public health guidances. They could form the missing link between an effective healthcare system in a deprived environment and one based on a specialist unable to reach for the community they are meant to serve. The limited evidence available suggests that community health workers in Africa are valuable support to community health programs and are cost-effective (18). They are easier to retain than highly qualified medical and paramedical staff and they respond well to incentives.

The deployment of community health workers to support emerging nephrologists in deprived environments within the developing world is the way forward to initiate preventive measures and attempt to reinforce curative ones. The international nephrology community will have to support the training and deployment of these community health workers. It will have to encourage emerging nephrologists to train and rely on these workers to deliver the care they aspire to within their community. It is imperative that both the emerging nephrologist and the community health worker appreciate their interdependence. It is also important that they combine effectively to produce the nucleus of an emerging nephrological service in a socially and economically deprived setting. Without such close interaction, neither would be able to discharge their responsibility of providing a basic medical and nephrological service.

Conclusion

The proposed evolutionary rather than creationist view of nephrologists may be most suitable for the emerging world, where a stepwise development program is justified and imposed by limited resources and skills. Such a vision is achievable only with the support of local, national, and international communities. The ISN and its COMGAN could play a lead role in establishing such global and ambitious program. Also, to train a growing number of highly specialized nephrologists has its limitations, as many find it frustrating to return to their country of origin and opt instead for a more lucrative career in the West. For that, regulations should be put in place to restrict the poaching of medical and nursing specialist from the developing countries. Multilateral agreements and compensations will have to be considered. Further, attention should be paid to a growing role for non-medically qualified community healthcare workers with limited aspirations and a commitment to their communities who could discharge many of the basic and key tasks of a nascent nephrological service.

REFERENCES

1. Lysaght MJ. Maintenance dialysis population dynamics: current trends and long-term implications. J Am Soc Nephrol 2002; 13:37–40.
2. Xue JL, Ma JZ, Louis TA, Collins AJ. Forecast of the number of patients with end-stage renal disease in United States to the year 2010. J Am Soc Nephrol 2001; 12:2753–2758.

3. De Vecchi AF, Dratwa M, Wiedmann ME. Healthcare systems and end-stage renal disease. An international review: costs and reimbursement of ESRD therapies. N Eng J Med 1999; 14:31–41.

4. Coresh J, Astor BC, Greene T, Eknoyan G, Levey AS. Prevalence of chronic kidney disease and decreased kidney function in the adult US population: Third National Health and Nutrition Examination Survey. Am J Kidney Dis 2003; 41:1–12.

5. Anonymous. K/DOQI clinical practice guidelines for chronic kidney disease, evaluation classification and stratification. Kidney disease outcome quality initiative. Am J Kidney Dis 2002; 39(suppl 2):S1–S246.

6. Chadban SJ, Briganti EM, Kerr PG, Dunstan DW, Welborn TA, Zimmet PZ, Atkins RC. Prevalence of kidney damage in Australian adults: the AusDiab Kidney Study. J Am Soc Nephrol 2003; 14:S131–S138.

7. Iseki K. The Okinawa screening program. J Am Soc Nephrol 2003; 7(suppl 2): S127–S130.

8. Iseki K, Ikemiya Y, Iseki C, Takishita S. Proteinuria and the risk of developing end stage renal disease. Kidney Int 2003; 63:1468–1473.

9. Iseki K, Ikemiya Y, Kinjo K, Inoue T, Iseki C, Takishita S. Body mass index and the risk of development of end-stage renal disease in a screened cohort. Kidney Int 2004; 65:1870–1876.

10. Hillege HL, Fidler V, Diercks GF, van Gilst WH, de Zeeuw D, et al. Prevention of Renal and Vascular End Stage Disease (PREVEND) Study Group. Urinary albumin excretion predicts cardiovascular and non-cardiovascular mortality in general population. Circulation 2002; 106:1777–1782.

11. Ramirez SPB, Hsu SI-H, McClellan W. Taking a public health approach to the prevention of end-stage renal disease: the NKF Singapore Program. Kidney Int 2003; (suppl 83):S61–S65.

12. Mani MK. Prevention of chronic renal failure at the community level. Kidney Int 2003; (suppl 83):S86–S89.

13. McDonald SP, Maguire GP, Hoy WE. Renal function and cardiovascular risk markers in a remote Australian Aboriginal community. Nephrol Dial Transplant 2003; 18(8):1555–1561.

14. Stidley CA, Shah VO, Narva AS, et al. A population-based, cross-sectional survey of the Zuni Pueblo: a collaborative approach to an epidemic of kidney disease. Am J Kidney Dis 2002; 39:358–368.

15. Brown WW, Peters RM, Ohmit SE, Keane WF, et al. Early detection of kidney disease in community settings. The Kidney Early Evaluation Program (KEEP). Am J Kidney Dis 2003; 42:22–35.

16. Hongoro C, McPake B. How to bridge the gap in human resources for health. Lancet 2004; 364:1451–1456.

17. Marchal B, Kegels G. Health workforce imbalances in times of globalization: brain drain or professional mobility? Int J Health Plann Manage 2003; 18(suppl 1):S89–S101.

18. Lehmann B, Friedman I, Sanders D. Review of utilization and effectiveness of community-based health workers in Africa. A joint learning initiative paper 4-1: human resources for health development, 2003. http://www.globalhealthtrust.org/doc/JLI%20WG%20Paper%204-1.pdf.

28

Education and Training in Nephrology in Africa

Saraladevi Naicker

*Division of Nephrology, University of the Witwatersrand,
Johannesburg, South Africa*

Rashad S. Barsoum

Kasr El Aini Medical School, Cairo University, Cairo, Egypt

Africa, a large and diverse continent with a population in excess of 750 million (1), has major diversity in nephrology education, ranging from countries with no formal education in nephrology at any level, as these countries do not have medical schools, to those that offer full and complete training in nephrology. Similarly, there are no nephrologists in many countries in Africa, with the largest numbers in Egypt, a maximum of 10 nephrologists per million of the population (Tables 1 and 2). An additional problem for Africa has been its medical emigration or "brain drain" to the more developed countries of the world, resulting in a severe loss of medical expertise from countries that cannot afford to lose their medical personnel (2).

NEPHROLOGY EDUCATION

Undergraduate

Those countries with Faculties of Medicine have formal teaching in nephrology for 9 to 50 hours, usually in the last 3 years of the undergraduate

Table 1 Countries with Specialist Training in Nephrology

	Egypt	Morocco	Tunisia	Nigeria	South Africa
Population (millions)	70	30	10	120	46
Number of nephrologists	700	125	50–60	50	50
Undergraduate nephrology course (hr)	24	20–24	25–30	50	20
Postgraduate/Internal Medicine course (years)	3	—		$2\frac{1}{2}$	4
Duration in nephrology (months)	24–36		6	3	3
Specialist training in nephrology (years)	2	4	4	$2\frac{1}{2}$	2
Examination	Ministry of Health Fellowship	National Diploma of University	Yes	Fellowship	Certificate of Colleges of Medicine
Degree	M.Sc.	—	M.Sc.		M.Sc./Ph.D. (optional)

Table 2 Countries Without Specialist Training in Nephrology

	Libya	Ethiopia	Tanzania	Kenya	Sudan	Congo Republic	Tchad	Botswana
Population (millions)	5.5	67	36.3	30	30	3.5	9.2	1.5
Number of nephrologists	50	7	2 (non-practicing)	16	15	3	0	0
Undergraduate nephrology teaching (hr)		9	42	20	15	36	36	0
Postgraduate nephrology teaching (months)	4	2	—	4	4	3	0	0

medical course. The teaching is in the form of lectures, seminars, clinico-pathological conferences, and tutorials.

Postgraduate

Internal Medicine

Following exposure to nephrology as an undergraduate, the majority of countries follow a 3 to 4-year postgraduate training course in Internal Medicine during which the trainee spends 3 to 6 months in a renal unit, acquiring basic skills in treating patients with kidney disease. During the training period in Internal Medicine, the trainee rotates through the majority of specialties in Internal Medicine, and is thus able to recognize and appropriately treat or refer patients for further management in the different specialties of medicine.

Specialization in Nephrology

After graduating from Internal Medicine, the future nephrologist undertakes training in an accredited institution for a further 2 to 3 years, culminating in examinations (postgraduate diploma) and/or a postgraduate research degree (e.g., M.Sc. or Ph.D.). The trainee spends time training in haemodialysis, peritoneal dialysis, renal transplantation and manages patients with chronic and acute renal failure, including intensive care patients and is involved in the care of patients with renal disease both in an in-patient and ambulatory setting. At the end of the training program in nephrology, the trainee is competent to provide an independent consulting and management service for the care of patients with renal disease. Table 1 outlines those few countries in Africa offering specialist training in nephrology; the majority of the countries of Africa are as those listed in Table 2, with some or no postgraduate medical training or no medical training at all, e.g., Botswana, Namibia, Swaziland, Lesotho, and others.

Additional training may be accessed from these or other countries in the form of fellowships, e.g., International Society of Nephrology fellowships currently offered to developing countries and taken up in Africa (Egypt and South Africa) or institutions in developed countries; government- or NGO-sponsored (e.g., WHO) training fellowships may be available to candidates in those countries that do not have in-house specialist training in nephrology. The young nephrologist often spends a variable period in a center of excellence in the developed world, acquiring further expertise in nephrology, either as a Fellow of the International Society of Nephrology or with other support.

NEPHROLOGY SYLLABUS

Undergraduate

The core syllabus includes anatomy, physiology, and embryology of the kidney as well as fluid and electrolyte disorders, acid–base disorders, urinary tract infections, glomerulonephritis, nephrotic syndrome, renal disease in the tropics, diabetes and the kidney, hypertension, acute and chronic renal failure, and prevention of progression of renal disease. In addition, systemic diseases and the kidney, drugs and the kidney, parasitic nephropathies, renal calculi, obstructive uropathy, renal tumors, and congenital and inherited renal diseases are covered.

Postgraduate

Internal Medicine

In addition to the above topics studied in greater depth, training in dialysis and renal transplantation as well as insertion of hemodialysis and peritoneal dialysis catheters and renal biopsies may be offered.

Specialization in Nephrology

The syllabus includes anatomy, physiology, and embryology of the kidney as well as fluid and electrolyte disorders, acid–base disorders, urinary tract infections, glomerulonephritis, nephrotic syndrome, renal disease in the tropics, diabetes and the kidney, hypertension, acute and chronic renal failure and prevention of progression of renal disease. In addition, systemic diseases and the kidney (including HIV, SLE), drugs and the kidney, parasitic nephropathies, renal calculi, obstructive uropathy, renal tumours, and congenital and inherited renal diseases are covered. The nephrology fellow is trained in ultrasound-guided renal biopsies and attends histopathology training and becomes adept in all of the above-mentioned procedures and topics related to dialysis and renal transplantation. The period of training culminates in an examination as well as a research dissertation (usually a Master's degree in most centers).

RECOMMENDATIONS FOR NEPHROLOGY TRAINING IN AFRICA

The traditional training of a nephrologist in Africa should continue with the intensive training in Internal Medicine (3–4 years) followed by a further 2 to 3 years of specialist nephrology training, as outlined above. This is obviously not feasible for the majority of the countries of Africa. Consideration should be given to intensive training for short periods directed to specific tasks, with the goal of providing nephrological services to the populations of these countries. Schools/Departments of Nephrology in the countries listed in Table 1 should consider offering short courses (for 3–12 months) in haemodialysis, peritoneal dialysis, renal transplantation, and prevention strategies. This is occurring to a limited extent under the ISN Fellowships program, especially with Egypt and South Africa serving as host countries; in addition governments in Africa are funding their physicians for short training periods in South Africa and Kenya. This serves the purpose of the training being "hands-on" and appropriate for the population of Africa and could be supplemented with further training in specific aspects of nephrology in more developed countries in the West. These efforts could be coordinated by an African School of Nephrology, with bases in the various countries of Africa that are currently training nephrologists; distance learning modules could be developed and practical training could then be carried out over a 3-month period, resulting in a "Diploma in Haemodialysis," for example.

CONCLUSION

The emphasis on the curative aspects of nephrology (diagnosis and treatment) has previously discouraged many young African physicians from undertaking training in nephrology, as it was not possible for these physicians to practice these aspects of nephrology in many countries of Africa. The questionnaire filled in by colleagues in different countries (as detailed below) reveals that preventive nephrology is now an important component of nephrology education at all levels, undergraduate and postgraduate, and is a priority for the ISN fellowship training program; this is very promising and, in time, should impact on the large burden of renal disease in Africa (3,4) and other developing countries.

ACKNOWLEDGMENTS

The authors are grateful to the following colleagues for generously supplying information about their regions:

1. Professor A. Afifi, Egypt
2. Professor M. Benghanem, Morocco
3. Professors A. el Matri and M. Ben Hamida, Tunisia
4. Professor W. Akinsola, Nigeria
5. Dr. A. Lahresh, Libya
6. Dr Y Tadesse, Ethiopia
7. Dr. L. Ezekiel, Tanzania
8. Professor O. Aboud, Sudan
9. Professor A. Assounga, Botswana, Congo Republic, and Tchad
10. Dr. A. Twahir, Kenya

REFERENCES

1. US Bureau of Census, Report WP/98, World Population Profile: 1998, US Government Printing Office, Washington, DC, 1999: page 140. In World Bank Annual Report, 2002.

2. World Health Organisation Report, 1998. In http://www.who.int/whr/1998/en/ whr98 en.pdf: page 140.
3. Naicker S. End stage renal disease in sub-Saharan and South Africa. Kidney Int 2003; 83(suppl):S119–S122.
4. Barsoum RS. End stage kidney disease in North Africa. Kidney Int 2003; 83(suppl):S111–S114.

29

Clinical Assessment, Investigation and Treatment of Renal Disease in Africa: A Practical Guide for Primary Care Physicians

J. Plange-Rhule and J. B. Eastwood

Departments of Renal Medicine and Transplantation, and Community Health Sciences, St. George's, University of London, London, U.K. and Department of Medicine, Komfo Anokye Teaching Hospital, Kumasi, Ghana

F. P. Cappuccio

Community Health Sciences, St. George's, University of London, London, U.K.

INTRODUCTION

Diseases of the kidneys and urinary tract are not uncommon in tropical Africa. However, the spectrum of disease is very different from that of the non-tropical more developed world. The reasons for this difference are two-fold: (a) the presence of bacterial, viral, parasitic, and other diseases of sub-Saharan Africa in this economically deprived region; and (b) the lack of those diseases that occur with age and affluence in more developed countries. An understanding of the principles involved in the genesis of renal diseases combined with knowledge of how to treat them should enable the health worker to manage many of the patients with disorders of the kidneys and urinary tract who seek medical help.

The countries of sub-Saharan Africa like many developing countries have very limited nephrological facilities. An added hindrance is the severe lack of doctors, nurses, and other health workers. Nevertheless, much can be done in the prevention of renal disease, particularly when secondary to diabetes mellitus or high blood pressure.

In Africa, nurses and other health workers are likely to be the health workers most involved in delivering the service (see Chapter 27—The Concept of the Emerging Nephrologist). Such workers may already be involved in community projects concerned with the detection and control of high blood pressure, and diabetes mellitus Urine testing will be an important aspect of these efforts.

This chapter is intended for nurses and other health workers as much as for doctors. It aims to provide them with a basic understanding of history-taking, diagnosis, and management of disorders affecting the kidneys.

HISTORY

The presentation of conditions of the kidneys differs from that of other systems where symptoms commonly draw attention to the organ involved. This is much less true of the kidneys, and a patient can be completely unaware that their tiredness and itching, for example, are caused by end-stage renal failure. Many forms of glomerulonephritis are silent though some produce macroscopic hematuria; others present as swollen feet. Renal involvement in conditions as diverse as diabetes mellitus, hypertension, sickle cell disease, tuberculosis, malaria, leprosy, and infections caused by hepatitis virus and HIV are likely to be silent and only detected by blood or urine testing, or by the finding of high blood pressure.

On the other hand, bacterial infection of the kidneys will produce symptoms referable to the urinary tract by causing frequency, dysuria, and sometimes macroscopic hematuria, loin pain and pain in the suprapubic region. Likewise, stone disease and parasitic infestations are likely to present with loin pain and lower urinary symptoms.

It is essential to take a focused, relevant history, and important to ascertain any recent or current acute febrile illness. It is vital also to ask about the ingestion of herbs and traditional remedies; some are associated with nephrotoxicity (see Chapter 6).

PRESENTATION

> **Box 1**
>
> - Proteinuria
> - Oedema
> - Oliguria – pre-renal, renal, post-renal
> - Polyuria
> - High blood pressure

A patient with renal disease will often come to notice because of swelling. Alternatively, the patient may be found to have to a raised blood pressure or protein in the urine. Occasionally, a change in urine volume is the presenting feature. Rarely a patient may present with anemia or pulmonary edema.

Edema

This is a common presenting symptom in Africa. Retention of fluid leads to the accumulation of fluid in dependent parts of the body (edema), especially the legs. The finding of heavy proteinuria will support a diagnosis of "nephrotic syndrome," which is defined as the combination of edema, proteinuria, and a low serum albumin. Causes include acute glomerulonephritis, other forms of glomerulonephritis and diabetes mellitus.

Oliguria and Polyuria

Sometimes, the presenting symptom is lack of urine. The so-called "obligatory" minimum volume of urine is 500 mL/day, which is based on the premise that the body needs to excrete 600 mOsm of solute per day, the maximum urine osmolarity achievable being 1200 mOsm/kg. For this reason, the term oliguria is applied to a urine volume of <400 mL in 24 hour. Anuria implies no urine at all, a circumstance that suggests obstruction within the urinary tract.

In Africa, the most likely cause of oliguria is hypovolemia, i.e., the cause is pre-renal (Table 1).

Symptoms of post-renal causes of oliguria include loin pain, pain on passing urine, macroscopic hematuria, frequency, hesitancy, and urgency. These suggest disease of the ureters or bladder/prostate, or urinary tract obstruction, particularly at the bladder neck. Chronic obstruction, it should be pointed out, usually causes polyuria.

If there is no evidence of pre-renal or post-renal cause, the cause may be primarily renal. Forms of rapidly progressive glomerulonephritis are

Table 1   Common Causes of Oligo-Anuria in Africa

Pre-renal	Extracellular fluid volume depletion (e.g., diarrhea, vomiting)
	Congestive cardiac failure
	Hemorrhage (e.g., ante-partum and post-partum hemorrhage)
	Sepsis
Renal	Rapidly progressive glomerulonephritis, renal vasculitis, etc.
	Nephrotoxic drugs
Post-renal	Schistosomiasis
	Nephrolithiasis
	Benign prostatic hypertrophy

uncommon but very important, as they are all potentially treatable with corticosteroids. Interstitial nephritis may be caused by drug allergy, ascending urinary tract infection such as brucellosis, and autoimmune disorders. A renal biopsy is needed to establish a primarily renal cause.

Polyuria is usually defined as a daily urine volume of more than 3 L, compared with a usual daily urine volume of 1.0–1.5 L (Table 2).

SIGNS

> **Box 2**
>
> - Volume status – JVP, peripheral perfusion
> - Body weight
> - Blood pressure

Volume Status

The best "bedside" sign for assessing volume status is the jugular venous pressure (JVP). With the patient lying at 45° and in a good light (preferably daylight), the diffuse distension of the lower neck that occurs with each expiration should be observed carefully. If no rhythmic distension is visible, the intra-abdominal pressure can be increased by gentle pressure in the center of the abdomen; the neck veins may then be visible. Lying the patient flatter may make the neck veins stand out better, but the reference point remains the manubrio-sternal joint. Only when the top of the column of venous blood can be seen, is it possible to make a judgment as to the state of hydration.

If the JVP is not visible even with the application of abdominal pressure, the patient may be fluid deplete. Other signs of fluid depletion are a low

Table 2 Causes of Polyuria

Solute-induced	Water-induced
Electrolyte	*Diabetes insipidus*
Sodium chloride	Head trauma
Saline-loading	Surgery
Frusemide	Resection of benign pituitary tumor
Sodium bicarbonate	Post-hypophysectomy
Sodium bicarbonate loss	Idiopathic
	Tuberculosis
	Sarcoidosis
	Post-encephalitis
Non-electrolyte	*Nephrogenic diabetes insipidus*
Glucose	Drugs
Urea	Lithium
Protein-loading	Electrolytes
	Hypokalaemia
	Hypercalcaemia
	Renal interstitial disease
	Sickle cell disease or trait
	Sjögren's syndrome
Both	*Neither*
Post urinary tract obstruction	Primary polydipsia
Post acute renal failure	Psychogenic

blood pressure, a rapid but low volume pulse, cold extremities, sunken eyes and facial features, and a decrease in body weight. When these signs are not found, a decrease in blood pressure while the patient is seated (or, if safe, standing) should be sought. A fall in either systolic or diastolic blood pressure of more than 20 mmHg should alert one to the possibility of volume depletion.

Volume overload is manifested by tachypnoea, crackles at the lung bases, raised JVP and oedema.

Body Weight

One of the most important (and simple) measurements in nephrology is the body weight, particularly in the assessment of the effect of treatment. Ordinary "standing" scales are adequate and measurement to the nearest 0.5 kg suffices in most clinical settings.

BP Measurement

Accurate measurement of blood pressure is very important in the management of patients with renal disease. The guidelines of the British Hypertension Society are given below (Tables 3 and 4). The aim of treatment of hypertension is to lower the BP to below 130/85 mmHg.

Mercury sphygmomanometers are very accurate and durable, and have the advantage of needing neither a source of electric power nor a battery.

Box 3
- Use properly maintained, calibrated and validated device (see for up-to-date information on validated devices)
- Measure sitting BP as a routine
- Measure standing BP at first visit in elderly and diabetic patients
- Remove tight clothing, support arm at level of heart, ensure hand relaxed; avoid talking during measurement
- Use cuff of appropiate size
- Squeeze all air out of the cuff before application and inflation
- Allow the patient to rest for at least 5 minutes before taking BP
- If using mercury sphygmomanmeter lower mercury column slowly (2 mm/sec)
- Read BP to nearest 2 mm Hg
- Measure diatolic as disappearance of sounds (Phase V)
- Take several readings - at least three
- Use the mean of the 2nd and 3rd readings
- Do not treat on the basis of an isolated reading

INVESTIGATIONS

Box 4

- Blood tests
- Urine tests
    - o   blood
    - o   protein
    - o   cells
    - o   casts
    - o   glucose

Blood Tests

Urea and creatinine are two substances whose plasma concentrations provide an indication of the state of renal function (glomerular filtration rate or GFR). Of the two, plasma creatinine is the more reliable in predicting

Table 3 Size of Bladder in BP Cuff

	Bladder		
	Width in cm	Length in cm	Arm circumference (cm)
Small adult/child	12	18	<23
Standard adult	12	26	<33
Large adult	12	40	<50
Adult thigh cuff	20	42	<53

renal function because its plasma level is stable throughout the day. By contrast, the blood level of urea varies according to protein intake, urine flow, and state of hydration.

In post-operative patients, the urea is sometimes raised out of proportion to the creatinine. The explanation is that under conditions of low urine flow, urea leaks back through the renal tubular epithelium and re-enters the circulation. This re-absorption of urea means that the normal urea clearance is 50–80 mL/min, i.e., substantially lower than the normal GFR of 80–120 mL/min. Figure 1 shows the relationship between serum creatinine and GFR.

Box 5

Increased

Raised urea
Hypovolaemia
Corticosteroids
Tetracyclines

Reduced creatinine
Muscle mass low

Decreased

Reduced urea
Inadequate intake
Reduced liver manufacture

Raised creatinine
Muscle mass high
Rhabdomyolysis

All drugs of the tetracycline group other than doxycycline and minocycline raise the blood urea and should be avoided in patients with chronic renal failure. However doxycycline and minocycline can be given in normal doses.

Glomerular Function

GFR is normally about 80–120 mL/min. A 24-hours urine collection for urinary creatinine estimation and a single sample of blood for plasma creatinine level are required for the calculation of creatinine clearance (C_{Cr}) using the standard clearance equation:

Table 4 Classification of Blook Pressure Levels

Category	Systolic (mmHg)	Diastolic (mmHg)
Optimal BP	<120	<80
Normal BP	<130	<85
High-normal BP	130–139	85–90
Grade 1 BP↑	140–159	90–99
Grade 2 BP↑	160–179	100–109
Grade 3 BP↑	≥180	≥110
Isolated systolic BP↑	140–159	
Isolated BP↑	≥160	<90

$$\text{GFR (mL/min)} = \text{Creatinine Clearance}(C_{cr}) = \frac{U_{Cr} \times V \times 1000}{P_{Cr} \times 1440}$$

where U_{Cr} = urinary concentration of creatinine; V = 24 hours urine volume; P_{Cr} = plasma creatinine concentration.

The inherent unreliability of 24-hours urine collections has led to the development of a number of formulae directed to predicting C_{Cr} using serum creatinine alone. One such formula is that devised by Cockcroft and Gault (1), which has been validated in sub-Saharan Africa (2). Another is the Modification of Diet in Renal Disease (MDRD formula) (3).

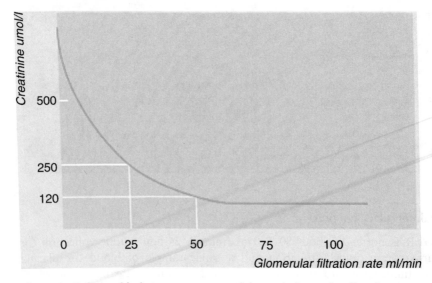

Figure 1 Relationship between serum creatinine and glomerular filtration rate.

FORMULAE FOR ESTIMATING GFR

Cockcroft and Gault (1976) (1)

$$C_{cr}(\text{mL/min}) = 1.23 \times \frac{(140 - \text{age}) \times \text{weight(kg)}}{\text{Serum creatinine(mol/L)}} \quad (\text{men})$$

$$C_{cr}(\text{mL/min}) = 1.04 \times \frac{(140 - \text{age}) \times \text{weight(kg)}}{\text{Serum creatinine(mol/L)}} \quad (\text{women})$$

MDRD Formula (1999) (3)

$$
\begin{aligned}
\text{GFR(mL/min)} = {} & 170 \times \text{Serum creatinine (mg/dL)}^{-0.999} \times \text{age}^{-0.176} \\
& \times 0.762 \text{ (if female)} \times 1.18 \text{(if Black)} \\
& \times \text{blood urea nitrogen}^{-0.17} \times \text{serum albumin}^{+0.318}
\end{aligned}
$$

Other methods not dependent on urine collection include the plasma clearance of ^{51}Cr-labelled EDTA but this is not generally available in sub-Saharan Africa.

URINE

Hematuria

The term "hematuria" on its own is meaningless clinically; it needs qualification.

Macroscopic hematuria (sometimes with clots) is the passage of blood that is visible to the naked eye. Confirmation microscopically will be necessary.

Microscopic hematuria indicates the presence of red cells on microscopic examination (see below).

Reagent strip hematuria depends on the detection of globin. Red cells, lysed red cells (hemolysis) and myoglobin will also give positive results. Microscopic examination should be sought for confirmation.

Proteinuria

The normal excretion of protein is 80 ± 24 (s.d.) mg/day, contributed to more or less equally by plasma and the lining and glands of the urinary tract. About a third of the protein in urine is albumin. The rest is made up of low molecular weight globulins such as β_2 microglobulin, immunoglobulins (principally IgG and IgA) and Tamm–Horsfall mucoprotein. Proteinuria increases during pregnancy. In addition, transient increases occur during febrile illnesses, following seizures and after exercise. Amounts up to 1 g a day do not indicate significant disease.

Pathological proteinuria is of four types:

Glomerular: Protein that leaks into the urine through damaged glomerular capillaries. This is typically caused by forms of glomerulonephritis, diabetes mellitus, and amyloidosis, i.e., diseases affecting primarily glomeruli. Urine protein usually amounts to 3–20 g/day.

Tubular: Protein that passes into the urine through normal tubular cells, or debris arising because of tubular damage. The usual range is 0.2–2.0 g/24 hr.

Overflow: High levels of low molecular weight substances in the blood overflowing into the urine. The glomerular filtration rate can be normal. Examples are immunoglobulin light chains (in myeloma), hemoglobin and myoglobin.

Selective: In individuals with the form of nephrotic syndrome known as minimal change nephropathy, the urine protein is composed mainly of albumin. If renal biopsy is not possible, calculation of the IgG clearance: transferrin clearance ratio can separate out those whose proteinuria is selective, i.e., composed mainly of albumin. If the IgG clearance:transferrin (surrogate for albumin) clearance ratio is <10%, the proteinuria is said to be "highly selective" and is suggestive of a corticosteroid sensitive condition, typically minimal change nephropathy.

Reagent strips are useful in the evaluation of urinary proteins. The test is based on detecting negatively charged proteins, especially albumin; positively charged proteins including immunoglobulins and Bence–Jones protein (light chains) are not detected. Albumin concentrations below 250 mg/L are not detectable.

Urine Microscopy

Cells

Red blood cells (Fig. 2). The normal range is 0–2 cells/high power field (equivalent to 1000–5000 erythrocytes/mL). The causes of red blood cells in urine are urinary tract infection, stones, bladder malignancy, certain types of glomerulonephritis, and polycystic kidney disease. Remember that red cells from extraneous sources, such as those resulting from balanitis, vulvitis, and menstrual blood, may contaminate the urine.

There is considerable variation in the appearance of red blood cells in urine depending on the site of origin of the cells. Generally, dysmorphic red cells (acanthocytes or budding yeast-like appearance) are glomerular in origin, so indicate glomerular disease (>20% dysmorphic). Red cells of non-glomerular origin are usually more uniform in size.

White blood cells (Fig. 3). The presence of white cells in the urine is suggestive of inflammation of the urinary tract and the type of white cells in the urine indicates the type of inflammation. Neutrophil polymorphs (pus cells) are the white cells commonly found in the urine. The presence

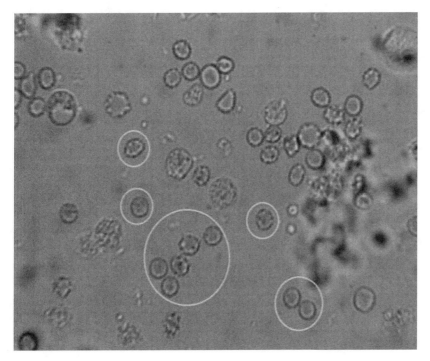

Figure 2 Red blood cells in urine.

of >5 white cells/high power field in spun urine indicates the presence of pyuria, which is the hallmark of bacterial infection of the urinary tract.

Both neutrophil polymorphs and lymphocytes are found in the urine of patients with tuberculosis of the urinary tract and also in chronic tubulo-interstitial disease; in both cases, the urine is sterile on conventional media. Sometimes, there are eosinophils in the urine of patients with acute tubulo-interstitial nephritis. White cells are also found in the urine of patients with renal calculi, papillary necrosis, and polycystic kidney disease.

Epithelial cells (*Fig. 4*). Epithelial cells from any part of the urinary tract may appear in the urine. Their importance is that their presence in a mid-stream urine indicates a poorly taken sample.

Other Cells. Sediments from spun urine may reveal malignant cells derived from tumors in the urinary tract.

Casts

Urinary casts are formed from the aggregation of cellular debris and glyco-proteins (for example Tamm–Horsfall protein) deposited in the tubule and may appear in urine. The different types of urinary casts seen provide some idea of the underlying pathology.

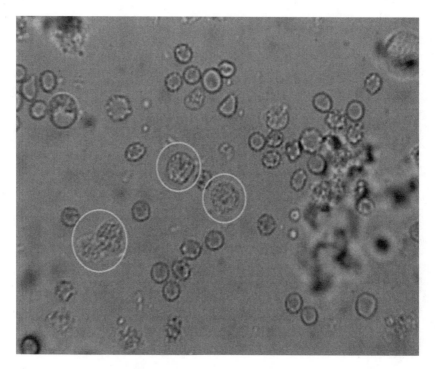

Figure 3 White blood cells in urine.

Hyaline casts (Fig. 5). These are formed from Tamm–Horsfall protein and are seen in the urine of patients with fever of any cause and sometimes following strenuous exercise. These casts do not indicate disease.

Red cell casts. Red cell casts indicate glomerular bleeding and are diagnostic of active glomerulonephritis.

White cell casts. White cell casts are seen in the urine of patients with acute or chronic inflammation of the renal parenchyma, usually of infectious origin.

Epithelial cell casts. Epithelial cells casts are formed from renal tubular epithelial cells. They are usually found in acute tubular necrosis.

Granular casts. Granular casts are derived from degenerating cellular casts of all types. Their presence in urine is always pathological. They are seen in glomerular disease with heavy proteinuria and a number of other conditions.

Other Findings in Urine

Urine microscopy may reveal crystals, bacteria and, especially in patients with terminal hematuria, the ova of *Schistosoma haematobium.*

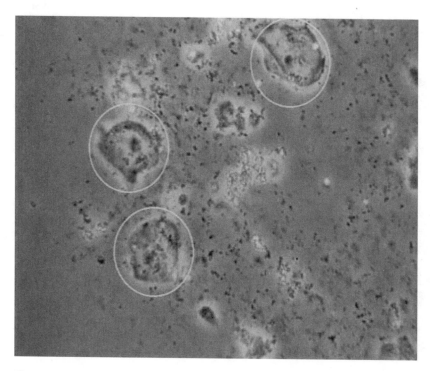

Figure 4   Epithelial cells in urine.

Urine Crystals. A variety of crystals may be seen in the urine in normal individuals and also in those with disease. Their presence depends on diet, urine pH, and the concentration of the urine. Typical examples are urate, phosphate, and oxalate crystals (Fig. 6). The presence of many of these does not indicate pathology. However, the presence of cystine crystals is always diagnostic of cystinuria.

Urine pH. Clinically, urine pH (normal 4.5–7.8 depending on the person's diet) is sometimes important in urinary tract infection. Urea-splitting bacteria such as Proteus mirabilis produce urine of very high pH (alkaline) and thereby lead to the formation of calcium-containing urinary tract calculi—sometimes staghorn "matrix" calculi. Uric acid and cystine stones are found in acidic urine. Acid urine is also found in patients with metabolic or respiratory acidosis.

Urine specific gravity. The specific gravity of urine ranges from 1.002 to 1.030. Urine specific gravity is important in determining the cause of polyuria; it is low (<1.005) in diabetes insipidus where there is loss of urine concentrating ability and also in psychogenic polyuria. It is increased (>1.020) in diabetes mellitus, and in individuals with volume depletion.

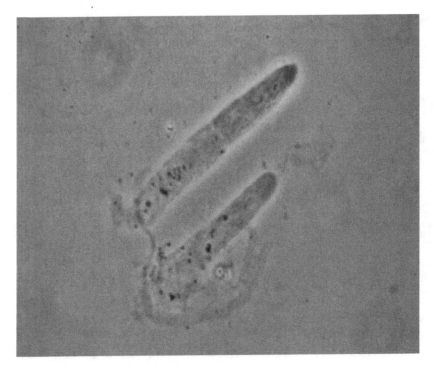

Figure 5   Hyaline casts in urine.

Reagent strips. Chemical test strips usually include leucocyte esterase and nitrite reductase portions. Urine from someone with a classical symptomatic urinary tract infection would be expected to show both tests as positive. Similarly, a strip negative for both elements would make a bacterial urinary infection very unlikely.

URINE REAGENT STRIP TESTING IN POSSIBLE
URINARY INFECTION (TABLE 5)

A problem arises when one test is positive and the other negative. For example, some acute bacterial urinary infections are associated with very few leucocytes; in this case the nitrite test would be positive but the leucocyte test negative. On the other hand, some organisms do not reduce nitrate to nitrite, so the test could be positive for leucocytes but negative for organisms. The same would happen if the patient had been on an antibiotic; the leucocyte test might be positive but the nitrite test could well be negative. There are, of course, other reasons why the urine might contain leucocytes in the absence of a urinary infection. Inflammation in any part of the urinary tract will give rise to leucocytes; for example, balanitis in the male and vulvitis in

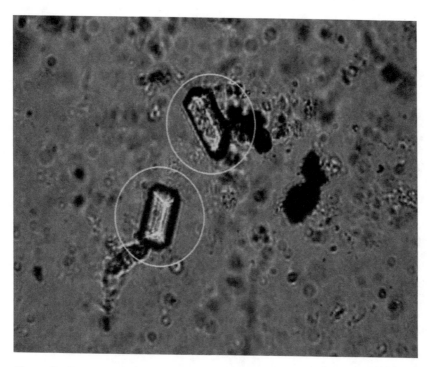

Figure 6 Crystals of magnesium ammonium phosphate in urine.

the female. Sometimes, renal calculi give rise to an increased number of leucocytes but usually there are increased numbers of red blood cells as well. In a patient with a "sterile pyuria," it is most important to consider tuberculosis of the renal tract (Box 6).

Table 5 Urine Testing in Possible Urinary Infection

Nitrite	Leucocytes	
	Positive	Negative
Positive	Urinary tract infection	Infection without WBC Nitrite from food Urine left in sunlight
Negative	Treated urinary tract infection Non-nitrite producing organism Tuberculosis	Urinary tract infection unlikely

It should be pointed out that reagent strips though useful in clinical management do not give any clue as to the organism involved.

Box 6
- Tuberculosis of the urinary tract
- *Chlamydia trachomatis* infection
- Chemically induced cystitis
- Renal calculi
- Coliform (or other pathogen) urinary tract infection but antibiotic inhibiting growth

*Remember white blood cells from the foreskin or vulva may contaminate the urine. If in doubt a supra-pubic sample using a needle of appropriate length will settle the matter

---

URINE CULTURE

Urine is usually culture on cystine lactose electrolyte-deficient (CLED) and blood agar media. A pure growth of a single organism in a concentration of $>10^8/L$ is indicative of urinary infection; inhibition of growth of an organism in the region of antibiotic discs gives information on the sensitivity of the particular organism to different antibiotic (Fig. 7).

SPECIALIST INVESTIGATIONS

Box 7

Urinary tract ultrasound
Plain X-ray film
Intravenous urogram
Doppler ultrasound
Renal arteriography
Renal biopsy

In much of sub-Saharan Africa, even the simplest forms of imaging are not available. Investigation of patients with renal disease is usually possible with simple plain x-rays and ultrasound examination. More complex forms of imaging are rarely necessary and usually unavailable.

Ultrasound

The ultrasound scan is useful in three main areas:

Evaluation of renal anatomy: Renal length and cortical thickness can be measured as well as the dimensions of the pelvi-calyceal system. Cysts

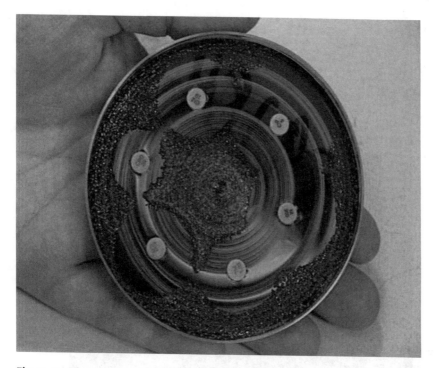

Figure 7 Blood agar medium with antibiotic discs. Degree of sensitivity of organism to particular antibiotic indicated by zones of inhibition (lucent areas) around the discs.

(simple, or multiple as in polycystic disease; Fig. 8) and solid masses, for example a tumor, can be identified. It is also possible to detect calcific densities such as calculi. These appear "bright," and cast an "acoustic" shadow.

Evaluation of renal echogenicity: Increase in renal echogenicity indicates an increase in fibrous tissue and often denotes a chronic process.

Evaluation of the bladder: It is important to examine the bladder ultrasonically in any patient with renal impairment. It could be considerably enlarged, have a thickened wall, or be dilated as a consequence of bladder neck obstruction. Alternatively, stones or tumor may be seen in the bladder. Ureters are not normally seen unless they are dilated.

In a patient with recurrent urinary infections, it is important to determine the ability of the patient to empty the bladder. Ultrasound performed before and after micturition will provide approximate urine volumes for the two examinations.

Plain Film and Intravenous Urogram (IVU)

On plain X-ray, it is sometimes possible to visualize soft tissues such as liver and kidneys, so it may be possible to measure renal length. Urinary

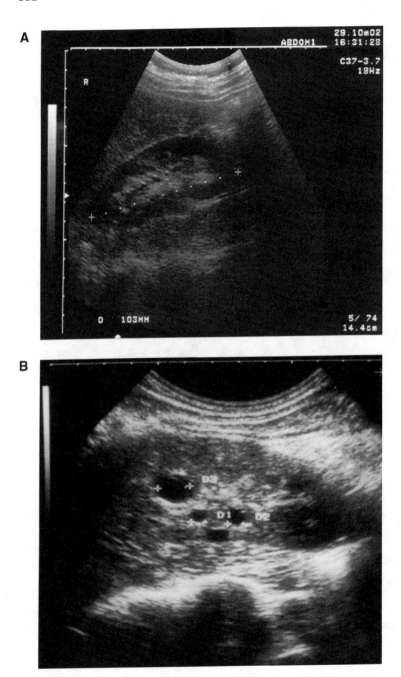

Figure 8 (A) Ultrasound of normal right kidney, the poles of which are denoted by white crosses. Note lack of echogenicity (*dark*) of renal cortex, which is less echogenic than the normal liver, which is visible adjacent to and above the kidney. (B) Right kidney shows a number of cysts as circular echo-poor (*black*) areas.

tract calculi, if more than 2 to 3 mm in diameter, can usually be seen on a plain film. IVU involves the injection of iodinated contrast medium into a vein in the arm. Usually, a preliminary film (full length) and immediate, 5, 10 and 20 minutes (full-length) films, and a pre- and post-micturition film are taken.

Intravenous urography is a very useful method for outlining the excretory pathway of the urinary tract (Fig. 9)—especially for abnormalities of the calyces (reflux nephropathy, renal tuberculosis, stones, and dilatation), pelvis (dilatation, stones), ureters (dilatation, stones double ureters), and bladder (dilatation, diverticula, stones, anatomical abnormalities, prostatic impression). It is less good for detecting abnormalities of the renal parenchyma.

Other

Doppler ultrasound. The most useful method for assessment of renal transplants is Doppler ultrasound. This modality combines conventional ultrasound with a Doppler probe. One can assess the anatomy of the kidney, its echogenicity and in the immediate post-operative period look for evidence of perinephric collections. Also, the renal pelvis and ureter can be assessed for evidence of dilatation.

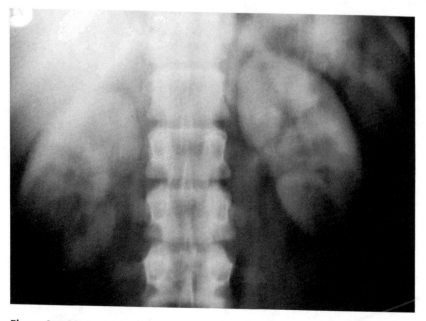

Figure 9a Normal intravenous urogram (IVU). Film taken immediately after contrast given, i.e., "nephrogram" phase of the IVU. The renal parenchyma becomes diffusely opaque as the contrast reaches the glomerular capillaries.

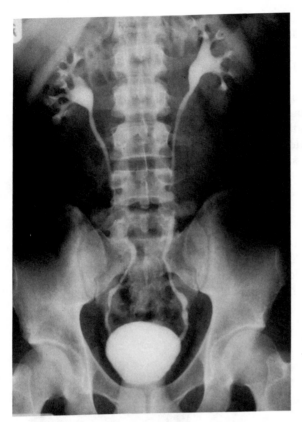

Figure 9b   Same patient as in Figure 9a. Full-length IVU film 20 minutes after contrast given. Film demonstrates the fact that the contrast has passed from the parenchyma into the pelvi-calyceal system, ureters, and bladder.

Renal artery stenosis. The Doppler probe is used in the assessment of the velocity of the renal arterial blood. Arterial stenosis produces high velocity. This condition produces hypertension and loss of function so it is important that it is recognized and treated.

Renal arteriography (Fig. 10). Renal artery stenosis—whether secondary to tropical aortitis or resulting from disease of the renal artery itself—is best defined by renal arteriography. Another abnormality that is sometimes detected is the aneurysms of polyangiitis nodosa.

Renal Biopsy

Percutaneous renal biopsy is an important investigative procedure in adults with renal disease. However, even in large centers where the procedure is carried out on a regular basis, there can be unforeseen hazards, the main

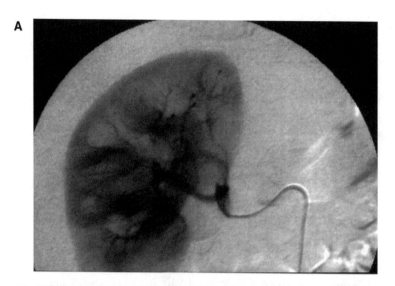

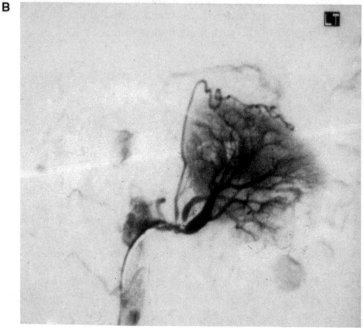

Figure 10 (A) Polyarteritis nodosa. Selective right renal arteriogram showing a number of arterial aneurysms (*black dots*) in the upper pole of the right kidney. (B) Renal arteriography shows stenosis of the main artery (*pair of arrows*) to small left kidney, and stenosis of the origin of the superior branch (*arrow*). Both vessels show post-stenotic dilatation. The features are typical of fibromuscular hyperplasia.

one being bleeding—either into peri-renal tissues or the urine. Figure 11 shows a slide of normal renal histology.

Indications. The procedure should be restricted to patients where knowledge of renal biopsy will affect management such as those with:

- nephrotic syndrome (where prednisolone treatment is considered);
- proteinuric states especially in the absence of other evidence of systemic disease, i.e., systemic lupus erythematosus (SLE), myelomatosis, amyloid, and vasculitides;
- suspected glomerular pathology in non-nephrotic patients.

In practice, renal biopsy will only influence management by determining whether or not the condition will respond to prednisolone.

Most patients with acute renal failure have relatively normal kidneys histologically in terms of vessels, glomeruli, and interstitium. Renal biopsy is only indicated if acute vasculitic disorders or acute interstitial nephritis are considered and prednisolone treatment contemplated.

Renal biopsy should only be carried out in centers with access to reliable interpretation of the histological appearances, and with facilities for the safe management of the pathology that is found.

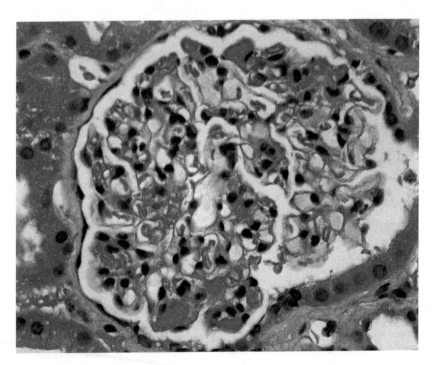

Figure 11 Normal glomerulus. Hematoxylin and eosin stain.

PREVENTION OF RENAL DISEASE

In the developing world, facilities for the treatment of end-stage renal disease are few. On the other hand, renal failure is common, and much is potentially preventable. In the present century, it is likely that diseases of affluence will overtake infectious diseases and disease of poverty as the major causes of renal disease. In other words, the pattern of renal disease will begin to resemble that of the developed world. Increasing urbanization is an important factor.

Foremost among the causes are diabetes mellitus and hypertension. Prevention of these conditions is a challenge for the next decades, as treatment of the primary conditions is unlikely to be available for the majority for many years.

TREATMENT OF RENAL CONDITIONS

In sub-Saharan Africa, renal problems may be primarily renal in origin or alternatively caused by urinary tract obstruction. In general, pre-renal causes—i.e., atheroma and other arterial problems—are unusual. Bilharzia, renal stones, and anatomical deformities are easily detectable and potentially treatable. Renal ultrasound is the cornerstone of diagnosis. Primary renal conditions include acute glomerulonephritis, forms of nephrotic syndrome, SLE, adult polycystic kidney disease, and drug-induced interstitial nephritis.

Acute deterioration in GFR is not uncommon. Severe volume depletion from diarrheal diseases, sepsis (e.g., typhoid fever), snake bite, hemolysis, and malaria in the non-immune are all potentially reversible. Fluid repletion, avoidance of nephrotoxic drugs, and prescription of appropriate antibiotics, all have a role in treatment.

PREVENTION OF DETERIORATION OF GFR IN INDIVIDUALS WITH ESTABLISHED CHRONIC KIDNEY FAILURE

There are a number of potential hazards in patients with chronic kidney failure (Table 6).

Volume (salt and water) depletion. In tropical regions, this is by far the commonest cause of a fall in GFR. Clinical assessment of volume is very important but can be misleading in a patient with fever and warm periphery. The best bedside sign of volume depletion is the JVP. In severe volume depletion, it may only be possible to see the top of the column of blood by laying the patient flat and exerting manual pressure on the abdomen. Central venous access can be hazardous in individuals whose veins are not distended, i.e., collapsed, so is best avoided in most patients.

Correct hypovolemia using intravenous 0.9% saline. If a diuresis does not occur despite achieving optimal intravascular volume, give fluid hourly

Table 6 Factors Adversely Affecting Renal Function in Patients with Chronic Renal Failure

Factor	Problem	Action
Salt and water depletion	Diarrhea, vomiting, fever, lack of access to H_2O, intercurrent infection, malaria, too much diuretic	Oral fluid, intravenous saline
Inadequately controlled BP	BP not measured, availability of drugs, cost of drugs, compliance	Close attention to BP control
Urinary tract obstruction	Diagnosis not considered, inadequate facilities for diagnosis and treatment	Exclude urinary tract obstruction in all patients
Drugs	Herbal remedies, tetracyclines, aminoglycosides, digoxin, non-steroidal anti-inflammatory drugs, ACE inhibitors (sometimes)	In all patients ask carefully about ingestion of drugs and traditional remedies. Check doses of all drugs given to patients with chronic renal failure
Urinary tract infection	Ascending infection causing bacterial interstitial nephritis	History, urine culture, investigate

on the basis of replacing measured losses plus estimated insensible losses (approximately 30 mL/hr) appropriate to the state of the patient. The goal is to achieve optimal (blood) volume; urine flow is of secondary importance. The use of a diuretic to increase urine flow in these circumstances is of no benefit to the glomerular filtration rate.

Patients should be advised to seek advice if they have a gastrointestinal upset or serious febrile illness lasting more than 24 hour.

Blood pressure. It is accepted that control of blood pressure is the most important aspect of management in patients with chronic renal failure. In diabetics, control of blood pressure is more important than control of blood sugar. The WHO recommends a target BP of 125/75 mmHg. This can be achieved in many patients by reduction of salt intake, and the use of thiazide diuretics, beta-blockers and calcium channel blockers. In general, ACE inhibitors and AII-receptor blockers are more expensive and probably no more effective than cheaper drugs.

Urinary tract obstruction. In all patients with chronic renal failure—especially in countries without dialysis—it is particularly important to consider whether there could be an element of urinary tract obstruction. If there is any doubt about the cause of the renal failure, the uncertainty can be removed by undertaking appropriate imaging, in this circumstance ultrasound examination.

Take care with drugs. The kidney is a major excretory route for drugs (Box 8). All types of antiinflammatory drugs (NSAIDS) can cause renal dysfunction and should be avoided as far as possible. In addition, they can potentially cause gastro-intestinal bleeding, which may be life-threatening. Look for and stop all nephrotoxic drugs that patient may have been taking. The timely stoppage of such drugs may prevent further deterioration in renal function.

Box 8 Characteristic of drug	**Examples**	**Action**
Wholly excreted by the kidney	Ethambutol, digoxin, aminoglycosides (streptomycin, gentamicin, vancomycin).	Use alternative drug if possible. If none available, measure blood level of prescribed drug. If in doubt seek suitable advice - pharmacist or physician.
Partially excreted by the kidney	Penicillins, cephalosporins, benzodiazepines (beware of oversedation).	Modify dose after consulting suitable formulary.
Not reliant on the kidney for excretion	Paracetamol, aspirin*, clindamycin, erythromycin, most anti-hypertensive drugs, loop diuretics (frusemide, bumetanide).	
Toxic metabolites	Pethidine, morphine, opioid analgesics (codeine and related drugs)**.	Avoid as much as possible. If no there is no satisfactory alternative use with great care.

*Remember that aspirin causes gastric irritation. Also the effect on platelet stickiness means that aspirin is best avoided in patients with advanced renal failure.
**Avoid if possible as respiratory depression is a very serious unwanted effect.

Infections (including urinary tract infections). In uncomplicated urinary tract infection, give oral ciprofloxacin 500 mg twice daily for 3 to 5 days. An alternative is a 5-day course of oral cefuroxime in a dose of 125 mg twice daily. It is useful to have the results of "dipstick" urine analysis before treatment because in patients who are not systemically unwell unnecessary treatment can be avoided by the finding of negative routine urine analysis.

In patients who are acutely ill, treatment should be started before routine urine analysis and culture results are available. In these ill patients, repeat urine culture should be done 1 week after completion of the course of antibiotic. Treatment is with intravenous ciproflocaxin (400 mg 12 hourly) or intravenous cefuroxime (750 mg 8 hourly) for 48 hour before changing to oral ciprofloxacin or cefuroxime when the patient is able to tolerate oral medication.

In all patients, a high oral fluid intake (about 2 L daily) should be encouraged. In some very ill patients, it may be necessary initially to give intravenous fluid.

Patients presenting with recurrent urinary tract infections should be investigated diligently, even in patients with a known cause of chronic renal failure, for evidence of urinary tract obstruction for example from renal stones, prostatic hypertrophy, anatomical urinary tract abnormalities, and problems with bladder emptying.

Fluid overload. A combination of fluid restriction and oral diuretics will usually produce a diuresis. Give frusemide 40 mg daily, doubling the dose every day or so until there is a satisfactory response. Sometimes a dose of 200 to 300 mg a day is required.

There is no substitute for a daily assessment of the patient's weight. Fluid charts are useful, however, for detecting a falling urine output. Remember that "input–output" charts, even when well kept, can be misleading. They are often only a rough estimate of fluid balance and do not take account of sweating, diarrhea, and other fluid losses.

Electrolyte disturbances. Hyperkalemia is common and results from reduced renal excretion of potassium, as a side effect of drugs (e.g., ACE inhibitors) and in acidosis. The clinical problems associated with raised serum potassium are cardiac arrhythmias, which include ventricular fibrillation, and asystole. Attempts should be made to lower potassium when serum K^+ exceeds 6.0 mmol/L. Give 10 mL of 10% calcium gluconate slowly IV if the ECG is abnormal. The dose can be repeated 30 to 60 minutes later. Alternatively, one can give 50 mL of 50% dextrose with 10 units of soluble human insulin, over 30 minute. This can be repeated if the hyperkalemia persists. Oral polystyrene sulfonate resin (calcium resonium), in a dose of 15 g four times daily, removes potassium from the body. All potassium-retaining drugs should be stopped.

URINARY TRACT STONES

Urinary tract stones are relatively common in the countries of the Sahel but rare in the tropical countries of sub-Saharan Africa. Recent surveys in Nigeria, Cameroon, Kenya, Tanzania, and South Africa, however, suggest that there has been an increase in the last 20 years. The estimated incidence rate in hospital series varies from 19.1 per 100,000 hospital admissions in Calabar, Nigeria, to 243 per 100,000 in Dar-es-Salaam, Tanzania. The male:female ratio varies from 2:1 to 5:1. Evidence from Sudan, Zambia, and Zaire suggests that causes other than *S. haematobium* are responsible.

Clinical Presentation

As stones form on the surface of renal papillae and within the collecting system, they do not give rise to symptoms. Accordingly, stones are often an incidental x-ray finding. Stones may cause macroscopic hematuria, and rank among the common causes of microscopic hematuria. Often, however, stones break loose and either occlude the pelvi-ureteric junction or, more commonly, enter the ureter causing pain and bleeding.

A stone can pass down the ureter without producing symptoms, but usually there is pain ("renal colic") and bleeding. The pain begins gradually, usually in the flank, and increases over 20 to 60 minutes to become very severe, the patient often requiring potent analgesics to gain relief. Later the pain spreads downwards and anteriorly toward the iliac fossa, testicles, penis, or vulva, indicating that the stone has passed to the lower third of the ureter (Fig. 12). When the stone reaches the segment of ureter within the bladder wall, it causes frequency, urgency, and dysuria, which may lead the clinician to suspect a urinary tract infection rather than a renal stone.

In any patient presenting with stones in the renal tract:

- deal first with the urgent clinical problem;
- after the acute episode, search for underlying metabolic abnormalities, as it may be possible to prevent the formation of further stones.

Investigation

Imaging

A plain x-ray of the abdomen will demonstrate most urinary tract stones (Fig. 13A). However, some urinary tract calculi are radiolucent. They are usually not seen on plain x-ray but are detectable on ultrasound. IVU is often very useful, as the stones will show up as negative images within the contrast (Fig. 13B). In the bladder, they may become encrusted with a calcific shell and be visible on plain film. Urinary tract dilatation is best seen on ultrasound examination, but this is not always available. In most cases, dilatation will also be detectable on IVU.

Metabolic

The commonest stones in Africa are composed of calcium oxalate (or calcium phosphate). They are radio-opaque and, if more than 2 to 3 mm in diameter, can be seen easily on plain abdominal films. Urate and cystine stones, on the other hand, both of which form in acid urine and are relatively uncommon in Africa, are radiolucent. Staghorn calculi and nephrocalcinosis are relatively unreported in Africa.

Very often it is not possible to identify an underlying metabolic disorder but hypercalcemia and hypercalciuria are not uncommon. Causes of

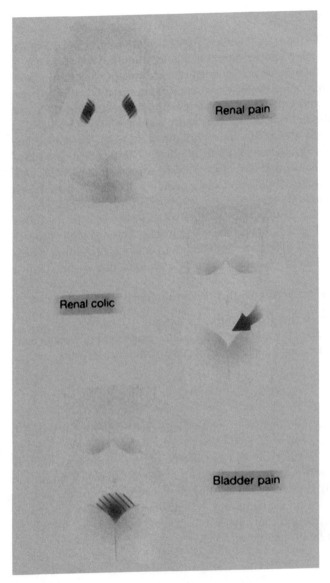

Figure 12   Distribution of pain in renal colic.

hypercalcemia include primary hyperparathyroidism, high calcium intake, and malignancy. Oxalate stones are occasionally found in patients with inflammatory bowel disease where the fat in the intestine becomes esterified with calcium, so leaving free oxalate available for absorption. It is useful to perform 24 hour urine collections for calcium, oxalate, urate, sodium, and potassium.

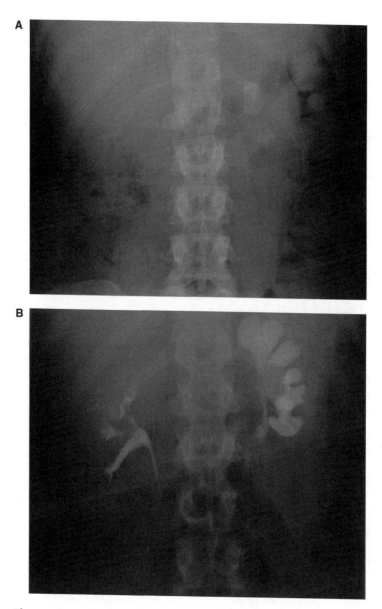

Figure 13 (A) Plain abdominal film to show radio-opaque stones in region of left kidney. (B) IVU film demonstrates the stones to lie in the left pelvi-calyceal system. The stones are relatively radiolucent and less dense than the surrounding contrast.

The life-time risk of recurrence of calcium stones is 100%. It is important, therefore, to consider simple measures to prevent the formation of further stones. Table 7 indicates important dietary changes known to be effective in preventing recurrence.

Management

In any patient presenting with typical symptoms, there are three potential problems:

- Pain
  - Diclofenac
  - Pethidine

- Infection
  - Urine culture

- Obstruction
  - Plain x-ray film
  - IVU

In any patient presenting with symptoms suggestive of a urinary tract calculus, it is important to attend to the three potential problems—pain, infection, and obstruction. The principles are to relieve the pain with oral analgesics and to ensure that the patient drinks liberal volumes of fluid, 3 to 4 L a day. The pain is best controlled with diclofenac sodium or pethidine though the place of smooth muscle relaxants is now much less certain.

Table 7   Formation of Calcium (Oxalate/Phosphate) Stones

Factor	Problem	Action in stone formers
Low fluid intake	Concentration of calcium in urine increases	Increase fluid intake
High salt intake	Increases urinary calcium excretion	Reduce salt intake
Low potassium intake	Increases urinary calcium excretion	Increase fruit and vegetable intake (particularly bananas, plantain, beans)
Low calcium intake	Increases oxalate absorption and urinary excretion	Do not reduce calcium excretion
Excessive intake of ascorbate or citrate	Increases urinary oxalate excretion	Limit the amount of citrus fruit, if excessive

If infection is suspected, urine culture will be crucial and the patient will need to be given an antibiotic. Plain film of the abdomen and urinary tract ultrasound gives important information on anatomy, and IVU will show any hold-up. Remember that some urinary tract calculi are radiolucent. They will not normally be visible on plain x-ray but are detectable on ultrasound. IVU is often very useful as the stones show up as negative images among the contrast. Fewer than 10% of patients need surgical intervention.

ACKNOWLEDGMENTS

We are grateful to Professor Anthony Coates and Kim Duffy of the Department of Medical Microbiology, and to Philip Harvey, Media Producer, Department of Media Services, St. George's Hospital Medical School, London SW17 0RE, for giving us permission to reproduce Figures 2–7.

REFERENCES

1. Cockcroft D, Gault MK. Prediction of creatinine clearance from serum creatinine. Nephron 1976; 16:31–41.
2. Sanusi A, Akinsola A, Ajayi A. Creatinine clearance estimation form serum creatinine values: evaluation and comparison of five predictive formulae in Nigerian patients. Afr J Med Sci 2000; 29:7–11.
3. Levey AS, Bosch JP, Lewis JB, Greene T, Rogers N, Roth D. A more accurate method to estimate glomerular filtration rate from serum creatinine: a new prediction equation. Modification of Diet in Renal Disease Study Group. Ann Intern Med 1999; 130:461–470.

FURTHER READING

Plange-Rhule J, Cappuccio FP, Eastwood JB. Body fluids. In: Parry EHO, et al. eds. Principles of Medicine in Africa. 3rd ed. Chapter 82. Cambridge: Cambridge University Press, 2004:1030–1038.
Plange-Rhule J, Cappuccio FP, Eastwood JB. The kidney. In: Parry EHO, et al. eds. Principles of Medicine in Africa. 3rd ed. Chapter 83. Cambridge: Cambridge University Press, 2004:1039–1079.

30

Meeting the Challenge: A Global View of Nephrology

John H. Dirks and Sheila Robinson

University of Toronto and Massey College, Toronto, Ontario, Canada

Chronic kidney disease is part of the growing global prevalence of non-communicable or chronic diseases. These include cardiovascular disease led by hypertension and diabetes, chronic respiratory disease, cancer, and mental illness. For the first time in history, the world has more deaths and disability from chronic and non-communicable disease than from communicable diseases. Indeed, chronic disease has replaced communicable disease as the main cause of mortality and morbidity in the 21st century (1). In 2005, this is true for every region of the world with the exception of Africa, with the death rates in developed and developing countries being comparable.

In 2002, there were approximately 32 million deaths from chronic disease. Of these, 17 million were from cardiovascular disease. This is predicted to rise to more than 50 million in 2020 (2). While deaths from communicable diseases remains around 20 million and starting to decline, cardiovascular disease will rise to 20 million in 2020 with two-thirds of these in the developing world where the steepest increase will occur. Simultaneously, the burden of diabetes will rise from 150 million in 2000 to 370 million in 2030, with three-quarters of these in the developing world. Since 30–40% of diabetes patients ware likely to develop diabetic nephrology and eventually renal failure over a period of 10 to 20 years, the burden of kidney failure will continue to increase. The United States will have over 600,000 patients by 2010 (3). Globally, it is predicted that the number of patients on dialysis will rise to 2.5 million by 2010. In 2002, individuals with kidney disease and other associated chronic diseases like diabetes and cardiovascular disease accounted for nearly 20% of the U.S. healthcare expenditures and RRT for nearly 8% (4). The attention by ISN and nephrologists in general in detecting early kidney disease becomes an important responsibility and challenge.

The development of chronic diseases including kidney disease is a lifelong process beginning with attention to birth weight and maternal care to avoid low birth weight. Genetics, ethnic factors, and perhaps gender are important early determinants. The issue of lifestyle and the environment also becomes important. ISN has developed a clear agenda for a broad preventive strategy. Emphasis on lifestyle changes to avoid or reduce obesity through dietary modification increased physical activity, and smoking cessation play a major role. Secondary prevention (through now well-proven studies that demonstrate that by controlling blood pressure and treating albuminuria using new angiotensin system blockade) reduces deterioration of renal function and cardiovascular risk. Significant measures to control glycemia, anemia, and Ca–P metabolism are also important. Finally, tertiary prevention of critical complications in the renal failure patients becomes necessary.

Chronic kidney diseases are emerging as a major global health problem. The incidence is increasing to the point that over 1 million people now die each year from renal disease and an estimated 60 million are estimated to have some level of kidney disease. This number likely underreports the true situation as recent research suggests that CKD patients often have cardiovascular disease and/or diabetes and their death may be attributed to these. Furthermore, current statistics indicate that the rate of RRT is 650 patients per million in the European Union and only 160 per million in Central and Eastern Europe. This probably says as much about the ability of each area to finance the treatment of renal disease as about the true numbers of patients. In developing countries in Africa, Asia, and South America, the reported prevalence would be even lower (5). In Ghana, for instance, there are only two trained nephrologists and consequently very few patients on dialysis. In Madagascar and Tanzania, there are no nephrologists at all. In these countries, lack of expertise and equipment means that people with chronic kidney disease die of uremia when their disease reaches the stage when they need some type of RRT.

In an effort to improve nephrology education and combat the epidemic of kidney disease, the International Society of Nephrology (ISN) launched a global outreach program in 1994 by establishing a developing countries commission (the Commission for the Global Advancement of Nephrology, or COMGAN) co-chaired by Barry Brenner and John Dirks. The goal was to bring nephrology education to developing and emerging countries in order to advance the practice of nephrology. While most people with kidney disease in the developed world can obtain RRT, it is in the developing world where the need for better renal care is most vital.

THE VISION

ISN COMGAN began by assessing educational and clinical needs in areas with inadequate renal care. This resulted in the development of education programs customized to meet the needs of each region. From the launch of the initial ISN Update CMEs in Moscow, St. Petersburg, and Tartu, Estonia, in June 1995, ISN COMGAN has grown remarkably. In 2004 alone, partnership meetings were organized with over 50 national and regional nephrology societies, bringing postgraduate education to 15,000 physicians in their own regions. Further, ongoing relationships have been established with the leaders and members of nephrology societies in over 70 countries, comprising more than 30,000 members.

Besides bringing Western nephrologists to emerging countries to train and educate local physicians ISN provides nephrologists from these countries the opportunity to study abroad. This is done through the ISN Fellowship Program, established in 1982 and directed by the Secretary General's office. As of 2004, this program has allowed over 367 fellows from 69 developing countries to obtain training for periods of 3 months to 2 years in 19 developed countries. Approximately 80% of these fellows have returned to their home countries to act as university teachers, clinicians in private practice and, to some extent, researchers.

The Fellowship Program has and continues to be a major contributor to the overall ISN mission to improve the level of renal patient care world worldwide. Of those who return to their home country, 61% teach, 67% care for patients, and 47% do research. The recently established Global Fellowship Club provides a forum for fellows from each region to join together to become ambassadors for ISN—recruiting new members, delivering the ISN mission, disseminating the ISN Guidelines, and assisting with regional meetings from which local physicians can benefit.

In 1997, ISN established a Sister Centre Program, which links individual nephrology centers in developing and developed countries. This has been successful only in part. However, the idea of sharing expertise and knowledge at an institution-to-institution level is a good one and it is hoped that with relatively small amounts of funding, this particular program could play a vital role in improving renal care with fairly minimal funding.

Knowledge materials including Kidney International, JASN, and others have also been made available though the ISN Treasurer's office as well as though an Informatics Committee, and this needs to be enhanced. Plans are underway for the creation of an educational website, which will allow both better access to information and ideally real time interaction with some of the world's foremost nephrologists.

In 2001, ISN made prevention of chronic kidney disease a global mission and rapid growth has occurred in the number of symposia and special meetings on prevention of CKD. In 2004, for example, 32 or 52 CMEs focused on or included major sessions on prevention. The prevention mission has also stimulated education and launched intervention studies in places such as China, Moldova, Bolivia, and Nepal, to name a few.

Finally, through COMGAN and its mission of prevention, ISN has developed relationships with a number of international health organizations geared to increasing the profile of kidney disease as a major non-communicable disease along with cardiovascular disease and diabetes. The costs of treating these three diseases are prohibitive in developed and impossible in less developed countries. By adopting an integrated approach to prevention working with other health organizations, ISN hopes to affect in a positive way the growing global inequity in patient care.

THE STRATEGY

CME Meetings

ISN COMGAN's first challenge within a developing country, which may have few or no local nephrologists, is to identify its educational and clinical needs. ISN COMGAN leaders from the developed world make contact with a local doctor or society and arrange a site visit. The purpose of these visits is to make contact with local nephrologists and/or primary care physicians, hospital administrators, members of the Department of Health, and make a tour of the hospitals. The local leader(s) will then become the liaison person(s) for further COMGAN activities. Recent site visits have been to Ghana, Nigeria, Uganda, Tanzania, Senegal, Myanmar, Indonesia, and Paraguay.

After the site visit, a small CME, usually subsidized by ISN, will be organized. The first one may be almost completely organized by ISN, often with the help of a single local or regional nephrologist, but gradually local physicians take over more and more of the planning and organization. Typically, ISN COMGAN sponsors and provides airfare for several international speakers, while the local organizing committee covers the local costs.

ISN COMGAN has organized 230 such outreach programs since 1995, reaching close to 60,000 physicians and healthcare workers in the developing and middle-income world. Participation in COMGAN programs ranges from 30 to 50 participants in the smaller courses to 500–3000 participants in larger national society meetings (map of where COMGAN has been).

The CME programs cover a broad range of topics dictated by local needs. Prevention, dialysis, and transplantation are three of the most requested. In the 52 CMEs conducted in 2004, for example, 22 have included major teaching sessions and workshops on prevention of kidney disease, 22 on dialysis, and 13 on transplantation. In general, ISN COMGAN programs focus emphasis on general nephrology, prevention of CKD, basic science, hemodialysis, peritoneal dialysis, transplantation, renal pathology, ARF, tropical nephrology, and renal registries. The ISN roster of just over 200 speakers includes most of the world's leading authorities in the field, which participate on a completely volunteer basis and offer state-of-the-art teaching.

One of the unique aspects of ISN is that it does not simply partner in a CME and then move on to another part of the world. Developing and maintaining an ongoing relationship between COMGAN and the local nephrologists is an integral part of its activity. Typically, CMEs will be organized every 1, 2, or 3 years in order to continue to provide top-ranked teaching faculty to the local community. Local leaders are identified and brought into the COMGAN network.

Early on, ISN COMGAN established regional sub-committees (Africa, Asia, Southeast Asia, East Asia, Latin America, Middle East, Eastern and Central Europe and, Russia/CIS, and Indonesia-Philippines-Pacific Islands) comprised mostly of local nephrologists. These committee members provide local insight and leadership to carry forward the agenda. They organize CMEs and nominate younger colleagues for fellowships in order to gradually increase the pool of well-trained nephrologists.

The Mission of Prevention

By 2002, it had become apparent that the most effective approach ISN could take was to concentrate its efforts on the prevention of progression of renal disease. The society adopted a global mission of prevention and since then the number of prevention-oriented meetings and prevention studies has grown steadily. The lack of expertise and equipment means prevention is the best and only hope for the populations in emerging countries. Even in high-income countries, costs are becoming prohibitive. Between 1990 and 2000, for instance, the number of people on dialysis maintenance has more than doubled, and it is expected to virtually double again by 2010 (6).

Without an effective and sustained approach to prevention, the increases in kidney disease and ultimately kidney failure will increase dramatically, particularly in emerging countries. The ISN COMGAN mission of prevention includes a basic approach that is repeated throughout the developing world:

- improving education of nephrologists, primary care doctors, and other health professionals;
- training that focuses on the areas of epidemiology, clinical pharmacology, and clinical trials;

- recognition of microalbuminaria and renal insufficiency as a marker for cardiovascular disease as well as kidney disease;
- activating research projects on early screening for renal disease;
- raising public awareness about kidney disease in the context of cardiovascular disease and diabetes.

Early in 2004, a special conference "Prevention of Renal Diseases in the Emerging World: Toward Global health Equity" was held in Bellagio. This was the most important prevention meeting undertaken by ISN COM-GAN, placing prevention, education, and equity at the forefront of ISN's work. It brought together 23 experts from WHO, the developed and the developing world to discuss recently obtained insights in the pathogenetic significance of chronic renal disease (CKD) to ischemic vascular injury in particular in relation to hypertensive and diabetes-related systemic cardiovascular disease.

Many diabetic patients will develop renal insufficiency requiring renal replacement therapy (RRT). The increase of both cardiovascular and diabetic disease is very pronounced in low-income countries, where RRT is too expensive and not widely available. However, even in the developed world, the growing economic burden of RRT is becoming unsustainable. Estimates as high as a trillion dollars per year are predicted at the end of the next decade.

Epidemiological analyses were presented at the Bellagio Conference revealing the growing worldwide inequity in renal replacement therapy for the millions of patients with end-stage renal disease and the need for early detection and prevention in order to avert the global threat of pandemic vascular disease. Multiple interventions such as dietary and other lifestyle changes like smoking cessation, and lowering of blood lipids, are all important as is designing programs for early detection, made possible by urinary albumin screening, blood pressure, and renal function measurement in populations at risk, followed by effective treatment in a clinical research. Recent U.S. and European studies have shown that drugs that lower albuminuria improve both renal and cardiac prognosis as well as reducing the risk of developing diabetes. Instituting screening programs for targeted populations is a cost-effective, and in the long run a cost-saving approach.

One such initiative, which took place earlier (between 1995 and 2000) among Australian Aboriginals, indicates the effectiveness of this approach. After an average of 3.4 years of follow-up with ACE inhibitor treatment, the incidence of ESRD was reduced by 63% and non-renal deaths by 50%. It has been estimated that at 2 years this program may have incurred savings of between AUS $800,000 and $4.1 million in the cost of dialysis either avoided or delayed (6).

Since the meeting in Bellagio, ISN has held a number of regional and national prevention meetings. A large meeting (over 1200 participants) was held in Hong Kong in June 2004, which resulted in a consensus statement focusing on three key areas: screening for chronic kidney disease; evaluation and estimating progression of chronic kidney disease; and measures to prevent the progression of chronic kidney disease. At a prevention meeting in Amsterdam in November 2004, the ISN called for national health organizations around the world to consider the urgent implementation of proactive albuminuria screening for the early detection of renal damage, followed by treatment to prevent further deterioration of the renal function. This will reduce the number of patients suffering from kidney failure, heart failure, and diabetes and their associated costs.

As part of its commitment to education and training in Latin America, ISN COMGAN will co-sponsor a conference in Chile in 2005 on identification and prevalence of ESRD, including surveillance and methodologies for local treatment, costs and feasibility of treatments, and educational strategies aimed at prevention.

Research and Prevention

The ISN COMGAN Research Subcommittee was established to compliment and extend the work being done through CMEs. In conjunction with its prevention mission, this subcommittee, under the leadership of Dr. Giuseppe Remuzzi has undertaken a number of detection and intervention programs for renal diseases, diabetes, and cardiovascular disease in the emerging world. These prevention programs have a consistent approach, yet are flexible enough to accommodate the local needs of a given country or region. Each project is consistent with the general mission and aims of ISN-COMGAN prevention programs.

Experience in Australia, Bolivia, and India have suggested that low-cost programs can be developed, which will reduce the burden disease in developing countries. Therefore, ISN has developed a proposal for "The Detection and Management of Chronic Kidney, Diabetic and Cardiovascular Disease in Developing Countries" or CKDC. Its aims are to help local physicians and healthcare workers establish their own prevention programs and to increase government and public awareness of the social and financial costs of these diseases. The CKDC agenda consist of two phases—detection and management. One of the important associated outcomes of the program will be the creation of a global database for kidney disease.

Programs are already being organized in Moldova, China, Sogod and Catmon (Philippines), Bolivia, and Nepal. Requests for educational/prevention programs have come from many other countries, including Paraguay, Morocco, Lithuania, Belorus, Ukraine, Saudi Arabia, and India. The program in China, where the exact incidence and prevalence of chronic renal failure, its costs, and patient outcomes are not known, will consist of a pilot mass screening (30,000 people) in the provinces of Guangdong, Hubei, and

Henan. It will be a community-based, prospective, observational, stratified mass screen, which will mainly focus on chronic kidney diseases with bundling screening with obesity, hypertension, diabetes, and dyslipidemia. The 12-month program will consist of pre-screening training courses for the doctors, nurses, and medical students who will be directly involved in the screening program, screening of subjects, input of data into the database, and finally data analyses and preparation of report/manuscript to ISN-COMGAN. Participants with a positive screening for renal diseases, hypertension, and diabetes should enter the intervention/treatment phase of the program. Patients with urinary tract infections will be treated and enrolled in a follow-up program. Those with high blood pressure and/or diabetes and/or albuminuric renal diseases will be enrolled in a formal research prevention program (7).

For these prevention programs, which are planning for a 5-year period, the COMGAN Research Committee is approaching national and local health authorities through its members directly involved in specific projects and local coordinators. In parallel, ISN is seeking funding and lower-cost medicines to start with these projects.

Education and Training Strategies

Training and education, which are at the heart of ISN COMGAN activities, extend beyond CMEs to a host of other activities. Over the past decade, ISN COMGAN, through its Education Advisory Committee, has developed a core curriculum for postgraduate training in nephrology. Its purpose is to give specific support to developing nations to aid the achievement of the minimum training standards embodied in the guidelines. These guidelines cover basic renal science; renal pathology, pathophysiology, immunology, and microbiology; clinical manifestations of renal disease and hypertension, investigation and diagnosis of renal disease and hypertension; treatment of renal disease and hypertension; and clinical epidemiology, prevention, and population health.

Developing International Links

ISN COMGAN has long believed that collaboration with other international health organizations would contribute to the mission of prevention. These relationships have resulted in a number of initiatives that have furthered the prevention agenda worldwide. In 2003, for example, the International Society of Nephrology (ISN) joined forces with the International Diabetes Federation (IDF) in a global campaign to heighten the understanding of negative impact of diabetes on the kidney. The two organizations published a report entitled "Diabetes and Kidney Disease: Time to Act" (available in English and Spanish and largely written by Bob Atkins and Giuseppe Remuzzi), which focuses on one of the most prevalent and costly long-term complications of diabetes—diabetic nephropathy.

ISN COMGAN has established a close working relationship with the International Society of Hypertension (ISH). ISH now sends speakers to a number of ISN prevention conferences. The International Pediatric Nephrology Association (IPNA) and ISN often send speakers to each other's meetings. IPNA has also stated its intent to undertake participation in the ISN Fellowship and Training Program. The World Heart Federation (WHF) would like to collaborate with ISN as they feel our experience in the training of physicians in low and middle-income countries is particularly impressive. Recently, ISN has undertaken talks with The Transplantation Society (TTS), and ISN leaders have been asked to contribute their perspective on future TTS programs. Talks are also underway regarding various joint activities such as CME meetings. An IFKF-ISN liaison committee has been established, which meets periodically to discuss and coordinate activities of mutual interest. One result has been a joint proposal for the establishment of a World Kidney Day, a project that is currently in process.

ISN COMGAN has had a number of interactions with WHO over the past 3 years and is now making formal application for admission into official relations with WHO.

CONTRIBUTIONS

COMGAN has contributed to world nephrology in a number of ways including:

1. increasing the number of CME meetings it partners/sponsors each year from seven in 1995 to 52 in 2004;
2. providing state-of-the-art teaching annually to 15,000 nephrologists, general and primary care physicians, nurses, and other healthcare workers, mostly in low- and middle-income countries;
3. the strengthened relationships with regional (i.e., ANSRT, SLANH, AFRAN, etc.) and national societies (for example, India, Turkey, Brazil, Mexico, and Thailand);
4. new relationships with nephrology societies worldwide, i.e., Ghana, Nigeria, Paraguay, Guatemala, Myanmar, Kenya, and Indonesia;
5. an increase in screening and prevention projects led by Giuseppe Remuzzi, the Research Chair, in developing countries (i.e., China, Moldova, Australia, South Africa, Bolivia, Cuba, Mexico, Nepal, India, etc.);
6. the improved practice reported by many developing world physicians;

7. assisted in developing ISN's reputation as a truly global organization by developing personal relationships with nephrologists from over 75 countries around the world;
8. improved teaching and the development of educational guidelines suited to the developing world;
9. the creation and strengthening of international linkages (i.e., WHO, ISH, IPNA, IDF, IFKF, WHF, World Bank) to increase global awareness of kidney disease;
10. the emergence of ISN as the world's largest medical sub-specialty education program;
11. the publication of a number of articles on prevention in nephrology and general medical journals as well as in the World Bank's Disease Control Priorities Project (DCPP2).

More specific outcomes are difficult to measure accurately, and can only be described anecdotally at this point from the many letters received. A physician in Tanzania, a country with no nephrologists, has gone to train as a nephrologist in South Africa after a site visit by COMGAN. Turkish nephrologists are now publishing in international journals and being invited to speak at major medical conferences. With encouragement from ISN COMGAN, Russia is trying to make changes to their medical education that will bring them more in line with Europe. Fired by the Bellagio conference on prevention, two Saudi nephrologists are presenting a document to their authorities to start a far-reaching program of prevention designed to meet their specific needs.

THE FUTURE

The success of the ISN COMGAN efforts to raise awareness and, in some regions, to impact on the level of nephrological care, has created the need to re-evaluate how best to use the limited resources available to this organization to achieve its stated goals in the coming decade. While CMEs have been and will remain at the heart of the ISN agenda, the next decade will bring new approaches and programs to meet the expanding needs of middle- and low-income countries. One such initiative, which is vital, is the establishment of a global kidney disease data center that would collate excellent CKD registry information and establish new registries for the full spectrum of kidney disease and act as an infrastructure for research studies in distant parts of the world.

The overall aim of these initiatives is to improve the ability of local and regional training programs to better train physicians, technicians, and nurses responsible for renal care. COMGAN will strengthen regional and national training centers as well as creating and/or strengthening local experts who could then train others in their own region. One example would be to send individual for 3 or 4 days at a time into an institution. They could have a checklist of measurable criteria for success and then revisit the same place over several years to see how things have improved.

Obviously, fellowships will only grow in importance. Not only do the recipients of fellowship training overwhelmingly return to their country of origin to elevate the level of care in their own institutions, they also become themselves the trainers for physicians and healthcare works in nearby regions.

COMGAN is now planning a volunteer program in which nephrologists who are born in developing countries but are now living and working in the Western countries will be encouraged to spend perhaps 1 month a year in their country of origin or in a country with the same language to activate specific teaching programs in undergraduate and postgraduate schools. If successful, this program could have a profound effect on a country like India, from which 1000 U.S.-based nephrologists have emigrated.

Finally, ISN is interested in establishing major kidney centers, hopefully in concert with diabetes and cardiovascular societies. Such "centers of excellence" will need to be well funded so as to enlist local physicians as clinicians and clinical scientists to train nephrologists and renal care staff. They, in turn, become a major source for epidemiological and research data collection, and will do important screening studies for healthcare progress in the developing world.

The effort of ISN COMGAN over the past decade has been a fulfilling one. Hundreds of nephrologists have given voluntarily of their time to build an ongoing and expanding network that, if nurtured, will improve kidney care in more than 100 countries in the next decade or more.

REFERENCES

1. World Health Report, 2002.
2. Yach D, Hawkes C, Linn Gould C, Hofman HJ. The global burden of chronic diseases: overcoming impediments to prevention and control. JAMA 2004; 291:2616–2622.
3. US Renal Data System USRDS. 2000 Annual Report. Bethesda, MD: NIH, NIDDKD, 2000.
4. Collins A. USRDS Powerpoint presentation, 2004.
5. Dirks J, Remuzzi G, Horton S, Schieppati A, Adibul Hasan Rizvi S. Diseases of the genitourinary system, DCPP2.
6. Program for Detection and Management of Chronic Kidney, Diabetic and Cardiovascular Disease in Developing Countries (CKDC Program), International Society of Nephrology, November 2004.
7. Peng L, Codreanu I, Zou H, Perico N, D'Amico G, Remuzzi G. Early Detection and Intervention Program for CKD in the People's Republic of China, June 2004 (draft).

Index

RIT - WALLACE LIBRARY
CIRCULATING LIBRARY BOOKS

OVERDUE FINES AND FEES FOR <u>ALL</u> BORROWERS

- Recalled = $1/ day overdue (no grace period)
- Billed = $10.00/ item when returned 4 or more weeks overdue
- Lost Items = replacement cost+$10 fee
- All materials must be returned or renewed by the duedate.